Pulmonology: A Case-Based Approach

Pulmonology: A Case-Based Approach

Edited by Gabriella Goodwin

hayle
medical

New York

Hayle Medical,
750 Third Avenue, 9th Floor,
New York, NY 10017, USA

Visit us on the World Wide Web at:
www.haylemedical.com

This book contains information obtained from authentic and highly regarded sources. Copyright for all individual chapters remain with the respective authors as indicated. All chapters are published with permission under the Creative Commons Attribution License or equivalent. A wide variety of references are listed. Permission and sources are indicated; for detailed attributions, please refer to the permissions page and list of contributors. Reasonable efforts have been made to publish reliable data and information, but the authors, editors and publisher cannot assume any responsibility for the validity of all materials or the consequences of their use.

ISBN: 978-1-63241-750-3

Trademark Notice: Registered trademark of products or corporate names are used only for explanation and identification without intent to infringe.

Cataloging-in-Publication Data

Pulmonology : a case-based approach / edited by Gabriella Goodwin.
   p. cm.
Includes bibliographical references and index.
ISBN 978-1-63241-750-3
1. Lungs--Diseases. 2. Respiratory organs--Diseases. 3. Lungs--Diseases--Case studies.
4. Respiratory organs--Diseases--Case studies. 5. Respiratory infections. I. Goodwin, Gabriella.
RC756 .P85 2019
616.24--dc23

Table of Contents

Preface

Pulmonology or respiratory medicine is a branch of internal medicine and an integral aspect of intensive care that is concerned with the provision of pulmonary care. It is especially significant in patients requiring life support or those suffering from conditions such as emphysema, asthma, tuberculosis, etc. Many complications can arise in the pulmonary health of an individual, which include, percussion of the lung fields, auscultation, clubbing or cyanosis, and palpation of the cervical lymph nodes, among others. A physical diagnosis and review of exposures to toxins, infectious agents, etc. as well as a thorough cardiac investigation are vital for making a diagnosis. Diagnostic tests such as pulmonary function tests, polysomnography, scintigraphy, bronchoscopy, etc. provide significant insights into the pulmonary condition. Medications can be oral or inhalatory. Oral medications include leukotriene antagonists and antibiotics, while inhalation medicines are steroids and bronchodilators. This book provides comprehensive insights into the field of pulmonology. From theories to research to practical applications, case studies related to all contemporary topics of relevance to this field have been included in this book. It includes contributions of experts and scientists, which will provide innovative insights into this field.

Significant researches are present in this book. Intensive efforts have been employed by authors to make this book an outstanding discourse. This book contains the enlightening chapters which have been written on the basis of significant researches done by the experts.

Finally, I would also like to thank all the members involved in this book for being a team and meeting all the deadlines for the submission of their respective works. I would also like to thank my friends and family for being supportive in my efforts.

Editor

Successful Pulmonary Endarterectomy in a Patient with Klinefelter Syndrome

E. Wierda,[1] H. J. Reesink,[2, 3, 4] H. Bruining,[5] O. M. van Delden,[6] J. J. Kloek,[7] and P. Bresser[3, 4, 7]

[1] Departments of Cardiology, Onze Lieve Vrouwe Gasthuis, 1090 HM Amsterdam, The Netherlands
[2] Department of Respiratory Medicine, St. Antonius Ziekenhuis, 3430 EM Nieuwegein, The Netherlands
[3] Department of Pulmonology, Academic Medical Center of the University of Amsterdam, 1105 AZ Amsterdam, The Netherlands
[4] Department of Respiratory Medicine, Onze Lieve Vrouwe Gasthuis, 1090 HM Amsterdam, The Netherlands
[5] Department of Psychiatry, Rudolf Magnus Institute of Neuroscience, 3584 CG Utrecht, The Netherlands
[6] Department of Radiology, Academic Medical Center of the University of Amsterdam, 1105 AZ Amsterdam, The Netherlands
[7] Department of Cardiothoracic Surgery, Academic Medical Center of the University of Amsterdam, Amsterdam, The Netherlands

Correspondence should be addressed to E. Wierda, e.wierda@olvg.nl

Academic Editors: L. Borderías, T. Kawashima, T. Kelesidis, M. Kreuter, J. Murchison, and M. Takao

Klinefelter syndrome (KS) is a frequent genetic disorder due to one or more supernumerary X chromosomes. KS is associated with an increased risk for venous thromboembolic events like deep venous thrombosis and pulmonary embolism. This paper describes a 37-year-old male patient with KS referred to our tertiary center with chronic thromboembolic pulmonary hypertension, and who was successfully treated by pulmonary endarterectomy.

1. Introduction

Klinefelter syndrome (KS; 47, XXY or higher aneuploidies) is a complex genetic disorder with highly variable endocrinological, metabolic, morphological, and neurobehavioral manifestations of altered X-chromosomal gene expression. Recent studies estimate the prevalence of KS 1 : 640 [1, 2], which makes it the most prevalent aneuploidy in males and also the most frequent cause of male infertility. KS is also associated with an increased risk for venous thromboembolic events (VTEs) like deep venous thrombosis (DVT) and pulmonary embolism (PE) [3]. Although the underlying mechanism is incompletely understood, it is thought to be related to a hypogonadism syndrome leading to an increased synthesis and activity of plasminogen activator inhibitor-1 (PAI-1) and thus a reduced fibrinolytic activity [3]. It might be hypothesized that patients with KS are also at higher risk to develop chronic thromboembolism and chronic thromboembolic pulmonary hypertension (CTEPH) [4]; however, no such case was reported before. Here, we report a case of a 37-year-old KS patient who suffered from CTEPH, and who was successfully treated by pulmonary endarterectomy.

2. Case Report

A 37-year-old male was referred to the CTEPH center of the Academic Medical Center of the University of Amsterdam for the analysis of suspected CTEPH. At the age of 30, he was diagnosed with KS by genetic counseling (karyotype 47, XXY). One year later, following a high energetic trauma complicated with osteomyelitis of the right femur, he presented with acute onset dyspnea. By computed tomographic (CT) pulmonary angiography, acute bilateral PE was diagnosed as sequelae of a DVT of the right leg. The patient's family history was negative for VTE. Anticoagulant treatment was instituted with vitamin K antagonists for total duration of six months, whereupon he recovered promptly.

Six years later, however, he started to suffer from slow onset dyspnea on exertion. Perfusion scintigraphy showed multiple segmental and subsegmental defects, consistent with possible pulmonary embolism. Since anticoagulant treatment for six months did not improve his complaints, he was referred to our hospital. At referral, the patient was in no respiratory distress at rest, with a peripheral oxygen saturation of 99%. He was mildly retarded and obese (body

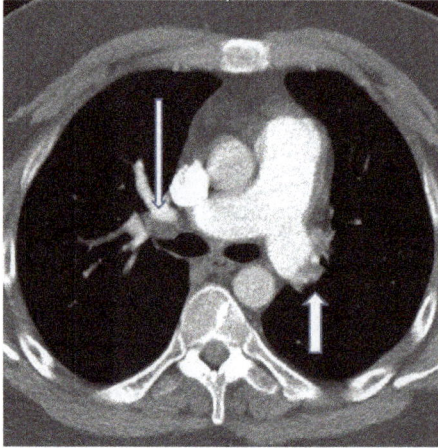

FIGURE 1: Computed tomography angiogram showing chronic thromboembolic clots in the central left and right pulmonary arteries (arrows).

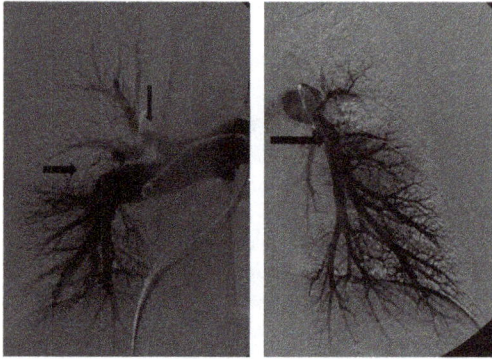

FIGURE 2: Distraction pulmonary angiogram of the right and left pulmonary artery demonstrating a web and acute stops in the right upper and lower lobe arteries as well as in the left lower lobe artery (arrows).

mass index 31.7), had a thickened neck, and a widened forehead with little hair growth. Systemic blood pressure was 120/80 mmHg. Cardiac and pulmonary examinations were normal, except for a split second heart tone. No peripheral oedema was observed. Laboratory tests were within normal range; NT pro-BNP:120 micrograms/mL ($N < 200$ pmol/l, [5]). No coagulation abnormalities were detected, except for Factor VIII which was slightly elevated 211% ($N < 150\%$). CT angiography demonstrated large, organized thrombi in the left main pulmonary artery, as well as in the right upper lobe multiple webs (Figure 1). Pulmonary angiography confirmed the diagnosis of proximal CTEPH with multiple webs on both sides and a central pouch in the left main pulmonary artery with diminished perfusion to the left upper lobe (Figure 2). Exercise capacity was decreased; the distance walked in the 6-minute walk test (6-MWD) was 480 meters (predicted value of 658 meters [6]). Echocardiography showed a dilated and hypertrophied right ventricle; systolic right ventricular function was normal (TAPSE 2.4 cm). Estimated systolic pulmonary

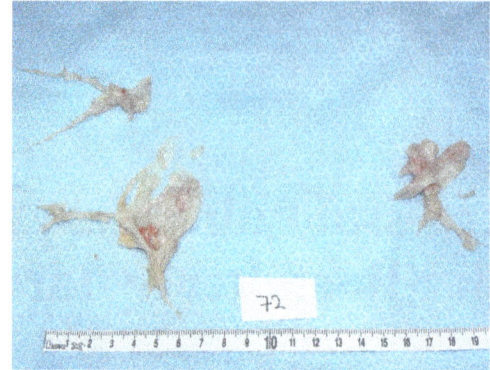

FIGURE 3: Chronic thromboembolic material obtained by pulmonary endarterectomy demonstrating central pouches from the right and left main pulmonary artery.

artery pressure (SPAP) was 65 mmHg ($N < 40$ mmHg). Left ventricular dimensions and function were normal. Right heart catheterisation demonstrated a pulmonary artery pressure of 59/29 mmHg, mean PAP of 43 mmHg ($N < 25$ mmHg), cardiac output of 6.0 L/min, pulmonary wedge pressure of 6 mmHg, mean right atrial pressure of 11 mmHg, and the calculated pulmonary vascular resistance (PVR) of 493 dynes$\cdot$s$\cdot$cm^{-5}.

The patient was diagnosed with proximal CTEPH. His functional impairment was classified as New York Heart Association (NYHA) III/IV; that is marked limitation in activity due to symptoms, even during less-than-ordinary activity. Without treatment, he had an estimated 5-year survival of less than 30% [7]. A multidisciplinary team consisting of a pulmonologist, a radiologist, and a thoracic surgeon considered the patient eligible for pulmonary endarterectomy (PEA). A PEA was performed, as previously described, under deep hypothermia and cardiac arrest [8]. The organized thrombi were successfully removed (Figure 3). Two days after surgery, mean PAP was 22 mmHg. The patient recovered promptly without any complication and could be dismissed after 2 weeks. At 1-year followup, the patient was in NYHA functional class I/IV (no symptoms, and no limitation in ordinary physical activity); subjectively, his exercise tolerance had fully normalised, and the 6-MWD had increased to 580 meters. Echocardiography at one year after surgery showed a normalized diameter of the right ventricle and an estimated systolic PAP of 27 mmHg. At 5-year followup, now, the patient is still in NYHA functional class I/IV, and he walked 630 meters in the 6-MWT.

3. Discussion

KS is associated with substantial morbidity [9] and increased mortality [10] with an increased relative risk of death due to diabetes, cardiovascular, respiratory, and gastrointestinal disorders [11]. KS is caused by chromosomal aneuploidy, in 80% of cases due to chromosome aberration 47 XXY [12]. The prototypic KS man has traditionally been described as tall, with small testes, and decreased verbal intelligence, but the clinical picture may range variably [9]. Here, we reported a patient with KS diagnosed at the age of 30, who developed symptomatic CTEPH six years after an acute pulmonary embolism.

CTEPH results from incomplete resolution of the vascular obstruction caused by pulmonary thromboembolism [13]. The incidence of CTEPH after acute pulmonary embolism is unknown but may be as high as 4% in patients after a first acute pulmonary embolism [13]. If left untreated, prognosis is poor and survival is related to the degree of pulmonary hypertension. Five-year survival in patients with a mean PAP above 30 mmHg is 30%, whereas patients with a mean PAP above 50 mmHg have a 5-year survival of only 10% [7]. Although specific pulmonary antihypertensive medication is currently available (such as endothelin-1 antagonists, phosfodiesterase-5 inhibitors, and prostanoids [14, 15]), PEA represents the therapy of choice for patients with surgically accessible thrombi [8, 16–18]. After surgery, most patients experience a substantial hemodynamic and functional improvement and have an excellent long-term survival [8, 16, 17, 19].

CTEPH manifested in this patient six years after the documented acute pulmonary embolism. Moreover, he had been fully asymptomatic for several years. Therefore, it is highly unlikely that it has been merely the consequence of this episode. Pengo et al. showed that CTEPH manifests itself within 2 years after an episode of pulmonary embolism [13]. Retrospectively, he did not recall any other acute episode. So, whether the development of CTEPH in our patient was caused by recurrent VTE, in situ thrombosis, or both remains unknown.

Thromboembolic disease is frequently observed in KS [3, 12]; however, the increased incidence of VTE is incompletely understood yet. The hypogonadism syndrome leads to an increased synthesis and activity of PAI-1 [20]. Plasma levels of PAI-1 are inversely correlated to the testosterone levels, and positively to the extent of obesity, as expressed by the BMI [21]. However, it is believed by most authors that additional thrombophilic conditions, such as Protein C deficiency [22], Factor V Leiden, or Factor II mutation, are mandatory to cause severe VTE [3, 23, 24]. Obesity that is also frequently observed in KS patients may serve as an additional independent risk factor for VTE in these patients [25]. In the present case, osteomyelitis in the absence of hormonal substitutional therapy may have triggered the initial DVT. Also, at referral to our hospital, Factor VIII levels were mildly elevated. Factor VIII is a well-recognised risk factor for single [26] and recurrent VTE [27]. Moreover, elevated levels of Factor VIII have been described in CTEPH patients [28].

As in VTE, elevation of PAI-1 activity is also considered to play a role in the pathogenesis of (postthrombotic) leg ulceration observed in KS patients [29, 30]. Postthrombotic venous ulceration is observed in up to 13% of KS patients [31]; in fact, this may trigger suspicion on KS [32]. In addition, the frequency of pulmonary embolism in KS is likely to be 5–17 times higher [3], and also a higher incidence of chronic thromboembolism in KS may be expected. This is important as most men with KS (64%) remain undiagnosed due to the highly variable and heterogeneous clinical presentation and insufficient professional awareness of this highly frequent syndrome [33]. Early diagnosis of KS might reduce the risk for VTE and timely androgen treatment will exert a favorable profibrinolytic effect [12]. Thus, both from the viewpoint of early detection as well as for early intervention, the association of KS with thromboembolic events needs to be more firmly acknowledged.

In conclusion, future studies are warranted to unravel the pathogenesis of VTE and the incidence of chronic thromboembolism in KS patients. However, given the increased incidence of VTE, in KS patients presenting with dyspnoea with or without a previous history of VTE, CTEPH must be considered. CTEPH is a life-threatening yet potentially curable form of pulmonary hypertension if diagnosed early in the course of the disease [16].

Abbreviations

KS:	Klinefelter syndrome
VTEs:	Venous thromboembolic events
DVT:	Deep venous thrombosis
PE:	Pulmonary embolism
CTEPH:	Chronic thromboembolic pulmonary hypertension (CTEPH)
CT:	Computed tomographic
NYHA:	New York Heart Association
PEA:	Pulmonary endarterectomy
PVR:	Pulmonary vascular resistance
6-MWT:	6-minute walking test.

References

[1] A. S. Herlihy, J. L. Halliday, M. L. Cock, and R. I. McLachlan, "The prevalence and diagnosis rates of Klinefelter syndrome: an Australian comparison," *Medical Journal of Australia*, vol. 194, no. 1, pp. 24–28, 2011.

[2] J. K. Morris, E. Alberman, C. Scott, and P. Jacobs, "Is the prevalence of Klinefelter syndrome increasing?" *European Journal of Human Genetics*, vol. 16, no. 2, pp. 163–170, 2008.

[3] W. A. Campbell and W. H. Price, "Venous thromboembolic disease in Klinefelter's syndrome," *Clinical Genetics*, vol. 19, no. 4, pp. 275–280, 1981.

[4] D. Bonderman, H. Wilkens, S. Wakounig et al., "Risk factors for chronic thromboembolic pulmonary hypertension," *European Respiratory Journal*, vol. 33, no. 2, pp. 325–331, 2009.

[5] J. L. Januzzi Jr., C. A. Camargo, S. Anwaruddin et al., "The N-terminal Pro-BNP investigation of dyspnea in the emergency department (PRIDE) study," *American Journal of Cardiology*, vol. 95, no. 8, pp. 948–954, 2005.

[6] S. Jenkins, N. Cecins, B. Camarri, C. Williams, P. Thompson, and P. Eastwood, "Regression equations to predict 6-minute walk distance in middle-aged and elderly adults," *Physiotherapy Theory and Practice*, vol. 25, no. 7, pp. 516–522, 2009.

[7] M. Riedel, V. Stanek, J. Widimsky, and I. Prerovsky, "Longterm follow-up of patients with pulmonary thromboembolism. Late prognosis and evolution of hemodynamic and respiratory data," *Chest*, vol. 81, no. 2, pp. 151–158, 1982.

[8] H. J. Reesink, J. T. Marcus, I. I. Tulevski et al., "Reverse right ventricular remodeling after pulmonary endarterectomy in patients with chronic thromboembolic pulmonary hypertension: utility of magnetic resonance imaging to demonstrate restoration of the right ventricle," *Journal of Thoracic and Cardiovascular Surgery*, vol. 133, no. 1, pp. 58–64, 2007.

[9] A. Bojesen, S. Juul, N. H. Birkebæk, and C. H. Gravholt, "Morbidity in Klinefelter syndrome: a Danish register study based on hospital discharge diagnoses," *Journal of Clinical Endocrinology and Metabolism*, vol. 91, no. 4, pp. 1254–1260, 2006.

[10] A. J. Swerdlow, C. D. Higgins, M. J. Schoemaker, A. F. Wright, and P. A. Jacobs, "Mortality in patients with Klinefelter syndrome in britain: a cohort study," *Journal of Clinical Endocrinology and Metabolism*, vol. 90, no. 12, pp. 6516–6522, 2005.

[11] A. J. Swerdlow, C. Hermon, P. A. Jacobs et al., "Mortality and cancer incidence in persons with numerical sex chromosome abnormalities: a cohort study," *Annals of Human Genetics*, vol. 65, no. 2, pp. 177–188, 2001.

[12] F. Lanfranco, A. Kamischke, M. Zitzmann, and P. E. Nieschlag, "Klinefelter's syndrome," *The Lancet*, vol. 364, no. 9430, pp. 273–283, 2004.

[13] V. Pengo, A. W. A. Lensing, M. H. Prins et al., "Incidence of chronic thromboembolic pulmonary hypertension after pulmonary embolism," *The New England Journal of Medicine*, vol. 350, no. 22, pp. 2257–2323, 2004.

[14] H. J. Reesink, S. Surie, J. J. Kloek et al., "Bosentan as a bridge to pulmonary endarterectomy for chronic thromboembolic pulmonary hypertension," *Journal of Thoracic and Cardiovascular Surgery*, vol. 139, no. 1, pp. 85–91, 2010.

[15] P. Bresser and S. Surie, "Medical therapy for chronic thromboembolic pulmonary hypertension," *Multidisciplinary Respiratory Medicine*, vol. 3, no. 6, pp. 434–439, 2008.

[16] C. J. Archibald, W. R. Auger, P. F. Fedullo et al., "Long-term outcome after pulmonary thromboendarterectomy," *American Journal of Respiratory and Critical Care Medicine*, vol. 160, no. 2, pp. 523–528, 1999.

[17] S. W. Jamieson, D. P. Kapelanski, N. Sakakibara et al., "Pulmonary endarterectomy: experience and lessons learned in 1,500 Cases," *Annals of Thoracic Surgery*, vol. 76, no. 5, pp. 1457–1464, 2003.

[18] G. Piazza and S. Z. Goldhaber, "Chronic thromboembolic pulmonary hypertension," *The New England Journal of Medicine*, vol. 364, no. 4, pp. 351–360, 2011.

[19] H. J. Reesink, M. N. van der Plas, N. E. Verhey, R. P. van Steenwijk, J. J. Kloek, and P. Bresser, "Six-minute walk distance as parameter of functional outcome after pulmonary endarterectomy for chronic thromboembolic pulmonary hypertension," *Journal of Thoracic and Cardiovascular Surgery*, vol. 133, no. 2, pp. 510–516, 2007.

[20] M. Lapecorella, R. Marino, G. De Pergola, F. A. Scaraggi, V. Speciale, and V. De Mitrio, "Severe venous thromboembolism in a young man with Klinefelter's syndrome and heterozygosis for both G20210A prothrombin and factor V Leiden mutations," *Blood Coagulation and Fibrinolysis*, vol. 14, no. 1, pp. 95–98, 2003.

[21] P. Caron, A. Bennet, R. Camare, J. P. Louvet, B. Boneu, and P. Sie, "Plasminogen activator inhibitor in plasma is related to testosterone in men," *Metabolism*, vol. 38, no. 10, pp. 1010–1015, 1989.

[22] L. R. Ranganath, L. Jones, A. G. Lim, S. R. Gould, and P. F. Goddard, "Thrombophilia in a man with long-standing hypogonadism," *Postgraduate Medical Journal*, vol. 73, no. 865, pp. 761–763, 1997.

[23] R. Kasten, G. Pfirrmann, and V. Voigtländer, "Klinefelter's syndrome associated with mixed connective tissue disease (Sharp's syndrome) and thrombophilia with postthrombotic syndrome," *Journal of the German Society of Dermatology*, vol. 3, no. 8, pp. 623–626, 2005.

[24] G. R. Mount and J. D. Roebuck, "Antiphospholipid syndrome in a 21-year-old with klinefelter syndrome," *Journal of Clinical Rheumatology*, vol. 15, no. 1, pp. 27–28, 2009.

[25] S. Eichinger, G. Hron, C. Bialonczyk et al., "Overweight, obesity, and the risk of recurrent venous thromboembolism," *Archives of Internal Medicine*, vol. 168, no. 15, pp. 1678–1683, 2008.

[26] J. O'Donnell, E. G. D. Tuddenham, R. Manning, G. Kemball-Cook, D. Johnson, and M. Laffan, "High prevalence of elevated factor VIII levels in patients referred for thrombophilia screening: role of increased synthesis and relationship to the acute phase reaction," *Thrombosis and Haemostasis*, vol. 77, no. 5, pp. 825–828, 1997.

[27] P. A. Kyrle, E. Minar, M. Hirschl et al., "High plasma levels of factor VIII and the risk of recurrent venous thromboembolism," *The New England Journal of Medicine*, vol. 343, no. 7, pp. 457–462, 2000.

[28] D. Bonderman, P. L. Turecek, J. Jakowitsch et al., "High prevalence of elevated clotting factor VIII in chronic thromboembolic pulmonary hypertension," *Thrombosis and Haemostasis*, vol. 90, no. 3, pp. 372–376, 2003.

[29] T. M. Zollner, J. C. J. M. Veraart, M. Wolter et al., "Leg ulcers in Klinefelter's syndrome—further evidence for an involvement of plasminogen activator inhibitor-1," *British Journal of Dermatology*, vol. 136, no. 3, pp. 341–344, 1997.

[30] E. J. Higgins, M. J. Tidman, G. F. Savidge, J. Beard, and D. M. MacDonald, "Platelet hyperaggregability in two patients with Klinefelter's syndrome complicated by leg ulcers," *British Journal of Dermatology*, vol. 120, no. 2, p. 322, 1989.

[31] W. A. Campbell, M. S. Newton, and W. H. Price, "Hypostatic leg ulceration and Klinefelter's syndrome," *Journal of Mental Deficiency Research*, vol. 24, no. 2, pp. 115–117, 1980.

[32] C. Spier, N. H. Shear, and R. S. Lester, "Recurrent leg ulcerations as the initial clinical manifestation of Klinefelter's syndrome," *Archives of Dermatology*, vol. 131, no. 2, p. 230, 1995.

[33] L. Abramsky and J. Chapple, "47,XXY (Klinefelter syndrome) and 47,XYY: estimated rates of and indication for postnatal diagnosis with implications for prenatal counselling," *Prenatal Diagnosis*, vol. 17, pp. 363–368, 1997.

Immunoadjuvant Therapy and Noninvasive Ventilation for Acute Respiratory Failure in Lung Tuberculosis

René Agustín Flores-Franco,[1] Dahyr Alberto Olivas-Medina,[1] Cesar Francisco Pacheco-Tena,[2] and Jorge Duque-Rodríguez[3]

[1]*Departamento de Medicina Interna, Christus Muguerza Hospital Del Parque, Calle Dr. Pedro Leal Rodriguez 1802, Colonia Centro, 31000 Chihuahua, CHIH, Mexico*
[2]*Facultad de Medicina, Universidad Autónoma de Chihuahua, Circuito Universitario Campus II, 31240 Chihuahua, CHIH, Mexico*
[3]*Servicios de Salud de Chihuahua, Sistema Estatal de Salud, Calle Tercera No. 604, Piso 3 Colonia Centro, 31000 Chihuahua, CHIH, Mexico*

Correspondence should be addressed to René Agustín Flores-Franco; rflores99@prontomail.com

Academic Editor: Javier de Miguel-Díez

Acute respiratory failure caused by pulmonary tuberculosis is a rare event but with a high mortality even while receiving mechanical ventilatory support. We report the case of a young man with severe pulmonary tuberculosis refractory to conventional therapy who successfully overcame the critical period of his condition using noninvasive ventilation and immunoadjuvant therapy that included three doses of etanercept 25 mg subcutaneously. We conclude that the use of etanercept along with antituberculosis treatment appears to be safe and effective in patients with pulmonary tuberculosis presenting with acute respiratory failure.

1. Introduction

In 2013, 9 million people became sick with tuberculosis and there were approximately 1.5 million tuberculosis-related deaths worldwide [1]. Acute respiratory failure (ARF) is considered an unusual complication of pulmonary tuberculosis (PT) with an estimated incidence of 1.5% in hospitalized patients and a mortality of 69%, mainly in cases that require mechanical ventilation [2]. Respiratory failure associated with PT may present with an acute form of a disease, such as miliary tuberculosis, acute respiratory distress syndrome (ARDS), and bronchopneumonia, or chronically as a consequence of respiratory, musculoskeletal, or surgical sequels [3]. Conventional treatment of acute disease includes immediate antituberculosis chemotherapy and, if required, mechanical ventilation. Noninvasive pressure support ventilation (NIPSV) and other adjuvant therapies have been useful and provided variable results [4–9]. Here, we present the case of a young patient with ARF, secondary to PT who

particularly benefited from a treatment that included these two modalities.

2. Case Report

A 21-year-old Tarahumara male was transferred from his community hospital with a 4-month history of cough, hemoptysis, progressive dyspnea, intermittent fever, and significant weight loss. On admission, he presented with a bad general condition, with the following vital signs: blood pressure of 90/60 mmHg, heart rate of 140 bpm, respiratory rate of 35 breaths per minute, and core body temperature of 99.5°F. The physical examination revealed a cachectic young man with evident signs of ARF including tachypnea, breathy speech, and accessory muscle use. Chest auscultation evidenced fine inspiratory crackles, mainly in the right apex. Arterial blood-gas (ABG) analysis while he breathed supplemental oxygen via a mask showed a pH of 7.37, PaO2 of 98 mmHg, PaCO2 of 36.5 mmHg, and HCO_3^- of 20.8 mEq/L.

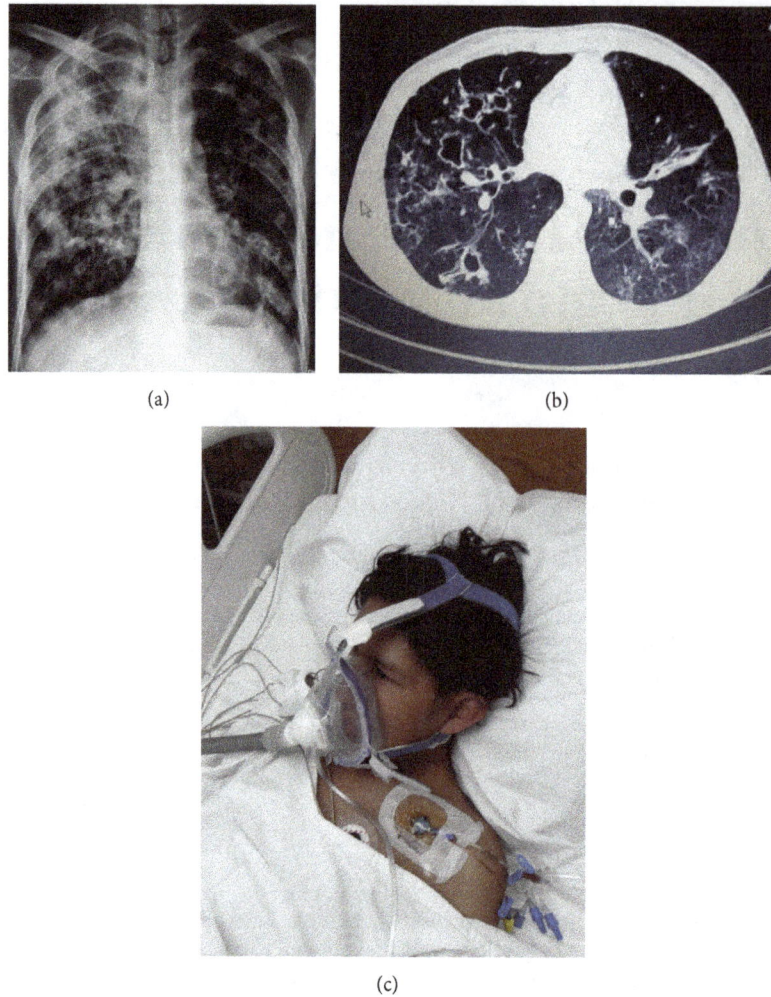

(a)

(b)

(c)

FIGURE 1: (a) Chest radiograph showing extensive multifocal consolidation and cavitation predominantly in the right upper lobe. (b) Computed tomography (CT) image scan obtained 5 weeks later shows the persistence of some caverns, nodules, and linear opacities but a significant improvement in areas of consolidation. (c) An oronasal mask was used to minimize air leakage and improve tolerance for noninvasive ventilation. Health personnel should not overlook the risk of tuberculosis transmission associated with short distances exposures.

Laboratory admission tests showed Hb of 11.1 g/dL, white blood count (WBC) of 11.6 cells/μL, neutrophils count of 10.9/μL, lymphocytes count of 0.2/μL, Na$^+$ of 136 mmol/L, Cl$^-$ of 98 mmol/L, K$^+$ of 4.02 mmol/L, Ca^{2+} of 7.6 mg/dL, glucose of 77 mg/dL, Cr of 0.36 mg/dL, blood urea nitrogen (BUN) of 6.1 mg/dL, uric acid of 3.7 mg/dL, cholesterol of 91 mg/dL, triglycerides of 98 mg/dL, and albumin of 2.1 g/dL. The HIV and hepatitis B and C tests were all negative. Sputum acid-fast stains were positive since his previous hospitalization and a real-time polymerase chain reaction (PCR) assay performed with another sputum sample confirmed the presence of *Mycobacterium tuberculosis* DNA. A chest X-ray showed diffuse alveolar and nodular opacities, as well an extensive right upper lobe cavitary disease (Figure 1). Based on the above findings, we calculated an APACHE II score of 13. The patient was treated with hydrocortisone 100 to 250 mg intravenously for 8 hours, and a daily regimen of intravenous amikacin 750 mg, and moxifloxacin 400 mg, along with antituberculosis treatment of 3 tablets of

a fixed-dose combination (DoTBal, SILANES Laboratories) of rifampicin 150 mg, isoniazid 75 mg, pyrazinamide 400 mg, and ethambutol 300 mg. The patient was admitted to the intensive care unit but on day 4 in the hospital, the increased work of breathing required the initiation of NIPSV with a single-limb-circuit bilevel ventilator (VPAP III, ResMed) through an oronasal interface at pressures of 8–12/4 cm H$_2$O. The DoTBal dose was increased to 4 tablets per day; however, the characteristic red color of the urine produced by rifampicin was no longer observed and the serum levels in a random sample were undetectable. Over the next 4 days despite slight improvement in PaCO2, it was not possible to wean the patient from NIPSV due to the persistent tachypnea. After a discussion regarding alternative therapies and under the respective observations of the local board of pharmacovigilance, the medical team decided as an extraordinary measure to administer etanercept (Enbrel, Wyeth Laboratories) 25 mg subcutaneously. The following day the patient showed a general improvement and an improved

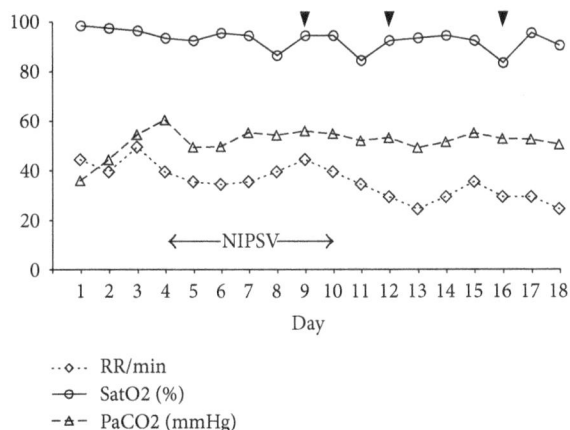

FIGURE 2: Changes in SatO2 and PaCO2 and respiratory rate (RR) in relation to the application of noninvasive pressure support ventilation (NIPSV) and 3 doses of etanercept 25 mg administered subcutaneously (black arrowheads).

respiratory condition (Figure 2). After 2 days, he could finally be separated from NIPSV and undergo continued care in an isolated hospital ward breathing supplemental oxygen via nasal prongs. Three days after the first dose of etanercept, a second dose was administered without significant changes in the clinical condition of the patient. However, 4 days after the second dose of etanercept, the patient experienced exacerbation of respiratory symptoms, malaise, and fever of 100.5°F (Figure 2). Due to the short half-life of etanercept, this scenario was attributed to a paradoxical reaction and resolved promptly with the administration of a final third dose of etanercept along with hydrocortisone 200 mg intravenously. Within a few days, the clinical condition of the patient allowed his transfer to a unit with long-term care facilities, and after a month with negative smears for acid-fast bacilli he was finally discharged to their community under a directly observed therapy (DOT) program.

3. Discussion

While advanced disease has become less common due to the availability of treatment, our ethnic minority group remains susceptible to advanced presentations of tuberculosis owing to recognized factors such as poverty, malnutrition, alcoholism, cultural aspects, and lack of access to health services [10]. In these patients, respiratory failure is explained by the dissemination of infection which leads to pneumonia, cavitation, miliary spread, lobar collapse, pneumothorax, or pleural effusion. The mortality of patients with active pulmonary tuberculosis who require mechanical ventilation is high and their most common indications occur in patients with ARDS, widespread fibrocavitary disease, and pneumonia.

In patients who are treated with regimens including rifampicin and isoniazid combination, a normalization of gas exchange is usually observed within 3-4 weeks; however, in some cases, normalization may not occur for months or never be achieved due to the extent of the sequels [11]. In Mexico, first-line antituberculosis drugs are only available as oral rather than intravenous preparations. Unfortunately, in patients with severe tuberculosis oral administration does not guarantee therapeutic levels of drug due to poor absorption as a consequence of a decreased gastric emptying time and decreased functional absorptive area in the intestines. This decreased absorption influences the pharmacokinetics and may contribute to the subtherapeutic plasma concentrations of these drugs, especially rifampin [12]. This argument is used to justify the use of the parenteral route of antituberculosis drugs, such as aminoglycosides, quinolones, and linezolid in critically ill tuberculosis patients [13].

Additionally, NIPSV has also been shown to be useful in patients with pulmonary tuberculosis. NIPSV may be indicated in patients with chronic respiratory failure due to severe sequels of tuberculosis and during exacerbations, such as in cases of COPD [3, 14]. However, the role of NIPSV in acute respiratory failure in patients with pulmonary tuberculosis is currently a debatable issue because some of these cases have recovered only with drug therapy. Recently, Agarwal et al. successfully used NIPSV for periods of 5–10 days in 3 patients with active pulmonary tuberculosis presenting nonhypercapnic respiratory failure and metabolic acidosis [4]. However, Valade et al. reported that among 53 patients with tuberculosis who were admitted to the intensive care unit, 27 (51%) required mechanical ventilation. Of these patients, 8 (15%) were initially treated with NIPSV but all of them eventually required tracheal intubation [5].

Granulomas are the hallmark of the host response to mycobacteria and represents bacteriostatic efforts to physically contain an infection that cannot be otherwise controlled by host defenses. The microenvironment generated inside the granuloma affects the metabolism, biosynthesis, and replication of the mycobacteria resulting in its semidormant state for prolonged periods. However, the granuloma may be associated with adverse effects on the host. During granuloma formation, initially infected macrophages die; the recruited macrophages then phagocytose the infected cell remnants and their bacterial contents promote the expansion of the mycobacteria population [15]. The physical effect as a barrier and the microenvironment generated within the granuloma reduce the bactericidal capacity of antituberculosis drugs, especially isoniazid [16]. Furthermore, the fully organized granuloma displaces parenchymal tissue and causes the development of perigranulomatous fibrosis, resulting in tissue damage [17]. The application of corticosteroids in patients with tuberculosis, especially in those with an extrapulmonary presentation of the disease, may inhibit the nonselective release of lymphokines and cytokines responsible for constitutional symptoms and tissue damage produced by granulomas [18]. In addition, disruption of the granuloma integrity by corticosteroids enhances the penetration of antituberculosis drugs [16, 19]. The beneficial effects of corticosteroids in patients with pulmonary tuberculosis and acute respiratory failure have been reported in cases of miliary tuberculosis and ARDS [20]. Nevertheless, corticosteroid therapy with tuberculosis remains controversial because of the retrospective nature of the research conducted to date. Therefore, recommendations should be established on an individual basis.

Tumor necrosis factor-alpha (TNF-α) is a potent proinflammatory cytokine that is expressed by macrophages and T cells and is considered essential for the formation and maintenance of granuloma [17]. Additionally, it is responsible for the systemic inflammatory response that is manifested by constitutional symptoms, including cachexia. Excessive production of TNF-α in active tuberculosis could contribute to tissue damage and lower concentrations, as observed in latent tuberculosis, would be responsible for maintaining the integrity of the granuloma, thus inhibiting the growth and spread of the mycobacteria [21]. In experimental models, the selective neutralization of TNF-α inhibits the formation of granulomas and reduces the microbicidal activity of macrophages and NK cells [16]. This would explain why patients with rheumatic diseases treated with an anti-TNF-α inhibitor have an increased risk of activation and dissemination of latent tuberculosis. The recognition of the important role of TNF-α in maintaining a semidormant state of mycobacteria has led to the development of screening and treatment guidelines for latent tuberculosis infection in patients receiving anti-TNF-α agents [22].

The role of anti-TNF-α therapy in cases of active tuberculosis is still subject to discussion. On the one hand, there is the disputed situation in which immunity is required for sterilization of the mycobacterial infection and delayed resolution of the granulomatous host response may adversely affect the resolution of infection [6, 7]. On the other hand, anti-TNF-α therapy has demonstrated an anecdotal prompt and beneficial effect in controlling steroid-resistant tuberculosis paradoxical reactions that occur after initiating antituberculosis treatment for severe tuberculosis with or without prior exposure to anti-TNF-α therapy [8, 9]. A paradoxical reaction in a patient with tuberculosis is defined as a worsening of the patient's conditions after initiation of antituberculous therapy and is attributed to the phenomenon of immunorestitution. The usefulness of anti-TNF-α therapy has also been demonstrated in two prospective studies that included HIV patients with newly diagnosed tuberculosis in whom an anti-TNF-α inhibitor accelerated the response to tuberculosis treatment [23, 24]. In those studies, patients received 8 doses of etanercept 25 mg subcutaneously twice weekly, starting on day 4 of the tuberculosis therapy. Similarly, as described for the use of corticosteroids, anti-TNF-α therapy may contribute to the response to tuberculosis therapy allowing the penetration of drugs into granulomas or improving their bactericidal activity against metabolically active bacilli. Unlike these studies, we did not seek to accelerate the sputum culture conversion or improve the medium and long-term prognosis. Our primary objective was to save the life of the patient and avoid possible therapeutic maneuvers with high risk of complications and significant mortality such as mechanical ventilation.

4. Conclusions

Mechanical ventilation in critically ill patients with PT is associated with a high mortality and thus studies are required to examine the benefits of NIPSV and immunomodulatory adjuvant treatment. Etanercept, which is associated with tuberculosis treatment, seems to be effective and safe in patients with active tuberculosis and should be seriously considered for use in patients with respiratory failure.

Abbreviations

ARF: Acute respiratory failure
PT: Pulmonary tuberculosis
ARDS: Acute respiratory distress syndrome
NIPSV: Noninvasive pressure support ventilation
ABG: Arterial blood-gas
BUN: Blood urea nitrogen
WBC: White blood count
PCR: Polymerase chain reaction
DOT: Directly observed therapy
TNF-α: Tumor necrosis factor-alpha.

References

[1] Centers for Disease Control and Prevention (CDC), *Tuberculosis. Data and Statistics*, 2015, http://www.cdc.gov/tb/statistics/.

[2] G. Hagan and N. Nathani, "Clinical review: tuberculosis on the intensive care unit," *Critical Care*, vol. 17, no. 5, article 240, 2013.

[3] J. M. Shneerson, "Respiratory failure in tuberculosis: a modern perspective," *Clinical Medicine*, vol. 4, no. 1, pp. 72–76, 2004.

[4] R. A. Agarwal, D. Gupta, A. Handa, and A. N. Aggarwal, "Noninvasive ventilation in ARDS caused by *Mycobacterium tuberculosis*: report of three cases and review of literature," *Intensive Care Medicine*, vol. 31, no. 12, pp. 1723–1724, 2005.

[5] S. Valade, L. Raskine, M. Aout et al., "Tuberculosis in the intensive care unit: a retrospective descriptive cohort study with determination of a predictive fatality score," *Canadian Journal of Infectious Diseases and Medical Microbiology*, vol. 23, no. 4, pp. 173–178, 2012.

[6] E. Vlachaki, K. Psathakis, K. Tsintiris, and A. Iliopoulos, "Delayed response to anti-tuberculosis treatment in a patient on infliximab," *Respiratory Medicine*, vol. 99, no. 5, pp. 648–652, 2005.

[7] R. S. Wallis, "Anti-tuberculosis treatment and infliximab," *Respiratory Medicine*, vol. 99, no. 12, pp. 1620–1622, 2005.

[8] T. K. Blackmore, L. Manning, W. J. Taylor, and R. S. Wallis, "Therapeutic use of infliximab in tuberculosis to control severe paradoxical reaction of the brain and lymph nodes," *Clinical Infectious Diseases*, vol. 47, no. 10, pp. e83–e85, 2008.

[9] R. S. Wallis, C. van Vuuren, and S. Potgieter, "Adalimumab Treatment of life-threatening tuberculosis," *Clinical Infectious Diseases*, vol. 48, no. 10, pp. 1429–1432, 2009.

[10] P. Narasimhan, J. Wood, C. R. Macintyre, and D. Mathai, "Risk factors for tuberculosis," *Pulmonary Medicine*, vol. 2013, Article ID 828939, 11 pages, 2013.

[11] M. M. Puri, S. Kumar, B. Prakash, K. Lokender, A. Jaiswal, and D. Behera, "Tuberculosis pneumonia as a primary cause of respiratory failure—report of two cases," *Indian Journal of Tuberculosis*, vol. 57, no. 1, pp. 41–47, 2010.

[12] C. F. N. Koegelenberg, A. Nortje, U. Lalla et al., "The pharma-cokinetics of enteral antituberculosis drugs in patients requiring intensive care," *South African Medical Journal*, vol. 103, no. 6, pp. 394–398, 2013.

[13] H. Cox and N. Ford, "Linezolid for the treatment of complicated drug-resistant tuberculosis: a systematic review and meta-analysis," *International Journal of Tuberculosis and Lung Disease*, vol. 16, no. 4, pp. 447–454, 2012.

[14] H. Aso, Y. Kondoh, H. Taniguchi et al., "Noninvasive ventilation in patients with acute exacerbation of pulmonary tuberculosis sequelae," *Internal Medicine*, vol. 49, no. 19, pp. 2077–2083, 2010.

[15] T. D. Bold and J. D. Ernst, "Who benefits from granulomas, mycobacteria or host?" *Cell*, vol. 136, no. 1, pp. 17–19, 2009.

[16] R. S. Wallis, "Reconsidering adjuvant immunotherapy for tuberculosis," *Clinical Infectious Diseases*, vol. 41, no. 2, pp. 201–208, 2005.

[17] R. S. Wallis and S. Ehlers, "Tumor necrosis factor and granu-loma biology: explaining the differential infection risk of etan-ercept and infliximab," *Seminars in Arthritis & Rheumatism*, vol. 34, no. 5, pp. 34–38, 2005.

[18] H. Mayanja-Kizza, E. Jones-Lopez, A. Okwera et al., "Immunoadjuvant prednisolone therapy for HIV-associated tuberculosis: a phase 2 clinical trial in Uganda," *Journal of Infectious Diseases*, vol. 191, no. 6, pp. 856–865, 2005.

[19] P. Muthuswamy, T.-C. Hu, B. Carasso, M. Antonio, and N. Dan-damudi, "Prednisone as adjunctive therapy in the management of pulmonary tuberculosis. Report of 12 cases and review of the literature," *Chest*, vol. 107, no. 6, pp. 1621–1630, 1995.

[20] Y. J. Kim, K. M. Pack, E. Jeong et al., "Pulmonary tuberculosis with acute respiratory failure," *European Respiratory Journal*, vol. 32, no. 6, pp. 1625–1630, 2008.

[21] M. A. Gardam, E. C. Keystone, R. Menzies et al., "Anti-tumour necrosis factor agents and tuberculosis risk: mechanisms of action and clinical management," *The Lancet Infectious Diseases*, vol. 3, no. 3, pp. 148–155, 2003.

[22] E. Díaz-Jouanen, C. Abud-Mendoza, M. A. Garza-Elizondo et al., "Guidelines in RA treatment: concepts on safety and recomendations using anti-TNF-alpha inhibitors," *Revista de Investigacion Clinica*, vol. 61, no. 3, pp. 252–266, 2009.

[23] R. S. Wallis, P. Kyambadde, J. Johnson, and L. Horter, "Adjunc-tive treatment with etanercept in HIV-1-associated tuberculo-sis," *Journal of the American Academy of Dermatology*, vol. 50, no. 3, p. P110, 2004.

[24] R. S. Wallis, P. Kyambadde, J. L. Johnson et al., "A study of the safety, immunology, virology, and microbiology of adjunctive etanercept in HIV-1-associated tuberculosis," *AIDS*, vol. 18, no. 2, pp. 257–264, 2004.

3

Metastatic Squamous Cell Carcinoma Component from an Adenosquamous Carcinoma of the Lung with Identical Epidermal Growth Factor Receptor Mutations

Jarred Burkart,[1] **Konstantin Shilo,**[2] **Weiqiang Zhao,**[2] **Efe Ozkan,**[3] **Amna Ajam,**[3] **and Gregory A. Otterson**[1]

[1]*Department of Internal Medicine, The Ohio State University College of Medicine, Columbus, OH 43210, USA*
[2]*Department of Pathology, The Ohio State University College of Medicine, Columbus, OH 43210, USA*
[3]*Department of Radiology, The Ohio State University College of Medicine, Columbus, OH 43210, USA*

Correspondence should be addressed to Gregory A. Otterson; greg.otterson@osumc.edu

Academic Editor: Nobuyuki Koyama

The case reported is a young "light" ex-smoker who initially had a localized adenosquamous carcinoma bearing an epidermal growth factor receptor (EGFR) sensitizing mutation. He first recurred six months after initial treatment within the brain with a pure squamous histology and the same EGFR mutation. Surgical resection and radiation rendered him disease-free. Subsequent isolated recurrence within the lung eighteen months later was a pure adenocarcinoma, again with the same identified EGFR mutation. These histologic changes (from adenosquamous to pure squamous to pure adenocarcinoma) have been described but not before in the absence of any selection pressure with EGFR tyrosine kinase inhibitors. This case points out the histologic "flexibility" of EGFR mutant lung cancers and the importance for appropriate molecular testing in nonsmokers with lung cancer of any histologic type.

1. Introduction

The identification of mutations within the epidermal growth factor receptor (EGFR), and the finding that these mutations make tumors exquisitely sensitive to EGFR tyrosine kinase inhibitors (TKIs), has revolutionized treatment of non-small-cell lung cancer (NSCLC). EGFR mutations are more common in never-smokers, in patients with Asian ethnicity, and in patients with adenocarcinoma histology [1]. We present the case of a young light ex-smoker (1-pack-year history of smoking) with an adenosquamous lung carcinoma that relapsed within the brain. The relapsed lesion showed pure squamous morphology and retained the exon 19 EGFR mutation in the absence of any preceding TKI treatment.

2. Case Presentation

The patient was a 43-year-old male who felt well until the onset of intermittent hemoptysis. A chest X-ray demonstrated a left upper lobe (LUL) mass. A Computed Tomography (CT) scan of the chest demonstrated a large LUL mass with satellite lesions and a 1 cm left lower lobe (LLL) nodule (Figure 1(a)). No mediastinal adenopathy or extrathoracic disease was noted, confirmed by Positron Emission Tomography (PET). Brain Magnetic Resonance Imaging (MRI) was negative. Following negative mediastinoscopy, the patient underwent a LLL segmental resection and LUL lobectomy, showing an adenosquamous carcinoma (Figures 1(b)–1(d)) with EGFRExon 19 in-frame (18 bp) deletion. This was detected using a Polymerase Chain Reaction- (PCR-) based Fluorescence Fragment Analysis assay. He received four cycles of adjuvant cisplatin and docetaxel for pT4N0 disease.

Six months after completion of adjuvant chemotherapy, the patient experienced headaches and altered mental status. A brain MRI showed an irregular frontal lobe lesion measuring 7 by 5 cm (Figures 2(a) and 2(b)). Craniotomy with resection revealed a metastatic poorly differentiated squamous cell carcinoma (Figures 2(c) and 2(d)) harboring the same EGFR mutation as the original tumor. The patient received postoperative focal radiotherapy. Given the absence

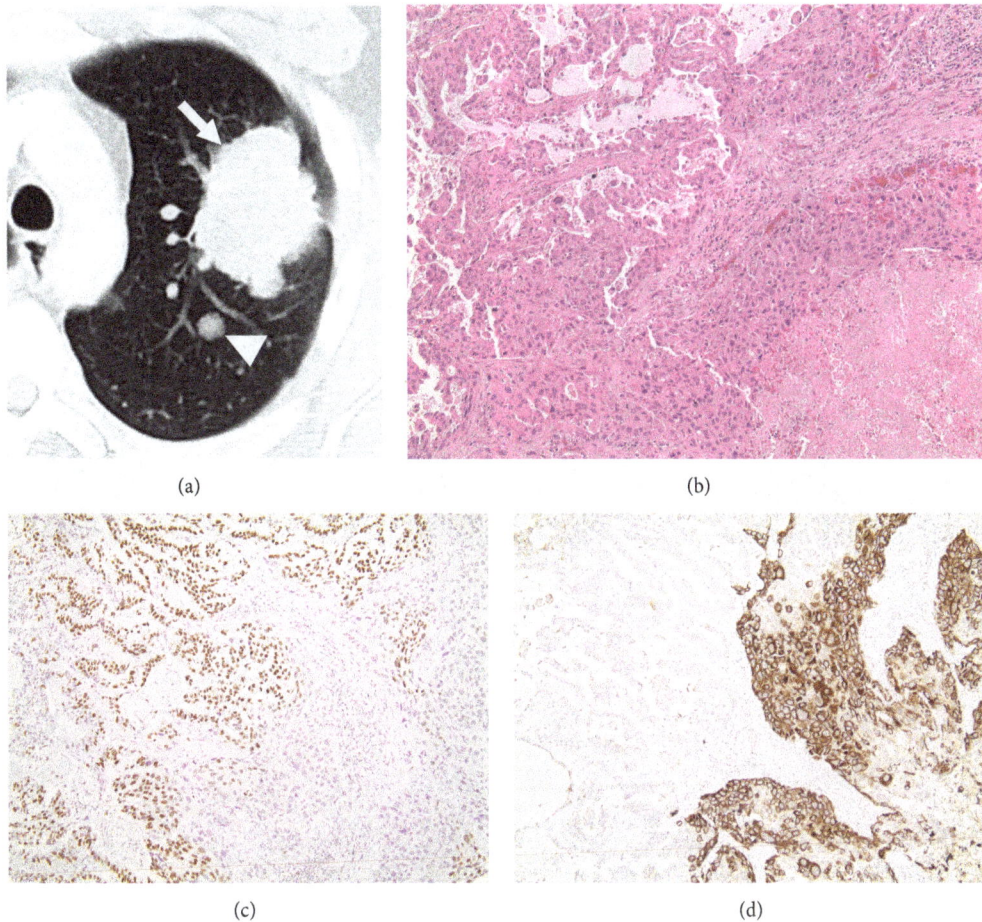

(a)

(b)

(c)

(d)

FIGURE 1: Radiologic and histologic features of lung cancer at initial presentation. (a) Contrast enhanced axial CT image shows a 6 cm lobulated left upper lobe mass (arrow) with irregular margins and pleural tags and a 1 cm satellite left upper lobe nodule (arrowhead). Histological examination shows (b) adenosquamous carcinoma with two distinct tumor components including (c) adenocarcinoma, immunoreactive with thyroid transcription factor-1 and (d) squamous cell carcinoma, immunoreactive with keratin CK5/6.

of systemic recurrence, no additional chemotherapy or EGFR directed therapy was administered.

Approximately eighteen months following resection of the brain metastatic disease, surveillance imaging demonstrated new left lung and hilar nodules (Figures 3(a) and 3(b)). The patient underwent left pneumonectomy. Histology demonstrated invasive mucinous adenocarcinoma (without squamous component) with the same EGFR exon 19 mutation. At this time, mutation analysis was completed using a next generation sequencing assay performed on the Ion AmpliSeq Cancer Hotspot Panel. The patient is currently in surveillance.

3. Discussion

Adenosquamous carcinomas are uncommon primary lung tumors. A report in 25 Korean patients with adenosquamous tumors showed that if an EGFR mutation is present (in 44% of their patients), it is present in both components. This finding supports a monoclonal derivation of this tumor (as opposed to a hypothetical "collision" tumor) [2]. An intriguing aspect of our case is the "evolution" of the tumor

first to a pure squamous histology in the brain metastatic site in the absence of any selective pressure by an EGFR tyrosine kinase inhibitor followed by a later local recurrence with pure adenocarcinoma histology. Histological transformation in patients with EGFR mutations treated with TKIs is a relatively newly described mechanism of TKI resistance; however, our patient had no prior exposure to TKIs [3].

This report also helps inform the strategy for mutational analysis. While the incidence of "actionable" EGFR or other mutations is infrequent in heavy smokers or squamous histology, the exclusion of these patients from testing would exclude a large proportion of patients with actionable mutations [4]. The National Comprehensive Cancer Network (NCCN) NSCLC and College of American Pathologists (ACP)/International Association for the Study of Lung Cancer (IASLC)/Association for Molecular Pathology (AMP) panels recommend testing in all nonsquamous histologies, in those with a never-smoking or light ex-smoking history, and in those with limited biopsy or cytology specimens. Neither panel excludes the possibility of molecular testing in patients with squamous histology, specifically to address the issues associated with limited biopsy samples and sometimes

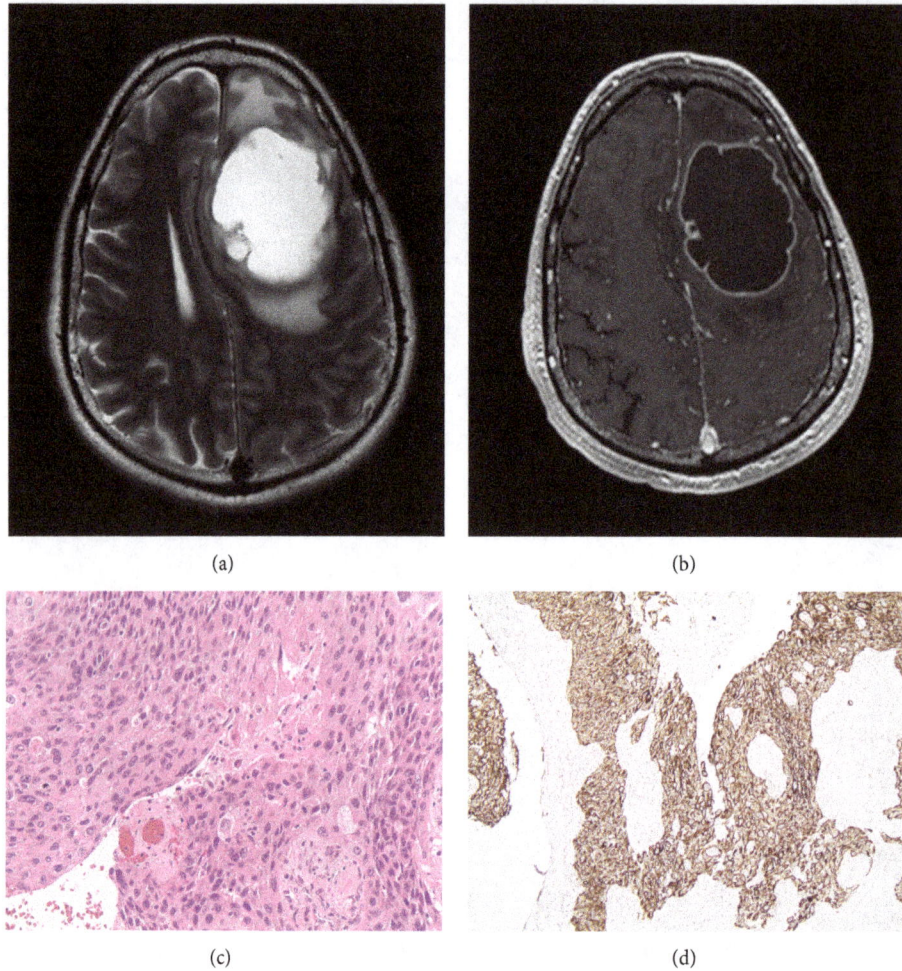

(a) (b)

(c) (d)

FIGURE 2: Radiologic and histologic features of brain metastasis. (a) Axial T2 weighted sequence demonstrates a large cystic mass in the left frontal lobe with surrounding edema, mass effect, and midline shift. (b) Axial postcontrasted T1 weighted sequence demonstrates an irregular cystic ring enhancing lesion with surrounding edema and mass effect. (c) Light microscopic examination shows squamous cell carcinoma (d) that is diffusely immunoreactive with keratin CK5/6.

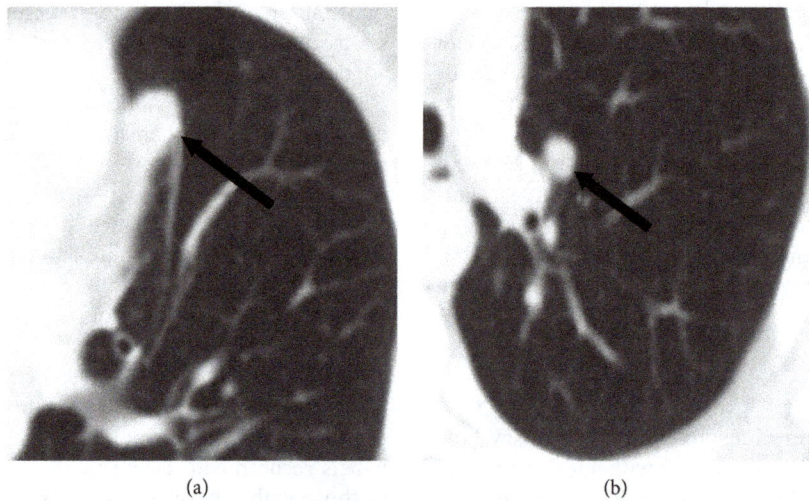

(a) (b)

FIGURE 3: Radiologic features of recurrent malignant lung disease. Contrast enhanced axial CT image shows (a) a 1.9 × 1.4 cm nodular paramediastinal opacity and (b) a left 1.1 × 0.9 cm perihilar nodule. Histological examination demonstrated pure adenocarcinoma with the same EGFR exon 19 mutation that was present in the original tumor.

equivocal nature of histologic diagnosis. Our case highlights these recommendations in the idea that our patient had a light smoking history and if the biopsy had "missed" the adenocarcinoma portion and returned a pure squamous cytology or histology, one might have concluded that the patient was unlikely to have an EGFR mutation.

4. Conclusion

This case points out that all nonsmoking lung cancer patients should have molecular testing for "actionable" mutations, regardless of histologic type.

Acknowledgment

The authors are thankful to Mr. Shawn Scally for help with microphotographs.

References

[1] T. J. Lynch, D. W. Bell, R. Sordella et al., "Activating mutations in the epidermal growth factor receptor underlying responsiveness of non-small-cell lung cancer to gefitinib," *The New England Journal of Medicine*, vol. 350, no. 21, pp. 2129–2139, 2004.

[2] S. M. Kang, H. J. Kang, J. H. Shin et al., "Identical epidermal growth factor receptor mutations in adenocarcinomatous and squamous cell carcinomatous components of adenosquamous carcinoma of the lung," *Cancer*, vol. 109, no. 3, pp. 581–587, 2007.

[3] L. V. Sequist, B. A. Waltman, D. Dias-Santagata et al., "Genotypic and histological evolution of lung cancers acquiring resistance to EGFR inhibitors," *Science Translational Medicine*, vol. 3, no. 75, Article ID 75ra26, 2011.

[4] S. P. D'Angelo, M. C. Pietanza, M. L. Johnson et al., "Incidence of EGFR exon 19 deletions and L858R in tumor specimens from men and cigarette smokers with lung adenocarcinomas," *Journal of Clinical Oncology*, vol. 29, no. 15, pp. 2066–2070, 2011.

4

Giant Right Intrathoracic Myxoid Fusocellular Lipoma

Petre V. H. Botianu,[1] **Anda Mihaela Cerghizan,**[2] **and Alexandru M. Botianu**[1]

[1]*Surgical Clinic 4, M5 Department, University of Medicine and Pharmacy of Tirgu Mures, Gheorghe Marinescu 1, 540139 Tirgu Mures, Romania*
[2]*Medical Clinic 3, M3 Department, University of Medicine and Pharmacy of Tirgu Mures, Revolutiei 35, 540043 Tirgu Mures, Romania*

Correspondence should be addressed to Petre V. H. Botianu; botianu_petre@yahoo.com

Academic Editor: Alan D. L. Sihoe

Intrathoracic lipomas are rare benign tumors; their behavior is not completely clear and their surgical removal may be challenging. We report a case of a giant right intrathoracic myxoid fusocellular lipoma compressing the lung, tracheobronchial tree, and esophagus which was removed through a posterolateral thoracotomy. Complete removal resulted in resolution of the chest pain and improvement of the dyspnea, with no recurrence at 4-year follow-up.

1. Introduction

Lipomas are common benign tumors of mesenchymal origin. They are usually located in the subcutaneous fat and are easy to treat; their surgical removal is usually simple, even for large tumors [1]. Intrathoracic location of this disease is much more rare and difficult to diagnose, and surgical removal may be challenging [2]. We report a patient with a large right intrathoracic lipoma that was completely removed through thoracotomy with complete resolution of the symptoms related to the compressive effect of the tumor.

2. Case Report

We report a 70-year-old male patient with a history of pleural effusion during childhood, stroke, nasopalpebral basocellular carcinoma excised 5 years before and severe heart disease resulting in NYHA III heart failure. His main actual complaints were pain and worsening dyspnea with no response to medical therapy. Chest X-ray (Figure 1) and CT scan (Figure 2) showed a large tumor located in the right hemithorax, with fatty densities and compressive effect. Bronchoscopy and upper digestive endoscopy showed an extrinsic compression of the trachea and right main bronchus, respectively, and esophagus, but without direct invasion of these structures. Due to the persistent pain and dyspnea the patient was referred to our unit for surgical removal of the tumor.

Surgery was performed using a large posterolateral thoracotomy. The approach was very difficult due to dense adhesions between the lung and the chest wall (probably secondary to the pleural effusion during childhood). A complete extrapulmonary tumor covered by the parietal pleura was found, with 3 vascular pedicles arising from the posterior intercostal vessels which required separate ligation. There was a cleavage plane that allowed the dissection of the tumor from the trachea, esophagus, and aorta and complete removal of the tumor (Figure 3).

The operative specimen measured 17 × 10 × 8 cm and weighed 1850 g (Figure 4(a)). Pathologic examination showed a myxoid fusocellular lipoma with no atypia (Figures 4(b) and 4(c)).

The postoperative course was complicated by a bronchopneumonia requiring prolonged antibiotic treatment. There was an obvious improvement of the dyspnea and resolution of the chest pain. At 4-year follow-up, there are no signs of recurrence.

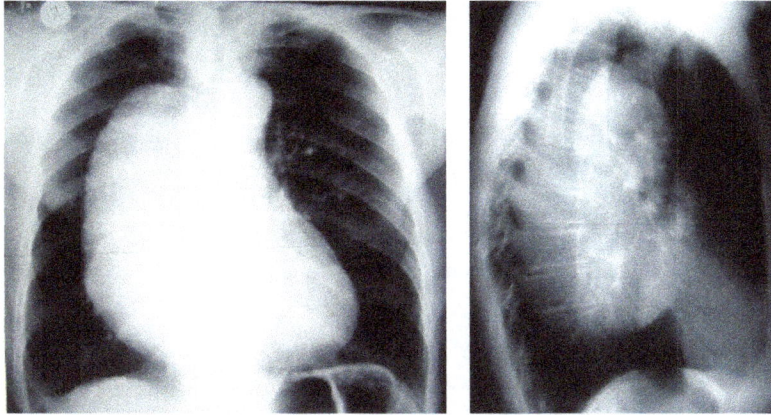

FIGURE 1: Preoperative chest X-ray showing a large intrathoracic tumor.

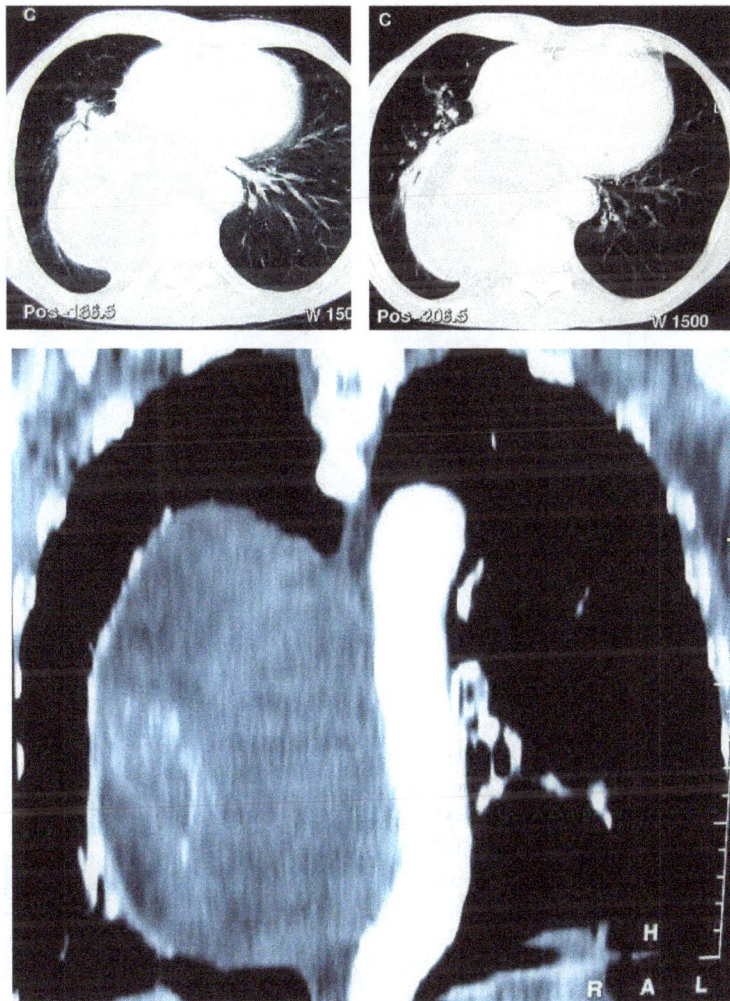

FIGURE 2: Preoperative CT scan: well-delineated mass with fatty densities and compression on the lung, trachea, right bronchus, and esophagus.

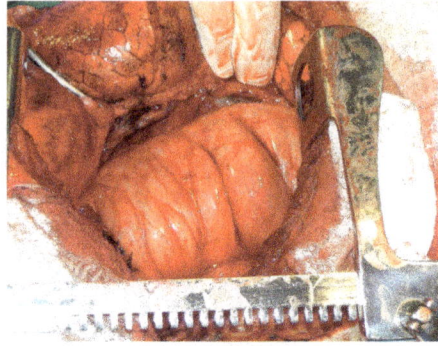

FIGURE 3: Intraoperative image showing the tumor completely dissected from the lung and covered by the parietal pleura.

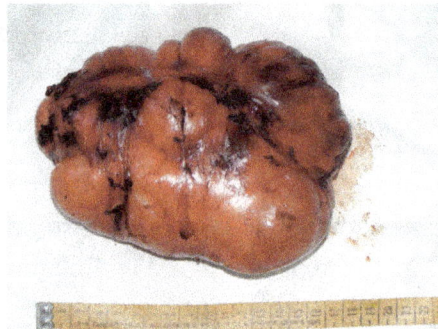

(a)

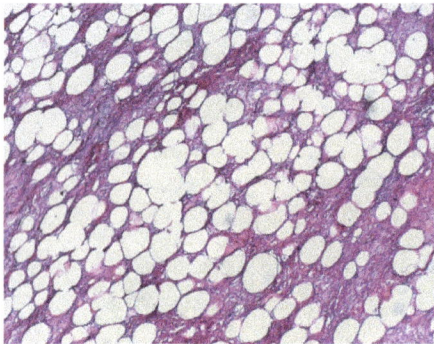

(b)

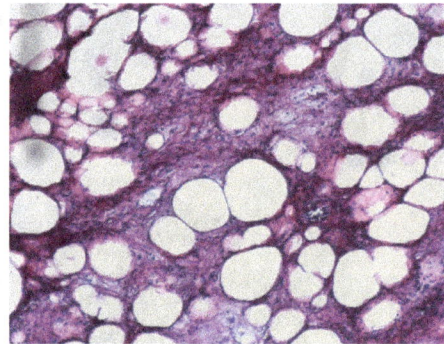

(c)

FIGURE 4: Operative specimen (a) and pathologic examination—hematoxylin-eosin 5x (b) and 10x (c) showing a myxoid spindle cell lipoma.

3. Discussions

According to their origin, intrathoracic lipomas may be classified as endobronchial, pulmonary, mediastinal (including cardiac), diaphragmatic, and pleural; an hourglass development through the intercostal space is also possible [3, 4]. In our case, due to the large dimensions of the tumor and the multiple adhesions from previous pleural effusion, the origin is not obvious. The fact that after the complete mobilization of the tumor the lung remained free and the presence of blood supply coming from the intercostal vessels strongly suggest a pleural lipoma, arising from the subpleural fatty tissue. Despite the large dimensions, the tumor had only an intrathoracic development.

The modern diagnosis of intrathoracic lipomas is based mainly on CT, which shows a well-delineated tumor with fatty densities [5]. However, there are other fat-containing masses that must be taken into consideration in the differential diagnosis, such as hamartoma, lipoid pneumonia, thymolipoma, lipoblastoma, teratoma, and teratocarcinoma. Most of the aforementioned lesions present with inhomogeneous densities, which allows for an easy differential diagnosis. Malignant lesions often present with an infiltrative aspect, invading the surrounding structures [6, 7]. However, even in the cases with a typical lipoma CT aspect, a malignant component is difficult to exclude (even on biopsy specimens), which is a plea for complete surgical removal of this kind of lesions [2]. For the lesions located near the diaphragm, diaphragmatic hernias and localized eventrations containing omentum, which is a fatty structure, must be also taken into consideration and excluded by careful 3D CT reconstructions or MRI examination [7].

Due to their rarity, the exact behavior of these tumors is not known. In the available literature, we were able to find only case reports and small series. Sakurai et al. emphasize that their clinical-pathological behavior is not always as straightforward as expected, with the possibility of liposarcoma or an infiltrative development [2]. Malignant transformation is a very rare possibility which should be also taken into consideration [8]. The difficult differentiation between benign lipoma and well-differentiated liposarcoma on small biopsy fragments is also a fact that must be taken into consideration as an argument for complete removal [9].

The indication for surgery is a matter of debate. Although it is a benign tumor, most authors advocate surgical removal due to the risks associated with the increasing of the dimensions and possible complications [2, 10, 11]. In our case, the indication for removal was based mainly on the obvious compression of the lung, with persistent dyspnea despite the aggressive medical treatment of the associated heart disease.

In selected cases, smaller tumors may be removed using a minimally invasive approach [12], but this was not the case in our patient.

4. Conclusions

Intrathoracic lipomas may represent a challenge despite their benign nature. A careful dissection and an adequate approach allow complete removal even in large tumors, with clinical improvement secondary to the removal of the compression.

References

[1] G. A. Salam, "Lipoma excision," *American Family Physician*, vol. 65, no. 5, pp. 901–905, 2002.

[2] H. Sakurai, M. Kaji, K. Yamazaki, and K. Suemasu, "Intrathoracic lipomas: their clinicopathological behaviors are not as straightforward as expected," *Annals of Thoracic Surgery*, vol. 86, no. 1, pp. 261–265, 2008.

[3] T. Sakellaridis, I. Panagiotou, S. Gaitanakis, and S. Katsenos, "Subpleural lipoma: management of a rare intrathoracic tumor," *International Journal of Surgery Case Reports*, vol. 4, no. 5, pp. 463–465, 2013.

[4] H. Çakmak and F. C. Bayram, "A giant intrathoracic and extrathoracic dumbbell-shaped lipoma," *European Journal of Cardiothoracic Surgery*, vol. 37, no. 3, p. 735, 2010.

[5] Y. I. Baris, A. F. Kalyoncu, A. Aydiner et al., "Intrathoracic lipomas demonstrated by computed tomography," *Respiration*, vol. 57, no. 2, pp. 77–80, 1990.

[6] S. C. Gaerte, C. A. Meyer, H. T. Winer-Muram, R. D. Tarver, and D. J. Conces Jr., "Fat-containing lesions of the chest," *Radiographics*, vol. 22, pp. S61–S78, 2002.

[7] M. Yildirim, E. Parlak, M. Köroglu, S. Köksal, M. Yildiz, and C. Gürses, "Diagnostics of periph erally located intrathoracic lipoma," *Acta Informatica Medica*, vol. 20, no. 2, pp. 129–130, 2012.

[8] P. Bicakcioglu, S. D. Sak, and A. I. Tastepe, "Liposarcoma of the chest wall. Transformation of dedifferentiated liposarcoma from a recurrent lipoma," *Saudi Medical Journal*, vol. 33, no. 8, pp. 901–903, 2012.

[9] A. Zidane, F. Atoini, A. Arsalane et al., "Parietal pleura lipoma: a rare intrathoracic tumor," *General Thoracic and Cardiovascular Surgery*, vol. 59, no. 5, pp. 363–366, 2011.

[10] C. Jayle, J. Hajj-Chahine, G. Allain, S. Milin, L. Soubiron, and P. Corbi, "Pleural lipoma: a non-surgical lesion?" *Interactive Cardiovascular and Thoracic Surgery*, vol. 14, no. 6, pp. 735–738, 2012.

[11] C. Asteriou, A. Lazopoulos, N. Giannoulis, I. Kalafatis, and N. Barbetakis, "Brugada-like ECG pattern due to giant mediastinal lipoma," *Hippokratia*, vol. 17, no. 4, pp. 368–369, 2013.

[12] S. Prasad, L. Ramachandra, S. Agarwal, and D. Sharma, "Successful management of pleural lipoma by video-assisted thoracoscopic surgery," *Journal of Minimal Access Surgery*, vol. 8, no. 1, pp. 19–20, 2012.

5

Pulmonary Nocardiosis in the Immunocompetent Host: Case Series

Inderjit Singh,[1] Frances Mae West,[1] Abraham Sanders,[1]
Barry Hartman,[2] and Dana Zappetti[1]

[1]Department of Medicine, Division of Pulmonary and Critical Care, Weill Cornell Medical College, New York, NY 10065, USA
[2]Department of Medicine, Division of Infectious Diseases, Weill Cornell Medical College, New York, NY 10065, USA

Correspondence should be addressed to Inderjit Singh; ins9021@nyp.org

Academic Editor: Manel Luján

Pulmonary nocardiosis is commonly recognized as an opportunistic infection in patients with predisposing immunosuppressive conditions. However, reports of pulmonary nocardiosis in the immunocompetent host are rare. Here, we report a case series of four patients with pulmonary nocardiosis without a predisposing condition.

1. Introduction

Nocardiosis is caused by Gram-positive, weakly acid-fast, filamentous aerobic actinomycetes. *Nocardia* species are ubiquitous in our environment. Human infection occurs from direct inoculation of skin or soft tissues or via direct inhalation of *Nocardia* species [1]. Nocardiosis is more likely to affect immunosuppressed patients particularly those with depressed cell-mediated immunity [2]. However, approximately one-third of patients with nocardiosis do not have a predisposing immunosuppressive condition [3].

2. Case 1

A 71-year-old female with chronic obstructive pulmonary disease (COPD) (Forced Expiratory Volume in one second of 29% predicted) presented with a one-month history of progressive exertional dyspnea, productive cough, and wheezing. Over the past 6 months, she received five courses of oral prednisone for recurrent COPD exacerbations. One week before admission, she received a 10-day course of Levofloxacin after her sputum culture grew pan-sensitive *Pseudomonas aeruginosa*. She was an ex-smoker of 105 pack-years.

On admission, her temperature was 36.5°C, blood pressure 153/68 mmHg, oxygen saturation on 2 liters 99%, pulse rate 110 beats/min, and respiratory rate 22 breaths/min. On respiratory exam, she had diffuse wheezing. Chest X-ray demonstrated hyperinflated lungs fields (Figure 1). Chest computed tomography (CT) performed 10 months earlier demonstrated severe centrilobular emphysema (Figure 1). She had leukocytosis on admission (13.3 × 10³/μL and 96% neutrophils).

Her admission sputum culture grew pan-sensitive *Pseudomonas aeruginosa* again. However, she continued to have ongoing wheezing and productive cough. Eventually, *Nocardia cyriacigeorgica* was identified on her acid-fast bacilli (AFB) sputum culture. She was started on Trimethoprim/Sulfamethoxazole (800/160 mg one tablet twice daily). Over the course of the next twelve months, she had repeated in-patient admission for worsening respiratory status. Subsequent sputum cultures repeatedly grew carbapenem-resistant *Acinetobacter baumannii*. *Nocardia* was never isolated again. She eventually died on home hospice care.

3. Case 2

A 68-year-old female with a history of left breast adenocarcinoma presented with a two-year history of productive cough and increasing dyspnea. She is an ex-smoker of 30 pack-years. She was diagnosed with breast cancer three years ago

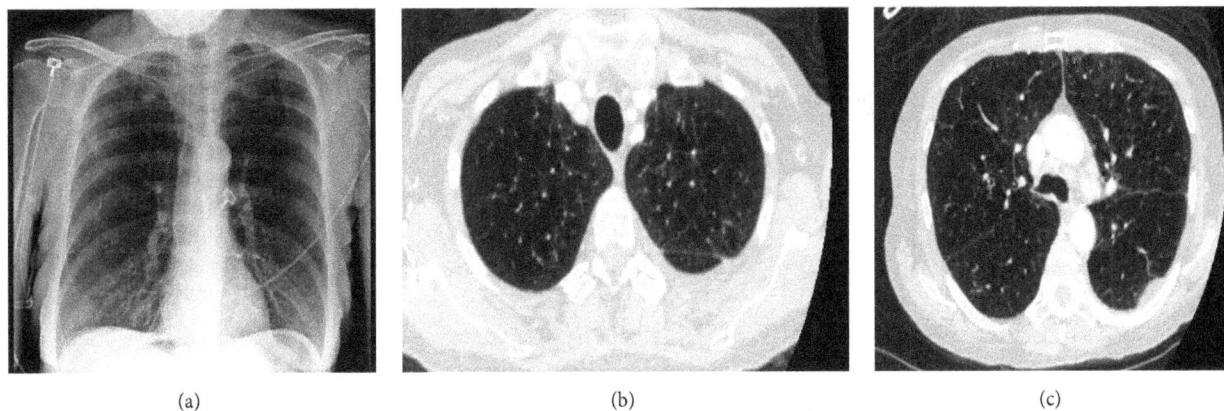

FIGURE 1: Chest X-ray and chest CT findings in Case 1. Chest X-ray findings on day of admission demonstrating hyperinflated lung fields. Chest CT findings 10 months before case presentation demonstrating severe centrilobular emphysema.

and underwent chemotherapy (Doxorubicin and Cyclophosphamide followed by Paclitaxel) followed by mastectomy and radiation therapy.

Her chest CT showed bronchiectasis and right sided tree-in-bud opacities (Figures 2(a) and 2(b)). The leading diagnosis at this stage was *Mycobacterium avium-intracellulare* complex (MAC) related lung disease. She was given a 14-day course of empiric Levofloxacin for treatment of bronchiectasis. Repeat chest CT eight weeks later showed waxing and waning parenchymal opacities with improvement in the right upper lobe but new nodular opacities involving the right middle lobe and lingula (Figure 2(c)). However, she continued to experience intermittent fevers with associated productive cough. Her sputum was sent for Gram stain and cultures grew *Nocardia cyriacigeorgica*.

She was treated with Trimethoprim/Sulfamethoxazole (800/160 mg DS twice daily). She improved clinically but developed urticarial rash. She was switched to inhaled Tobramycin (300 mg twice daily for 8 weeks) and oral Linezolid (600 mg twice daily). She improved clinically with radiographic resolution of disease (Figures 2(d) and 2(e)).

4. Case 3

A 75-year-old woman with COPD (Forced Expiratory Volume in one second of 32% predicted) and chronic MAC colonization with bronchiectasis presented with two-month history of progressive exertional dyspnea, productive cough, and constitutional symptoms. Several days before her presentation, she was started empirically on Amoxicillin/Clavulanate. An expectorated sputum sample grew MAC. Notably, in the past, a routine sputum culture grew *Nocardia cyriacigeorgica*; however, she was not treated due to stable symptoms. She presented to the emergency room because her symptoms persisted.

On initial evaluation, she was afebrile with right basilar rhonchi. Laboratory investigations were notable for leukocytosis ($12 \times 10^3/\mu L$ and 79% neutrophils). Her chest X-ray showed stable bilateral nodular opacities (Figures 3(a) and 3(b)). She was treated empirically with Trimethoprim/Sulfamethoxazole for the previously identified *Nocardia*

cyriacigeorgica. Chest CT showed bronchiectasis with bilateral lower lobe tree-in-bud infiltrates (Figures 3(c) and 3(d)). She underwent bronchoscopy with lavage which revealed no growth and bronchial wash that grew MAC. Her antibiotics were discontinued. She was treated with diuretics for worsening pulmonary hypertension. She clinically improved.

Following discharge, she developed worsening exertional dyspnea and cough. Sputum culture at that time grew *Nocardia cyriacigeorgica* and *Pseudomonas putida*. She was given Levofloxacin for treatment of the latter. However, she continued to complain of dyspnea and productive cough. Repeat echocardiogram showed improvement in her pulmonary hypertension. Her sputum culture again grew *Nocardia cyriacigeorgica*. She was then started on Trimethoprim/Sulfamethoxazole. During subsequent office visits, she reported subjective improvement in her respiratory status. She continued treatment with Trimethoprim/Sulfamethoxazole for eleven months and subsequent sputum cultures have not grown *Nocardia* spp.

5. Case 4

A 77-year-old woman with a history of bronchiectasis and MAC colonization presented with increasing sputum production. She is an ex-smoker with a 10-pack-year smoking history. She had a history of breast cancer treated with mastectomy and hormonal therapy. Three years ago, she underwent left lower lobectomy for lung adenocarcinoma. MAC infection was diagnosed on bronchoscopy eight years earlier and treated with triple drug therapy with symptom resolution. Subsequent sputum cultures revealed continued colonization with MAC. One week prior to presentation, she developed fever and cough and was prescribed Levofloxacin. Her fever resolved, but she continued to have persistent cough despite a short course of oral corticosteroid treatment.

On presentation, she was afebrile with room air oxygen saturation of 97%. Her chest radiograph is shown in Figure 4. An expectorated sputum sample was obtained for culture. The sputum culture grew multiple organisms, including *Pseudomonas aeruginosa*, *Staphylococcus aureus*, *Chryseobacterium indologenes*, MAC, and *Nocardia nova*. She was treated

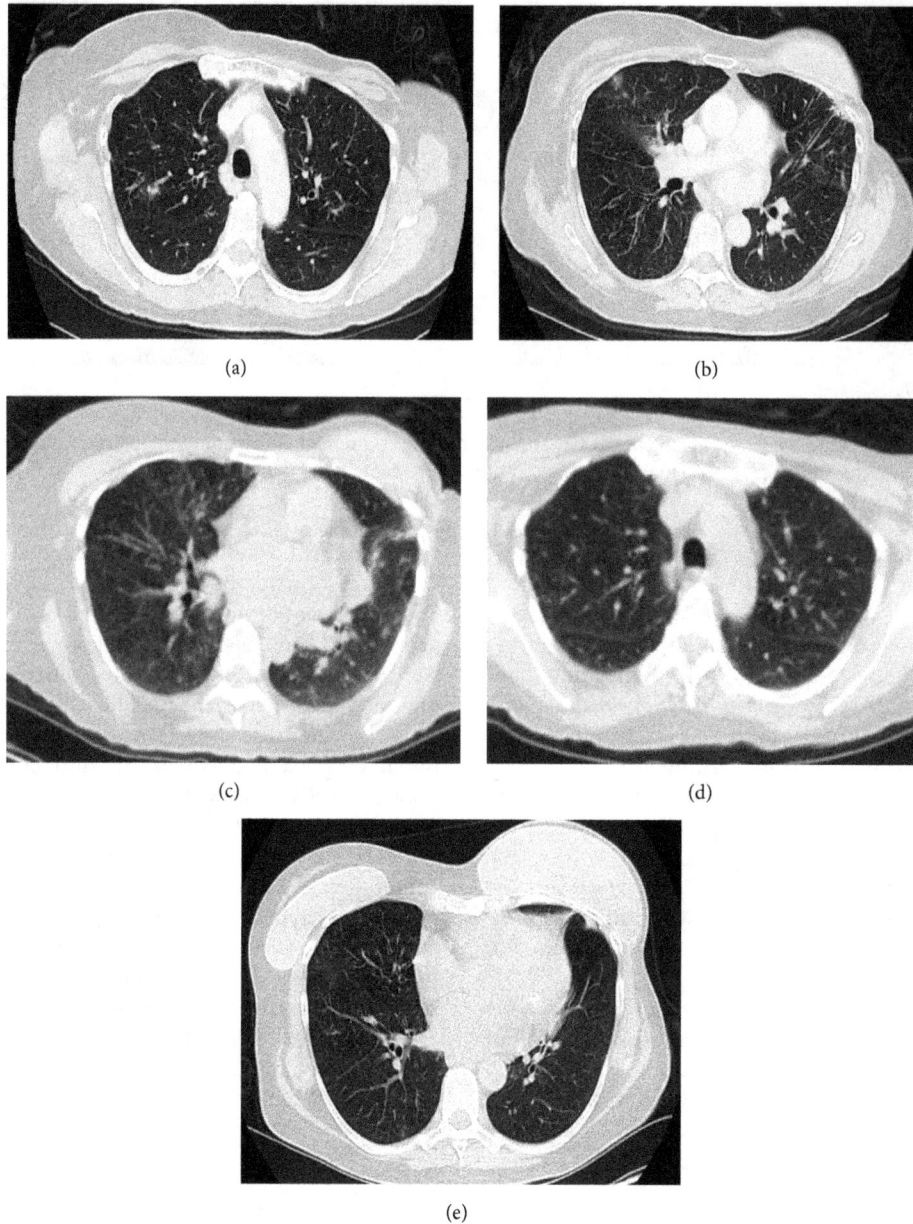

FIGURE 2: Chest CT findings in Case 2. Right upper and middle lobes nodular opacities (a) and lingular bronchiectasis (b). Waxing and waning opacities involving the right upper and middle lobes and lingula (c). Interval resolution of right middle lobe (d) and lingular opacities (e).

for bronchiectasis exacerbation with Levofloxacin, which relieved her fever and cough. She is being actively monitored for pulmonary nocardiosis with symptom monitoring and repeat sputum cultures. She has remained asymptomatic and has not been treated for *Nocardia* so far.

6. Discussion

Pulmonary nocardiosis is the most common manifestation of *Nocardia* infection. The estimated annual incidence of pulmonary nocardiosis in the United States is between 500 and 1000 cases [4]. The majority of patients have impaired cell-mediated immunity, including those with underlying malignancies and human immunodeficiency virus infection, solid-organ or hematopoietic stem cell transplant recipients, and those receiving long term corticosteroids and medications that suppress cell-mediated immunity [1]. Preexisting pulmonary disorders such as COPD [5], bronchiectasis [6], and MAC lung disease [6] are additional risk factors. In this patient population, an intrinsic defect in airway clearance and bacterial colonization of the lower airways alter ciliary motility and hasten epithelial destruction, facilitating nocardial infection. Most cases of pulmonary nocardiosis in COPD patients occur with concurrent corticosteroid use [5, 7, 8].

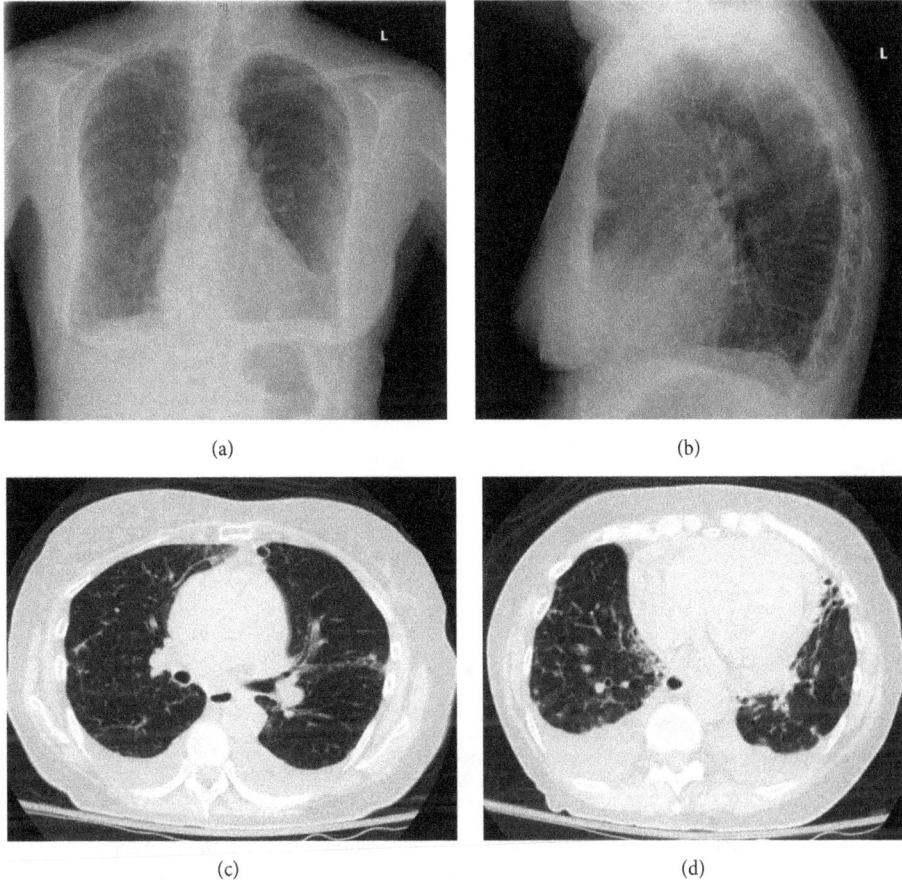

(a)

(b)

(c)

(d)

FIGURE 3: Chest X-ray and chest CT findings in Case 3. Chest X-ray showing stable bilateral nodular opacities and lower lobe predominant interstitial reticular thickening with new small bilateral pleural effusions (a, b). CT of the chest reveals bronchiectasis in the right middle and lingular lobes (c) and tree-in-bud nodular infiltrates in the bilateral lower lobes with new bilateral moderate pleural effusions.

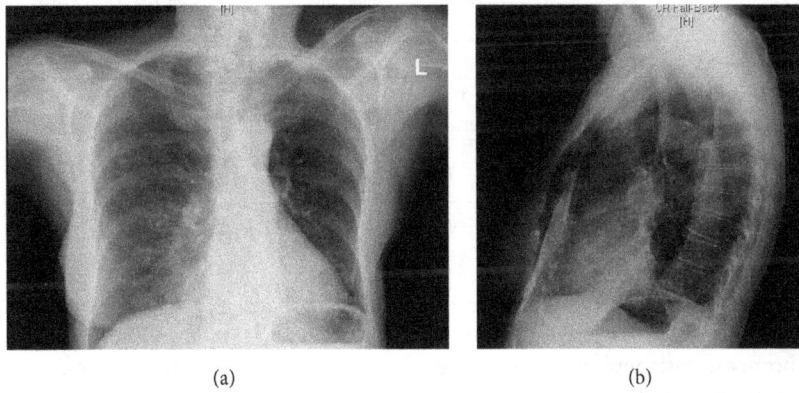

(a)

(b)

FIGURE 4: Chest X-ray findings in Case 4. Chest X-ray shows prior left lower lobectomy, stable bilateral nodules, and new consolidation versus atelectasis of the lingula.

Table 2 highlights the predisposing conditions that may have contributed to pulmonary nocardiosis in our patients.

Clinical and radiographic features of pulmonary nocardiosis often resemble those of fungal and mycobacterial disease [8]. The identification of *Nocardia* from asymptomatic immunocompetent patients should be interpreted cautiously.

The clinical status of the patient in Case 4 is being closely monitored; the decision of treatment will depend on the development of symptomatic disease. The patient in Case 4 represents *Nocardia* colonization rather than infection because her presentation of fevers and productive cough resolved following institution of Levofloxacin. Following her

TABLE 1: Antimicrobial susceptibilities of *Nocardia* species isolated from sputum cultures.

Antibiotic	*Nocardia cyriacigeorgica*			*Nocardia nova*
	Case 1 MIC (μg/mL)	Case 2 MIC (μg/mL)	Case 3 MIC (μg/mL)	Case 4 MIC (μg/mL)
Amikacin	≤8 S	≤1	≤1 S	≤8 S
Amoxicillin/Clavulanate	16/8 Int.	32/16 R	4/2 S	>32/16 R
Azithromycin	64 Int.	Not available	Not available	≤16 S
Cefepime	8 S	Not available	Not available	≤4 S
Cefotaxime	≤8 S	Not available	Not available	≤8 S
Ceftriaxone	≤8 S	8 S	≤4	≤8 S
Ciprofloxacin	>8 R	4 R	>4 R	>8 R
Clarithromycin	8 Int.	>16 R	8 R	≤25 R
Clofazimine	≤0.5 S	Not available	Not available	0.5 S
Doxycycline	Not available	4 Int.	8 R	Not available
Gentamicin	≤2 S	Not available	Not available	16 R
Imipenem	≤2 S	4 S	≤2 S	≤2 S
Kanamycin	16 R	Not available	Not available	16 R
Linezolid	2 S	2 S	2 S	≤1 S
Minocycline	≤1 S	2 Int.	>8 R	4 S
Moxifloxacin	Not available	4 R	4 R	Not available
Tobramycin	≤2 S	≤1 S	≤1 S	>16 R
Trimethoprim/Sulfamethoxazole	≤0.5/9.5 S	≤0.25/4.8 S	0.5/9.5 S	2/38 S

MIC: minimum inhibitory concentration; S: sensitive; R: resistant; Int: intermediate.

TABLE 2: Patient demographics, predisposing condition, and treatment course.

	Case 1	Case 2	Case 3	Case 4
Age (years)	73	69	79	78
Sex	Female	Female	Female	Female
Predisposing condition	COPD and concurrent steroid use	Bronchiectasis	COPD and MAC colonization with bronchiectasis	MAC colonization
Pathogen	*Nocardia cyriacigeorgica*	*Nocardia cyriacigeorgica*	*Nocardia cyriacigeorgica*	*Nocardia nova*
Treatment	Trimethoprim/ Sulfamethoxazole	Inhaled Tobramycin and oral Linezolid	Trimethoprim/ Sulfamethoxazole	Observation
Duration	6 months	8 weeks	11 months	Continued observation

COPD: chronic obstructive pulmonary disease; MAC: *Mycobacterium avium-intracellulare* complex.

treatment course, she continues to remain asymptomatic. In Case 2, the constitutional symptoms and chest CT features of nodular opacities and bronchiectasis resemble MAC lung disease; thus clinicians often overlook the less common pulmonary nocardiosis. Taken together, the protracted incubation period along with its nonspecific presentation and radiographic features makes the diagnosis of pulmonary nocardiosis challenging.

The diagnosis of pulmonary nocardiosis requires isolation and identification of the organism in respiratory secretions. Sputum cultures are positive in approximately 90% of patients. If patients are unable to expectorate, bronchoscopy with bronchoalveolar lavage can be considered. The diagnostic yield with bronchoalveolar lavage was reported as 100 percent in one study [9]. However, in Case 3, the bronchoalveolar lavage specimen was not diagnostic. Staining with modified acid-fast and Gram stains allows for a presumptive diagnosis to be made. Currently, *Nocardia* genus has over 50 species that have been characterized using various phenotypic and molecular techniques [8]. Molecular techniques such as polymerase chain reaction (PCR) testing, restriction enzyme analysis, and 16s ribosomal-DNA sequencing have enhanced the identification of the different *Nocardia* spp. *Nocardia* species in all cases were isolated using the 16s ribosomal-DNA sequencing technique.

Accurate *Nocardia* spp. identification is important because of the variation in antibiotic susceptibilities seen between the various *Nocardia* spp. (Table 1) [10]. In vitro susceptibility testing should therefore complement the identification of *Nocardia* isolates from clinical specimens.

The treatment of choice for pulmonary nocardiosis is Trimethoprim/Sulfamethoxazole (divided doses of 5 to 10 mg/kg per day of the Trimethoprim component are recommended). Alternative agents include Amikacin, Imipenem, Meropenem, Ceftriaxone, Cefotaxime, Minocycline, Moxifloxacin, Levofloxacin, Linezolid, Tigecycline, Amoxicillin/Clavulanate, and Tobramycin. The duration of treatment varies and depends on patient's clinical response because susceptibility testing does not always correlate with clinical outcome. In a prior case series of patient with nocardiosis, a favorable response was reported in 89% of patients with susceptible strains and in 75% with Trimethoprim/Sulfamethoxazole-resistant strains [11]. Along with emerging Trimethoprim/Sulfamethoxazole-resistant strains, it is reasonable to consider combination therapy and alternative agents with a proven clinical response to treat nocardiosis [12]. Immunocompetent patients with pulmonary nocardiosis are treated for at least six to twelve months [1]. There have not been any randomized controlled trials to determine the optimal agent(s), route of administration, or treatment duration for patients with pulmonary nocardiosis.

The mortality rate from pulmonary nocardiosis in immunosuppressed patients is approximately 40% [13, 14]. This increases to 64% in those with disseminated disease and 100% in those with central nervous system (CNS) involvement [13]. Patients with pulmonary nocardiosis should therefore be considered for brain imaging and blood culture testing to assess possible disseminated or CNS disease.

7. Conclusion

This case series highlights the notion that pulmonary nocardiosis should be included in the differential diagnosis even among immunocompetent patients. It is important to recognize the predisposing factors in this patient group and to differentiate nocardial infection from colonization. A high index of clinical suspicion together with close collaboration with the microbiology laboratory allows for more accurate diagnosis in order to initiate appropriate therapy with the purpose of reducing mortality.

References

[1] J. W. Wilson, "Nocardiosis: updates and clinical overview," *Mayo Clinic Proceedings*, vol. 87, no. 4, pp. 403–407, 2012.

[2] P. F. Long, "A retrospective study of nocardia infections associated with the acquired immune deficiency syndrome (AIDS)," *Infection*, vol. 22, no. 5, pp. 362–364, 1994.

[3] B. L. Beaman, J. Burnside, B. Edwards, and W. Causey, "Nocardial infections in the United States, 1972-1974," *Journal of Infectious Diseases*, vol. 134, no. 3, pp. 286–289, 1976.

[4] M. A. Aidê, S. S. Lourenço, E. Marchiori, G. Zanetti, and P. J. J. Mondino, "Pulmonary nocardiosis in a patient with chronic obstructive pulmonary disease and bronchiectasis," *Jornal Brasileiro de Pneumologia*, vol. 34, no. 11, pp. 985–988, 2008.

[5] M. Anderson and T. J. Kuźniar, "Pulmonary nocardiosis in a patient with chronic obstructive pulmonary disease—case report and literature review," *Pneumonologia i Alergologia Polska*, vol. 80, no. 6, pp. 565–569, 2012.

[6] K. Yagi, M. Ishii, H. Namkoong et al., "Pulmonary nocardiosis caused by *Nocardia cyriacigeorgica* in patients with *Mycobacterium avium* complex lung disease: two case reports," *BMC Infectious Diseases*, vol. 14, article 684, 2014.

[7] E. R. Lederman and N. F. Crum, "A case series and focused review of nocardiosis: clinical and microbiologic aspects," *Medicine*, vol. 83, no. 5, pp. 300–313, 2004.

[8] R. Martínez, S. Reyes, and R. Menéndez, "Pulmonary nocardiosis: risk factors, clinical features, diagnosis and prognosis," *Current Opinion in Pulmonary Medicine*, vol. 14, no. 3, pp. 219–227, 2008.

[9] R. Menéndez, P. J. Cordero, M. Santos, M. Gobernado, and V. Marco, "Pulmonary infection with Nocardia species: a report of 10 cases and review," *European Respiratory Journal*, vol. 10, no. 7, pp. 1542–1546, 1997.

[10] Y. Glupczynski, C. Berhin, M. Janssens, and G. Wauters, "Determination of antimicrobial susceptibility patterns of *Nocardia* spp. from clinical specimens by Etest," *Clinical Microbiology and Infection*, vol. 12, no. 9, pp. 905–912, 2006.

[11] M. V. Minero, M. Marín, E. Cercenado, P. M. Rabadán, E. Bouza, and P. Muñoz, "Nocardiosis at the turn of the century," *Medicine*, vol. 88, no. 4, pp. 250–261, 2009.

[12] R. Schlaberg, R. C. Huard, and P. Della-Latta, "Nocardia cyriacigeorgica, an emerging pathogen in the United States," *Journal of Clinical Microbiology*, vol. 46, no. 1, pp. 265–273, 2008.

[13] R. Martínez Tomás, R. Menéndez Villanueva, S. Reyes Calzada et al., "Pulmonary nocardiosis: risk factors and outcomes," *Respirology*, vol. 12, no. 3, pp. 394–400, 2007.

[14] B. Mari, C. Montón, D. Mariscal, M. Luján, M. Sala, and C. Domingo, "Pulmonary nocardiosis: clinical experience in ten cases," *Respiration*, vol. 68, no. 4, pp. 382–388, 2001.

6

Thoracic Primitive Neuroectodermal Tumor: An Unusual Case and Literature Review

Kubra Erol Kalkan,[1] Ahmet Bilici,[2] Fatih Selcukbiricik,[2] Nurcan Unver,[3] and Mahmut Yuksel[4]

[1] Department of Internal Medicine, Sisli Etfal Education and Research Hospital, 34377 Istanbul, Turkey
[2] Department of Medical Oncology, Sisli Etfal Education and Research Hospital, 34377 Istanbul, Turkey
[3] Department of Pathology, Yedikule Education and Research Hospital, 34020 Istanbul, Turkey
[4] Department of Nuclear Medicine, Medical Park Bahcelievler Hospital, 34160 Istanbul, Turkey

Correspondence should be addressed to Ahmet Bilici; ahmetknower@yahoo.com

Academic Editors: H. Dutau, G. Hillerdal, T. Koizumi, D. T. Merrick, and A. Turna

We describe herein a rare case of a primary primitive neuroectodermal tumor (PNET) in the mediastinum of a 75-year-old man. Grossly, the tumor was located in the left upper anterior mediastinum. Transcutaneous fine-needle biopsy (TCNB) revealed small round-cell proliferation. The expression immunohistochemical analysis was confirmed the diagnosis of PNET. He was successfully treated with chemotherapy and is alive with no sign of recurrence for 17 months after the diagnosis.

1. Introduction

PNET represents a family of tumors which shows varying degrees of neuronal differentiation most often presenting as a bone or soft tissue mass in the trunk or axial skeleton in adolescents and young adults [1]. Infrequently, PNETs have been described in other organs, such as the kidney, gonads, pancreas, and myocardium. Intrapulmonary PNET is very rare, PNET is a highly malignant neoplasm and it is composed of small, round, uniform cells [2]. Diagnosis of the tumor is confirmed using various immunohistochemical studies and detecting the presence of a translocation, t(11;22) through fluorescent in situ hybridization (FISH) [3]. PNET can be treated with various combinations of radical surgical resection, neoadjuvant and adjuvant chemotherapy, and irradiation. The chemotherapy of choice for these tumors consists of combinations of doxorubicin, ifosfamide, cyclophosphamide, and vincristine [4].

2. Case Report

A 75-year-old man was admitted to our Department of Medical Oncology because of dry cough which started 1 month ago in July 2011. Chest X-ray showed a left paramediastinal mass. Computed tomography (CT) of the chest demonstrated a 30 × 90 mm in diameter in the upper anterior mediastinal mass with pleural effusion around the left lower lobe. A diagnostic work up was started because of possible primary lung malignancy. FDG-PET-CT scan revealed intense and homogenous hypermetabolic activity at the upper anterior paramediastinal region (standardized uptake value (SUV): 7). Furthermore, there was hypermetabolic lesions at the left basal pleura which was compatible with metastases (Figure 1). Thereafter, a percutaneous needle biopsy was performed. Histopathologic examination of the biopsy specimen indicated malignant, small, round-cell tumor. Some of the cells had irregularly vacuolated cytoplasm secondary to glycogen deposition, which was positive for Periodic Acid Schiff (PAS) stain. In addition, the glycoprotein p30/32 (CD99), which is encoded by the MIC2 gene, is strongly expressed on the surface of the tumor cells (Figure 2). The chromosome rearrangement t(11;22)(q24;q12); t(21;22)(q22;q12); t(21;22)(q22:q21) could not be identified. The morphologic characteristics and the immunohistochemistry (positive for CD99) were compatible with PNET.

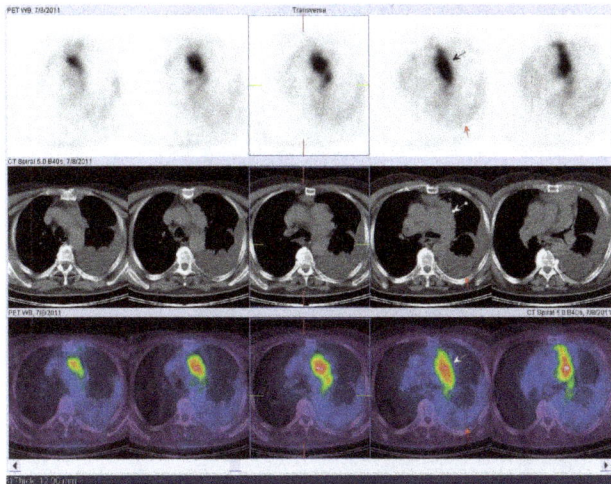

FIGURE 1: PET/CT scan shows intense and homogenous hypermetabolic activity at the upper anterior paramediastinal region (SUV: 7) and there was hypermetabolic lesions at the left basal pleura, which was compatible with metastases.

After the diagnosis of PNET was made, he was treated with combination chemotherapy including cisplatin $75 \, \text{mg/m}^2$, day 1–3, and etoposide $100 \, \text{mg/m}^2$, day 1–3, every three weeks. A partial response was achieved after three cycles of chemotherapy and the chemotherapy was continued with the same protocol. PET/CT scan revealed that there was a nearly complete response of mediastinal mass after six courses of chemotherapy (Figure 3). There was no evidence of clinical relapse after completion of six courses of chemotherapy. While the patient was well, follow-up chest CT scan showed a $40 \times 25 \, \text{mm}$ mass in size as maximal diameter in the left upper lobe anterior segment invading the pleura five months after the competition of chemotherapy. PET/CT scan was carried out to investigate further the presence of metastatic disease. It revealed increased FDG uptake within the mass (a SUVmax; 9.1) with no evidence of distant metastasis. Thereafter, the chemotherapy with doxorubicin $60 \, \text{mg/m}^2$, day 1, every three weeks, was started due to disease progression. After three and six courses of chemotherapy, chest CT scan demonstrated complete regression of the mass. He had no specific symptom and was remained to remission during a followup of four months.

3. Discussion

Peripheral PNETs are small round-cell malign neoplasms of neuroectodermal origin and are considered a member of the Ewing/PNET family of tumors. PNETs most frequently arise from the soft tissues and the bones, but rarely have been reported in other sites, such as ovary, uterus, testis, kidney, and pancreas [12].

In the thoracic region, these tumors are more commonly seen originating from the chest wall ("Askintumor"). Initially, Askin et al. reported 20 cases of malignant small cell tumor of the thoracopulmonary region in childhood (Askin tumor) in 1976 [13]. Primary pulmonary PNETs are uncommon

tumors. Fewer than 15 primary PNETs in the lung have previously been described in the literature. Weissferdt and Moran recently described six primary PNETs of the lung [4]. Review of the literature shows a male preponderance (M : F = 1.8 : 1) with a mean age of 28.2 (8–56) years [5]. Cough, fever, dyspnea, hemoptysis, and chest pain were presenting symptoms. The tumors were described as large (3.6–9.6 cm) and mostly arising from the peripheral lung parenchyma [4]. Our case was older in age than those of previous reported patients in the literature, while he was compatible with respect to presenting symptoms. The cases of primary pulmonary PNET in the literature are summarized in Table 1.

The differential diagnosis of PNET of the lung includes small cell carcinoma and other small round-cell tumors, such as malignant lymphoma, Langerhans' cell histiocytosis, granulocytic sarcoma, rhabdomyosarcoma, classical neuroblastoma, and synovial sarcoma [2]. Histochemical and immunohistochemical studies are performed to confirm the diagnosis. Careful histological evaluation and the use of several immunohistochemical (IHC) markers and antibodies such as O13, HBA-71, and 12E7 (the MIC2 gene product) that recognizes the cell surface antigen, defined by the cluster of CD99, facilitate the diagnosis. Although not specific for PNET or Ewing sarcoma, CD99 is generally present in these tumors [14]. Malignant lymphoma is distinguished from pPNETs, which do not stain for LCA. Small cell carcinoma is distinguished with the consistent positive immunoreactivity to cytokeratins, and reactivity for IHC markers such as chromogranin and TTF-1 supports the diagnosis of small cell carcinoma [15]. In addition, the IHC expression of muscle-specific markers such as desmin, myogenin, or myo-D1 is characteristic of rhabdomyosarcoma. The identification of a nonrandom t(11;22)(q24;q12) chromosome rearrangement has been reported in these aggressive malignant tumors [9, 14, 15]. This translocation was demonstrated in five cases of pulmonary PNET whereas in our case it could not be demonstrated [7].

PNET is a highly malignant tumor with a very poor prognosis. The treatment of choice for these tumors was various combinations of radical surgical resection, neoadjuvant and adjuvant chemotherapy, and irradiation [16]. Resection and adjuvant chemotherapy with or without radiation were administered in seven patients while neoadjuvant chemotherapy and resection with or without adjuvant chemotherapy were administered in six patients, and five patients underwent resection only. The 2-year survival rates are 33%, 66%, and 33%, respectively. Five of the six patients administered neoadjuvant chemotherapy were alive with a follow-up ranging from 11 to 34 months [4]. The present case was treated only with chemotherapy due to inoperable disease, after that complete response was obtained. To our knowledge, this is the first report of inoperable thoracic PNET treated with chemotherapy, and complete regression of the mass is demonstrated and the patient is alive with a followup of 17 months.

This report constitutes the first case of PNET of the lung successfully treated with chemotherapy in the literature. In patients with mediastinal mass, primary PNET of the

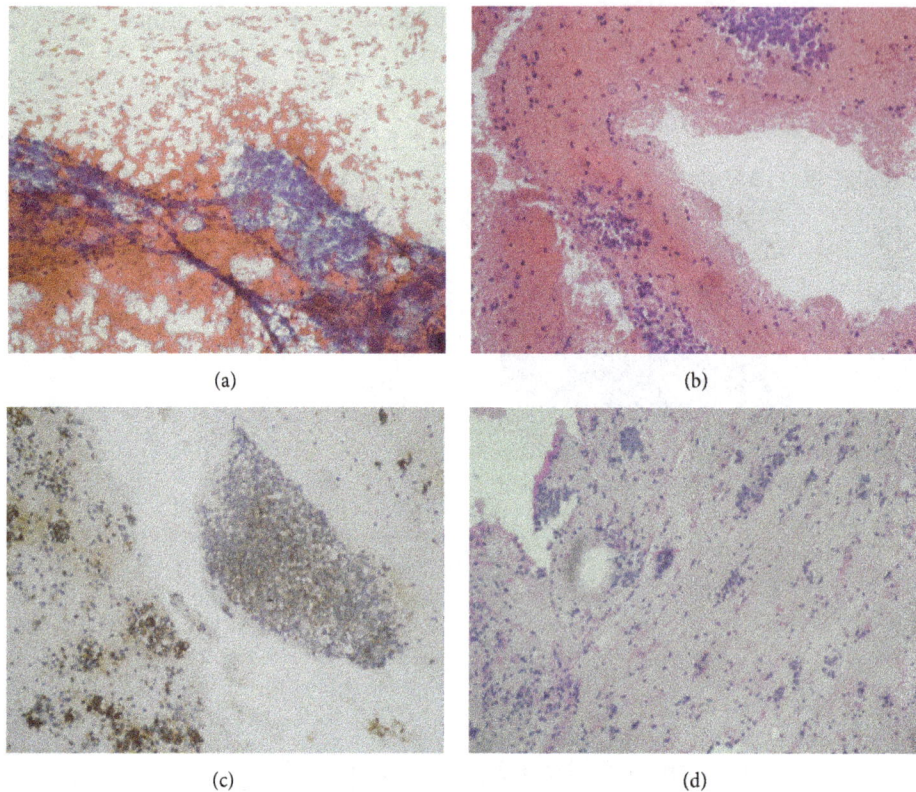

FIGURE 2: (a) Cytologic features, cellular aspirate PAP stained (original magnification, ×200).JPG; (b) Hematoxylin and Eosin stained cell block section shows a cluster of uniform cells with fine, pale chromatin and a moderate amount of cytoplasm (original magnification, ×200) 2.JPG; (c) CD99 EMA immunohistochemistry shows strong membranous staining (original magnification, ×400).JPG; (d) Periodic Acid Schiff (PAS) stain, ×200.JPG.

TABLE 1: Primary pulmonary primitive neuroectodermal tumor patients in the literature.

Case	Year	Sex	Age	Tumor location	Treatment	Followup	Reference
1	1998	F	25	LLL	Resection only	DOD at 24 months	[2]
2	1998	M	15	LLL	Resection only	A&W at 24 months	[2]
3	2000	F	30	RLL	Neoadjuvant CT/resection/adjuvant CT	A&W at 16 months	[5]
4	2000	M	41	LUL	Neoadjuvant CT/resection	A&W at 22 months	[5]
5	2001	F	26	L hilum	Neoadjuvant CT/resection/adjuvant CRT	DOD at 8 months	[6]
6	2001	M	18	RML	Resection only	DOD at 24 months	[7]
7	2001	F	17	RLL	Resection/adjuvant CRT	DOD at 9 months	[8]
8	2007	M	8	RUL	Resection/neoadjuvant CT	A&W at 9 months	[9]
9	2009	F	22	Lung, NOS	Neoadjuvant CT/resection/adjuvant CRT	A&W at 32 months	[10]
10	2009	F	28	Lung, NOS	Resection/adjuvant CRT	A&W at 18 months	[10]
11	2009	M	22	Lung, NOS	Resection/adjuvant CRT	DOD at 18 months	[10]
12	2009	M	47	Lung, NOS	Neoadjuvant CT/resection/adjuvant CT	A&W at 34 months	[10]
13	2010	M	44	RUL	Resection/adjuvant CT	DOD at 5 months	[11]
14	2012	M	22	RUL	Resection only	NK	[4]
15	2012	M	27	LUL	Resection/adjuvant CT	DOD at 24 months	[4]
16	2012	F	29	LUL	Resection/adjuvant CT	DOD at 36 months	[4]
17	2012	M	31	RLL	Resection/adjuvant CT	DOD at 54 months	[4]
18	2012	M	29	RUL	Resection only	NK	[4]
19	2012	F	56	RML	Neoadjuvant CT/resection/adjuvant CT	A&W at 11 months	[4]
20	2013	M	75	LUL	CT only	A&W at 17 months	This case

M: male, F: female, NK: not known, RUL: right upper lobe, LUL: left upper lobe, RLL: right lower lobe, RML: right middle lobe, L: left, NOS: not otherwise specified, CT: chemotherapy, RT: radiotherapy, CRT: chemoradiation, A&W: alive and well, DOD: dead of disease.

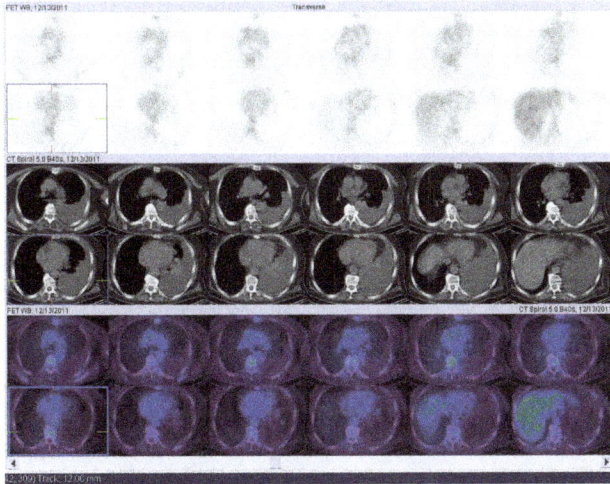

FIGURE 3: After six cycles of chemotherapy, PET/CT revealed nearly complete response of mediastinal mass.

mediastinum should be considered in differential diagnosis of the mediastinal mass as primary lung cancer. In this situation, our case highlights the eliminating of patients with mediastinal mass from the other small round-cell tumors; the treatment options in these tumors are markedly different because PNETs are more chemosensitive tumors.

References

[1] Y. B. Thyavihally, H. B. Tongaonkar, S. Gupta et al., "Primitive neuroectodermal tumor of the kidney: a single institute series of 16 patients," *Urology*, vol. 71, no. 2, pp. 292–296, 2008.

[2] S. Tsuji, M. Hisaoka, Y. Morimitsu et al., "Peripheral primitive neuroectodermal tumour of the lung: report of two cases," *Histopathology*, vol. 33, no. 4, pp. 369–374, 1998.

[3] E. Cambruzzi, E. E. Guerra, H. C. Hilgert et al., "Primitive neuroectodermal tumor of the liver: a case report," *Case Reports in Medicine*, vol. 2011, Article ID 748194, 4 pages, 2011.

[4] A. Weissferdt and C. A. Moran, "Primary Pulmonary Primitive Neuroectodermal Tumor (PNET): a clinicopathological and immunohistochemical study of six cases," *Lung*, vol. 190, pp. 677–683, 2012.

[5] F. Imamura, T. Funakoshi, S. I. Nakamura, M. Mano, K. Kodama, and T. Horai, "Primary primitive neuroectodermal tumor of the lung: report of two cases," *Lung Cancer*, vol. 27, no. 1, pp. 55–60, 2000.

[6] F. J. Baumgartner, B. O. Omari, and S. W. French, "Primitive neuroectodermal tumor of the pulmonary hilum in an adult," *Annals of Thoracic Surgery*, vol. 72, no. 1, pp. 285–287, 2001.

[7] A. G. Kahn, A. Avagnina, J. Nazar, and B. Elsner, "Primitive neuroctodermal tumor of the lung," *Archives of Pathology & Laboratory Medicine*, vol. 125, pp. 397–399, 2001.

[8] Y. Mikami, M. Nakajima, H. Hashimoto et al., "Primary pulmonary primitive neuroectodermal tumor (PNET). A case report," *Pathology Research and Practice*, vol. 197, no. 2, pp. 113–119, 2001.

[9] D. Takahashi, J. Nagayama, Y. Nagatoshi et al., "Primary Ewing's sarcoma family tumors of the lung—a case report and review of the literature," *Japanese Journal of Clinical Oncology*, vol. 37, no. 11, pp. 874–877, 2007.

[10] A. Demir, M. Z. Gunluoglu, N. Dagoglu et al., "Surgical treatment and prognosis of primitive neuroectodermal tumors of the thorax," *Journal of Thoracic Oncology*, vol. 4, no. 2, pp. 185–192, 2009.

[11] K. Hancorn, A. Sharma, and M. Shackcloth, "Primary extraskeletal Ewing's sarcoma of the lung," *Interactive Cardiovascular and Thoracic Surgery*, vol. 10, no. 5, pp. 803–804, 2010.

[12] T. Takeuchi, H. Iwasaki, Y. Ohjimi et al., "Renal primitive neuroectodermal tumor: an immunohistochemical and cytogenetic analysis," *Pathology International*, vol. 46, no. 4, pp. 292–297, 1996.

[13] F. B. Askin, J. Rosai, R. K. Sibley, L. P. Dehner, and W. H. Mc Alister, "Malignant small cell tumor of the thoracopulmonary region in childhood. A distinctive clinicopathologic entity of uncertain histogenesis," *Cancer*, vol. 43, no. 6, pp. 2438–2451, 1979.

[14] C. F. Stephenson, J. A. Bridge, and A. A. Sandberg, "Cytogenetic and pathologic analysis of Ewing's sarcoma and neuroectodermal tumors," *Human Pathology*, vol. 23, pp. 1270–1277, 1992.

[15] T. V. Colby, M. N. Koss, and W. D. Travis, *Tumors of the Lower Respiratory Tract (Atlas of Tumor Pathology, 3rd Series, Fascicle 13)*, AFIP, Washington, DC, USA, 1995.

[16] M. A. Applebaum, J. Worch, R. Goldsby et al., "Clinicalfeaturesandoutcomes in patients with extraskeletal Ewingsarcoma," *Cancer*, vol. 117, pp. 3027–3032, 2011.

7

Successful Flexible Bronchoscopic Management of Dynamic Central Airway Obstruction by a Large Tracheal Carcinoid Tumor

Vijay Hadda, Karan Madan, Anant Mohan, Umasankar Kalai, and Randeep Guleria

Department of Pulmonary Medicine and Sleep Disorders, All India Institute of Medical Sciences, New Delhi 110029, India

Correspondence should be addressed to Vijay Hadda; vijayhadda@yahoo.com

Academic Editor: Hiroshi Niwa

Typical carcinoid of the trachea presenting as an endoluminal polypoidal mass is a rare occurrence. Herein, we report a case of a 34-year-old female patient who presented with features of central airway obstruction. Flexible bronchoscopy demonstrated a large pedunculated growth arising from the lower end of the trachea near carina which was flopping in and out of the main tracheal lumen and the proximal right bronchus leading to dynamic airway obstruction. Successful electrosurgical excision (using a snare loop) of the polypoidal growth was performed using the flexible bronchoscope itself. The patient had immediate relief of airway obstruction and histopathological examination of the polyp demonstrated features of typical carcinoid (WHO Grade I neuroendocrine tumor).

1. Introduction

Endobronchial benign tumors of the respiratory tract are rare [1, 2]. Carcinoids are among the commonest endobronchial benign tumors; however, primary typical carcinoids of the trachea are uncommon [1, 2]. Due to slow growth rate, symptoms are often mistaken for bronchial asthma and a delay in diagnosis is usual. Hemoptysis may not be present in all the patients. Trepopnea is an underrecognized form of dyspnea where patient is having breathing difficulty in only one lateral decubitus position. We report a case of a young female patient who presented with trepopnea and with a normal chest X-ray examination. CT scan followed by a bronchoscopic examination of the airways demonstrated the presence of a large pedunculated tracheal tumor which was successfully removed with endobronchial electrocautery with a snare loop using flexible bronchoscopy. Primary tracheal tumors are rare neoplasms which can be missed due to paucity of symptoms and difficulty in detecting them with chest radiographs.

2. Case Presentation

A 34-year-old lady presented with history of shortness of breath of four-month duration and shortness of breath used to be worse on lying in the left lateral position (trepopnea). She also complained of dull aching central chest pain and dry cough for the same duration. In addition, she also complained of recurrent seasonal episodes of sneezing and nasal obstruction associated with headache. There was no history of fever, wheeze, and hemoptysis or weight loss. General physical examination revealed expiratory stridor. Respiratory rate was 24/min and oxygen saturation while breathing at room air was 95%. Examination of the respiratory system and rest of the systemic examination was normal.

Chest radiograph was normal. In a young female in view of trepopnea and expiratory stridor, intrathoracic (tracheal/major bronchial) obstruction was suspected and contrast enhanced computed tomography (CT) scan of the thorax was performed. In view of symptoms suggestive rhinosinusitis CT of paranasal sinuses was also performed. CT scan of the thorax showed presence of endoluminal polypoidal growth arising from the posterior wall of the tracheal bifurcation measuring 13 mm in anteroposterior diameter and 13 mm in the transverse diameter (Figure 1). The growth was not enhancing postcontrast administration. There was no mediastinal lymph node enlargement and both lungs appeared normal.

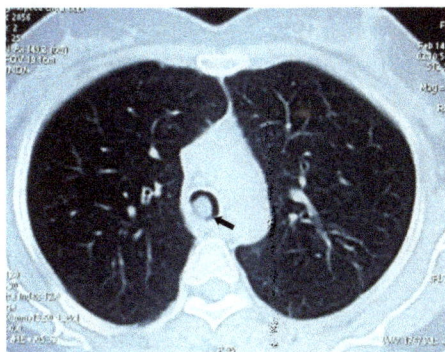

FIGURE 1: CT scan of the thorax showing a endoluminal polypoidal growth (arrow) arising from the posterior wall of the tracheal bifurcation.

Flexible fiberoptic bronchoscopy (FOB) was performed for further assessment. It revealed a large fleshy polypoidal growth with well-defined narrow stalk arising from the posterior wall of the lower trachea (Figure 2(a)). The growth was flopping in and out of the right main bronchus and trachea leading to dynamic airway obstruction of either of the two main bronchi. The major bronchi and the distal bronchial segments were normal.

In view of the respiratory distress (central airway obstruction), a decision to attempt flexible bronchoscopic removal of the polyp was taken. Facility for rigid bronchoscopy was standby, in case there was any difficulty during flexible bronchoscopic removal. Olympus BF-1T-180 video bronchoscope (with a 3 mm working channel) via oral route was used. An electrosurgical snare loop (SD 7C-1, Olympus) was used for electrosurgical excision. The snare loop was used to encircle and firmly tighten around the neck of the polypoidal growth and electrosurgical excision was performed. The mass got avulsed from its base completely and stuck on to the snare loop and the same was removed in toto along with the flexible bronchoscope (Figure 2(b)). The procedure was done under conscious sedation using lidocaine nebulization and intravenous injection of midazolam 2 mg, fentanyl 50 microgram, and Phenergan (promethazine) 25 mg. There was no procedural complication/bleeding. Patient had immediate relief of symptoms of breathlessness and trepopnea in the same day.

The histopathology of the tracheal growth was suggestive of carcinoid (Figure 3). A DOTANOC Positron Emission Tomographic CT scan was performed later which demonstrated no areas of abnormal tracer uptake. Patient is under regular follow-up and follow-up bronchoscopic examination has been normal.

3. Discussion

Carcinoids arise from the Kulchitsky cells disseminated in the bronchopulmonary mucosa [1]. These tumors are uncommon and account for approximately 2% of all bronchopulmonary tumors [3, 4]. Most of bronchopulmonary carcinoids (75–90%) are localized to central airways whereas smaller proportion (10–25%) is peripheral [3, 4]. According to WHO

2004, neuroendocrine tumors of the lung are divided into three main entities: carcinoid tumors (typical/atypical), large cell neuroendocrine carcinomas (LCNEC), and small cell carcinomas (SCC) [5]. These are further classified as well differentiated (low grade) typical, moderately differentiated (intermediate grade) atypical, and poorly differentiated (high grade) LCNEC and SCC based on the appearance, mitotic rate, Ki-67 index, and presence of necrosis [5].

Typical carcinoid tumors, which represent 90% of carcinoid lung neoplasms, occur mostly in young patients. Among patients with typical carcinoids metastases to lymph node (5%–15%) and distant sites (3%) are uncommon at presentation. In comparison, atypical carcinoids though rare (0.1%-0.2%) lung tumors, however, lymph node (40%–50%) or distant (20%) metastasis are common at presentation [6]. Bagheri et al. reported that the most common site of involvement was the left main bronchus (25%) while tracheal involvement was seen in 5% [7]. Tracheal carcinoids most commonly arise from the distal one third of the trachea from the posterior noncartilaginous fibrous membrane as in our case. The usual symptoms are dyspnea, wheezing, and hemoptysis; however, our patient presented with unusual symptom of trepopnea which has never been reported in the literature previously. Trachea being a blind spot in the chest radiograph and the symptoms of wheeze and stridor are misinterpreted as asthma; there remains a delay in the diagnosis of primary tracheal tumor. 68Ga-DOTATOC PET/CT is a useful imaging investigation for the evaluation of pulmonary carcinoids with sensitivity of 96% and 100% specific while 18F-FDG PET/CT scan suffers from low sensitivity and specificity in differentiating the pulmonary carcinoids from other tumors [8].

Carcinoid tumors, when localized, are primarily treated surgically. With surgical removal the five-year survival is 97% and 78% for typical and atypical carcinoid tumors, respectively [2]. The histology and lymph node involvement were the main prognostic factors for these patients [2]. However, for patients with metastatic disease there is little to offer as metastatic tumors are generally not sensitive to chemotherapy or radiotherapy.

Bronchoscopic ablation is a useful and efficacious modality for the removal of endobronchial tumors [1, 4, 9]. The indications of endobronchial ablative therapy include an endobronchial tumor occupying more than 50% of the lumen of large airways associated with dyspnea and hemoptysis related to the lesion, lesions preventing the mucociliary clearance and causing recurrent pneumonitis or intractable cough. Only absolute contraindication of endobronchial ablative therapy is the extrinsic compression of the airways. Both flexible as well as rigid bronchoscope may be used for endobronchial ablation. In patients with significant airway obstruction and especially patients who are in respiratory failure, rigid bronchoscopy is the preferred modality for removal. The large lumen of the ventilating rigid bronchoscope allows ventilation to continue while airway procedures are being simultaneously performed. Removal of the endobronchial growths can be accomplished by either coring out the tumor using the beveled tip of the rigid bronchoscope or by application of endobronchial ablative modalities like laser,

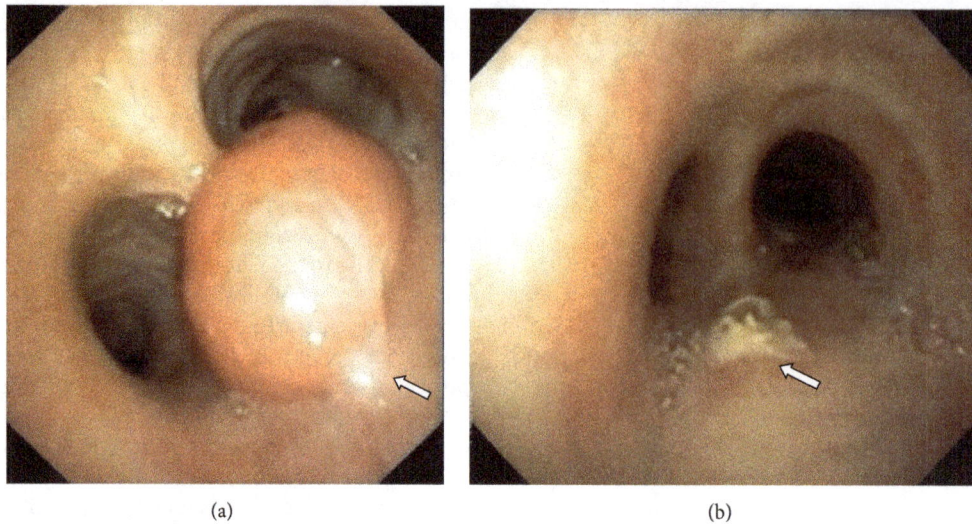

(a)   (b)

FIGURE 2: (a) Flexible bronchoscopic image showing a large fleshy polypoidal growth with well-defined narrow stalk (arrow) arising from the posterior wall of the lower trachea. (b) The electrosurgical excision successfully removed the tumor in toto (b). There was no bleed or gross evidence of residual tumor at the intervention site (arrow).

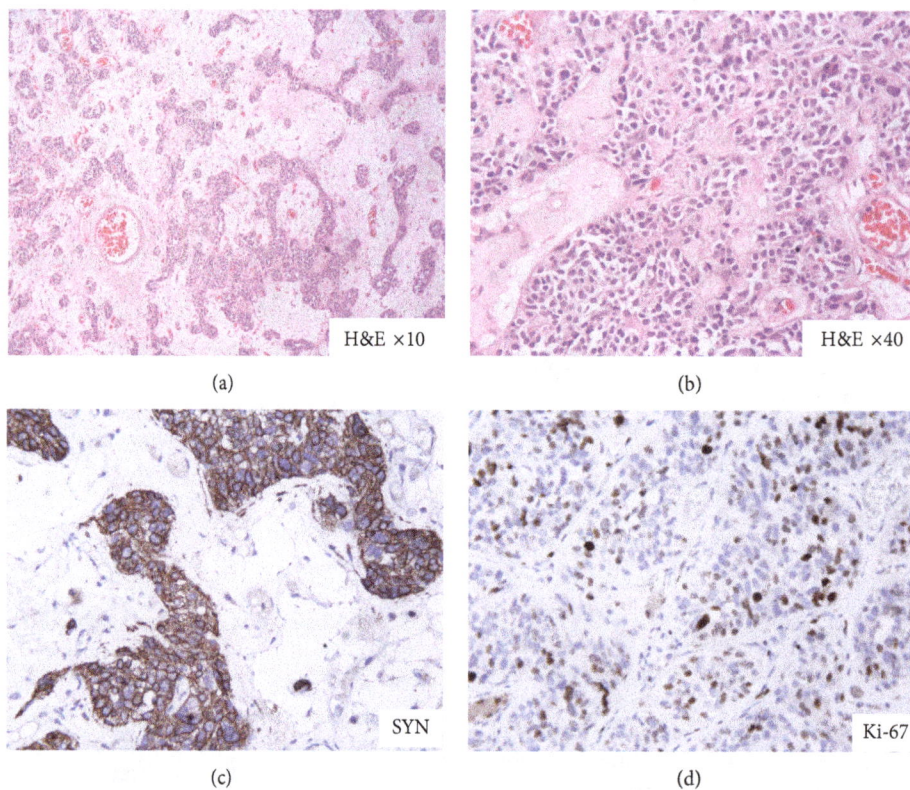

FIGURE 3: Histopathology of the ablated tumor showing features of carcinoid. Tumor cells are arranged in nests with rich vascular stroma (a). They show salt and pepper type of nuclear chromatin (b). Immunohistochemistry shows positivity for synaptophysin (c) with increased proliferating (KI 67 labelling) index (d).

electrocautery, cryotherapy, and so forth [3, 9, 10]. Flexible bronchoscopic removal of endobronchial tumors can also be performed efficaciously especially in the hands of trained operators. We performed endobronchial removal, since CT scan was suggestive of isolated endobronchial lesion without extension through the cartilaginous area. However, it must be kept in mind that inadvertent complications may arise during flexible bronchoscopic removal like tumor displacement, significant bleeding, and so forth which might necessitate urgent rigid bronchoscopy.

4. Conclusion

Central airway tumors are mimickers of bronchial asthma and chest X-ray can be normal; hence, CT should be considered in patients who have symptoms of stridor or trepopnea. Tracheal carcinoid without extension to the mediastinum can be successfully removed using flexible bronchoscopy and electrocautery but needs close follow-up of the excision site for recurrence.

References

[1] V. E. Gould, R. I. Linnoila, V. A. Memoli, and W. H. Warren, "Neuroendocrine components of the bronchopulmonary tract: hyperplasias, dysplasias, and neoplasms," *Laboratory Investigation*, vol. 49, no. 5, pp. 519–537, 1983.

[2] M. García-Yuste, J. M. Matilla, A. Cueto et al., "Typical and atypical carcinoid tumours: analysis of the experience of the Spanish multi-centric study of neuroendocrine tumours of the lung," *European Journal of Cardio-Thoracic Surgery*, vol. 31, no. 2, pp. 192–197, 2007.

[3] F. Davini, A. Gonfiotti, C. Comin, A. Caldarella, F. Mannini, and A. Janni, "Typical and atypical carcinoid tumours: 20-year experience with 89 patients," *Journal of Cardiovascular Surgery*, vol. 50, no. 6, pp. 807–811, 2009.

[4] N. Rekhtman, "Neuroendocrine tumors of the lung," *Archives of Pathology and Laboratory Medicine*, vol. 134, no. 11, pp. 1628–1638, 2010.

[5] W. D. Travis, E. Brambilla, H. K. Muller-Hermelink, and C. C. Harris, *World Health Organization Classification of Tumours . Pathology and Genetics of Tumours of the Lung, Pleura, Thymus and Heart*, IARC Press, Lyon, France, 2004.

[6] B. I. Gustafsson, M. Kidd, A. Chan, M. V. Malfertheiner, and I. M. Modlin, "Bronchopulmonary neuroendocrine tumors," *Cancer*, vol. 113, no. 1, pp. 5–21, 2008.

[7] R. Bagheri, M. Mashhadi, S. Z. Haghi, A. Sadrizadh, and F. Rezaeetalab, "Tracheobronchopulmonary carcinoid tumors: analysis of 40 patients," *Annals of Thoracic and Cardiovascular Surgery*, vol. 17, no. 1, pp. 7–12, 2011.

[8] B. Venkitaraman, S. Karunanithi, A. Kumar, G. C. Khilnani, and R. Kumar, "Role of 68Ga-DOTATOC PET/CT in initial evaluation of patients with suspected bronchopulmonary carcinoid," *European Journal of Nuclear Medicine and Molecular Imaging*, vol. 41, no. 5, pp. 856–864, 2014.

[9] K. Madan, R. Agarwal, A. Bal, and D. Gupta, "Bronchoscopic management of a rare benign endobronchial tumor," *Revista Portuguesa de Pneumologia*, vol. 18, no. 5, pp. 251–254, 2012.

[10] K. Madan, R. Agarwal, A. Aggarwal, and D. Gupta, "Therapeutic rigid bronchoscopy at a tertiary care center in North India: initial experience and systematic review of Indian literature," *Lung India*, vol. 31, no. 1, pp. 9–15, 2014.

8

Primary Tubercular Chest Wall Abscess in a Young Immunocompetent Male

Shweta Sharma,[1] R. K. Mahajan,[1] V. P. Myneedu,[2] B. B. Sharma,[3] and Nandini Duggal[1]

[1] Department of Microbiology, Dr. Ram Manohar Lohia Hospital and PGIMER, New Delhi 110001, India
[2] SAG Grade, Department of Microbiology, LRS, Institute of Tuberculosis and Respiratory Disease, Delhi 110030, India
[3] Department of Radiology, Dr. Ram Manohar Lohia Hospital and PGIMER, New Delhi, India

Correspondence should be addressed to Shweta Sharma; drshwetamicro@gmail.com

Academic Editor: Alan D. L. Sihoe

Chest wall tuberculosis is a rare entity especially in an immunocompetent patient. Infection may result from direct inoculation of the organisms or hematogenous spread from some underlying pathology. Infected lymph nodes may also transfer the bacilli through lymphatic route. Chest wall tuberculosis may resemble a pyogenic abscess or tumour and entertaining the possibility of tubercular etiology remains a clinical challenge unless there are compelling reasons of suspicion. In tuberculosis endemic countries like India, all the abscesses indolent to routine treatment need investigation to rule out mycobacterial causes. We present here a case of chest wall tuberculosis where infection was localized to skin only and, in the absence of any evidence of specific site, it appears to be a case of primary involvement.

1. Introduction

Tuberculosis (TB) is a major public health problem with associated high morbidity and mortality if not treated adequately, especially in the developing countries like India which accounts for one-fourth of the global incident TB cases annually. In 2012, out of the global annual incidence of 8.6 million TB cases, 2.3 million were estimated to have occurred in India [1]. As per the WHO Global Report on tuberculosis in 2013, 20% of all the freshly diagnosed cases in India are extrapulmonary. The report also highlights that of 300,000 cases of MDR in the world, India alone has the burden of 64,000 cases [1, 2]. Chest wall tuberculosis is rare form of extrapulmonary TB and accounts for 1–5% of all musculoskeletal TB, which itself is very rare [3]. Sternum remains the most common site to be involved though rib shafts, costochondral junctions, and vertebral bodies can also be involved. Chest wall TB may result from direct inoculation or hematogenous/lymphatic spread or as an extension of underlying pleurapulmonary disease or infection of bony structures. Diagnosis of chest wall tuberculosis is often arduous since clinical presentation may resemble pyogenic abscess and since MOTT are important causes of skin infections failure to respond to conventional ATT may further complicate the diagnosis. Here we are presenting a case of primary tubercular abscess in the chest wall of a 16-year-old boy where the bacilli appeared to have got directly deposited on the damaged skin from an open case of tuberculosis in the family and evolve into a fully developed abscess.

2. Case Report

A 16-year-old male presented to the surgical OPD with a painful swelling in the sternal region. Swelling was pea sized (1×1 cm) two months back which gradually increased to the present size of 6×7 cm. There was history of intermittent fever and loss of appetite for the last 5-6 weeks. The boy recalled getting the skin over his sternum abraded with a metallic religious locket which he used to wear around his neck. There were no respiratory complaints or past history of tuberculosis. There was family history of pulmonary tuberculosis in his brother, who was put on anti-tubercular therapy (ATT) about two weeks before this boy reported to our institution.

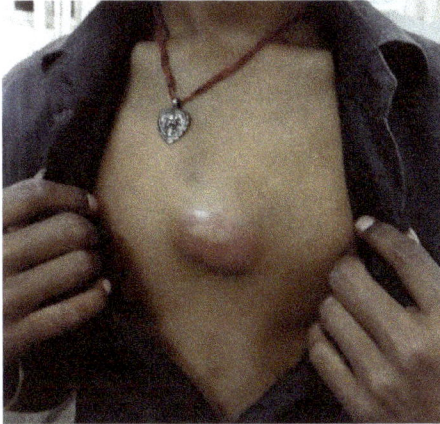

FIGURE 1: Showing large solitary well defined lesion over sternum.

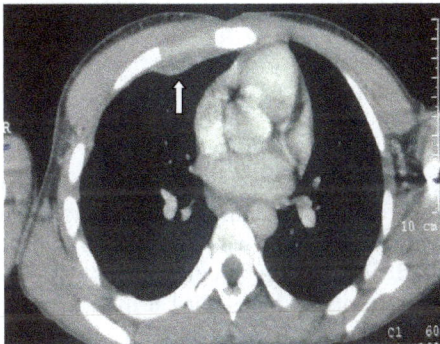

FIGURE 2: Axial CECT image at lesion level in mediastinal window showing well loculated eliptical hypodense collection with peripheral enhancement on the anterior chest wall with no evidence of mediastinal lymphadenopathy.

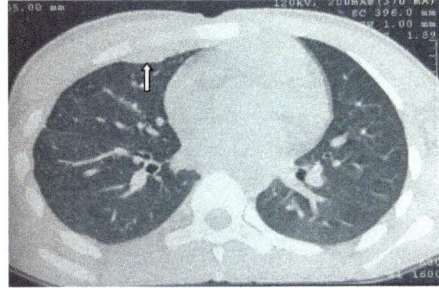

FIGURE 3: Axial CT image at lesion level in lung window showing no evidence of lung parenchymal involvement.

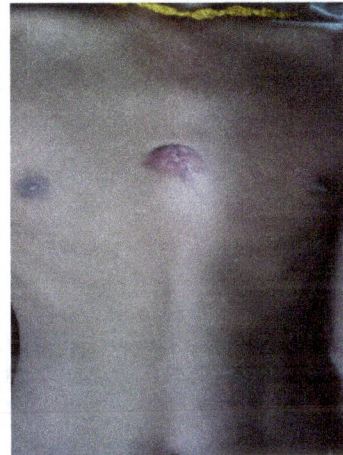

FIGURE 4: Showing the healed lesion on follow-up examination after 4 months of ATT.

On examination, the patient was average built, afebrile, and with normal pulse and blood pressure. Respiratory system examination was normal. Local examination revealed a large solitary lesion over sternum of 6 × 7 cm in dimensions. The lesion was soft, fluctuating, tender, warm, with well-defined margins, movable, and not attached to underlying bony structures (Figure 1). There was no involvement of the regional lymph nodes. Since the lesion appeared inflamed, patient was given oral antibiotic—amoxicillin—clavulanic acid combination (Augmentin) for five days. After completion of the antibiotic schedule, when it was observed that the abscess has increased in size, a detailed work up including; incision and drainage of the abscess and CT (computed tomography) chest was planned to assess the extension of the abscess into the surrounding area.

His haemogram, liver, and renal functions were within reference ranges. Serology for HIV was nonreactive. X-ray chest did not show any abnormality. On the basis of his routine laboratory investigations, incision and drainage (I&D) of the abscess was undertaken on the emergency basis. The drained pus material was sent to the microbiology laboratory for pyogenic culture and Ziehl Neelsen (ZN) staining. There was no growth of any pyogenic organism after

48 hrs of incubation but acid fast bacilli (AFB) were seen in ZN stain. Patient was subjected to CT investigation after I&D had been done. Both plain and contrast enhanced CT (CECT) were done with a proper protocol. Axial contrast enhanced CT in the mediastinal window showed loculated hypodense collection of 1.8 × 1.7 cm in the anterior chest wall in the right parasternal location with peripheral enhancement with no evidence of erosion of ribs or sternum (Figure 2). Also there was no evidence of either lung parenchymal lesion or mediastinal lymphadenopathy (Figure 3). Ultrasound abdomen was within normal limits. Urine sample was negative for AFB. Pus sample was also sent to the LRS Institute of Tuberculosis and Respiratory Diseases (National Reference Laboratory) for culture and sensitivity of *Mycobacterium tuberculosis*. Sample grew *M. tuberculosis* on LJ (Lowenstein Jensen) medium after one week of incubation. In-line probe assay (GenoType MTBDRplus, Hain Life Science), the isolate, was identified as *M. tuberculosis* and found to be sensitive to isoniazid (H) and rifampicin (R) and to other first line drugs, that is, pyrazinamide (Z) and ethambutol (E) by Bactec MGIT (Mycobacteria Growth Indicator Tube) 960 system.

The patient was put on Category I treatment (ATT) which consists of an intensive phase of H, R, Z, and E administered under direct supervision thrice weekly on alternate days for 2 months, followed by a continuation phase of H and R thrice

(a)   (b)

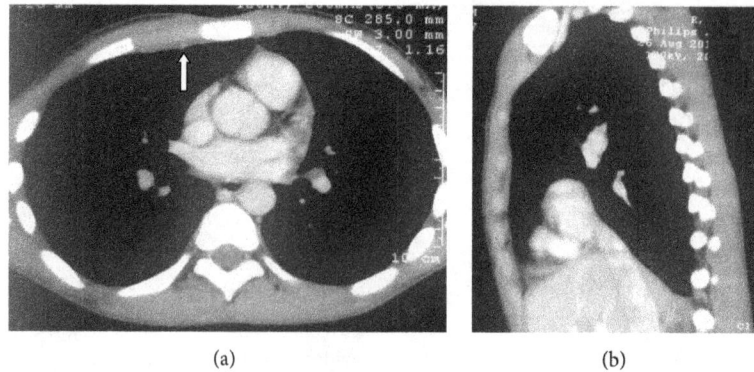

FIGURE 5: (a) Axial CECT image at lesion level in mediastinal window after 4 months of treatment showing considerable decrease in the collection with no peripheral enhancement. (b) The reconstructed CECT coronal image of the same patient.

weekly on alternate days for 4 months. On follow-up after 4 months, patient responded well to treatment and the abscess resolved drastically (Figures 4 and 5).

3. Discussion

Three mechanisms are described in the pathogenesis of chest wall abscess: direct extension from pleural or pulmonary parenchymal disease, hematogenous dissemination of a dormant tuberculous focus, or direct extension from lymphadenitis of the chest wall [4, 5]. Primary tuberculosis of the chest wall is rare and diagnosis in most of the cases is demanding and effortful because the lesions grossly simulate pyogenic abscess or tumour and do not respond to conventional therapeutic interventions. This patient was also prescribed amoxy-clavulanic acid combination for five days but the lesion increased in size though the inflammatory component was relieved. In this particular case, the abscess appeared to be the result of direct inoculation of the organism into the abraded skin because there is history of trauma in the area of lesion with a metallic locket which the boy would wear regularly. The patient comes from low socioeconomic status and used to share bed with his brother, an open case of pulmonary tuberculosis. It is hypothesized that infective droplets from his brother appeared to have settled in the damaged skin to set up infection and develop into an abscess.

Chest wall abscess usually occurs as a solitary lesion, most frequently at the margins of the sternum and in the shafts of the ribs [6]. In the present case, the abscess was present in the upper part of the chest in the sternal region. Chest X-ray of the patient was within normal limits, without any hilar adenopathy. Also the contrast enhanced CT scan suggested the lesion in the subcutaneous and muscle tissue (between the pectoralis muscles) without any involvement of the pleura or underlying bony structures or adjacent lymph nodes. This suggests that the primary focus was neither in the pleura or pulmonary parenchyma, nor in the bony structures and adjacent lymph nodes.

AFB in the aspirated pus signalled the tubercular etiology of the lesion but site of the lesion mandates that the organism is cultured and identified up to the species level because *Mycobacteria* other than tuberculosis (MOTT) are more frequently associated with skin lesions and are one of the significant causes of the treatment failure to ATT [7]. This lesion grew *Mycobacterium tuberculosis* in culture and was susceptible to all the first line drugs in the line probe assay and Bactec MGIT culture and sensitivity system. There is controversy regarding the duration of treatment of chest wall tuberculosis; few reports suggest good response with antitubercular drugs only, while others suggest wide surgical debridement along with antitubercular drugs. However, Revised National Tuberculosis Control Programme (RNTCP) recommends a standard 6-month regimen with 2 months of intensive phase (HRZE) and 4 months of continuation phase (HR) [1]. Patient was started on 1st line drugs for 6 months and on follow-up patient responded well to the treatment and the size of the abscess reduced drastically.

Primary tubercular involvement of extrapulmonary site like chest wall abscess is extremely rare. Demonstration of acid fast bacilli should not form the basis of starting antitubercular treatment; rather the organism requires to be identified up to the species level to exclude the possibility of MOTT as the causative agents which would require separate treatment protocol. In country like India that has massive pool of tuberculosis cases and in the background of priority to pick up open cases, there is a possibility that extrapulmonary tuberculosis may be missed or misdiagnosed. Identification of extrapulmonary isolates would be absolutely essential for instituting right therapeutic intervention but with limited facilities for mycobacterial culture and sensitivity some kinds of linkages are required to provide support services to sites engaged in handling tuberculosis patients.

References

[1] "TB INDIA 2014 Revised National TB Control Programme Annual status report," Central TB Division, Directorate General of Health Services, Ministry of Health and Family Welfare, 2014.

[2] Multidrug-resistant tuberculosis (MDR-TB), World Health Organisation, 2013, http://www.who.int/tb/.

[3] A. Mathlouthi, S. Ben M'Rad, S. Merai et al., "Tuberculosis of the thoracic wall. Presentation of 4 personal cases and review of the literature," *Revue de Pneumologie Clinique*, vol. 54, no. 4, pp. 182–186, 1998.

[4] M. Sakuraba, Y. Sagara, and H. Komatsu, "Surgical treatment of tuberculous abscess in the chest wall," *Annals of Thoracic Surgery*, vol. 79, no. 3, pp. 964–967, 2005.

[5] K. D. Cho, D. G. Cho, M. S. Jo, M. I. Ahn, and C. B. Park, "Current surgical therapy for patients with tuberculous abscess of the chest wall," *Annals of Thoracic Surgery*, vol. 81, no. 4, pp. 1220–1226, 2006.

[6] H. E. Burke, "The pathogenesis of certain forms of extrapulmonary tuberculosis; spontaneous cold abscesses of the chest wall and Pott's disease," *The American Review of Tuberculosis*, vol. 62, no. 1 B, pp. 48–67, 1950.

[7] C. Piersimoni and C. Scarparo, "Extrapulmonary infections associated with nontuberculous mycobacteria in immunocompetent persons," *Emerging Infectious Diseases*, vol. 15, no. 9, pp. 1351–1358, 2009.

9

Lipoid Pneumonia in a Gas Station Attendant

Gladis Isabel Yampara Guarachi, Valeria Barbosa Moreira, Angela Santos Ferreira, Selma M. De A. Sias, Cristovão C. Rodrigues, and Graça Helena M. do C. Teixeira

Department of Pulmonology, Faculty of Medicine, Fluminense Federal University, Pedro Antonio University Hospital, Rua Marques de Paraná, 303 Center, 24033-900 Niterói, RJ, Brazil

Correspondence should be addressed to Gladis Isabel Yampara Guarachi; gypneumo@gmail.com

Academic Editor: Fabio Midulla

The exogenous lipoid pneumonia, uncommon in adults, is the result of the inhalation and/or aspiration of lipid material into the tracheobronchial tree. This is often confused with bacterial pneumonia and pulmonary tuberculosis due to a nonspecific clinical and radiologic picture. It presents acutely or chronically and may result in pulmonary fibrosis. We describe here a case of lipoid pneumonia in a gas station attendant who siphoned gasoline to fill motorcycles; he was hospitalized due to presenting with a respiratory infection that was hard to resolve. The patient underwent bronchoscopy with bronchoalveolar lavage, which, on cytochemical (oil red O) evaluation, was slightly positive for lipid material in the foamy cytoplasm of alveolar macrophages. Due to his occupational history and radiographic abnormalities suggestive of lipoid pneumonia, a lung biopsy was performed to confirm the diagnosis. The patient was serially treated with segmental lung lavage and showed clinical, functional, and radiological improvement.

1. Introduction

The occurrence of exogenous lipoid pneumonia (LP) in healthy adults is infrequent, occurring mainly in occupational accidents, resulting in microaspiration of lipid formulations [1, 2]. These oily substances are not cleared by the lung and inhibit the cough reflex and function of the muciliary apparatus, which facilitates aspiration, even in normal individuals [3]. They are also responsible for recurrent acute respiratory infections. Diagnosis is often difficult because it mimics other common pulmonary diseases, such as bacterial pneumonia and pulmonary tuberculosis [1].

The objective of this work was to report on the clinical course and treatment of a case of exogenous LP in a gas station attendant who siphoned gasoline in filling motorcycles.

2. Case Report

A 41-year-old man, gas station attendant for 14 years, reported that he frequently siphoned gasoline while filling vehicles, mainly motorcycles (Figure 1). One year ago start makes dry cough and nonspecific pain insidiously in the lower third of the left hemithorax, with progressive worsening of symptoms. He denied any history of fever or weight loss. He sought medical attention, where he was hospitalized for 15 days for treatment of community-acquired pneumonia. Since there was no improvement, empirical treatment for pulmonary tuberculosis was implemented, also without response, and he was therefore referred to the Respiratory Outpatient Clinic of Hospital Universitario Antonio Pedro (HUAP) with the same symptoms, besides dyspnea on exertion. He denied prior history of tobacco use and other pulmonary diseases.

Physical examination revealed good general condition, afebrile, with crackling rales at the lung bases and clubbing. Hemogram and blood chemistries were normal and the PPD was negative. A chest radiograph revealed consolidations in the lung bases. High resolution computed tomography (HRCT) of the chest showed, despite the extensive nonhomogeneous consolidations in the posterior segments of both lower lobes, ground-glass opacities and areas of fibrosis with bronchiectasis in the lung parenchyma (Figures 2(a) and 2(b)). Spirometry revealed moderate restrictive ventilatory disturbances and 6-minute walk distance was 420 m (maximum and minimum: 608 and 455 m).

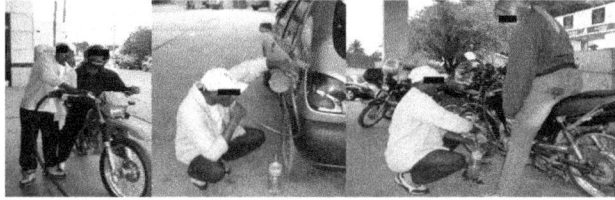

FIGURE 1: Patient siphoning excess gasoline in filling vehicles due to wrong information provided by the clients.

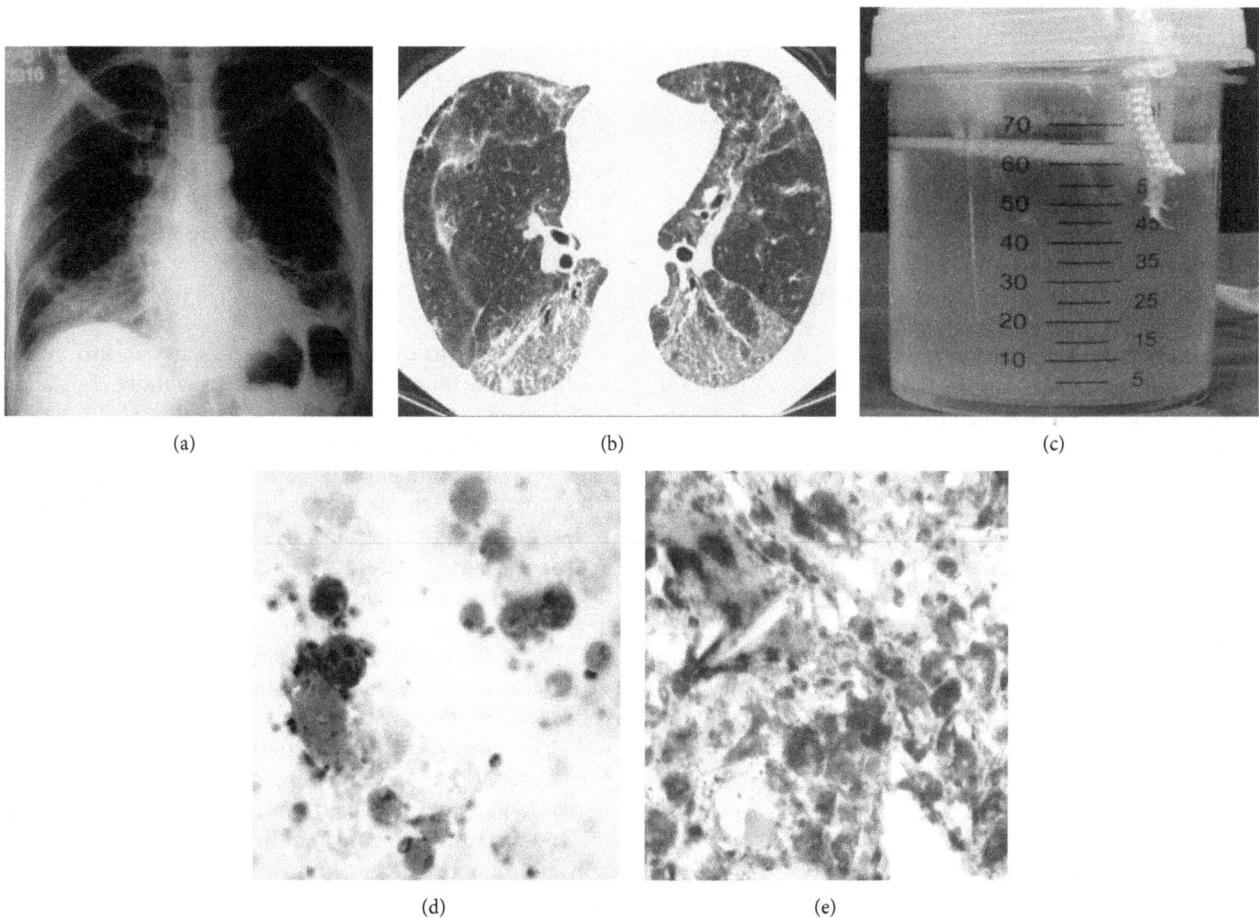

(a) (b) (c)

(d) (e)

FIGURE 2: (a) PA chest radiograph: consolidations at lung bases. (b) Chest HRCT: nonhomogeneous consolidations, ground-glass opacities, areas of fibrosis with parenchymal beams, and bronchiectasis traction. (c) Segmental pulmonary lavage fluid: cloudy with halo of fatty supernatant. (d) Bronchoalveolar lavage fluid: presence of macrophages with foamy cytoplasm showing positive oil red O staining. (e) Histopathologic section of lung (oil red O, 400x) showing orange-colored lipid contents "lipid laden macrophages."

The patient was subjected to bronchofibroscopy with bronchoalveolar lavage, where cytology revealed pleocytosis with a predominant increase in the percentage of lymphocytes (57%). Microbiological (BK, fungi, and bacteria) and cytopathologic studies were negative. Cytochemical evaluation with oil red O showed weak positive staining, which called for a lung biopsy. Histopathologic assessment of the lung fragment revealed distortion of the pulmonary architecture with fibrosis and multinucleated giant cells with cholesterol clefts and intra-alveolar and interstitial macrophages showing foamy cytoplasm stained with oil red O "lipid laden macrophages," confirming the lipid nature, compatible with exogenous LP (Figure 2(c)).

The patient underwent segmental pulmonary lavage (Table 1) series made with warm physiological saline 0.9% with a volume of 100 mL per segment in the areas of greater commitment demonstrated by tomography of chest high-resolution, three segments per procedure. The aim of the lung lavage segment was to improve respiratory symptoms and changes in cellularity of the liquid were made ten sessions, once a week, associated with the use of corticosteroids (prednisone 1 mg/kg/day orally) for one year to wean gradual,

TABLE 1: Global and specific cytology of bronchoalveolar lavage fluid, segmental and sequential (evolution), after 10 sessions.

	Total cells/mm^3	Macrophages %	Lymphocytes %	Neutrophils %	Eosinophils %
Normal range	200 to 250	85 to 92	6 to 12	1 to 3	<1
Before	382	30	57	10	3
After	152	70	24	5	1

taking it to present significant clinical and radiological improvement (Figure 2(e)).

3. Discussion

LP was described for the first time by Laughlen in 1925, where, according to its origin, it can be endogenous, exogenous, or idiopathic [1, 3].

The rarer endogenous form is found associated with pulmonary fat embolism, alveolar proteinosis, and lipid deposit diseases such as alveolar phospholipoproteinosis, Niemann-Pick disease, Wegener granulomatosis, and undifferentiated connective tissue disease. The idiopathic form, also rare, has been described in healthy smokers [1–3].

The exogenous form is often more common in children and the elderly, and it is related to the use of mineral oil for the treatment of intestinal constipation.

Mineral oil, inert material for our body, reduces glare from coughing or choking, facilitating aspiration, even in the absence of risk factors. In the lung, mineral oil is phagocytized by the macrophages and fills the alveoli, remaining in the alveolar walls and reaching the interlobular septa through lymphatic channels, which results in foreign body-type granulomas localized in the pulmonary interstitium, and later, with repeated aspirations, this can develop into pulmonary fibrosis and loss of lung function and volume [1, 4].

Exogenous PL can present in the acute or chronic form. The acute form is described in children and the elderly in the treatment of intestinal constipation.

The chronic form is less frequent and occurs as a consequence of continuous aspiration of various materials in the work area (contact with oil vapors, kerosene, and/or others), as in the case described here, in which the patient, a gas station attendant, siphoned excess gasoline (petroleum derivate like mineral oil).

Other related exposures, also not very common, include the inhalation of nasal preparations for nasopharyngeal obstruction and chronic use of Vicks Vaporub [1–5].

The differentiation between the exogenous and endogenous forms is made not only by the clinical history compatible with the ingestion and/or aspiration of oils, in the case of the exogenous form, but also by the distinct histologic characteristics, that is, the detection of extracellular lipid material, the appearance of intracytoplasmic vacuoles, the distribution of macrophages in the lung tissue, and the physicochemical characteristics of the oil [1, 4]. The degree of damage and pulmonary fibrosis depends on the quantity of free fatty acid and the rapidity of the process of hydrolysis at the alveolar level. The different characteristics of the oils can be detected according to histochemical reactions: mineral oil in exogenous PL shows a positive reaction as a yellow or orange color by staining with Sudan IV and oil red O, while in endogenous PL, staining shows a positive reaction with a red color [4].

In exogenous PL, the clinical manifestations are nonspecific, varying according to the age of the patient and the form of exposure (acute or chronic). Usually, patients present with cough and dyspnea [4]. Fever, weight loss, chest pain, and hemoptysis are less frequent manifestations [1, 3, 4]. The majority of exogenous PL cases are initially treated as bacterial pneumonia and occasionally also as pulmonary tuberculosis due to clinical, laboratory, and nonspecific radiologic findings [1, 4, 6].

In the present case report, the patient was also initially treated for pneumonia and tuberculosis without clinical and radiologic improvement.

The radiologic alterations of exogenous PL are nonspecific, varying from perihilar opacity to extensive areas of consolidations with air bronchogram, which occur mainly in the lower and posterior lobes of the lungs, resulting in similar appearance as lobar pneumonia [6]. Accordingly, it is important to include exogenous PL in the differential diagnosis of the chronic, repeated, or delayed pneumonia.

HRCT is the best imaging method for the diagnosis of exogenous LP, where its main finding is alveolar consolidation with negative density (−30 to −150 Hounsfield units), frequently associated with the presence of fat, ground-glass opacities, abnormalities of the interstitium, and nodular lesions (small poorly defined centrilobular nodules) [4, 6].

The diagnosis is confirmed by clinical history of ingestion and/or aspiration of mineral oil and the presence of alveolar macrophages with foamy cytoplasm and positive cytochemical staining with Sudan or oil red O in the sputum, bronchoalveolar lavage fluid, and gastric lavage fluid or tissue. In the patient reported here, the diagnosis of exogenous LP was suspected because of his occupational history and confirmed by histopathologic examination of the lung fragment, which showed cytochemical staining with oil red O, indicating the presence of lipid material in the cytoplasm of the macrophages "lipid laden macrophages."

There is general consensus that the principal approach in the treatment of exogenous LP is the immediate suspension of mineral oil in cases of children and the elderly. However, in adults, staying away from the work area and further exposure is urged, such as for the patient described here.

The use of corticosteroids is still controversial in the treatment of PL, where they are recommended in the more serious cases, as a strategy to block inflammation and the development of fibrosis [3, 4].

Later studies suggested that the principal measure would be the mechanical removal of the oil present in the lungs, in view that natural defense mechanisms, such as mucociliary activity and cough are harmed devido the presence of mineral oil, preventing its removal. There are reports of PL treated successfully utilizing total pulmonary lavage in patients who did not respond to treatment with high doses of corticosteroids. Sias et al. [4] utilized multiple segmental pulmonary lavages in 10 children with PL obtaining clinical and radiologic improvement. Multiple segmental pulmonary lavages have the advantage of not needing general anesthesia and can be done in cases in which total pulmonary lavage shows more risk than benefit for the patients.

The patient in the present case report was subjected to sequential segmental pulmonary lavage combined with systemic corticotherapy, resulting in clinical, functional, and radiologic improvement.

The scheme used steroids with prednisone 1 mg/kg/day, orally during gradual weaning year every three months (60 mg, 40 mg, 20 mg, and 10 mg), which showed good results.

4. Conclusion

Chronic exogenous PL in healthy adults is an unusual condition and its diagnosis can be delayed, since the clinical picture and radiologic changes can mimic bacterial pneumonia and tuberculosis. The occupational history is of extreme importance and should always be investigated. Avoidance of the exposure to mineral oils is the main treatment of exogenous LP. Other treatment options described in literature include whole lung lavage, lobar or segmental lavage, and corticosteroids for selected severe cases.

References

[1] S. M. A. Sias, P. A. Daltro, E. Marchiori et al., "Clinic and radiological improvement of lipoid pneumonia with multiple bronchoalveolar lavages," *Pediatric Pulmonology*, vol. 44, no. 4, pp. 309–315, 2009.

[2] A. P. L. de Albuquerque Filho, "Pneumonia lipóide exógena: importância da história clínica no diagnóstico," *Jornal Brasileiro de Pneumologia*, vol. 32, pp. 596–598, 2006.

[3] G. P. Alaminos, R. A. Colodro, G. M. J. Menduiña, S. F. Báñez, and C. G. Pérez, "Neumonía lipoidea exógena. Presentación de un nuevo caso," *Anales de Medicina Interna*, vol. 22, pp. 283–284, 2005.

[4] S. M. A. Sias, P. A. Daltro, E. Marchiori et al., "Clinic and radiological improvement of lipoid pneumonia with multiple bronchoalveolar lavages," *Pediatric Pulmonology*, vol. 44, no. 4, pp. 309–315, 2009.

[5] C. D. Brown, K. Hewan-Lowe, A. S. Kseibi, and Y. Y. Huang, "Exogenous lipoid pneumonia secondary to an occupational exposure in a furniture factory," *Chest*, vol. 126, no. 4, p. S997, 2004.

[6] E. Marchiori, G. Zanetti, D. L. Escuissato et al., "Pneumonia lipoídica em adultos: aspectos na tomografia de alta resolução," *Radiologia Brasileira*, vol. 40, no. 5, pp. 315–319, 2007.

10

Untreated Active Tuberculosis in Pregnancy with Intraocular Dissemination: A Case Report and Review of the Literature

Shadi Rezai,[1] Stephen LoBue,[2] Daniel Adams,[2] Yewande Oladipo,[2]
Ramses Posso,[1] Tiffany Mapp,[1] Crystal Santiago,[1] Manisha Jain,[1]
William D. Marino,[3] and Cassandra E. Henderson[1,4]

[1]Department of Obstetrics and Gynecology, Lincoln Medical and Mental Health Center, Bronx, NY 10451, USA
[2]St. George's University, School of Medicine, Grenada
[3]Coney Island Hospital, Pulmonary Medicine, Brooklyn, NY 11235, USA
[4]Cornell Medical College, NY 10065, USA

Correspondence should be addressed to Cassandra E. Henderson; cassandra.henderson@nychhc.org

Academic Editor: Tun-Chieh Chen

Background. Tuberculosis (TB) is a disease that affects hundreds of millions of people across the world. However, the incidence in developed countries has decreased over the past decades causing physicians to become unfamiliar with its unspecific symptoms. Pregnant individuals are especially difficult because many symptoms of active TB can mimic normal physiological changes of pregnancy. We present a case report of a 26-year-old multiparous woman, G4P3003, at 38-week gestation with a history of positive PPD who emigrated from Ghana 6 years ago. She came to the hospital with an initial complaint of suprapubic pain, pressure, and possible leakage of amniotic fluid for the past week. Patient also complained of a productive cough for the past 3 to 4 months with a decrease in vision occurring with the start of pregnancy. Visual acuity was worse than 20/200 in both eyes. Definitive diagnosis of active TB was delayed due to patient refusal of chest X-ray. Fortunately, delay in diagnosis was minimized since patient delivered within 24 hours of admission. Active TB was confirmed with intraocular dissemination. Patient had optic atrophy OS (left eye) and papillitis, choroiditis, and uveitis OD (right eye) due to TB infiltration. Fetus was asymptomatic and anti-TB therapy was started for both patients.

1. Introduction

According to the most recent World Health Organization (WHO) data from 2014, around 3.3 million women contract tuberculosis (TB) a year with a total mortality of about 510,000 [1]. Out of 510,000 people who died, 180,000 were HIV positive [1]. Worldwide, TB is the third leading cause of morbidity and premature mortality in women of reproductive age from 15 to 44 years old [2–4].

However, approximately one-third of the world's population or approximately 900 million women have latent tuberculosis infection (LTBI) [1]. Pregnant women with LTBI are more likely to progress to active tuberculous disease than men [5].

The prevalence of active TB among pregnant women ranges from 0.06% to 0.25% in low-burden countries compared to 0.07% and 0.5% in high-burden countries. Prevalence was found to increase in high-burden countries to 0.7% and 11% when coinfected with HIV [6].

In 2014, Southeast Asia and the Western Pacific Regions had the greatest incidence of TB, accounting for 58% of new cases globally [1]. However, Africa carried the most severe burden, with an average of 281 cases per 100,000 compared with a global average of 133 per 100,000 [1]. Particularly, the prevalence of TB in Ghana is very high with 282 infected with TB per 100,000 [1].

Although the prevalence of TB has decreased in the United States, immigrant populations from high-burden

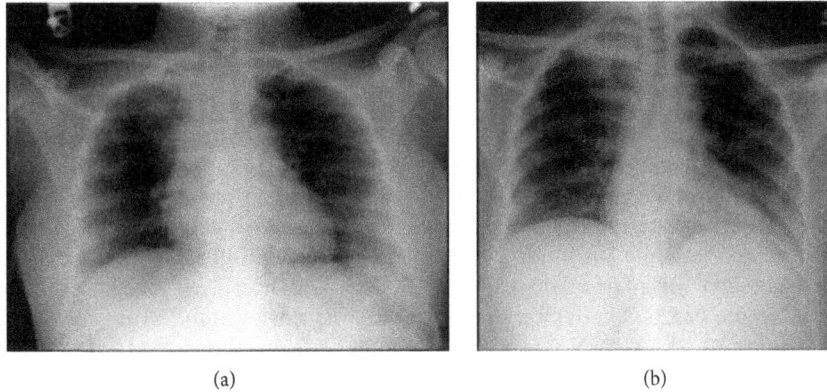

(a)

(b)

FIGURE 1: Chest imaging prior to anti-TB therapy and during TB therapy. (a) CXR showing nodular opacity in the apex of the lung fields and (b) CXR showing increased density in the right upper lobe.

areas as well as those with immunodeficiency have significantly increased risks [1, 7].

2. Presentation of Case

A 26-year-old multiparous woman from Ghana, with a history of positive PPD (purified protein derivative) test and gestational diabetes, presented to labor and delivery at 38-week gestation with complaints of suprapubic pain, pressure, and possible leakage of amniotic fluid.

The patient's suprapubic pain had occurred for a week and was associated with vomiting. The patient also complained of a productive cough for the past 3 to 4 months with a decrease in vision occurring at the start of pregnancy. She reported good fetal movement and denied vaginal bleeding. She also denied the use of alcohol, tobacco, and illicit drugs. The patient had a history of positive PPD with a normal chest X-ray in 2009. Treatment never occurred as the patient was lost to follow-up.

Physical examination revealed a frequent productive cough with urinary incontinence. The patient had a visual acuity worse than 20/200 in each eye and was referred to ophthalmology. Ophthalmology diagnosed her with optic atrophy OS (left eye) and papillitis, choroiditis, and uveitis OD (right eye). She was prescribed ophthalmic prednisolone and cyclopentolate for the uveitis and timolol for secondary glaucoma due to the uveitis. However, the patient refused all eye medications stating that headaches and eye pain occurred with use.

The patient was also evaluated by pulmonology for chronic cough. Initial imaging was delayed due to patient refusal. The mother believed that imaging would be harmful to the fetus and would not consent to the procedure.

Day one after admission the patient delivered a healthy infant of 2960 grams at 38 weeks via vacuum assisted vaginal delivery. APGAR score was 9/9 with no perinatal complications. After the patient delivered, a chest X-ray (CXR) showed right nodular opacity in the apex of the lung field measuring 1.6×1.0 cm (Figure 1(a)). *Mycobacterium tuberculosis* was confirmed by positive AFB smear and culture leading to the diagnosis of active TB.

The baby was isolated from the mother and fed with formula due to increased likelihood of TB transmission. Physical examination performed on the newborn revealed no anatomic, visual, or neurologic deficits. As a safety precaution, the infant was initiated on isoniazid oral suspension of 0.1 mg and pyridoxine oral suspension of 29 mg daily (10 mg/kg/day).

Immediately following maternal diagnosis of active TB, the patient was isolated and started on an antituberculosis regimen comprising of isoniazid and pyridoxine 300 mg once daily, rifampin 300 mg twice daily, pyrazinamide 500 mg three times daily, and ethambutol 1,200 mg daily to be completed on a 6-month course. However, ethambutol was discontinued due to the patient's history of left optic nerve atrophy, which may progress due to ethambutol toxicity.

Prior to being discharged, a CXR was done on April 7, 2015, which revealed increased density in the right upper lobe that appeared to be more prominent compared to the previous imaging (Figure 1(b)). On April 13, 2015, the patient was cleared for discharge after the documentation of three consecutive partially negative AFB smears and culture. She was released to the care of a public health advisor at the Department of Health who will provide follow-up care.

3. Discussion

Tuberculosis (TB) is a contagious, airborne pathogen, listed as the second leading cause of death from an infectious agent [1]. Its mortality rate as an infectious agent is second only to HIV [1]. TB is also one of the top causes of mortality in women from 15 to 44 years old [2–4]. However, within this demographic, the most susceptible group of women are pregnant individuals. Pregnant women with latent tuberculosis infection (LTBI) are more likely to progress to active tuberculous disease than men [5].

The increased rate of progression of LTBI to active infection is supported by immunological changes associated with pregnancy. For one, pregnancy is linked with upregulation of potent anti-inflammatory hormones such as cortisol [8]. A progressive increase of circulating CRH, ACTH, and free cortisol levels has been documented in the third trimester

[8]. One study documented a gradual increase in total plasma cortisol and 24-hour urinary free cortisol with levels peaking during the third trimester to levels threefold higher than those in nonpregnant controls [9].

Increased levels of glucocorticoids suppress innate and cellular immune responses [10–13]. Previous studies have indicated that glucocorticoids inhibit T-helper 1 (Th1) and enhance T-helper 2 (Th2) cytokine secretion, thus impeding the effectiveness of cellular immunity on intracellular organisms such as Mycobacterium tuberculosis [10–13]. A downregulation of Th1 inhibits the production of interferon-gamma (IFN-y) and Interleukin 12 (IL-12). IFN-y is a vital macrophage activating cytokine involved in cellular immunity against Mycobacterium tuberculosis [14]. Individuals become highly susceptible to mycobacteria infection when IFN-y production is absent or decreased [15]. A decrease in IL-12 also hinders activation of natural killer cells which are also important for fighting intracellular pathogens [4, 16].

Although progression of latent tuberculosis infection (LTBI) to an active infection is more common in pregnancy, the clinical diagnosis is often delayed. For one, manifestations of active TB may go unnoticed due to overlap of normal physiological changes in pregnancy [17, 18]. Symptoms such as fatigue, sweating, shortness of breath, and low grade fever are similar to the physiological symptoms seen in pregnancy [17, 18].

However, patients from TB endemic nations should have increased clinical suspicion for active or latent TB. Endemic areas include India, Indonesia, Nigeria, Ghana, South Africa, Pakistan, and China [1]. Our patient had many nonspecific symptoms common in pregnancy. However, the chronic productive cough coupled with endemic travel history led us to have a high clinical suspicion of TB.

Nevertheless, a definitive diagnosis was delayed. Chest radiographs with abdominal shields are often delayed until after delivery due to maternal concerns for fetal health [19]. Our patient also adamantly refused imaging for concern of fetal safety. However, a tuberculin skin test is a safe and effective diagnostic tool for TB in pregnancy. Patient exhibiting night sweats, evening pyrexia, hemoptysis, weight loss, history of travel from an endemic area, and chronic productive cough for over 3 weeks duration should have a tuberculin skin test [20, 21]. Most immigrants from TB endemic countries in Asia and Africa were vaccinated against certain strains of TB with the Bacillus Calmette-Guerin (BCG) vaccine. BCG vaccine will produce a false positive PPD, a negative Quanti FERON, and a negative chest X-ray [21, 22]. Unfortunately many physicians are unaware that the protocol for screening and treatment of BCG vaccinated patients is identical to the protocol for non-BCG vaccinated patients [22].

A delay in treatment may allow active pulmonary TB to disseminate, becoming extrapulmonary tuberculosis (EPTB). EPTB may affect cardiovascular system, skin, central nervous system, gastrointestinal tract, genitourinary tract, and eyes [23]. The prevalence of EPTB is not well documented but approximately 15% of the cases are extrapulmonary tuberculosis in low incidence countries such as the United States and Great Britain [24]. Once again EPTB symptoms may be vague including fatigue, malaise, nausea/vomiting, and anorexia. Many of these symptoms overlap with pregnancy and are difficult to discern from an activated TB infection [4, 25].

The incidence of ocular TB is unknown due to lack of uniform diagnostic criteria [26]. Initially ocular TB was considered to be very rare but a study in Spain from 1997 showed that 18 out of 100 people with confirmed systemic tuberculosis had ocular manifestations [27]. Ocular lesions included choroiditis, papillitis, retinitis, vasculitis, dacryoadenitis, and scleritis [27]. However, more recent studies in other countries found intraocular TB to be much lower. A study in Japan found a rate of uveitis due to TB to be 6.9% out of 189 patients [28]. Yet in China only 4% of uveitis was due to TB [29]. A study in Riyadh, Saudi Arabia, had an incidence of 10.5% of cases [30]. However, larger studies in India found the incidence of ocular TB to be significantly lower with variability occurring among the same center. One study in South India of 1,005 patients with active pulmonary and extrapulmonary TB reported ocular manifestation in only 1.39% of patients [31]. Another study from the same center reported ocular tuberculosis contributed to only 0.39% of uveitis seen in 1,273 patients [32].

The most common clinical presentation of ocular TB is posterior uveitis [27]. Other common ocular symptoms which have been noted include anterior uveitis, intermediate uveitis, retinitis, choroiditis, retinal vasculitis, optic neuropathy, neuroretinitis, endophthalmitis, and panophthalmitis [27]. The involvement of the optic nerve from TB can manifest as an optic nerve tubercle, papillitis, papilledema, optic neuritis, retrobulbar neuritis, neuroretinitis, or optochiasmatic arachnoiditis [26]. In this case report, our patient had papillitis, choroiditis, posterior uveitis OD (right eye), and optic atrophy OS (left eye). The funduscopic examination results were consistent with pathology caused by hematogenous dissemination of TB to the eyes, with subsequent posterior segment inflammation and optic neuropathy. MRI of the head without IV contrast revealed no dissemination to the brain.

Yet, one of the most concerning complications with EPTB during pregnancy is vertical transmission to the fetus. Active TB in pregnancy is associated with increased fetal risks including prematurity, low birth weight, growth retardation, and low Apgar scores [4, 5, 33].

One study in Sub-Saharan Africa analyzed 107 pregnant women with TB, of which 50% had systemic TB, showing that 46% of newborns were premature, 66% had low birth weight, and 49% had intrauterine growth restriction [34]. 16% also had vertical transmission of TB from mother to infant [34]. However, it is important to note that, of the 107 patients, 82 were coinfected with HIV-1. Although HIV-1-infected mothers and their exposed newborns had significantly lower CD4 counts, there was no association between perinatal maternal viral load, CD4 count, and vertical transmission of TB [34].

However, another study in India noted a vertical transmission of TB in only 9% of infants born to mothers of active TB and HIV coinfection [35]. This study found TB to be strongly associated with postpartum maternal and infant death [35]. Smaller gestational sizes and increased infant morbidity and mortality were also seen from studies in South Asia and Mexico [33, 36–38]. One case report documented a disseminated TB inducing a spontaneous abortion [39].

Nevertheless, the fetus may be asymptomatic even in disseminated TB [40, 41]. Our patient delivered a healthy, full term infant, with no complications. Regardless of the infant being asymptomatic, treatment should begin immediately for both the mother and infant.

Almost half of children born to mothers with active TB will become infected within the first year if they are not given appropriate chemoprophylaxis [42]. Asymptomatic infants should be started on isoniazid (INH) 10 to 15 mg/kg po once/daily and discharged home at the normal time. Infants who will be breastfed should receive pyridoxine 1 to 2 mg/kg once daily [42]. A PPD skin test should be done when the baby is 3 or 4 months of age. If the baby screens negative and the mother has been compliant with her course of anti-TB treatments, INH treatment for the baby is discontinued [42]. However, if the baby screens positive, chest X-ray and cultures for acid-fast bacilli are taken. If active disease is excluded, treatment with INH is continued for a total of 9 months. If cultures become positive for TB at any time, the baby should be treated for active TB.

Treatment of TB in neonates slightly varies depending on whether TB is congenital or acquired after birth. Treatment of congenital TB requires isoniazid 10 to 15 mg/kg po, rifampin 10 to 20 mg/kg po, pyrazinamide 30 to 40 mg/kg po, and an aminoglycoside such as amikacin [42]. Pyridoxine is also given in neonates exclusively breastfed [42]. Acquired TB after birth requires treatment once/day with isoniazid 10 to 15 mg/kg po, rifampin 10 to 20 mg/kg po, and pyrazinamide 30 to 40 mg/kg [42]. A fourth drug such as ethionamide, ethambutol, or an aminoglycoside can be added if drug resistance or TB meningitis is suspected [42]. After the first 2 months of treatment, all drugs are stopped besides isoniazid and rifampin which are continued for a 6- to 12-month course depending on the disease category [42].

Most first-line medications used in the treatment of TB are proven to be safe for use during the antenatal and postpartum breastfeeding period [17]. Treatment of EPTB follows the same scheme as active pulmonary TB. Isoniazid (INH), rifampin (RIF), and ethambutol (EMB) are used daily for 2 months. After 2 months, ethambutol is discontinued. INH and RIF are administered daily for 7 months for a total of 9 months of treatment. Streptomycin is potentially ototoxic to the fetus and should not be used unless rifampin is contraindicated [42]. Also, pyrazinamide (PZA) is not recommended to be used because its effect on the fetus is unknown.

However, due to optic neuropathy associated with ethambutol [26], our patient was started on ethambutol and discontinued to prevent any further damage to the eyes. Some slow responding cases of TB require a prolonged course of 12 months of pharmacotherapy [17]. In addition, women with TB involvement of the meninges, pericardium, or eye may benefit from the addition of oral corticosteroids or ophthalmic corticosteroids to the treatment regimen [26].

4. Conclusions

TB is also one of the top causes of mortality of women of reproductive ages from 15 to 44 [2–4]. However, within this demographic, the most susceptible group of women are pregnant individuals. Pregnant women with latent tuberculosis infection (LTBI) are more likely to progress to developing active tuberculous disease than men [5]. Although progression of latent tuberculosis infection (LTBI) to an active infection is more common in pregnancy, the clinical diagnosis is often delayed. For one, manifestations of active TB may go unnoticed due to overlap of normal physiological changes in pregnancy [17, 18]. Symptoms such as fatigue, sweating, shortness of breath, and low grade fever are similar to the physiological symptoms seen in pregnancy [17, 18].

Our patient was an immigrant from Ghana who presented with vague symptoms. She had suprapubic pain associated with nausea, vomiting, chronic productive cough for 3 to 4 months, and a significant decrease in vision bilaterally. Radiological imaging was initially delayed 24 hours until after gestation due to maternal fear of infant safety. One day into the postpartum a diagnosis of active TB with intraocular dissemination was supported based on findings of chest X-ray, positive QuantiFERON test, and positive AFB culture and smear.

Based on this case report we present several learning objectives. For one, clinicians should be alert for tuberculosis in women that have lived in endemic areas including India, Indonesia, Nigeria, Ghana, South Africa, Pakistan, and China. A high clinical suspicion for TB should be employed for all pregnant females emigrating from these endemic areas. Secondly the importance of radiologic imaging needs to be explained to the patient in order to prevent diagnostic delay. Delay is most often due to cultural and communication barriers. Thus, more time needs to be spent reassuring and addressing the concerns of the mother that may result in any delay in treatment. Evidence has shown that prenatal diagnosis and treatment of TB result in a better outcome for the mother and infant [42]. Lastly, all first-line medications used in the treatment of TB are proven to be safe for use during the antenatal and postpartum breastfeeding period [5]. Asymptomatic infants should always be treated if TB is in question with the mother.

Acknowledgment

Special thanks are due to Ms. Judith Wilkinson, Medical Librarian, from Lincoln Medical and Mental Health Center Science Library for assistance in finding of the reference articles.

References

[1] World Health Organization, *Global Tuberculosis Report 2014*, WHO, Geneva, Switzerland, 2014.

[2] P. C. Clark, M. W. Yencha, and A. K. Hart, "Management of isolated extrapulmonary tuberculosis in a pregnant patient," *Annals of Otology, Rhinology & Laryngology*, vol. 113, no. 8, Article ID 15330145, pp. 648–651, 2004.

[3] H.-C. Lin, H.-C. Lin, and S.-F. Chen, "Increased risk of low birthweight and small for gestational age infants among women with tuberculosis," *BJOG: An International Journal of Obstetrics & Gynaecology*, vol. 117, no. 5, pp. 585–590, 2010.

[4] D. Zenner, M. E. Kruijshaar, N. Andrews, and I. Abubakar, "Risk of tuberculosis in pregnancy: a national, primary care-based cohort and self-controlled case series study," *American Journal of Respiratory and Critical Care Medicine*, vol. 185, no. 7, pp. 779–784, 2012.

[5] M. Bates, Y. Ahmed, N. Kapata, M. Maeurer, P. Mwaba, and A. Zumla, "Perspectives on tuberculosis in pregnancy," *International Journal of Infectious Diseases*, vol. 32, pp. 124–127, 2015.

[6] J. S. Mathad and A. Gupta, "Tuberculosis in pregnant and postpartum women: epidemiology, management, and research gaps," *Clinical Infectious Diseases*, vol. 55, no. 11, pp. 1532–1549, 2012.

[7] Centers for Disease Control and Prevention, "Decrease in reported tuberculosis cases—United States, 2009," *Morbidity and Mortality Weekly Report*, vol. 59, no. 10, pp. 289–294, 2010.

[8] B. Allolio, J. Hoffmann, E. A. Linton, W. Winkelmann, M. Kusche, and H. M. Schulte, "Diurnal salivary cortisol patterns during pregnancy and after delivery: relationship to plasma corticotrophin-releasing-hormone," *Clinical Endocrinology*, vol. 33, no. 2, pp. 279–289, 1990.

[9] C. Jung, J. T. Ho, D. J. Torpy et al., "A longitudinal study of plasma and urinary cortisol in pregnancy and postpartum," *Journal of Clinical Endocrinology and Metabolism*, vol. 96, no. 5, pp. 1533–1540, 2011.

[10] F. Ramírez, D. J. Fowell, M. Puklavec, S. Simmonds, and D. Mason, "Glucocorticoids promote a Th2 cytokine response by CD4$^+$ T cells in vitro," *Journal of Immunology*, vol. 156, no. 7, pp. 2406–2412, 1996.

[11] R. H. DeKruyff, Y. Fang, and D. T. Umetsu, "Corticosteroids enhance the capacity of macrophages to induce Th2 cytokine synthesis in CD4+ lymphocytes by inhibiting IL-12 production," *The Journal of Immunology*, vol. 160, no. 5, pp. 2231–2237, 1998.

[12] M. H. Blotta, R. H. DeKruyff, and D. T. Umetsu, "Corticosteroids inhibit IL-12 production in human monocytes and enhance their capacity to induce IL-4 synthesis in CD4+ lymphocytes," *The Journal of Immunology*, vol. 158, no. 12, pp. 5589–5595, 1997.

[13] I. J. Elenkov, D. A. Papanicolaou, R. L. Wilder, and G. P. Chrousos, "Modulatory effects of glucocorticoids and catecholamines on human interleukin-12 and interleukin-10 production: clinical implications," *Proceedings of the Association of American Physicians*, vol. 108, no. 5, pp. 374–381, 1996.

[14] H. L. Collins and S. H. E. Kaufmann, "The many faces of host responses to tuberculosis," *Immunology*, vol. 103, no. 1, pp. 1–9, 2001.

[15] E. Jouanguy, R. Doffinger, S. Dupis, A. Pallier, F. Altare, and J. L. Casanova, "IL-12 and IFN-gamma in host defense against mycobacteria and *Salmonella* in mice and men," *Current Opinion in Immunology*, vol. 11, pp. 346–351, 1999.

[16] H. T. Nguyen, C. Pandolfini, P. Chiodini, and M. Bonati, "Tuberculosis care for pregnant women: a systematic review," *BMC Infectious Diseases*, vol. 14, article 617, 2014.

[17] C. L. Nhan-Chang and T. B. Jones, "Tuberculosis in pregnancy," *Clinical Obstetrics & Gynecology*, vol. 53, no. 2, pp. 311–321, 2010.

[18] H. T. Nguyen, C. Pandolfini, P. Chiodini, and M. Bonati, "Tuberculosis care for pregnant women: a systematic review," *BMC Infectious Diseases*, vol. 14, no. 1, 2014.

[19] R. F. C. Doveren and R. Block, "Tuberculosis and pregnancy: a provincial study (1990–1996)," *Netherlands Journal of Medicine*, vol. 52, no. 3, pp. 100–106, 1998.

[20] S. Janssen, X. Padanilam, R. Louw et al., "How many sputum culture results do we need to monitor multidrug-resistant-tuberculosis (MDR-TB) patients during treatment?" *Journal of Clinical Microbiology*, vol. 51, no. 2, pp. 644–646, 2013.

[21] C. C. Dobler, Q. Luu, and G. B. Marks, "What patient factors predict physicians' decision not to treat latent tuberculosis infection in tuberculosis contacts?" *PLoS ONE*, vol. 8, no. 9, Article ID e76552, 2013.

[22] J. Salazar-Schicchi, V. Jedlovsky, A. Ajayi, P. W. Colson, Y. Hirsch-Moverman, and W. El-Sadr, "Physician attitudes regarding bacille Calmette-Guérin vaccination and treatment of latent tuberculosis infection," *International Journal of Tuberculosis and Lung Disease*, vol. 8, no. 12, pp. 1443–1447, 2004.

[23] S. K. Sharma, A. Mohan, A. Sharma, and D. K. Mitra, "Miliary tuberculosis: new insights into an old disease," *The Lancet Infectious Diseases*, vol. 5, no. 7, pp. 415–430, 2005.

[24] D. Hillemann, S. Rüsch-Gerdes, C. Boehme, and E. Richter, "Rapid molecular detection of extrapulmonary tuberculosis by the automated genexpert MTB/RIF system," *Journal of Clinical Microbiology*, vol. 49, no. 4, pp. 1202–1205, 2011.

[25] J. J. Parker, R. S. Svingos, D. N. Reeder, and E. Grieser, "A rare cause of blindness," *The Journal of Emergency Medicine*, vol. 45, no. 2, pp. e27–e30, 2013.

[26] V. Gupta, A. Gupta, and N. A. Rao, "Intraocular tuberculosis—an update," *Survey of Ophthalmology*, vol. 52, no. 6, pp. 561–587, 2007.

[27] E. Bouza, P. Merino, and P. Muñoz, "Ocular tuberculosis. A prospective study in a general hospital," *Medicine*, vol. 76, pp. 53–61, 1997.

[28] T. Wakabayashi, Y. Morimura, Y. Miyamoto, and A. A. Okada, "Changing patterns of intraocular inflammatory disease in Japan," *Ocular Immunology and Inflammation*, vol. 11, no. 4, pp. 277–286, 2003.

[29] I. W. Abrahams and Y. Q. Jiang, "Ophthalmology in China. Endogenous uveitis in a Chinese ophthalmological clinic," *Archives of Ophthalmology*, vol. 104, no. 3, pp. 444–446, 1986.

[30] S. M. M. Islam and K. F. Tabbara, "Causes of uveitis at The Eye Center in Saudi Arabia: a retrospective review," *Ophthalmic Epidemiology*, vol. 9, no. 4, pp. 239–249, 2002.

[31] J. Biswas and S. S. Badrinath, "Ocular morbidity in patients with active systemic tuberculosis," *International Ophthalmology*, vol. 19, no. 5, pp. 293–298, 1995.

[32] J. Biswas, S. Narain, D. Das, and S. K. Ganesh, "Pattern of uveitis in a referral uveitis clinic in India," *International Ophthalmology*, vol. 20, no. 4, pp. 223–228, 1996.

[33] N. Jana, K. Vasishta, S. C. Saha, and K. Ghosh, "Obstetrical outcomes among women with extrapulmonary tuberculosis," *The New England Journal of Medicine*, vol. 341, no. 9, pp. 645–649, 1999.

[34] T. Pillay, A. W. Sturm, M. Khan et al., "Vertical transmission of *Mycobacterium tuberculosis* in KwaZulu Natal: impact of HIV-1 co-infection," *International Journal of Tuberculosis and Lung Disease*, vol. 8, no. 1, pp. 59–69, 2004.

[35] A. Gupta, U. Nayak, M. Ram et al., "Postpartum tuberculosis incidence and mortality among HIV-infected women and their infants in Pune, India, 2002–2005," *Clinical Infectious Diseases*, vol. 45, no. 2, pp. 241–249, 2007.

[36] N. Jana, K. Vasishta, S. K. Jindal, B. Khunnu, and K. Ghosh, "Perinatal outcome in pregnancies complicated by pulmonary tuberculosis," *International Journal of Gynecology and Obstetrics*, vol. 44, no. 2, pp. 119–124, 1994.

[37] H.-C. Lin, H.-C. Lin, and S.-F. Chen, "Increased risk of low birthweight and small for gestational age infants among women with tuberculosis," *BJOG*, vol. 117, no. 5, pp. 585–590, 2010.

[38] S. N. Tripathy and S. N. Tripathy, "Tuberculosis and pregnancy," *International Journal of Gynecology and Obstetrics*, vol. 80, no. 3, pp. 247–253, 2003.

[39] Y. Jacquemyn, C. Van Casteren, M. Luijks, and C. Colpaert, "Disseminated tuberculosis in pregnancy unknown to doctors in Western Europe case presentation: 'part of the routine study in infertility," *BMJ Case Reports*, vol. 2012, 2012.

[40] K. L. Ard, B. T. Chan, D. A. Milner Jr., P. E. Farmer, and S. P. Koenig, "Peritoneal tuberculosis in a pregnant woman from Haiti, United States," *Emerging Infectious Diseases*, vol. 19, no. 3, pp. 514–516, 2013.

[41] F. Z. F. Alaoui, M. Rachad, H. Chaara, H. Bouguern, and M. A. Melhouf, "Peritoneal tuberculosis in pregnancy: a case report," *The Pan African Medical Journal*, vol. 12, article 65, 2012.

[42] M. T. Caserta, "Perinatal Tuberculosis (TB)," Infections in Neonates, April 2015, http://www.merckmanuals.com/professional/pediatrics/infections-in-neonates/perinatal-tuberculosis-tb.

11

Recurrent Pleural Effusions Occurring in Association with Primary Pulmonary Amyloidosis

Lauren Tada,[1] Humayun Anjum,[2] W. Kenneth Linville,[3] and Salim Surani[4,5]

[1]Corpus Christi Medical Center, 7002 William Drive, Corpus Christi, TX 78412, USA
[2]Pulmonary & Critical Care, Bay Area Medical Center, 7002 William Drive, Corpus Christi, TX 78412, USA
[3]Pathology Department, Bay Area Medical Center, 7002 William Drive, Corpus Christi, TX 78412, USA
[4]Texas A&M University, 1177 West Wheeler Avenue, Aransas Pass, TX 78336, USA
[5]University of North Texas, 1177 West Wheeler Avenue, Suite 1, Aransas Pass, TX 78336, USA

Correspondence should be addressed to Salim Surani; srsurani@hotmail.com

Academic Editor: Gunnar Hillerdal

Recurrent pleural effusions occurring in association with immunoglobulin light chain amyloidosis and not associated with amyloid cardiomyopathy are rare. These portend an overall poor prognosis with mean survival time of approximately 1.8 months. We hereby report a case of a 59-year-old Caucasian female with recurrent pleural effusions and an ultimate diagnosis of pulmonary amyloidosis in association with plasma cell myeloma. The optimal treatment for recurrent pleural effusions in amyloidosis has not been determined; however, our patient responded to therapy with Cyclophosphamide-Bortezomib- (Velcade-) Dexamethasone (CyBorD) and had no repeat hospitalizations or recurrence of pleural effusion at four-month follow-up after initiation of therapy.

1. Introduction

Amyloidosis is a rare disorder of protein misfolding and deposition in various organs and tissues [1]. Primary amyloidosis often occurs in association with a plasma cell dyscrasia, whereas secondary amyloidosis tends to occur in association with longstanding chronic inflammatory diseases. The most common primary amyloidosis is immunoglobulin light chain (AL) amyloidosis. There are variable presentations which have been observed clinically with this disorder and commonly involved organ systems including renal, cardiac, gastrointestinal, neurologic, musculoskeletal, hematologic, and dermatologic [2]. Pulmonary manifestations are rare, and only 1-2% of patients with systemic amyloidosis develop persistent pleural effusions. This is important clinically because the presence of pleural effusions has been documented to portend an overall poor prognosis with mean survival time of 1.8 months when untreated [3]. Early diagnosis is critical because of these implications; however, a diagnostic challenge exists where a high clinical suspicion must be present and patients must undergo invasive biopsy and screening in order to secure an accurate diagnosis.

We hereby present a case report of a 59-year-old female with persistent pleural effusions and diagnosis of primary pulmonary amyloidosis in association with plasma cell myeloma.

2. Case Report

A 59-year-old Caucasian female with history of recurrent bilateral pleural effusions was admitted with worsening dyspnea and a nonproductive cough present over the course of one week. She had undergone outpatient right-sided thoracentesis on the day prior to admission, with drainage of 1500 mL of pleural fluid.

The recurrent pleural effusions had been occurring for three months prior to this presentation, and she had undergone thoracentesis twice for the right-sided pleural effusion and six times for the left-sided pleural effusion without any conclusive diagnosis. Results from all of thoracentesis procedures were suggestive of transudative effusions and cultures were negative.

On physical exam, this patient was mildly dyspneic but without retractions or accessory muscle use. There were

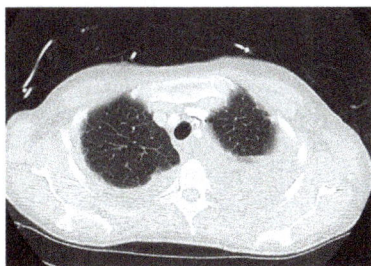

FIGURE 1: CT scan of the chest showing bilateral pleural effusions.

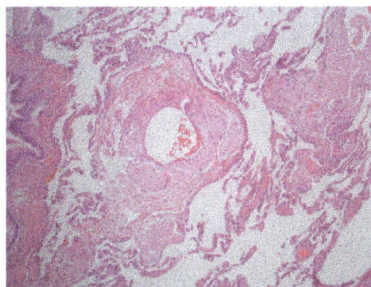

FIGURE 2: Thickened intrapulmonary vessel with adjacent interstitial eosinophilic amorphous material confirmed to be amyloid on Congo Red. (H&E, 100x).

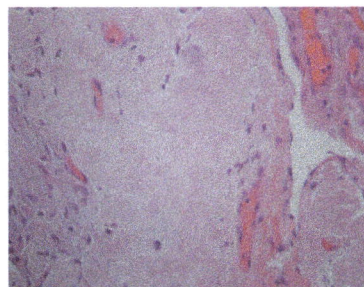

FIGURE 3: Intrapulmonary interstitial deposits of eosinophilic amorphous material that showed apple-green birefringence under polarized light on Congo Red stains (H&E, 400x).

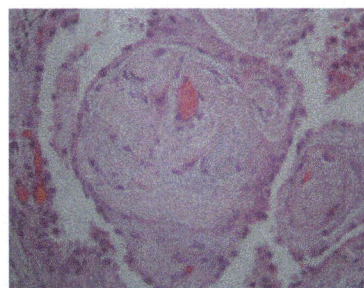

FIGURE 4: Pulmonary endothelial lined small vascular structure surrounded by amyloid deposits and marginated by a rim of reactive Type II pneumocytes (H&E, 400x).

decreased breath sounds at both lung bases. Temperature was 98.5°F, heart rate was 94/min, respiratory rate was 18/min, blood pressure was 97/55 mm Hg, and oxygen saturations were 99% on room air. Complete blood count and basic metabolic panel showed WBC 8.6 thou/μL, Hb 14.1 g/dL, Hct 44.2 g/dL, Plt 356 thou/μL, sodium of 140 mmol/L, potassium of 4 mmol/L, chloride of 101 mmol/L, bicarbonate 32 mmol/L, BUN 13 mg/dL, Creatinine 0.8 mg/dL, and glucose 112 mg/dL. Serum immunofixation electrophoresis showed small lambda monoclonal protein and no Bence-Jones proteinuria. Chest X-ray taken at the time of admission demonstrated a moderate to large left-sided pleural effusion as well as a right lower lobe consolidation. CT scan of chest showed bilateral pleural effusions, greater on the left side (Figure 1). During her hospitalization, the patient underwent thoracentesis which showed WBC 484 mm^3, RBC 38 mm^3, lymphocyte count of 99%, monocyte count of 1%, glucose of 106 mg/dL, total bilirubin of 2.4 gm/dL, lactate dehydrogenase (LDH) of 80 U/L, amylase 19 U/L, cholesterol of 45 mg/dL, triglyceride 17 mg/dL, and adenosine deaminase of 2.3 U/L, and the cultures for routine, acid fast bacilli, and fungus were negative. Cytology demonstrated benign findings with numerous lymphocytes present. The patient underwent biopsy of the left upper lobe of the lung as well as chemical pleurodesis for her recurrent left-sided pleural effusion. Lung biopsy showed diffuse pulmonary amyloidosis, and Congo Red staining was positive confirming the diagnosis (Figures 2–4). Biopsy of the pleura was negative for any pathologic findings.

The patient underwent hematology/oncology evaluation. Echocardiogram showed left concentric ventricular hypertrophy. Rheumatoid factor and thyroid stimulating hormone

levels were normal. Follow-up immunoglobulin and electron microscopy as well as bone marrow biopsy were performed and favored plasma cell myeloma over primary amyloidosis. There were 6% plasma cells on aspirate smears and 15–20% on CD138 immunohistochemical staining of biopsy and clot sections. Flow cytometry showed 1.4% of monoclonal plasma cells typical of a plasma cell dyscrasia.

The patient was started on Cyclophosphamide, Dexamethasone, and Bortezomib (Velcade) therapy and was discharged in stable condition with outpatient follow-up. She had no recurrent pleural effusions at four-month follow-up.

3. Discussion

Amyloidosis is a rare disorder that involves the formation of abnormal protein fibrils and deposition of these fibrils within various organs and tissues throughout the body. Amyloid fibrils are composed of low molecular weight protein subunits, which are normally soluble in the plasma [1, 4]. There are over 20 protein subunits recognized as those which may induce fibrillogenesis. All have a predominantly beta-pleated sheet configuration, which lends them the ability to bind Congo Red stain and demonstrate a characteristic apple-green birefringence by polarized microscopy.

Amyloidosis can be primary or secondary, systemic or localized, and inherited or acquired. AL amyloidosis is caused by immunoglobulin light chain fibril formation and deposition and is typically thought of as primary amyloidosis. It may occur alone or in association with a plasma cell dyscrasia. AA amyloidosis is caused by fibril formation by the acute phase reactant, amyloid A. This is typically seen in association with chronic diseases of inflammation and is therefore generally thought of as a secondary amyloidosis. Heritable forms of amyloidosis also occur and are generally referred to as AF amyloidosis, or familial amyloidosis. As the name implies, these disorders tend to be familial and associated with consistent patterns of clinical manifestation within families. The incidence of AL amyloidosis is unknown, but has been reported to be about 6 to 10 cases per million person-years [4]. The mean age of diagnosis is 64, and 65–70% of patients affected are male.

AL amyloidosis is a systemic disorder that presents with a variety of clinical manifestations depending on the predominantly affected organ system. Commonly involved organ systems include renal, cardiac, gastrointestinal, neurologic, musculoskeletal, hematologic, and dermatologic. Pulmonary involvement has rarely been reported, and published literature has suggested that only 1-2% of patients with systemic amyloidosis develop persistent pleural effusions. We have presented a patient with primary pulmonary AL amyloidosis whose initial presentation was for recurrent bilateral pleural effusions in order to contribute to the current literature for such patients. Our patient was also female and therefore provides information which may later serve as a reference for those who are in the minority of individuals affected by this disease.

Diagnostic criteria have been established by the Mayo Clinic and International Myeloma Working Group and require four criteria to be met for the diagnosis of AL amyloidosis. These include (1) amyloid deposition with distinct organ system involvement, (2) documentation of the presence of amyloid deposition by Congo Red staining, (3) evidence that the amyloid itself is formed by immunoglobulin light-chains, and (4) evidence of a monoclonal plasma cell proliferative disorder. This may be observed with serum or urine M protein, an abnormal serum free light chain ratio, or clonal plasma cells noted within the bone marrow [4]. Our patient met all four criteria and once again provided a unique presentation when compared with previously reported cases of AL amyloidosis.

In one retrospective analysis, medical records were examined for AL amyloidosis patients that had isolated respiratory system involvement between 1990 and 2011 [5]. Of the 13 cases identified during that time period, 9 male patients and 4 female patients were identified as having high mortality with a mean disease course of 46.5 months. Various presentations were recorded further indicating the diagnostic challenge that came with these cases. These included tracheal stenosis, bronchial stenosis, atelectasis, pulmonary nodules, lung consolidation, and lymph node enlargement.

Another published study compared persistent pleural effusions occurring in AL amyloidosis patients with cardiac involvement and those occurring in AL amyloidosis without cardiac involvement. Pleural involvement in this study indicated limited survival where the untreated persistent pleural effusions that occurred alone conferred a median survival of 1.8 months and where untreated persistent pleural effusions that occurred in association with cardiac involvement

resulted in a mean survival of 6 months. These findings were found to be statistically significant with a p value of 0.031 [3]. Survival after chemotherapy and stem cell transplantation was noted to be comparable between groups with a mean survival of 21.8 months in the persistent pleural effusion group and 15.6 months in the group with persistent pleural effusion in association with cardiac involvement. These findings signal a poor prognosis where pleural effusions are present and untreated. It has been reported that parenchymal lung involvement occurs in approximately 28% of patients with AL amyloidosis; however, this does not appear to affect survival [3].

Various case reports have been published for pleural effusions presenting in cases of AL amyloidosis, and the presentations have been just as varied as amyloidosis has proven to be as a disease overall. There have been case reports of transudative as well as exudative pleural effusions (which appear to occur in about the same frequency) [6–8] and pleural effusions of various compositions. There have been different theories about the underlying pathogenesis of pleural effusions that occur in patients with AL amyloidosis based on these observations. The most common presentation of pleural effusions in AL amyloidosis patients occurs in association with amyloid-induced cardiomyopathy, and this suggests that there is pleural fluid accumulation that occurs as a result of ventricular dysfunction. Another possibility is that nephrotic syndrome causes low oncotic pressure in the serum and therefore formation of pleural effusions [3]. It has also been postulated that pleural effusions may result from impaired fluid resorption [9]. One case report of amyloidosis, which manifested with the parietal pleura being covered with brown nodules, seemed to support this theory, as the localized presence of amyloid would have resulted in occlusion of stomata on the parietal pleura where fluid resorption occurs. Still another theory is that severe inflammation that occurs from amyloid deposition might result in increased permeability of the pleural capillaries at the pleura. This has been given as one possible explanation for exudative pleural effusions that have been observed in AL amyloidosis [6].

It should be noted that pleural effusions might occur in AL amyloidosis as well as AA amyloidosis and Senile Systemic Amyloidosis [10–13]. Case reports have been published with pleural effusions present for each of these amyloidosis subtypes, and pleural fluid caused by AL amyloidosis has typically been documented to be composed of lymphocytic fluid with only two case reports of chylous fluid published in the current literature [14]. No clear association has been made for the pleural fluid composition and its occurrence, however. Our patient had pleural fluid of the lymphocytic type, and further studies will need to be undertaken to further elucidate this clinical finding.

Current treatment guidelines for AL amyloidosis involve the use of chemotherapy and autologous stem cell transplantation [15]. In the past, melphalan and prednisone were shown to prolong survival in patients with primary amyloidosis [16]. This combination treatment has been documented to increase median survival by approximately 17 months; however, there has not typically been regression of organ dysfunction or cure. The Amyloid Program at Boston University School of Medicine treated patients with systemic AL amyloidosis using high-dose intravenous melphalan and autologous stem cell transplantation and observed hematologic cure in 62% of patients with a 65% improvement in organ function providing some hope for improved survival in these patients [17]. The treatment of persistent pleural effusions from AL amyloidosis in particular has been more of a challenge, however, and generally requires optimizing cardiac filling pressure, symptomatic relief often with serial drainage as in our patient, and consideration of chemical pleurodesis for effusions that are refractory to other treatments. The optimal treatment for this specific condition has not been determined. There have been two case reports that have explored other chemotherapeutic regimens that have had good results for systemic amyloidosis patients with pleural effusions. In one study, a patient who had previously been receiving intermittent melphalan and prednisone therapy for 7 years was treated with vincristine, adriamycin, and dexamethasone (VAD) therapy with prevention of recurrence of his pleural effusions for the six months that he was on treatment, with return of his pleural effusions only after cessation of therapy [18]. Ultimately, this patient underwent chemical pleurodesis and continued melphalan and prednisone therapy with no increase in his pleural effusions at four-year follow-up.

In another published report, a patient that had diffuse parenchymal pulmonary amyloidosis was treated with melphalan, prednisolone, and Bortezomib chemotherapy [19]. This patient was subsequently noted to have normalization of her serum monoclonal protein levels as well as improvement over her overall pulmonary function and oxygenation with a 16.2% increase in vital capacity and 18.1% improvement in the diffusing capacity for carbon monoxide (DLCO). Similarly, there was a case report of a patient with recurrent pleural effusions and a subsequent diagnosis of AL amyloidosis which were treated with Cyclophosphamide-Bortezomib-(Velcade-) Dexamethasone (CyBorD) therapy with normalization of her serum protein immunoglobulin and no further recurrence of her pleural effusion at 8 months. Improvement in pulmonary function and oxygenation was also observed with this regimen. This is the treatment that our patient received after the diagnosis of AL amyloidosis, and, at the time of this report, there have been no repeat hospitalizations at 4 months [8].

4. Conclusion

Pleural effusions occur rarely in cases of systemic amyloidosis and have variable pleural fluid compositions. Because they portend a poor prognosis with a mean survival of 1.8 months when they occur in patients with AL amyloidosis, prompt diagnosis is critical in order to initiate treatment, which may improve pulmonary function and oxygenation and ultimately improve survival. This case provides an additional report of pleural effusions as they presented in a patient with AL amyloidosis and documents a current case being treated with CyBorD therapy.

References

[1] D. C. Seldin and M. Skinner, "Amyloidosis," in *Kelly's Textbook of Rheumatology*, D. F. A. Longo, D. Kasper, S. Hauser, J. Jameson, and Loscalzo, Eds., McGraw-Hill, 2012.

[2] P. S. P. Gorevic and P. Romain, *Overview of Amyloidosis*, 2011, http://www.uptodate.com/contents/overview-of-amyloidosis.

[3] J. L. Berk, J. Keane, D. C. Seldin et al., "Persistent pleural effusions in primary systemic amyloidosis: etiology and prognosis," *Chest*, vol. 124, no. 3, pp. 969–977, 2003.

[4] S. G. R. Rajkumar, R. Kyle, and R. Connor, *Clinical Presentation, Laboratory Manifestations and Diagnosis of Immunoglobulin Light Chain (AL) Amyloidosis*, 2014, http://www.uptodate.com/contents/clinical-presentation-laboratory-manifestations-and-diagnosis-of-immunoglobulin-light-chain-al-amyloidosis-primary-amyloidosis.

[5] H. Chu, L. Zhao, Z. Zhang, T. Gui, X. Yi, and X. Sun, "Clinical characteristics of amyloidosis with isolated respiratory system involvement: a review of 13 cases," *Annals of Thoracic Medicine*, vol. 7, no. 4, pp. 243–349, 2012.

[6] N. Fujimoto, H. Masuoka, H. Kosaka, S. Ota, M. Ito, and T. Nakano, "Primary amyloidosis with pulmonary involvement which presented exudative pleural effusion and high fever," *Internal Medicine*, vol. 42, no. 8, pp. 756–760, 2003.

[7] B. Erickson, G. Dhaliwal, M. C. Henderson, E. Amsterdam, and J. Rencic, "Effusive reasoning," *Journal of General Internal Medicine*, vol. 26, no. 10, pp. 1204–1208, 2011.

[8] S. Karim and Y.-S. Chang, "An unusual cause of pleural effusion," *The New Zealand Medical Journal*, vol. 126, no. 1378, pp. 79–81, 2013.

[9] F. Bontemps, I. Tillie-Leblond, M. C. Coppin et al., "Pleural amyloidosis: thoracoscopic aspects," *The European Respiratory Journal*, vol. 8, no. 6, pp. 1025–1027, 1995.

[10] N. Alappan, J. Dobkin, and P. Klapper, "A rare cause of pleural effusion," *American Journal of Respiratory and Critical Care Medicine*, vol. 185, article A5191, 2012.

[11] Y. Shimizu, K. Endou, Y. Hashizume et al., "Massive pleural effusion due to pleural AA amyloidosis," *American Journal of Respiratory and Critical Care Medicine*, vol. 186, no. 12, pp. e19–e20, 2012.

[12] M. O. Al-Qadi, E. J. Brown, T. E. Noonan, and M. A. Khan, "Persistent large pleural effusion due to senile systemic transthyretin amyloidosis," *American Journal of Respiratory and Critical Care Medicine*, vol. 185, Article ID A5900, 2012.

[13] H. G. M. Seth, S. Desai, V. Sein, B. Shinar, and M. Mathews, "Persistent pleural effusion in systemic AL amyloidosis," *American Journal of Respiratory and Critical Care Medicine*, vol. 187, Article ID A6132, 2013.

[14] T. S. Panchabhai, S. P. Kellie, S. P. Slone, R. S. Cavallazzi, R. L. Perez, and Y. M. Cua, "Bilateral chylothorax as a sentinel presentation of primary Al amyloidosis," *American Journal of Respiratory and Critical Care Medicine*, vol. 185, article A5190, 2012.

[15] S. Mahmood, G. Palladini, V. Sanchorawala, and A. Wechalekar, "Update on treatment of light chain amyloidosis," *Haematologica*, vol. 99, no. 2, pp. 209–221, 2014.

[16] R. A. Kyle, M. A. Gertz, P. R. Greipp et al., "A trial of three regimens for primary amyloidosis: colchicine alone, melphalan and prednisone, and melphalan, prednisone, and colchicine," *The New England Journal of Medicine*, vol. 336, no. 17, pp. 1202–1207, 1997.

[17] J. L. Berk, A. O'Regan, and M. Skinner, "Pulmonary and tracheobronchial amyloidosis," *Seminars in Respiratory and Critical Care Medicine*, vol. 23, no. 2, pp. 155–165, 2002.

[18] T. Araoka, H. Takeoka, K. Nishioka et al., "Successful management of refractory pleural effusion due to systemic immunoglobulin light chain amyloidosis by vincristine adriamycin dexamethasone chemotherapy: a case report," *Journal of Medical Case Reports*, vol. 4, article 322, 2010.

[19] H. Higo, K. Fujiwara, H. Watanabe et al., "Diffuse parenchymal pulmonary amyloidosis showing an objective response to bortezomib-based chemotherapy," *Internal Medicine*, vol. 53, no. 16, pp. 1809–1812, 2014.

12

Right Heart Transvalvular Embolus with High Risk Pulmonary Embolism in a Recently Hospitalized Patient: A Case Report of a Therapeutic Challenge

Gyanendra Kumar Acharya,[1] **Ajibola Monsur Adedayo,**[1] **Hejmadi Prabhu,**[2]
Derek R. Brinster,[3] **and Parvez Mir**[4]

[1] *Department of Internal Medicine, Wyckoff Heights Medical Center, Brooklyn, NY 11237, USA*
[2] *Division of Cardiology, Department of Internal Medicine, Wyckoff Heights Medical Center, Brooklyn, NY 11237, USA*
[3] *Department of Cardiothoracic Surgery, Lenox Hill Hospital, North Shore-Long Island Jewish Health System,*
New York, NY 10075, USA
[4] *Division of Pulmonary and Critical Care Medicine, Department of Internal Medicine, Wyckoff Heights Medical Center,*
Brooklyn, NY 11237, USA

Correspondence should be addressed to Gyanendra Kumar Acharya; achgyanen@hotmail.com

Academic Editor: Akif Turna

Thrombus-in-transit is not uncommon in pulmonary embolism but Right Heart Transvalvular Embolus (RHTVE) complicating this is rare. A 54-year-old obese male with recent hospitalization presented with severe dyspnea and collapse. Initial investigations revealed elevated d-dimer and troponin. CTA showed saddle pulmonary embolus and bedside echocardiogram revealed right ventricular (RV) pressure overload and dilatation (RV > 41 mm), McConnell's sign, and mobile echodensity attached to tricuspid valve. Patient was immediately resuscitated and promptly transferred for surgical embolectomy under cardiopulmonary bypass. A long segment of embolus traversing through the tricuspid valve and extensive bilateral pulmonary artery embolus were removed. IVC filter was placed for a persistent right lower extremity DVT. Hypercoagulable work-up was negative. Patient continued to do well after discharge on Coumadin. Open embolectomy offers great promises where there is no consensus in optimal management approach in such patients. Bedside echocardiogram is vital in risk stratification and deciding choice of advanced PE treatment.

1. Introduction

Right-heart-thrombus is not uncommon in acute massive pulmonary embolism (PE) and appears to increase mortality substantially [1, 2]. It requires emergency treatment, but there is no consensus regarding optimal management. Our patient presented with massive PE along with a unique echocardiographic finding of a long Right Heart Transvalvular Embolus (RHTVE) traversing the tricuspid valve. In appropriate settings, such patients would benefit from emergency surgical embolectomy.

2. Case Presentation

54-year-old obese male presented to ER with episodic dyspnea and collapse without loss of consciousness associated with palpitation, chest discomfort, and diaphoresis. He was recently hospitalized for colonic diverticular abscess that was drained. Medical history includes hypertension, CAD, and asthma. He denied smoking/illicit drugs. Examination was remarkable for tachycardia, hypotension, and mild hypoxia. Laboratory findings revealed elevated lactic acid, troponin, d-dimer, and abnormal EKG (Table 1, Figure 1). Urgent CT

TABLE 1: Baseline laboratory findings in the patient at presentation.

SN	Tests	Values	Reference value
		CBC	
	WBC	12.60	$4.50–10.9\,K/mm^3$
	RBC	4.92	$3.8–5.2 \times 10^6/mm^3$
(1)	Hb	14.2	12.2–15 gm/dL
	Platelets	212.0	$130–400 \times 10^3/mm^3$
	ESR	30.0	0–35 mm/hr
		Chemistry	
	Sodium	137.0	136–145 mmol/L
	Potassium	4.9	3.5–5.1 mmol/L
(2)	BUN	16.0	6–20 mg/dL
	Creatinine	1.0	0.6–1.1 mg/dL
	LDH	482.0	100–190 IU/L
	Troponin I	0.122	0–0.1 ng/ml
	Lactic acid	5.0	0.5–2.2 mmol/L
		Basic coagulation profile	
	PT	13.8 sec	9.70–13.20 sec
(3)	INR	1.21	0.86–1.16 (ratio)
	PTT	35.3	20.30–36.00 sec
	d-dimer	7205.26	400–560 ng/mLFEU

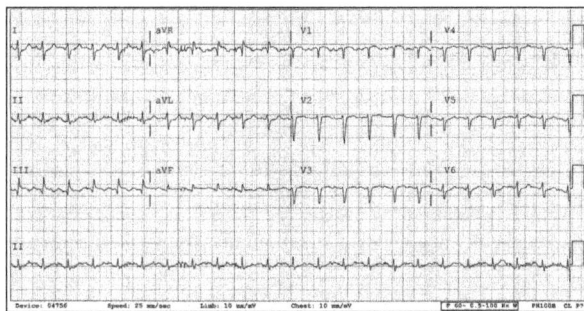

FIGURE 1: 12-lead EKG showing right ventricular strain pattern.

angiogram showed extensive bilateral pulmonary embolus (Figure 2), and bedside echocardiogram revealed right ventricular (RV) pressure overload with enlarged RV (>41 mm) and mobile echodensity attached to tricuspid valve that appeared to extend into right atrium and ventricle, RHTVE (Figure 3).

Patient was resuscitated with intravenous fluid, 40% Ventimask, and anticoagulated with intravenous heparin. After interdisciplinary discussion, patient was transferred to the nearest tertiary facility for open embolectomy with cardiopulmonary bypass. On follow-up with the tertiary center, a long segment of blood clot traversing the right atrium and ventricle (Figure 4(b)) and extensive bilateral pulmonary artery embolus (Figure 4(a)) were removed. Additionally, IVC filter was placed for a continued right lower extremity thrombus extending from common femoral to the posterior tibial vein. Work-up for hypercoagulable studies was negative. He was discharged on Coumadin and continues to do well on follow-up with us.

3. Discussion

Thrombus-in-transit is not an unusual presentation in high risk PE [3]. This case chronicles a rare large embolus traversing through tricuspid valve from right atrium to right ventricle and we termed this as Right Heart Transvalvular Embolus (RHTVE). High risk PE may be massive or submassive. It often results from embolization of proximal deep vein thrombus in the lower extremities. Massive PE is characterized by sustained hypotension with SBP <90 for at least 15 minutes or requiring intravenous vasopressor(s). It may also be a state of bradycardia with heart rate <40 associated with signs and symptoms of shock or pulselessness. Submassive PE is that without hypotension associated with RV dysfunction (right bundle branch block/right heart strain, McConnell's sign, or elevated BNP) or evidence of myocardial injury (troponin >0.1) [4].

Pulmonary artery pressure increases abruptly once the embolus occludes > 30–50% of the total cross-sectional area of pulmonary arterial bed. This anatomical obstruction and reactive vasoconstriction induced by release of thromboxane A2 and serotonin together increase pulmonary vascular resistance [5]. The RV adapts via frank-sterling mechanism to maintain BP by generating counterpressure (persistent contraction) against rising pulmonary artery pressure, this adaptation is limited, and soon RV dilatation ensues precipitating hemodynamic instability [5]. Secondly, the resulting ventilation perfusion mismatch and decreased cardiac output contribute to hypotension, hypoxemia, and eventual respiratory failure [5]. Hypoxemia and increased myocardial demand may explain the lactic acidemia and elevated troponin in our patient.

Investigators have associated massive and submassive PE with 52.4% and 14.7% 90-day mortality, respectively [6]. One study concluded that hemodynamically unstable PE is associated with >25% in-hospital mortality [7]. Echocardiographic and CTPA findings of RV dysfunction were shown as independent predictors of 30-day mortality while elevated troponin increases short-term risk of death up to fivefold [8–10]. Resuscitative measures, with judicious intravenous fluid administration to stabilize SBP and 40% Ventimask to decrease work of breathing, provided the critical window for urgent CTA and echocardiogram. Echocardiogram served as a cornerstone for both diagnosis and risk stratification (identified RHTVE).

Currently, there is no randomized trial that supports or contravenes open embolectomy; it remains a vital treatment option in advanced management of PE. Open embolectomy has its attendant risks and complications but early surgical referral can skew outcome favorably [11]. Investigators have suggested open embolectomy as a reasonable option provided that patients are identified before onset of cardiac arrest [11–14]. Our patient presented with massive PE and a unique Echo finding of RHTVE. After interdisciplinary consultations, we concluded that surgical option would not only recover the thrombus in right heart and central branches of pulmonary artery before further deterioration, but also avert the possibilities of failed thrombolysis. We opted for invasive approach (open embolectomy with cardiopulmonary bypass) for

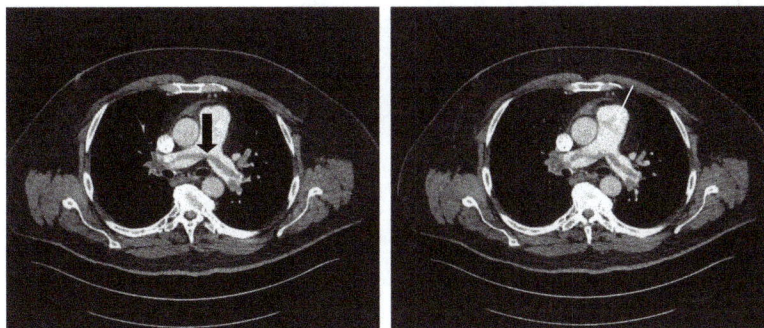

FIGURE 2: Computed Tomographic Pulmonary Angiogram (CTPA) showing massive saddle pulmonary embolus (bold arrow) with hypodense area at the root of pulmonary artery consistent with other emboli (white arrow).

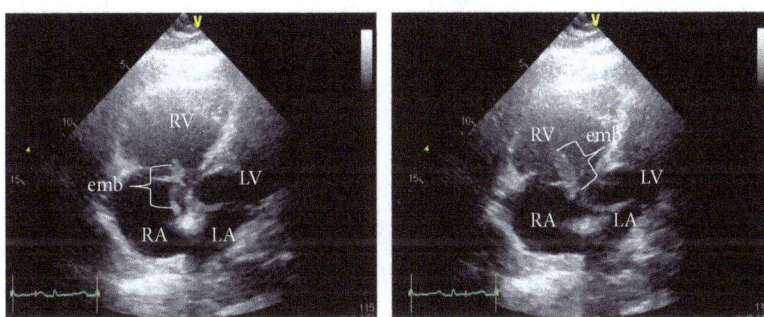

FIGURE 3: Transthoracic echocardiogram, apical 4-chamber view, showing RV pressure overload with enlarged RV diameter (>41 mm) and a long echodensity (embolus) attached to TV extending in both RA and RV (RHTVE); LA: left atrium; RV: right ventricle; RA: right atrium; LV: left ventricle; TV: tricuspid valve; emb: embolus; RHTVE: Right Heart Transvalvular Embolus.

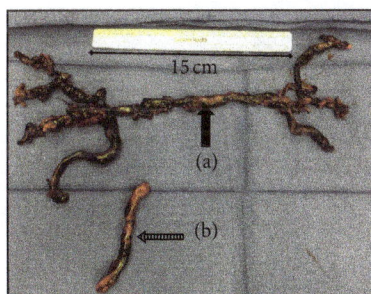

FIGURE 4: Postoperative demonstration of (a) a large (~25 cm) pulmonary embolus *en bloc* (bold arrow) retrieved from the right and left pulmonary arteries; (b) a long segment of embolus (doted arrow) traversing along tricuspid valve (TV). Both of them were removed in the same open embolectomy under cardiopulmonary bypass procedure.

the following reasons. Bedside 2D echocardiogram revealed a long embolus traversing through the tricuspid valve on the background of massive saddle embolus extending in main branches of pulmonary artery. The right ventricle was already on massive pressure overload with dilatation and shifting of ventricular septum towards left ventricle. Further clot burden to pulmonary artery (by imminent dislodging the transvalvular clot) would have been catastrophic in the patient. So it was decided to immediately transfer the patient to operating

room for open embolectomy under cardiopulmonary bypass procedure. Clot propagation was still ongoing as evidenced by presence of large thrombus in the femoral and tibial veins (IVC filter was placed). This could continue to be deposited distally. Catheter-directed thrombolysis may be complicated by deposition of fragments in terminal branches of the pulmonary arteries, which may result in chronic pulmonary embolism/hypertension. Other treatment approaches may still be complicated with cardiac arrest with even higher mortality. The benefits outweighed the risk. Open embolectomy offers great promises in selected patients who are relatively stable (absence of cardiac arrest) where there is no consensus yet in optimal management approach.

In conclusion, bedside echocardiogram is vital in risk stratification and deciding choice of advanced PE treatment. High risk PE patients with RHTVE can benefit from emergent open embolectomy with cardiopulmonary bypass.

Abbreviations

BNP: Brain natriuretic peptide
BUN: Blood urea nitrogen
CAD: Coronary artery disease
CBC: Complete blood count
CT: Computed tomography
CTA: Computed tomographic angiogram
CTPA: Computed Tomographic Pulmonary Angiogram

Echo:	Echocardiogram
EKG:	Electrocardiogram
emb:	Embolus
ER:	Emergency room
INR:	International normalized ratio
IVC:	Inferior vena cava
LA:	Left atrium
LDH:	Lactate dehydrogenase
LV:	Left ventricle
PE:	Pulmonary embolism
PT:	Prothrombin time
PTT:	Partial thromboplastin time
RA:	Right atrium
RBC:	Red blood cells
RHTVE:	Right Heart Transvalvular Embolus
RV:	Right ventricle
SBP:	Systolic blood pressure
TV:	Tricuspid valve
WBC:	White blood cells.

References

[1] G. Kronik, "The European cooperative study on the clinical significance of right heart thrombi," *European Heart Journal*, vol. 10, no. 12, pp. 1046–1059, 1989.

[2] A. Torbicki, N. Galié, A. Covezzoli et al., "Right heart thrombi in pulmonary embolism: results from the International Cooperative Pulmonary Embolism Registry," *Journal of the American College of Cardiology*, vol. 41, no. 12, pp. 2245–2251, 2003.

[3] F. Casazza, A. Bongarzoni, F. Centonze, and M. Morpurgo, "Prevalence and prognostic significance of right-sided cardiac mobile thrombi in acute massive pulmonary embolism," *American Journal of Cardiology*, vol. 79, no. 10, pp. 1433–1435, 1997.

[4] M. R. Jaff, M. S. McMurtry, S. L. Archer et al., "Management of massive and submassive pulmonary embolism, iliofemoral deep vein thrombosis, and chronic thromboembolic pulmonary hypertension: a scientific statement from the american heart association," *Circulation*, vol. 123, no. 16, pp. 1788–1830, 2011.

[5] S. V. Konstantinides, A. Torbicki, G. Agnelli et al., "ESC guidelines on the diagnosis and management of acute pulmonary embolism," *European Heart Journal*, vol. 35, no. 43, pp. 3033–2069, 3069a–3069k, 2014.

[6] N. Kucher, E. Rossi, M. D. Rosa, and S. Z. Goldhaber, "Massive pulmonary embolism," *Circulation*, vol. 113, no. 4, pp. 577–582, 2006.

[7] W. Kasper, S. Konstantinides, A. Geibel et al., "Management strategies and determinants of outcome in acute major pulmonary embolism: results of a multicenter registry," *Journal of the American College of Cardiology*, vol. 30, no. 5, pp. 1165–1171, 1997.

[8] N. Kucher, E. Rossi, M. De Rosa, and S. Z. Goldhaber, "Prognostic role of echocardiography among patients with acute pulmonary embolism and a systolic arterial pressure of 90 mm Hg or higher," *Archives of Internal Medicine*, vol. 165, no. 15, pp. 1777–1781, 2005.

[9] C. Becattini, G. Agnelli, F. Germini, and M. C. Vedovati, "Computed tomography to assess risk of death in acute pulmonary embolism: a meta-analysis," *European Respiratory Journal*, vol. 43, no. 6, pp. 1678–1690, 2014.

[10] C. Becattini, M. C. Vedovati, and G. Agnelli, "Prognostic value of troponins in acute pulmonary embolism: a meta-analysis," *Circulation*, vol. 116, no. 4, pp. 427–433, 2007.

[11] P. D. Stein and F. Matta, "Case fatality rate with pulmonary embolectomy for acute pulmonary embolism," *American Journal of Medicine*, vol. 125, no. 5, pp. 471–477, 2012.

[12] N. Meneveau, M.-F. Séronde, M.-C. Blonde et al., "Management of unsuccessful thrombolysis in acute massive pulmonary embolism," *Chest*, vol. 129, no. 4, pp. 1043–1050, 2006.

[13] M. Leacche, D. Unic, S. Z. Goldhaber et al., "Modern surgical treatment of massive pulmonary embolism: results in 47 consecutive patients after rapid diagnosis and aggressive surgical approach," *Journal of Thoracic and Cardiovascular Surgery*, vol. 129, no. 5, pp. 1018–1023, 2005.

[14] B. Sareyyupoglu, K. L. Greason, R. M. Suri, M. T. Keegan, J. A. Dearani, and T. M. Sundt, "A more aggressive approach to emergency embolectomy for acute pulmonary embolism," *Mayo Clinic Proceedings*, vol. 85, no. 9, pp. 785–790, 2010.

13

A Behcet's Disease Patient with Right Ventricular Thrombus, Pulmonary Artery Aneurysms, and Deep Vein Thrombosis Complicating Recurrent Pulmonary Thromboembolism

Selvi Aşker,[1] **Müntecep Aşker,**[2] **Özgür Gürsu,**[3] **Rıdvan Mercan,**[4] **and Özgür Bülent Timuçin**[5]

[1] *Department of Chest Disease, Van Training and Research Hospital, Van, Turkey*
[2] *Department of Cardiology, Van Training and Research Hospital, Van, Turkey*
[3] *Department of Cardiovascular Surgery, Van Training and Research Hospital, Van, Turkey*
[4] *Division of Rheumatology, Department of Internal Medicine, Gazi University, Ankara, Turkey*
[5] *Department of Ophthalmology, İstanbul Hospital, Van, Turkey*

Correspondence should be addressed to Selvi Aşker; selviasker@mynet.com

Academic Editors: A. Sihoe and N. Tanabe

Intracardiac thrombus, pulmonary artery aneurysms, deep vein thrombosis, and pulmonary thromboembolism are rarely seen symptoms of Behcet's disease. A 20-year-old female patient was admitted for complaints of cough, fever, palpitations, and chest pain. On the dynamic thorax computed tomograms (CT) obtained because of significantly enlarged hilar structures seen on chest radiograms, aneurysmal dilatation of the pulmonary artery segments bilaterally, chronic thrombus with collapse, and consolidation substances compatible with pulmonary embolism involving both lower lobes have been observed. It is learned that, four years ago, the patient had been diagnosed with Behcet's disease and received colchicine treatment but not regularly. The patient was hospitalized. On the transthoracic echocardiogram, a thrombosis with a dimension of 4.2×1.6 cm was recognized in the right ventricle. On abdomen CT, aneurysmal iliac veins and deep vein thrombus on Doppler ultrasonograms were diagnosed. At the controls after three months of immunosuppressive and anticoagulant therapies, some clinical and radiological improvements were recognized. The patient suspended the treatment for a month and the thrombus recurred. We present our case in order to show the effectiveness of immunosuppressive and anticoagulant therapies and rarely seen pulmonary thromboembolism in recurrent Behcet's disease.

1. Introduction

Behcet's disease (BD) is a multisystem disorder presenting with recurrent buccal aphthosis, genital ulcer, and uveitis with hypopyon [1]. Pulmonary involvement in Behcet's disease is rare, occurring in 1 to 7.7% of the patients [2, 3]. Pulmonary artery aneurysms, arterial and venous thrombosis, pulmonary infarction, recurrent pneumonia, bronchiolitis obliterans organised pneumonia, and pleurisy are the main features of pulmonary involvement in Behcet's disease [4]. Cardiac involvement causes coronary artery disease, recurrent pericarditis, myocardiopathy, and endocardiac abnormalities. Intracardiac thrombus formation is very uncommon

[5]. We present a Behcet's disease patient with intracardiac thrombus, pulmonary artery aneurysms, and deep vein thrombosis complicating recurrent pulmonary embolism.

2. Case Report

A twenty-year-old woman was admitted to the hospital with complaints of cough, fever, palpitations, and chest pain. It was learned that, four years ago the patient had been diagnosed with Behcet's disease and received irregular colchicine treatment. During interviews, we learned that, he had recurrent oral and genital ulcers. On examination, there was no

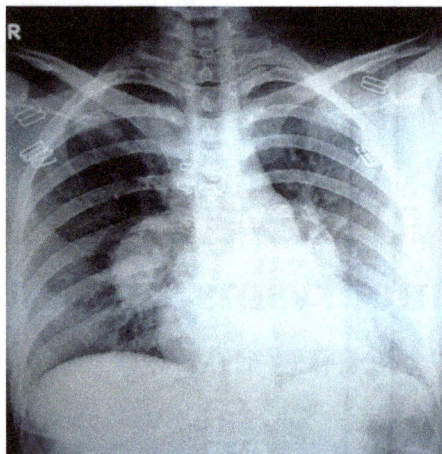

FIGURE 1: Chest radiogram demonstrating bilateral hilar enlargement and patchy infiltration.

pathological finding except for high temperature (38.5°C). Her chest radiogram showed bilateral, hilar enlargement and peripheral but localized patchy infiltration (Figure 1). Initial diagnosis of pulmonary artery aneurysm and pulmonary emboli were especially associated with the hilar enlargement and previous diagnosis of Behcet's disease. Accordingly, dynamic contrasted CT was obtained. On dynamic thorax computed tomograms of both pulmonary arteries, aneurysmal dilatation and chronic thrombus involving all interior lmen of both pulmonary arteries were detected. Consolidated substances were determined on posterobasal segment of the left pulmonary lower lobe with a dimension of 3 × 2 cm related to, newly formed emboli (Figures 2 and 3).

On concurrent transthoracic echocardiograms (TTE) a bulk with a dimension of 4.5 × 1.6 cm was determined in the right ventricle explaining symptoms of thrombus (Figure 4). On cardiac MRI, a mass lesion was detected in the right ventricle with the dimensions of 4.5 × 1.5 cm concordant with the thrombus. Thrombus was determined in the bilateral femoral veins by venous Doppler ultrasonography of the lower extremities. Hematologic parameters of the patient were within the normal limits. Thrombophilia panel was reported as normal. The patient was referred to an ophthalmologist who found evidence of active uveitis.

Pulsed immunosuppressive therapy was administered to the patient. She was quickly relieved of her symptoms after a combination therapy with methylprednisolone, cyclophosphamide, and low-molecular-weight heparin (LMWH).

Significant improvement of the laboratory parameters of the patient was obtained (Table 1). Dynamic thorax CT was repeated at the end of the 3rd month of the treatment. Partial dissolution of the thrombi and pulmonary defects were observed. Besides, an irregular hypodense defect with irregular contours with its largest diameter comparatively regressed from 3 cm to 2 cm was observed. The diameter of the pulmonary truncus which was previously 29 mm measured 23 mm on control CT, and minimisation of the mass lesion in the right ventricle was observed (Figures 3(a), 3(b),

4(a), and 4(b)). Doppler USG demonstrated disappearance of the previously detected thrombus in femoral veins.

The patient was admitted again to the hospital on the 6th month of the treatment with complaints of leg pain, headache and palpitations. It was learned that she had quitted anticoagulant therapy 1 month ago. Doppler USG manifested evidence of recurrent DVT ischemic gliotic changes which were unobserved before being seen on brain MR angiograms. Anticoagulant treatment of the patient was repeated.

During a follow-up period of 10 months, the patient is still under treatment and doing well.

3. Discussion

Intrathoracic manifestations of Behcet's disease consist mainly of thromboembolism of the superior vena cava and/or other mediastinal veins, aneurysms of the aorta and pulmonary arteries, pulmonary infarct and hemorrhage, pleural effusion, and rarely, myocardial and pericardial involvement, cor pulmonale, and mediastinal or hilar lymphadenopathy [6]. Pulmonary infarction is a stage in the natural course of the disease. Pulmonary vasculitis and thromboses of pulmonary vessels may cause infarctions, focal or diffuse hemorrhages, and focal areas of atelectasis [6–8]. Although vascular involvement is seen only in 25% of the patients, it is the most common cause of mortality in Behcet's disease [6, 9, 10]. New imaging technologies, especially, dynamic thorax CT, can be helpful in the demonstration of thrombus of the systemic veins, heart and pulmonary arteries [8]. Dynamic thorax CT revealed a right ventricular thrombus in our patient. The thrombus was confirmed by echocardiography. Thromboembolism stemming from a cardiac cavity has been previously deemed to be relatively uncommon [9]. A review by Moğulkoç et al. regarding intracardiac thrombi in 25 patients with Behcet's disease was previously published [5]. The authors noted that they had seen pulmonary embolism in 13 patients (52%). In seven of these 13 patients, thrombophlebitis was observed in the major vessels which might have been the source of the embolism. Although deep venous thrombosis of the lower extremities frequently accompanies pulmonary artery aneurysms, pulmonary thromboembolism is very rare in Behcet's disease because the thrombi in inflamed veins are strongly adherent [11]. In a review study done by Houman et al. on 113 Behcet's disease patients, vein involvement had been detected in 49 patients (43.3%), and deep vein thrombus had been observed in 44 of them (38.9%). Deep vein thrombosis was more frequently observed among males (40 males and 4 females) [12]. Another review consisting of reports of Turkish authors revealed one intracardiac thrombus out of 56 (1.78%) Behcet's disease patients [13]. Recently, two Behcet's disease patients with intracardiac thrombi and pulmonary artery aneurysms have been reported [14, 15]. Luo et al. analyzed the clinical characteristics of Behcet's disease with intracardiac thrombus [16]. The data of 8 patients diagnosed with Behcet's disease with intracardiac thrombi in Peking Union Medical College Hospital from January 1990 to January 2011 were studied retrospectively. Intracardiac thrombus associated

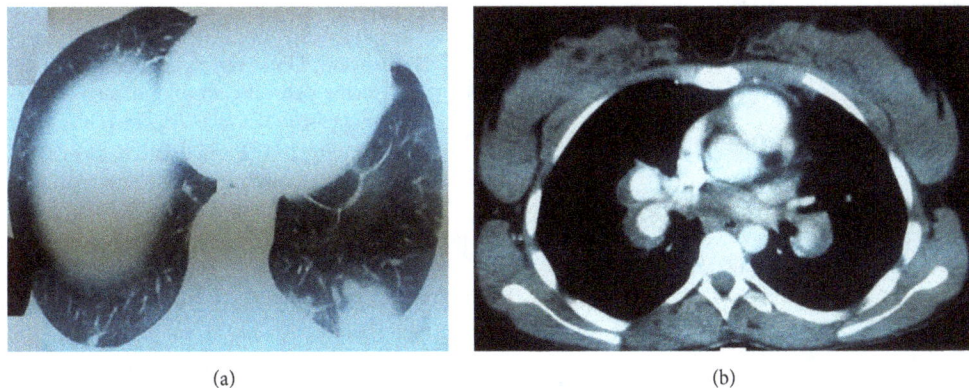

(a)   (b)

FIGURE 2: Thorax computed tomogram showing consolidated substances related to emboli in the posterobasal segment of the left pulmonary lower lobe (a), pulmonary artery thrombus and aneurysmal dilatation of the pulmonary artery (b).

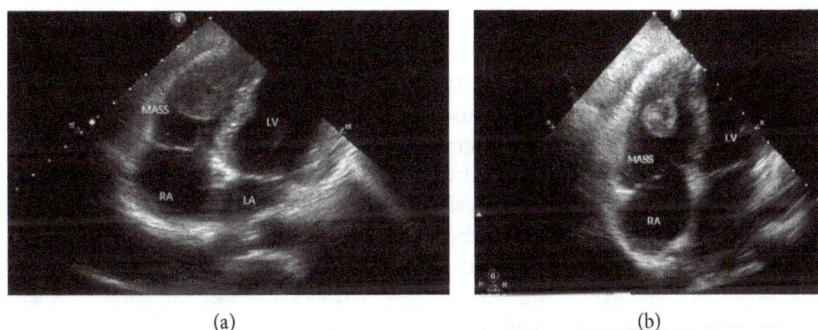

(a)   (b)

FIGURE 3: Thrombus in the right ventricle as seen on transthoracic echocardiogram (a), partial minimisation of the thrombus after the treatment (b).

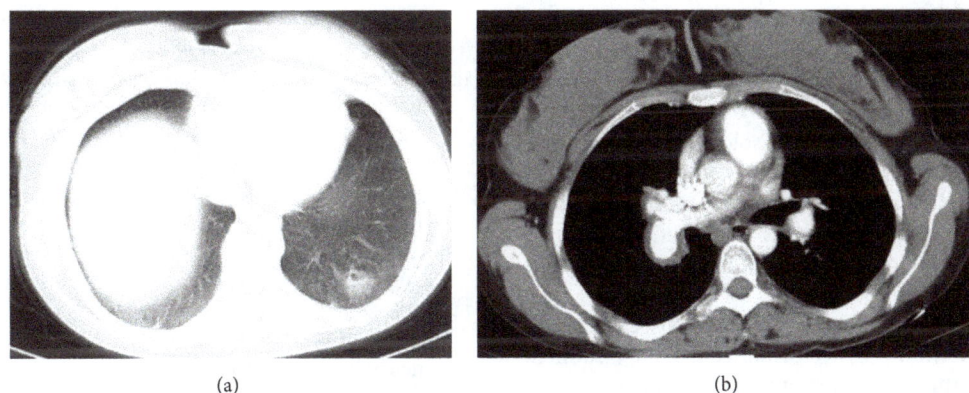

(a)   (b)

FIGURE 4: Minimisation of the consolidated substance related to the emboli on CT after the treatment (a), partial dissolution of the thrombus and minimisation of its PA diameter (b).

with Behcet's disease most commonly occurs in young men and usually involves the right side of the heart [16].

The pathologic mechanism of microvascular thrombus formation in vasculitis is believed to be caused by endothelial cell ischemia or disruption that leads to enhanced platelet aggregation [4, 5]. Decreased release of vascular tissue plasminogen activator has been reported in systemic and cutaneous vasculitis [9]. Impaired fibrinolysis as a result of endothelial cell injury from deposited immune complexes is another possible mechanism. Prolonged euglobulin lysis times and abnormal fibrin concentrations were found in several types of vasculitis, including Behcet's disease [6, 8]. In the present case, intracardiac thrombus, deep vein thrombosis, and pulmonary embolism were detected. Considering the possible mechanisms leading to thrombus, and recurrent emboli due to intracardiac thrombus and deep vein thrombosis, immunosuppressive and antithrombotic medications were started. Warfarin was not the preferred

TABLE 1: Laboratory findings after and before the treatment.

	Pretreatment	Posttreatment
Hemoglobin (g/dL)	12.6	12.2
White blood cell (WBC) (/mL)	16.5	7.6
Erythrocyte sedimentation rate (ESR) (mm/h)	55	10
C-reactive protein (CRP) (mg/dL)	94	1
Fibrinogen (mg/dL)	501	290
D-dimer (ng/dL)	699	233

treatment option due to the risk of bleeding. Although the first line treatment is medical, thrombus can become massive and may demand surgical treatment.

We presented infarct centers and new emboli centers on peripheral divisions showing chronic thrombus observed related to the repeated emboli on pulmonary arteries. During the follow-up, there was in change on thrombus divisions. Newly formed emboli were not observed and infarct centers regressed. This situation showed the effectiveness of the treatment. Our patient's pulmonary artery pressure was not high. Since pulmonary artery aneurysm decreases the load on the right side of the heart, rise in the pulmonary artery pressure might be observed in cases with severe pulmonary embolism. There was cardiac and deep vein thrombus inside the right ventricle of our patient. As these two diagnoses might cause recurrent embolisms *per se*, anticoagulant treatment needs to be used concomitantly with the immunosuppressive treatment. Some publications have asserted that these patients were subjected to bleeding episodes, and anticoagulant treatment is contraindicated for them. On the contrary, we saw that this treatment prevented occurrence of recurrent embolisms.

We have initiated methylprednisolone and cyclophosphamide combination therapy as suggested for the management of other severe forms of systemic vasculitis. We added an anticoagulant treatment into this combination. We have observed clinical and radiological improvement with this treatment.

We kindly deemed suitable to present this case report in order to show the necessity of anticoagulant treatment to be added to the immunosuppressive therapy in such complicated cases.

Acknowledgment

The authors declare that they have no affiliation with or financial involvement in any organization or entity with a direct financial interest in the subject matter or materials discussed in the paper.

References

[1] H. Behçet, "Über rezidivierende, aphtöse, durch ein virus verursachte gescwüre am mund, auge und an den genitalien," *Dermatologische Wochenschrift*, vol. 105, pp. 1152–1157, 1937.

[2] J. D. O'Duffy, J. A. Carney, and S. Deodhar, "Behçet's disease. Report of 10 cases, three with new manifestations," *Annals of Internal Medicine*, vol. 75, pp. 561–570, 1971.

[3] F. Erkan, "Pulmonary involvement in Behçet's disease," *Current Opinion in Pulmonary Medicine*, vol. 5, pp. 314–318, 1999.

[4] F. Erkan, A. Gül, and E. Tasali, "Pulmonary manifestations of Behçet's disease," *Thorax*, vol. 56, pp. 572–578, 2001.

[5] N. Moğulkoç, I. M. Burgess, and P. W. Bishop, "Intracardiac thrombus in Behçet's disease," *Chest*, vol. 118, pp. 479–587, 2000.

[6] A. Tunacı, Y. M. Berkmen, and E. Gökmen, "Thoracic involvement in Behçet's disease: pathologic, clinical, and imaging features," *American Journal of Roentgenology*, vol. 164, pp. 51–56, 1995.

[7] M. Tunaci, B. Ozkorkmaz, A. Tunaci, A. Gül, G. Engin, and B. Acunaş, "CT findings of pulmonary artery aneurysms during treatment for Behçet's disease," *American Journal of Roentgenology*, vol. 172, pp. 729–733, 1999.

[8] J. M. A. Joong Mo Ahn, J.-G. Im, J. W. Ryoo et al., "Thoracic manifestations of Behcet syndrome: radiographic and CT-findings in nine patients," *Radiology*, vol. 194, no. 1, pp. 199–203, 1995.

[9] Y. Koç, I. Güllü, G. Akpek et al., "Vascular involvement in Behçet's disease," *The Journal of Rheumatology*, vol. 19, pp. 402–410, 1992.

[10] T. Chajek and M. Fainaru, "Behcet's disease. Report of 41 cases and a review of the literature," *Medicine*, vol. 54, no. 3, pp. 179–196, 1975.

[11] V. Hamuryudan, S. Yurdakul, F. Moral et al., "Pulmonary artery aneurysms in Behçet's syndrome: a report of 24 cases," *British Journal of Rheumatology*, vol. 33, pp. 48–51, 1994.

[12] M. H. Houman, I. Ben Ghorbel, I. Khiari Ben Salah, M. Lamloum, M. Ben Ahmed, and M. Miled, "Deep vein thrombosis in Behçet's disease," *Clinical and Experimental Rheumatology*, vol. 19, no. 5, pp. S48–S50, 2001.

[13] E. S. Uçan, G. Kıter, Ö. Abadoğlu, C. Karlıkaya, S. Akoğlu, and U. Bayındır, "Thoracic manifestations of Behçet's disease: reports of the Turkish authors," *Turkish Respiratory Journal*, vol. 2, pp. 29–44, 2001.

[14] A. Kaya, Ç. Ertan, Ö. U. Gürkan et al., "Behçet's disease with right ventricle thrombus and bilateral pulmonary artery aneurysms. A case report," *Angiology*, vol. 55, pp. 573–575, 2004.

[15] N. Düzgün, C. Anıl, F. Özer, and T. Acican, "The disappearence of pulmonary artery aneurysms and intracardiac thrombus with immunosuppressive treatment in a patient with Behçet's disease," *Clinical and Experimental Rheumatology*, vol. 20, supplement 26, pp. 556–557, 2002.

[16] L. Luo, Y. Ge, Z. Y. Liu, Y. T. Liu, and T. S. Li, "A report of eight cases of Behçet's disease with intracardiac thrombus and literatures review," *Zhonghua Nei Ke Za Zhi*, vol. 50, no. 11, pp. 914–917, 2011.

14

Pancoast's Syndrome due to Fungal Abscess in the Apex of Lung in an Immunocompetent Individual: A Case Report and Review of the Literature

Anirban Das, Sabyasachi Choudhury, Sumitra Basuthakur, Sibes Kumar Das, and Angshuman Mukhopadhyay

Department of Pulmonary Medicine, Medical College, Kolkata, West Bengal, India

Correspondence should be addressed to Anirban Das; dranirbandas_chest@rediffmail.com

Academic Editor: Akif Turna

Malignant tumours in the apices of the lungs, especially bronchogenic carcinoma (Pancoast tumours), are the most common cause of Pancoast' syndrome which presents with shoulder or arm pain radiating along the medial aspect of forearm and weakness of small muscles of hand with wasting of hypothenar eminence due to neoplastic involvement of C8 and T1 and T2 nerve roots of brachial plexus. There are a number of benign conditions which may lead to Pancoast's syndrome; fungal abscess located in the apex of lung is one of them. Oral or intravenous antifungals are the treatment of choice in this case and complete recovery is usual, whereas, surgical resection followed by chemoradiotherapy is the treatment of choice in case of Pancoast's syndrome due to lung cancers. Hence, tissue diagnosis is mandatory. Here, we report a case of apical fungal abscess causing Pancoast's syndrome in an immunocompetent individual of 35 years of age to raise the awareness among the clinicians regarding this rare clinical entity.

1. Introduction

Pancoast's syndrome is characterized by the pain in superior extremity and weakness and wasting of the small muscles of hand. Sometimes, it may be associated with ipsilateral Horner's syndrome. In 1924, it was first described by Henry Pancoast [1, 2]. This syndrome is most commonly caused by a malignant tumour located at the superior pulmonary sulcus of the thorax, known as Pancoast tumour. Squamous cell carcinoma of lung is the most common histological type causing Pancoast's syndrome [3]. Bronchogenic carcinoma is responsible for over 80% of cases [4]. Other malignant causes of Pancoast's syndrome are non-Hodgkin's lymphoma, pleural mesothelioma, multiple myeloma, solid tumour metastases (liver, cervix, urinary bladder, and kidneys), adenoid cystic carcinoma, malignant neurogenic tumours, thyroid carcinoma, and so forth [3, 5, 6]. Benign causes of Pancoast's syndrome are rarely reported in the literature. Here, we report a case of fungal abscess located in the apex of lung causing Pancoast's syndrome in an immunocompetent housewife of thirty-five years of age.

2. Case Report

A thirty-five-year-old nonsmoker, nondiabetic female presented with low grade, intermittent fever and a shooting type of pain in left shoulder and arm radiating through medial aspect of left forearm and hand for 4 months. The pain was gradually progressive and was associated with weakness and wasting of hypothenar muscles. Severity of the shoulder pain was more at night, and it was not relieved by simple analgesic. There was history of cough and scanty, mucoid expectoration for the same duration. There was no history of shortness of breath, hemoptysis, and heaviness of the chest. History of anorexia, significant weight loss, night sweats, and fatigue were present.

General examination revealed anemia, but no clubbing, and enlarged superficial lymph node. Her pulse rate was 100 beats/minute, respiratory rate 16 breaths/minute, temperature 100°F, and blood pressure 110/70 mmHg. Examination of eye revealed left sided Horner's syndrome only, that is, presence of partial ptosis, enophthalmos, miosis, in association with anhidrosis over the left hemifacial region, and loss of

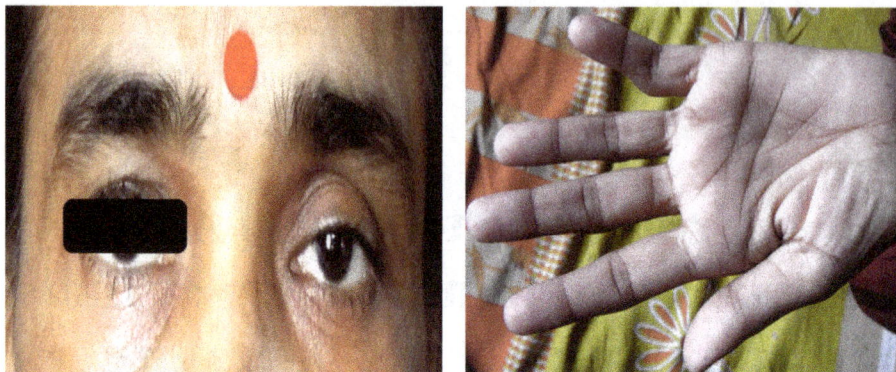

FIGURE 1: Photograph showing left sided partial ptosis and enophthalmos with wasting of hypothenar eminence of left hand.

ciliospinal reflex with preservation of pupillary light reflex and corneal reflex on the same side (Figure 1). Examination of left superior extremity revealed only the weakness of small muscles of the left hand (grade III power) and wasting of hypothenar eminence on left side (Figure 1). Examination of respiratory system revealed central mediastinum and dull percussion note over clavicles, second and third intercostal spaces over midclavicular line, and suprascapular areas on both sides. There were diminished vesicular breath sounds and decreased vocal resonance over both infraclavicular and suprascapular areas. Examination of other systems did not reveal any abnormality.

Complete hemogram and blood biochemistry were within normal limit, except that hemoglobin concentration was 8.3 g/dL. Blood for anti-HIV-1 and anti-HIV-2 antibodies was negative. Spontaneous and induced sputum for acid fast bacilli and malignant cells was negative. Mantoux test (5 TU) was positive (11 mm induration), indicating integrated cell mediated immunity. Chest X-ray-posteroanterior view (P.A. view) showed bilateral pleural based alveolar air space consolidation in upper zone. Sputum for fungal smear was negative. Contrast enhanced computed tomography (CECT) scan of thorax showed two ill-defined, heterogeneous, mildly enhanced, partly necrotic, pleural based lesions in the apicoposterior segments of both upper lobes (Figure 2). There was no rib erosion. CT-guided fine needle aspiration cytology (FNAC) from both lesions showed suppurative inflammation and no acid fast bacilli, and malignant cell was detected. Gram stain, pyogenic culture, fungal smear, and mycobacterial culture of FNAC materials were negative. Fibreoptic bronchoscopy revealed no endobronchial lesion and bronchoalveolar lavage (BAL) fluid did not show any abnormality. Finally, CT-guided tru-cut biopsy tissue taken from the lesions of both sides showed branching filamentous fungi with septate hyphae branching at acute angles (lactophenol cotton blue stain), suggestive of bilateral fungal abscesses in upper lobes, out of which the left one resulted in Pancoast's syndrome (Figure 3). Finally, fungal culture of biopsy tissue showed growth of fungus with septate hyphae having finger-like branching at acute angles, suggestive of growth of *Aspergillus fumigatus*. Hence, the diagnosis was bilateral upper lobe

lung abscesses due to *Aspergillus*, out of which the left one causes Pancoast's syndrome. The patient was treated with itraconazole tablet, 200 mg (two tablets, each of 100 mg) twice daily for six weeks. Six weeks of treatment with oral antifungals resulted in radiological resolution of both apical lesions (Figure 4), along with clinical recovery of left sided Pancoast's syndrome and Horner's syndrome, documented on followup.

3. Discussion

Pancoast's syndrome is characterized by shoulder and arm pain which is radiated to ulnar aspect of arm and forearm, Claude Bernard-Horner's syndrome, and weakness and atrophy of ipsilateral hypothenar muscles. Destruction of adjacent vertebral bodies or first, second, and third ribs with dense white apical shadow is detected on chest radiograph. It is due to involvement of C8 and T1 and T2 nerve roots of brachial plexus (lower brachial plexopathy) and paravertebral cervical sympathetic trunk above the stellate ganglion. Excruciating chest pain may be due to erosion of ribs and anterior chest wall. Pancoast tumours, that is, apical lung cancers and other malignancies, are predominant causes of Pancoast's syndrome. Besides them, few benign tumours like solitary pleural fibroma and infective conditions like fungal abscess caused by *Aspergillus, Cryptococcus, Mucor*, or *Allescheria boydii*, apical tuberculosis, hydatid cyst, and bacteria (e.g., *Staphylococci, Pseudomonas, Actinomyces*, and *Nocardia*) are reported to cause Pancoast's syndrome in the literature [7–9].

Immunosuppressed patients (diabetes, HIV infection, congenital immunodeficiency, postchemotherapy, neutropenia, etc.) are susceptible to invasive fungal infections which may cause Pancoast's syndrome due to direct or vascular invasion of bones, soft tissues, and nerves at thoracic inlet [10]. But, surprisingly, in our case bilateral apical *Aspergillus* abscesses were seen of which the left one was producing Pancoast's syndrome without any evidence of immunosuppression.

CECT thorax or magnetic resonance imaging of neck is essential to demonstrate anatomical details of the lesion

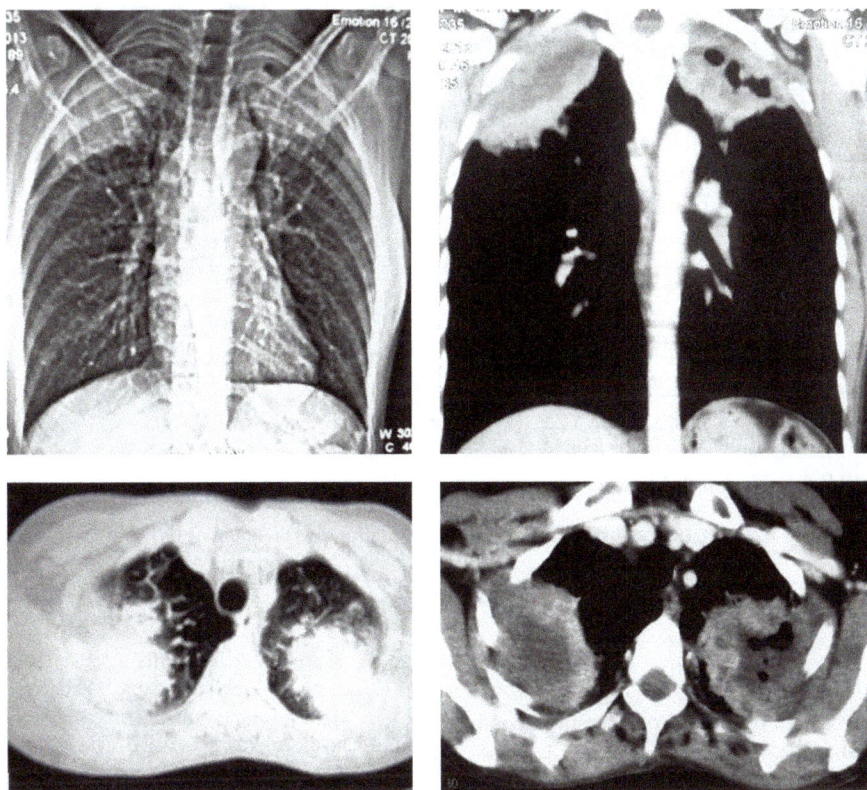

FIGURE 2: CECT thorax showing heterogeneous, pleural based lung masses in upper lobes of both sides.

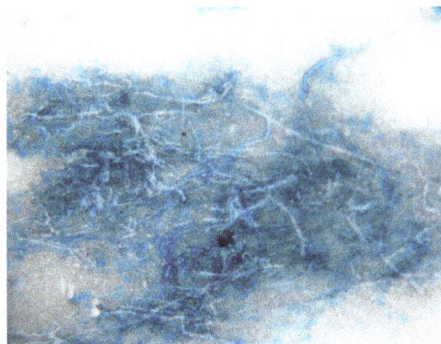

FIGURE 3: Microphotograph of histopathological examination of CT-guided tru-cut biopsy showing branching filamentous fungi with septate hyphae with finger-like branching at acute angles (lactophenol cotton blue stain, 40x).

and the locoregional extension of the lesion into the surrounding soft tissues, especially that of brachial plexus [11].

Fungal staining of sputum smear and fungal culture of sputum or bronchial washing obtained by fibreoptic bronchoscopy is frequently negative due to peripheral location of the infiltrate. Integrated defense mechanisms of lung parenchyma contain the infection in immunocompetent individuals, thus making the isolation of fungus from sputum and bronchial aspirate difficult. So in this situation, CT-guided tru-cut biopsy of peripherally located fungal abscess is essential to detect *Aspergillus* infection. *Aspergillus* hyphae are narrow with septate branches at 45° angles. Finally, fungal

culture of the biopsy material shows the growth of *Aspergillus* to confirm the diagnosis as in our case.

Pancoast's syndrome due to fungal etiology can successfully be treated by antifungals like oral itraconazole or voriconazole [12]. Intravenous amphotericin B is an alternative [12]. Surgical excision followed by chemoradiotherapy is the standard treatment for Pancoast's syndrome, caused by superior sulcus tumours, and prognosis is definitely guarded. Hence, tissue diagnosis by image-guided tru-cut biopsy is essential in any case of Pancoast' syndrome to confirm the etiology, as reversible etiology like fungal abscess is associated with complete resolution of the syndrome by administration of antifungals only.

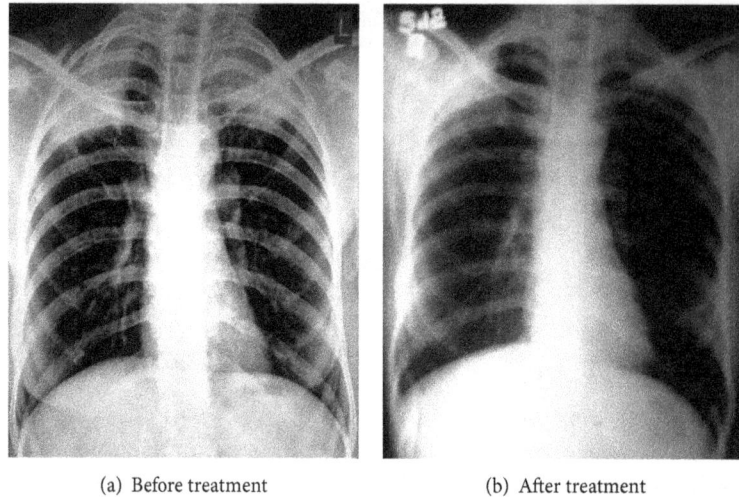

(a) Before treatment

(b) After treatment

FIGURE 4: CXR-P.A. views showing pretreatment bilateral apical consolidations with necrosis (a) and posttreatment almost complete resolution of the lesions (b).

References

[1] H. K. Pancoast, "Importance of careful roentgen-ray investigationsof apical chest tumors," *The Journal of the American Medical Association*, vol. 83, no. 18, pp. 1407–1411, 1924.

[2] H. Pancoast, "Superior pulmonary sulcus tumor: tumor characterizedby pain, Horner's syndrome, destruction of bone andatrophy of hand muscles," *The Journal of the American Medical Association*, vol. 99, pp. 1391–1396, 1932.

[3] V. C. Archie and C. R. Thomas Jr., "Superior sulcus tumors: a mini-review," *The Oncologist*, vol. 9, no. 5, pp. 550–555, 2004.

[4] R. Comet, M. Monteagudo, S. Herranz, X. Gallardo, and B. Font, "Pancoast's syndrome secondary to lung infection with cutaneous fistulisation caused by Staphylococcus aureus," *Journal of Clinical Pathology*, vol. 59, no. 9, pp. 997–998, 2006.

[5] C.-F. Chang, W.-J. Su, T.-Y. Chou, and R.-P. Perng, "Hepatocellular carcinoma with Pancoast's syndrome as an initial symptom: a case report," *Japanese Journal of Clinical Oncology*, vol. 31, no. 3, pp. 119–121, 2001.

[6] N. Panagopoulos, V. Leivaditis, E. Koletsis et al., "Pancoast tumors: characteristics and preoperative assessment," *Journal of Thoracic Disease*, vol. 6, no. 1, pp. S108–S115, 2014.

[7] J. J. Fibla, J. C. Penagos, and C. León, "Pseudo-pancoast syndrome caused by a solitary fibrous tumor of the pleura," *Archivos de Bronconeumologia*, vol. 40, no. 5, pp. 244–245, 2004.

[8] H. D. White, B. A. A. White, C. Boethel, and A. C. Arroliga, "Pancoast's syndrome secondary to infectious etiologies: A not so uncommon occurrence," *The American Journal of the Medical Sciences*, vol. 341, no. 4, pp. 333–336, 2011.

[9] R. Comet, M. Monteagudo, S. Herranz, X. Gallardo, and B. Font, "Pancoast's syndrome secondary to lung infection with cutaneous fistulisation caused by *Staphylococcus aureus*," *Journal of Clinical Pathology*, vol. 59, no. 9, pp. 997–998, 2006.

[10] M. Bansal, S. R. Martin, S. A. Rudnicki, K. M. Hiatt, and E. Mireles-Cabodevila, "A rapidly progressing Pancoast syndrome due to pulmonary mucormycosis: a case report," *Journal of Medical Case Reports*, vol. 5, article 388, 2011.

[11] G. Manenti, M. Raguso, S. D'Onofrio et al., "Pancoast tumor: the role of magnetic resonance imaging," *Case Reports in Radiology*, vol. 2013, Article ID 479120, 5 pages, 2013.

[12] B. Vahid and P. E. Marik, "Fatal massive hemoptysis in a patient on low-dose oral prednisone: chronic necrotizing pulmonary aspergillosis," *Respiratory Care*, vol. 52, no. 1, pp. 56–58, 2007.

15

Delayed Recurrence of Atypical Pulmonary Carcinoid Cluster: A Rare Occurrence

Salim Surani,[1] Jennifer Tan,[2] Alexandra Ahumada,[3,4] Saherish S. Surani,[5] Sivakumar Sudhakaran,[6] and Joseph Varon[7,8]

[1] *Pulmonary, Critical Care & Sleep Medicine, Texas A&M University, Corpus Christi, 1177 West Wheeler Avenue, Suite 1, Aransas Pass, TX 78336, USA*

[2] *Corpus Christi Medical Center, 7101 South Padre Island Drive, Corpus Christi, TX 78412, USA*

[3] *Universidad Autonoma de Baja California, Avenue Álvaro Obregón Sn, Nueva, 21100 Mexicali, BC, Mexico*

[4] *Dorrington Medical Associates, 2219 Dorrington Street, Houston, TX 77030, USA*

[5] *Pulmonary Associates, 1177 West Wheeler Avenue, Aransas Pass, TX 78336, USA*

[6] *Texas A&M University Health Science Center, 8447 State Highway 47, Bryan, TX 77807, USA*

[7] *The University of Texas Health Science Center, 7000 Fannin Street, Houston, TX 77030, USA*

[8] *University General Hospital, 7501 Fannin Street, Houston, TX 77054, USA*

Correspondence should be addressed to Salim Surani; srsurani@hotmail.com

Academic Editor: Akif Turna

Carcinoid is one of the most common tumors of the gastrointestinal tract followed by the tracheobronchial tree. Bronchial carcinoid compromises 20% of total carcinoid and accounts for 1–5% of pulmonary malignancies. Carcinoid can be typical or atypical, with atypical carcinoid compromises 10% of the carcinoid tumors. Carcinoid usually presents as peripheral lung lesion or solitary endobronchial abnormality. Rarely it can present as multiple endobronchial lesion. We hereby present a rare case of an elderly gentleman who had undergone resection of right middle and lower lobe of lung for atypical carcinoid. Seven years later he presented with cough. CT scan of chest revealed right hilar mass. Flexible bronchoscopy revealed numerous endobronchial polypoid lesions in the tracheobronchial tree. Recurrent atypical carcinoid was then confirmed on biopsy.

1. Introduction

The most common location of carcinoid tumors is the gastrointestinal tract, followed by the tracheobronchial tree [1]. Bronchial carcinoids are low-grade neuroendocrine malignant tumors that comprise 1–5% of all lung neoplasms [2–4]. It used to be felt as a benign tumor but when distant metastases happen, it tends to be less aggressive than the noncarcinoid lung malignancies [5–7].

In 2004, new criteria divided lung carcinoids into different groups: typical and atypical carcinoids, large cell neuroendocrine carcinoma, and small cell lung carcinoma [8]. Of the bronchial carcinoids, the typical is much more common than the atypical type (90% versus 10%) [9]. We hereby present a case of 63-year-old male who presented with recurrence of carcinoid seven years after curative resection of his carcinoid.

2. Case Report

63-year-old nonsmoker male presented to the office with chronic cough of 2-month duration. The cough was dry with no sputum production. Patient denies dyspnea, wheezing, hemoptysis, night sweat, and weight loss. Seven years prior to this presentation the patient had resection of right middle and lower lobe for the solitary atypical bronchoscopic biopsy proven endobronchial carcinoid just below the right minor carina. On pathology the patient's lesion confirmed atypical carcinoid. The hilar and mediastinal nodes were negative for any tumor and the margins as well were free of any

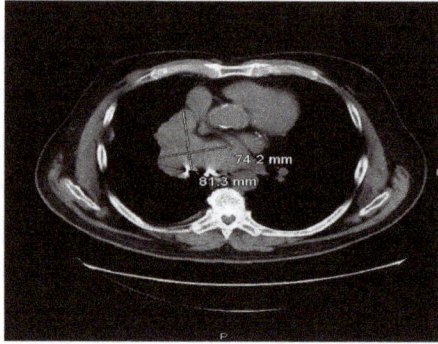

FIGURE 1: CT Scan of chest showing right hilar mass.

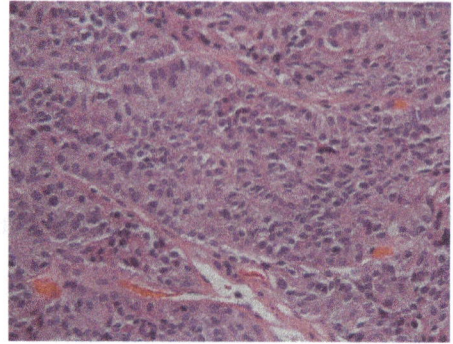

FIGURE 3: High magnification image showing well-differentiated cells forming tubular and glandular structure without atypia.

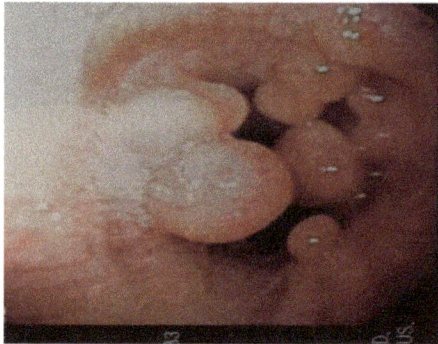

FIGURE 2: Bronchoscopic images of right main stem bronchi showing multiple polypoid lesions, which on biopsy confirmed carcinoid.

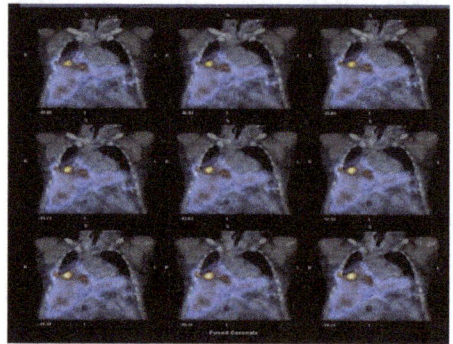

FIGURE 4: Octreotide scan showing abnormal activities in the right hilum and carinal area as well as liver suggestive of metastatic carcinoid.

tumor. Computerized tomography (CT) scan and positron emission tomography (PET) scan showed no evidence of any local or distant spread. Patient besides the previous history of carcinoid also had history of hypertension and coronary heart disease. Patient was not on any angiotensin converting enzyme inhibitor (ACE) or angiotensin receptor blocker (ARB) for the control of his blood pressure. Physical examination revealed decreased breath sound in the right lower chest. No wheezing or rhonchi were heard in both lungs.

In view of his chronic cough, the patient underwent X-ray of the chest, which showed some hilar fullness. A computed tomography (CT) scan of chest revealed a new 8.1 × 7.4 cm right hilar mass, with no evidence of disease noted in trachea or left lung and no evidence of any endobronchial lesions (Figure 1). PET scan showed right hilar mass that was not FDG-avid. Flexible video bronchoscopy showed numerous polypoid masses in vocal cords, trachea, and left and right mainstem bronchus (Figure 2). Biopsy of one of the lesions in the right mainstem bronchus showed a well-differentiated tumor consisting of neuroendocrine-appearing cells forming small tubular and glandular-like structures, without significant atypia or mitotic activity, consistent with carcinoid (Figure 3). Chromogranin and synaptophysin stains for neuroendocrine tumor are positive and Ki-67 stain for mitotic activity is relatively low. The patient underwent Octreotide scan which showed extensive metastatic carcinoid, including osseous metastasis, liver metastasis, right hilar, subcarinal,

right pleural involvement, right chest wall, and subcutaneous tumor behind right chest (Figure 4). Patient was then started on octreotide intramuscular injections every 4 weeks. Three months after diagnosis, patient is doing well and is asymptomatic.

3. Discussion

Carcinoid tumors are neuroendocrine tumors that typically arise from gastrointestinal tract and the bronchus. Bronchial carcinoid tumors comprise approximately 20% of all carcinoid tumors and approximately 1–5% of all lung malignancies in adults [10, 11]. Carcinoid tumors can secrete many different types of products, the most common of which are serotonin, histamine, tachykinins, kallikrein, and prostaglandins. These products cause the classic symptoms associated with carcinoid tumors: diarrhea and cutaneous flushing [12]. Bronchial carcinoid tumors can be asymptomatic or can cause causes wheezing, dyspnea, cough, hemoptysis, and recurrent pneumonia due to bronchospasm and obstruction [13].

Due to the variability of clinical presentation of bronchial carcinoid, there can be a delay in diagnosing or even misdiagnosis. The differential diagnosis of a patient with symptoms of bronchial obstruction, bronchospasm, and hemoptysis is wide; it includes an obstructing bronchial carcinoma, endobronchial metastasis, hamartomas, aspirated foreign body, asthma, and COPD.

While the 24-hour urinary excretion of 5-hydroxyindol-eacetic acid (HIAA) is a useful initial diagnostic test for carcinoid tumors arising in the midgut (jejunoileal, appendiceal, and ascending colon), it is not as helpful for carcinoid tumors arising in the foregut (gastroduodenal and bronchus) or hindgut (transverse, descending, and sigmoid colon and rectum), as they secrete less serotonin [14]. Therefore the diagnosis of bronchial carcinoid tumors sometimes can be challenging. Chest X-ray and CT scan can detect bronchial carcinoid tumors, and the diagnosis can be confirmed by bronchoscopic biopsy for central lesions and CT-guided needle biopsy for peripheral lesions. Bronchial carcinoid commonly appears as a pinkish to reddish vascular mass, attached to the bronchus by a broad base, but can have a polypoid appearance as well. While an experienced bronchoscopist can make a diagnosis based on appearance, biopsy aids in diagnosis; cytology from bronchial brushing is often not helpful [15].

There are several differences between these two groups; in atypical carcinoids, the age of presentation tends to be much higher as in our patient's case. In one study the mean was 51 years for atypical versus 43 years for typical [16, 17]. In this case, the age of presentation was 70 years old, which is higher than the average age reported in the literature. Also, in these tumors the stage is more advanced and they are larger at the time of diagnosis, which could be explained because they are located mostly in the periphery and produce fewer symptoms [7, 18]. They have been found to have a more aggressive behavior and are most likely to metastasize [19].

Bronchial carcinoids have not been found to have any associations to smoking cigarettes or exposure to tobacco smoke [16, 20].

They can present with symptoms or be asymptomatic. In several studies, 17–52% of patients presented symptoms. In our case, the patient had nonresolving cough, which was found to be the most common symptom besides hemoptysis. Other reported problems were recurrent pulmonary infection, fever, and dyspnea. Carcinoid syndrome associated with bronchial carcinoid is very rare and in most studies it was not present; only a retrospective study reported that it happened in one patient [7, 16, 20–22].

In asymptomatic patients, the disease is usually diagnosed with a simple chest X-ray, which would show a radiopaque mass [23]. Our patient underwent CT scan of the chest after abnormality was seen on the chest X-ray. The best method of diagnosis is fiberoptic bronchoscopy with biopsy, which is what our patient underwent after seeing abnormalities on the CT scan [19, 21] though the caution needs to be undertaken for any bleed, which can compromise the airway, and rigid bronchoscopy can be option too in those circumstances. In one study, mucosal infiltration and obstruction of the lumen were the two most common macroscopic features found during bronchoscopy; polypoid lesion was not as common, and it is what we found in this case [16]. Besides diagnosis, bronchoscopy can also aid in surgical planning, since it can provide spatial information for the surgeon and also could give an idea whether it is possible to resect the tumor or not [19, 24].

The management is very straightforward; surgery is the mainstay for the treatment of bronchial carcinoid, whether it is typical or atypical. Our patient did not undergo surgery as the lesion was involving trachea, vocal cords, and both mainstem bronchi. With the typical carcinoids, it is possible to remove less tissue, that is, bronchial sleeve resection, since they are not as aggressive, but, with the atypical, lobectomy and pneumonectomy are the most common options [19, 25]. For entirely intraluminal endobronchial carcinoid tumors without evidence of bronchial wall involvement or suspicious lymphadenopathy, bronchoscopic resection can be curative. Care must be taken, as potential bleeding during biopsy or resection can lead to airway compromise with flexible bronchoscopy, and for this reason rigid bronchoscopy may be preferable. Once diagnosis is established, the preferred treatment of choice for bronchial carcinoid is surgical resection, with bronchoplastic techniques (i.e., sleeve, wedge, or flap resection) in order to preserve lung parenchyma [26]. The role of adjuvant therapy of a bronchial carcinoid is a topic of controversy, as there are no prospective trials addressing the benefit of chemotherapy with or without radiation therapy for resected bronchial carcinoids. For patients with carcinoid syndrome, control of the symptoms caused by tumor's secretion of peptide and amines can be achieved by somatostatin receptor analogues such as octreotide.

The most important prognostic factor for bronchial carcinoid is the histology. As we had already discussed, typical carcinoids have a better prognosis and less rate of recurrence than atypical carcinoids [19]. In our case, the patient had atypical carcinoid and it recurred after 7 years of being asymptomatic.

The 5-year survival ranges from 89 to 92% in the typical carcinoid group and from 66.7 to 75% in the atypical carcinoid group. The 10-year survival was 82–88.9% for typical and 50–56% for atypical, as we should expect, given the more aggressive behavior in the latter group [16, 20].

However, as bronchial carcinoid tumors are a spectrum consisting of more indolent tumor to more aggressive tumors with the potential to metastasize or recur locally, long-term follow-up is needed as local or distant recurrence may occur many years after the initial diagnosis and treatment as in this case [7]. There is not a consensus on the optimal surveillance strategy after treatment. Some proposed strategies include high-resolution CT (with or without flexible bronchoscopy) annually for the more indolent "typical" bronchial carcinoids; for the more aggressive "atypical" bronchial carcinoids, it is every 6 months for the first 2 years and then annually [27].

4. Conclusion

The most important prognostic factor for bronchial carcinoid is the histology. As we had already discussed, typical carcinoids have a better prognosis and less rate of recurrence than atypical carcinoids [19]. In our case, the patient had atypical carcinoid and it recurred after 7 years. The 5-year survival ranges from 89 to 92% in the typical carcinoid group and from 66.7 to 75% in the atypical carcinoid group. The 10-year survival was 82–88.9% for typical and 50–56% for atypical, as we should expect, given the more aggressive behavior in the latter group [16, 20]. It is important to recognize that the carcinoid can recur after curative resection after several years. Clinical vigilance is necessary especially in the patients with atypical carcinoid.

References

[1] J. L. Buck and L. H. Sobin, "Carcinoids of the gastrointestinal tract," *Radiographics*, vol. 10, no. 6, pp. 1081–1095, 1990.

[2] D. G. Davila, W. F. Dunn, H. D. Tazelaar, and P. C. Pairolero, "Bronchial carcinoid tumors," *Mayo Clinic Proceedings*, vol. 68, no. 8, pp. 795–803, 1993.

[3] D. H. Harpole, J. M. Feldman, S. Buchanan, W. G. Young, and W. G. Wolfe, "Bronchial carcinoid tumors: a retrospective analysis of 126 patients," *The Annals of Thoracic Surgery*, vol. 54, no. 1, pp. 50–55, 1992.

[4] G. Cardillo, F. Sera, M. Di Martino et al., "Bronchial carcinoid tumors: nodal status and long-term survival after resection," *Annals of Thoracic Surgery*, vol. 77, no. 5, pp. 1781–1785, 2004.

[5] M. B. Beasley, F. B. J. M. Thunnissen, E. Brambilla et al., "Pulmonary atypical carcinoid: predictors of survival in 106 cases," *Human Pathology*, vol. 31, no. 10, pp. 1255–1265, 2000.

[6] D. R. A. Swarts, F. C. S. Ramaekers, and E.-J. M. Speel, "Molecular and cellular biology of neuroendocrine lung tumors: evidence for separate biological entities," *Biochimica et Biophysica Acta—Reviews on Cancer*, vol. 1826, no. 2, pp. 255–271, 2012.

[7] P. L. Filosso, O. Rena, G. Donati et al., "Bronchial carcinoid tumors: surgical management and long-term outcome," *The Journal of Thoracic and Cardiovascular Surgery*, vol. 123, no. 2, pp. 303–309, 2002.

[8] N. Rekhtman, "Neuroendocrine tumors of the lung," *Archives of Pathology & Laboratory Medicine*, vol. 134, no. 11, pp. 1628–1638, 2010.

[9] M. L. R. de Christenson, G. F. Abbott, W. M. Kirejczyk, J. R. Galvin, and W. D. Travis, "Thoracic carcinoids: radiologic-pathologic correlation," *Radiographics*, vol. 19, no. 3, pp. 707–736, 1999.

[10] I. M. Modlin, K. D. Lye, and M. Kidd, "A 5-decade analysis of 13,715 carcinoid tumors," *Cancer*, vol. 97, no. 4, pp. 934–959, 2003.

[11] E. M. Bertino, P. D. Confer, J. E. Colonna, P. Ross, and G. A. Otterson, "Pulmonary neuroendocrine/carcinoid tumors: a review article," *Cancer*, vol. 115, no. 19, pp. 4434–4441, 2009.

[12] J. Strosberg, "Neuroendocrine tumours of the small intestine," *Best Practice and Research: Clinical Gastroenterology*, vol. 26, no. 6, pp. 755–773, 2012.

[13] S. Fischer, M. Kruger, K. McRae, N. Merchant, M. S. Tsao, and S. Keshavjee, "Giant bronchial carcinoid tumors: a multidisciplinary approach," *Annals of Thoracic Surgery*, vol. 71, no. 1, pp. 386–393, 2001.

[14] G. Aggarwal, K. Obideen, and M. Wehbi, "Carcinoid tumors: what should increase our suspicion?" *Cleveland Clinic Journal of Medicine*, vol. 75, no. 12, pp. 849–855, 2008.

[15] M. Aron, K. Kapila, and K. Verma, "Carcinoid tumors of the lung: a diagnostic challenge in bronchial washings," *Diagnostic Cytopathology*, vol. 30, no. 1, pp. 62–66, 2004.

[16] L. Schrevens, J. Vansteenkiste, G. Deneffe et al., "Clinical-radiological presentation and outcome of surgically treated pulmonary carcinoid tumours: a long-term single institution experience," *Lung Cancer*, vol. 43, no. 1, pp. 39–45, 2004.

[17] M. El Jamal, A. G. Nicholson, and P. Goldstraw, "The feasibility of conservative resection for carcinoid tumours: is pneumonectomy ever necessary for uncomplicated cases?" *European Journal of Cardio-Thoracic Surgery*, vol. 18, no. 3, pp. 301–306, 2000.

[18] W. H. Warren, M. Welker, and P. Gattuso, "Well-differentiated neuroendocrine carcinomas: the spectrum of histologic subtypes and various clinical behaviors," *Seminars in Thoracic and Cardiovascular Surgery*, vol. 18, no. 3, pp. 199–205, 2006.

[19] T. N. Machuca, P. F. G. Cardoso, S. M. Camargo et al., "Surgical treatment of bronchial carcinoid tumors: a single-center experience," *Lung Cancer*, vol. 70, no. 2, pp. 158–162, 2010.

[20] G. Fink, T. Krelbaum, A. Yellin et al., "Pulmonary carcinoid: Presentation, diagnosis, and outcome in 142 cases in Israel and review of 640 cases from the literature," *Chest*, vol. 119, no. 6, pp. 1647–1651, 2001.

[21] C. Madrid-Carbajal, M. García-Clemente, A. Pando-Sandoval, H. C. Martín, T. González-Budiño, and P. Casan-Clarà, "Bronchial carcinoid tumor: study of 60 patients," *Medicina Clínica*, vol. 141, no. 2, pp. 73–76, 2013.

[22] C. F. Thomas Jr., H. D. Tazelaar, and J. R. Jett, "Typical and atypical pulmonary carcinoids: outcome in patients presenting with regional lymph node involvement," *Chest*, vol. 119, no. 4, pp. 1143–1150, 2001.

[23] R. Nessi, P. B. Ricci, S. B. Ricci, M. Bosco, M. Blanc, and C. Uslenghi, "Bronchial carcinoid tumors: radiologic observations in 49 cases," *Journal of Thoracic Imaging*, vol. 6, no. 2, pp. 47–53, 1991.

[24] D. M. McMullan and D. E. Wood, "Pulmonary carcinoid tumors," *Seminars in Thoracic and Cardiovascular Surgery*, vol. 15, no. 3, pp. 289–300, 2003.

[25] M. Mezzetti, F. Raveglia, T. Panigalli et al., "Assessment of outcomes in typical and atypical carcinoids according to latest WHO classification," *Annals of Thoracic Surgery*, vol. 76, no. 6, pp. 1838–1842, 2003.

[26] B. I. Gustafsson, M. Kidd, A. Chan, M. V. Malfertheiner, and I. M. Modlin, "Bronchopulmonary neuroendocrine tumors," *Cancer*, vol. 113, no. 1, pp. 5–21, 2008.

[27] C. Thomas and J. Jett, *Bronchial Carcinoid Tumors: Treatment and Prognosis*, UpToDate, 2013.

16

An Osteolytic Metastasis of Humerus from an Asymptomatic Squamous Cell Carcinoma of Lung: A Rare Clinical Entity

Anirban Das, Sudipta Pandit, Sibes k. Das, Sumitra Basuthakur, and Somnath Das

Department of Pulmonary Medicine, Medical College, 88 College Street, Kolkata, West Bengal 700 073, India

Correspondence should be addressed to Anirban Das; dranirbandas¯chest@rediffmail.com

Academic Editor: Shinichiro Ohshimo

Advanced lung cancer is complicated by skeletal metastases either due to direct extension from adjacent primaries or, more commonly, due to haematogenous dissemination of neoplastic cells. Lumber spine is the most common site for bony metastases in bronchogenic carcinoma. Proximal lone bones, especially humerus, are unusual sites for metastases from lung primaries. Small cell and large cell varieties of lung cancer are most commonly associated with skeletal dissemination. It is also unusual that an asymptomatic squamous cell carcinoma of lung presents with painful, soft tissue swelling with osteolytic metastasis of humerus which is reported in our case. Systemic cytotoxic chemotherapy, local palliative radiotherapy, adequate analgesia, and internal fixation of the affected long bone are different modalities of treatment in this advanced stage of disease. But the prognosis is definitely poor in this stage IV disease.

1. Introduction

The skeleton is a common site for metastases from epithelial tumours. Most common malignancies which present with bone metastases are carcinomas of prostate, breast, and lung [1]. Approximately one-third of the patients with bronchogenic carcinoma present with symptoms due to extrathoracic metastases [2]. In lung cancers, axial skeleton is more commonly involved than extremities [3]. Spine, ribs, pelvis, skull, and proximal long bones like femur or humerus are the bony sites for the metastases of lung cancers [3]. Thoracolumbar vertebrae are most common site for skeletal metastases in lung cancers [4]. A very few reports of metastasis to humerus in bronchogenic carcinoma are available in the literature. Here we report a rare case of bronchogenic carcinoma metastasizing to humerus and, surprisingly, the patient presented with a painful swelling of the left arm without any respiratory symptom.

2. Case Report

A fifty-five-year-old normotensive, nondiabetic, male smoker presented with progressively increasing soft tissue swelling in the left upper arm with intractable pain which was increasing at night for last 3 months. He also complained of weakness of left upper limb and difficulty to move the part of the limb distal to the swelling. There was history of significant weight loss, loss of appetite, and extreme fatigue, but no fever. There was no respiratory symptom or any history of contact with the patient with smear positive pulmonary tuberculosis.

General examination of the patient revealed anaemia and clubbing but no superficial lymphadenopathy. His axillary temperature was 37°C, respiratory rate 16 breaths/minute, pulse rate 84 beats/minute, and blood pressure 110/70 mmHg. Systemic examination revealed no abnormality except a tender soft tissue swelling located in the midhumerus of left side, firm in consistency, irregular in shape, and 7.5 cm × 5 cm in size with indistinct margins. Skin overlying the swelling was reddened, warm, edematous, and nodular with prominence of superficial veins but had no discharging sinus. Movements of the shoulder joints were normal. Movement of the part of the limb distal to the swelling was restricted. Biceps, triceps, and supinator jerks were absent in left side. But there was no sensory loss.

Complete hemogram and blood biochemistry including serum calcium (9.1 mg/dL) and alkaline phosphatase were normal. Chest X-ray (CXR) posteroanterior (P.A.) view showed a spiculated nodule in the left midzone with an osteolytic lesion in middle of the left humerus (Figure 1). Fine needle aspiration cytology (FNAC) of the osteolytic lesion revealed sheets, clumps, and dense malignant cells having hyperchromatic, pleomorphic nuclei with inconspicuous nucleoli and squamoid differentiation at places on the hemorrhagic background. Few cells showed individual keratinization, suggestive of metastatic squamous cell carcinoma (Figure 2(a)). Contrast enhanced computed tomography (CECT) scan of thorax showed a spiculated nodule in left upper lobe with osteolytic lesion in the midhumerus on the left side (Figure 3). CT-guided FNAC of the left lung nodule showed clusters of malignant epithelial cells with nuclear pleomorphism, hyperchromasia, distinct nucleoli, moderate amount of cytoplasm, and distinct cell boundary, suggestive of nonsmall cell carcinoma and squamous cell variety. (Figure 2(b)). Ultrasound of the abdomen revealed no abnormality. ^{99m}TcRadionuclide bone scan revealed an increased uptake of radiotracer over the midhumerus on left side only, suggestive of metastatic bony lesion to left humerus (Figure 4). So, the final diagnosis was squamous cell carcinoma of upper lobe of left lung with osteolytic metastasis to left humerus, that is, stage IV disease of bronchogenic carcinoma. Palliation of the symptoms was the only option. With consultation of the radiotherapy department of our institution, palliative radiotherapy (total dose: 30 Gy in 10 fractions) was given to the osteolytic lesion of the left midhumerus with an aim to relieve the pain and reduce the size of the lesion. First cycle of chemotherapy comprising of cisplatin + etoposide was given intravenously following radiotherapy. Although chemoradiotherapy was a very good option for palliation of the malignant bone pain, in our patient, size of the primary lung tumour was gradually increasing (as evidenced by serial CXRs) and pain of the osteolytic lesion of left humerus was not relieved, though the size of the lesion reduced marginally. As a whole, therapeutic benefits on primary and metastatic tumours were very poor, probably due to squamous cell histology which is a chemo- and radiotherapy resistant variant of lung cancer. On the other hand, the part of the limb distal to the metastatic lesion was totally nonfunctioning. This is why below shoulder amputation of the left upper limb was planned. Preoperative magnetic resonance imaging (MRI) of left upper extremity showed destructive and expansile osteolytic lesion in the junction of upper and midthird of the shaft of the left humerus, marrow edema, and surrounding soft tissue infiltration (Figure 5). After first cycle of chemotherapy amputation of upper limb was done in the department of orthopaedics, and histopathological examination of resected specimen showed metastatic squamous cell carcinoma of the bone (Figure 6). He succumbed to his illness after second cycle of chemotherapy.

3. Discussion

Clinical presentations of bronchogenic carcinoma are variable and of four types. The majority of patients present with

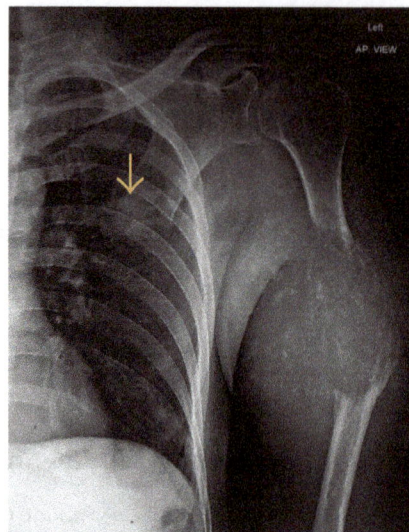

FIGURE 1: CXR-PA view showing osteolytic lesion in left midhumerus and a spiculated nodule in left midzone.

new onset respiratory symptom or worsening of preexisting respiratory state (cough, hemoptysis, postobstructive pneumonia, hoarseness of voice, superior vena caval obstruction, atelectasis, etc.). A very few patients have no respiratory symptoms and an opacity on chest radiograph is detected incidentally. A third group develops nonspecific symptoms of malignancy, like malaise, anorexia, and weight loss or symptoms due to paraneoplastic syndrome. The last group presents with symptoms due to distant metastasis (bone pain, focal neurological deficits, cranial nerve palsy, symptoms due to raised intracranial tension, jaundice, abdominal pain, lymphadenopathy, metastatic nodules in contralateral lung, pleural effusion, etc.) with or without pulmonary symptoms [2]. Asymptomatic adrenal metastases or metastases to skin or skeletal muscles are seen as atypical presentations of lung cancers. Hence, this group with stage IV diseases has poor prognosis. When the patients present with extrathoracic symptoms with no respiratory manifestation, as occurring in our case, there is delay in the diagnosis, even misdiagnosis, and survival of the patients is further compromised.

In our case, the patient initially presented to orthopaedic department for the painful swelling in proximal humerus. Later, we detected the small, irregular primary tumour in left lung on chest radiograph during routine evaluation for the nature of the bony tumour, whether it was secondary or primary. In this scenario, a question was raised: which one was secondary? Is it from the humerus to lung or lung to humerus? Initially, it was thought that possibility of first condition was high, as painful swelling of the humerus was predominant manifestation, and the lung lesion was solitary, asymptomatic, and very small. But the irregular margin of the lung lesion and solitary number go against the possibility of lung metastasis. Usually pulmonary metastases are multiple, round in shape with very smooth margin, although solitary pulmonary metastasis is not unusual. FNAC of the lung mass and the swelling of the left humerus solved the problem, and

(a)

(b)

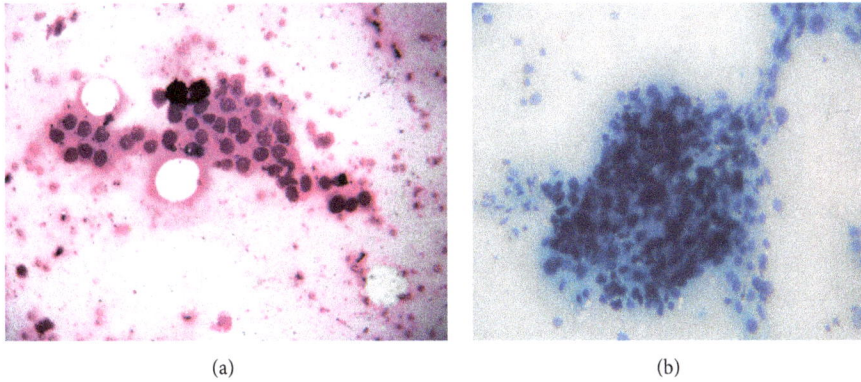

FIGURE 2: (a) Microphotograph of FNAC of osteolytic lesion of left humerus showing metastatic squamous cell carcinoma (MGG stain, 10x). (b) Microphotograph of FNAC of left lung nodule showing squamous cell carcinoma (MGG stain, 10x).

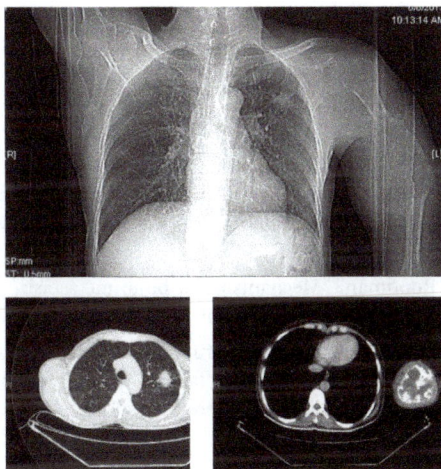

FIGURE 3: CECT thorax showing a spiculated nodule in the left upper lobe with osteolytic lesion in middle of the humerus on the left side.

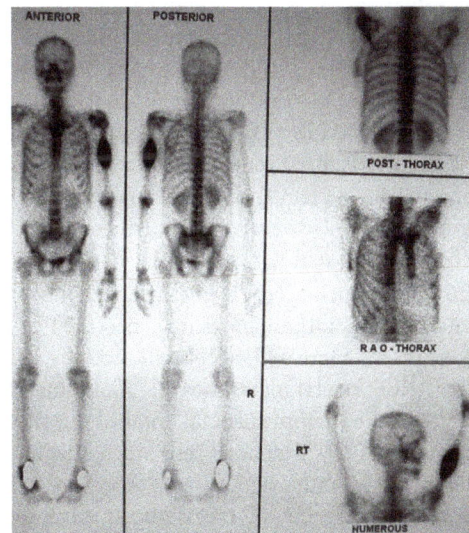

FIGURE 4: ^{99m}TcRadionuclide bone scan showing an increased uptake of radiotracer over the midhumerus of left side, suggestive of metastatic bony lesion.

FIGURE 5: MRI of left upper extremity showing osteolytic lesion in left humerus with marrow edema and soft tissue infiltration.

final tissue diagnosis was squamous cell carcinoma of left lung with metastasis to left humerus. Absence of respiratory symptoms delayed the diagnosis in our case. But the age of the patient and history of heavy smoking raised the suspicion of primary lung malignancy in this setup. Due to overlapping histological characteristics it is sometimes impossible to differentiate between primary and metastatic lung cancer. Immunohistochemistry stain may be helpful in this situation. Cytokeratin 7 is useful for differentiation between adenocarcinoma of lung colon cancer metastasis which stains cytokeratin 20 [5]. With the advent of gene expression arrays and proteomic classification of tumours, molecular classification is an emerging tool to assist in determining whether a lung nodule is primary or secondary [6]. Another important message from this case is that, in any case of painful bone tumour, possibility of metastatic bone disease is much more than primary, because secondary tumours of bone are far more common than primaries. Small cell carcinoma of lung may present with metastatic manifestations with a small, asymptomatic lung primary, but

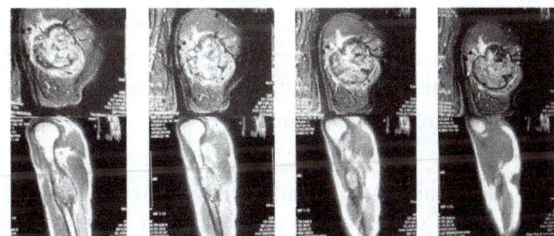

it is very uncommon in squamous cell variety. Our case was a unique one in this respect also.

Bone metastases are of three types: osteolytic (associated with increased osteoclast activity and hypercalcaemia),

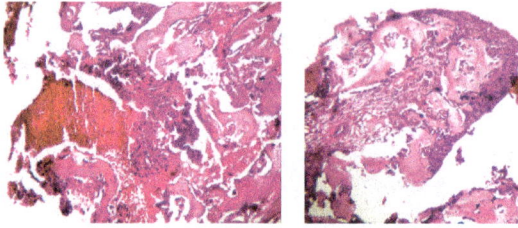

FIGURE 6: Microphotograph of HPE of resected specimen of left humerus showing metastatic squamous cell carcinoma (H&E stain, 10x).

osteoblastic (associated with increased activity of osteoblasts and new bone formation with raised serum alkaline phosphatase), and mixed [7]. Skeletal metastases in lung cancers are predominantly osteolytic; purely osteolytic lesion is seen only in multiple myeloma [8]. On the other hand, purely osteoblastic metastases are uncommon. Regardless of osteolytic or osteoblastic phenotype of bone metastases, osteoclastic proliferation and hypertrophy is present [9]. Bone pain is the main presentation of skeletal metastases from lung cancers. However, pathological fractures, bony swelling with soft tissue invasion, and erosion of the bones are other manifestations. Plain X-ray is adequate for detection of osteolytic metastases. However an osteolytic metastasis is not detected on conventional X-ray until there is a 30–50% loss of bone [10]. Radionuclide (^{99m}Tc-methylene diphosphonate) bone scans (bone scintigraphy) show increased uptake of radioisotope due to increased osteoblastic activity and blood flow at the site of skeletal metastases [11]. Computed tomography delineates the anatomical details of the bone metastases better than plain X-ray. Magnetic resonance imaging (MRI) is superior to bone scintigraphy with respect to sensitivity, specificity, and the extent of metastatic involvement [10]. MRI is also useful for detection of invasion of adjacent soft tissue and vascular invasion and especially useful to exclude cord compression in vertebral metastases [12]. [18F]-fluorodeoxyglucose positron emission tomography (FDG-PET) is another promising method for detection of bone metastases but is less sensitive than MRI in detection of osteal metastases [10]. FNAC is used to confirm the diagnosis of skeletal metastases with 100% cytodiagnostic accuracy [12]. A biopsy should be done to confirm the histopathological type of metastatic carcinomas of bones.

The patient had stage IV lung cancer with poor prognosis. Palliative local radiotherapy may be given to the painful metastases of the humerus to relieve the pain (as it was refractory to nonopioid and opioid analgesics) and also to reduce the size of the lesion with intent to unite the pathological fracture of the humerus with the help of internal fixation [13, 14]. Cytotoxic chemotherapy consisting of cisplatin and gemcitabine may be given for palliation. Bisphosphonates like zoledronic acid may be used to treat hypercalcaemia [15]. Curative resection of both the tumours in a case of primary lung cancer with a solitary metastasis to adrenal gland or brain is very much successful [16], but it may not be applicable in other solitary metastases like bone, as in our case.

References

[1] D. J. Jacofsky, D. A. Frassica, and F. J. Frassica, "Metastatic disease to bone," *Hospital Physician*, vol. 40, pp. 21–28, 2004.

[2] R. J. Fergusson, "Lung cancer," in *Crofton and Douglas's Respiratory Diseases*, A. Seaton, D. Seaton, and A. G. Leitch, Eds., vol. 2, pp. 1077–1122, Blackwell Science, Oxford, UK, 5th edition, 2000.

[3] R. Capanna and D. A. Campanacci, "The treatment of metastases in the appendicular skeleton," *Journal of Bone and Joint Surgery B*, vol. 83, no. 4, pp. 471–481, 2001.

[4] K. Singh, D. Samartzis, A. R. Vaccaro, G. B. J. Andersson, H. S. An, and J. G. Heller, "Current concepts in the management of metastatic spinal disease: the role of minimally invasive approaches," *Journal of Bone and Joint Surgery B*, vol. 88, no. 4, pp. 434–442, 2006.

[5] P. Cagle, "Differential diagnosis between primary and metastatic carcinomas," in *Lung Tumours: Fundamental Biology and Clinical Management*, C. Brambilla and E. Brambilla, Eds., pp. 127–137, Marcel Dekker, New York, NY, USA, 1999.

[6] A. Vachani, M. Nebozhyn, S. Singhal et al., "A 10-gene classifier for distinguishing head and neck squamous cell carcinoma and lung squamous cell carcinoma," *Clinical Cancer Research*, vol. 13, no. 10, pp. 2905–2915, 2007.

[7] G. D. Roodman, "Mechanisms of bone metastasis," *The New England Journal of Medicine*, vol. 350, pp. 1655–1664, 2004.

[8] J. Y. Hung, D. Horn, K. Woodruff, T. Prihoda, C. Lesaux, and J. Peters, "Colony—stimulating factor 1 potentiates lung cancer bone metastasis," *Laboratory Investigation*, vol. 94, pp. 371–381, 2014.

[9] K. G. Halvorson, M. A. Sevcik, J. R. Ghilardi, T. J. Rosol, and P. W. Mantyh, "Similarities and differences in tumor growth, skeletal remodeling and pain in an osteolytic and osteoblastic model of bone cancer," *Clinical Journal of Pain*, vol. 22, no. 7, pp. 587–600, 2006.

[10] N. Ghanem, M. Uhl, I. Brink et al., "Diagnostic value of MRI in comparison to scintigraphy, PET, MS-CT and PET/CT for the detection of metastases of bone," *European Journal of Radiology*, vol. 55, no. 1, pp. 41–55, 2005.

[11] N. Lawrentschuk, I. D. Davis, D. M. Bolton, and A. M. Scott, "Diagnostic and therapeutic use of radioisotopes for bony disease in prostate cancer: current practice," *International Journal of Urology*, vol. 14, no. 2, pp. 89–95, 2007.

[12] C. Lee and C. Jung, "Metastatic spinal tumor," *Asian Spine Journal*, vol. 6, no. 1, pp. 71–87, 2012.

[13] F. Ampil and R. Baluna, "Humeral metastasis in patients with stage IV non-small-cell lung cancer portends a short life expectancy," *Journal of Palliative Medicine*, vol. 12, no. 10, pp. 869–870, 2009.

[14] A. J. Bauze and M. T. Clayer, "Treatment of pathological fractures of the humerus with a locked intramedullary nail," *Journal of Orthopaedic Surgery*, vol. 11, no. 1, pp. 34–37, 2003.

[15] C. M. Perry and D. P. Figgitt, "Zoledronic acid: a review of its use in patients with advanced cancer," *Drugs*, vol. 64, no. 11, pp. 1197–1211, 2004.

17

Community-Acquired Pneumonia and Empyema Caused by *Citrobacter koseri* in an Immunocompetent Patient

Miguel Angel Ariza-Prota, Ana Pando-Sandoval, Marta García-Clemente, Ramón Fernández, and Pere Casan

Hospital Universitario Central de Asturias (HUCA), Instituto Nacional de Silicosis (INS), Área del Pulmón, Facultad de Medicina, Universidad de Oviedo, 33011 Oviedo, Spain

Correspondence should be addressed to Miguel Angel Ariza-Prota; arizamiguel@hotmail.com

Academic Editor: Daniel Curcio

Citrobacter species, belonging to the family Enterobacteriaceae, are environmental organisms commonly found in soil, water, and the intestinal tracts of animals and humans. *Citrobacter koseri* is known to be an uncommon but serious cause of both sporadic and epidemic septicemia and meningitis in neonates and young infants. Most cases reported have occurred in immunocompromised hosts. The infections caused by *Citrobacter* are difficult to treat with usual broad spectrum antibiotics owing to rapid generation of mutants and have been associated with high death rates in the past. We believe this is the first case described in the literature of a community-acquired pneumonia and empyema caused by *Citrobacter koseri* in an immunocompetent adult patient.

1. Introduction

The genus *Citrobacter* belongs to the family of *Enterobacteriaceae* and comprises 11 different species of facultative anaerobic, motile, Gram-negative bacilli, which are oxidase negative and typically utilize citrate as the sole carbon source [1]. Among *Citrobacter* species, the most commonly isolated from human clinical specimens are *C. koseri* (formerly named *C. diversus*), *C. freundii*, *C. youngae*, *C. braakii*, and *C. amalonaticus* [1]. *Citrobacter* infections typically occur in hospital settings in patients with multiple comorbidities and seldom cause disease in the general population [2]. Neonates and immunocompromised hosts are highly susceptible to *Citrobacter* infections, which are mainly caused by *Citrobacter freundii* and *Citrobacter koseri*. *C. freundii* is usually associated with hepatobiliary tract infections, while *C. koseri* causes neonatal meningitis and brain abscess with high mortality rates [3].

In the environment, *Citrobacter* are commonly found in water, soil, and food and as occasional colonizers of the gastrointestinal tract of animals and humans [4]. Although *Citrobacter* strains colonizing the human gastrointestinal tract were traditionally considered to have low virulence [5], they can be the source of several types of infections [6], such as urinary tract, respiratory, intra-abdominal, wound, bone, bloodstream, and central nervous system infections [7–9]. We believe this is the first report of community-acquired pneumonia and empyema caused by *Citrobacter koseri* in an immunocompetent adult patient.

2. Case Presentation

A 72-year-old Spanish male was admitted to our hospital, 6 months ago, after two weeks of marked general syndrome (asthenia, hyporexia, and 3 Kg weight loss), accompanied with cough and mucopurulent sputum, moderate dyspnea, fever, night sweats, and right pleuritic chest pain. He had a 25-pack-year history of smoking and was diagnosed with arterial hypertension (HTN) in 2001. He worked as an architect and had no surgical background or other medical backgrounds of interest. He was taking Enalapril at the time.

The clinical findings were the following: body temperature 38°C; blood pressure 108/65 mmHg; heart rate 90 beats/min; respiratory rate 24 breaths/min; and oxygen saturation 93% (room air). The physical examination was normal, except for pulmonary auscultation, where diminished respiratory sounds and crackles were found bilaterally at the bases of both lungs. Laboratory tests revealed $24,800 \times 10^9$ L white blood cell count with 88% neutrophils; 12.3 g/dL haemoglobin; the C-reactive protein (CRP) level that was 29 mg/L; procalcitonin (PCT) level 0.92 ng/mL; N-terminal probrain natriuretic peptide (NT-proBNP) level that was 400 pg/mL; glucose 129 mg/dL; and platelet count, arterial blood clotting, and the rest of biochemical tests that were within normal ranges. The arterial blood gases showed PaO_2 69 mmHg, $PaCO_2$ 36 mmHg, pH 7.38, and standard HCO_3 37 mEq/L (room air).

The chest X-ray revealed bilateral alveolar infiltrates with associated right pleural effusion (Figure 1). Urinary antigen for pneumococcus and *Legionella*, sputum cytology, mycobacterial culture, and serologic HIV tests were negative. Antibiotic treatment with piperacillin/tazobactam and levofloxacin was initiated on admission. A chest and abdomen computed tomography (CT) scan was performed two days after admission. The CT scan showed a right lower lobe alveolar consolidation with air bronchogram and in the left lower lobe and posterior segment of the left upper lobe similar lesions were identified in relation to a bilateral pneumonic process with associated loculated right pleural effusion and diffuse pleural thickening related to empyema (Figure 2). A subdiaphragmatic lesion was discarded. A diagnostic thoracocentesis was performed obtaining purulent fluid (empyema was confirmed). The pleural fluid biochemistry showed 430,000 white blood cells; 3000 red blood cells; glucose level 44 mg/dL; 22 g/L proteins; and pH of 6,99. A CT-guided pigtail catheter was correctly placed extracting 500 mL of purulent fluid (Figure 3). The patient showed clinical improvement with disappearance of the fever. The pleural fluid culture identified *Citrobacter koseri* and no other pathogen was isolated. The isolate was sensitive to amoxicillin clavulanic acid and piperacillin/tazobactam (resistant to ampicillin). The bacilloscopy, PCR *M. tuberculosis* (XPERT MTB/RIF), and mycobacterial cultures were negative.

After 12 days of intravenous antibiotic treatment, piperacillin/tazobactam and levofloxacin were suspended, and treatment with oral amoxicillin clavulanic acid (1000 mg/ 62,5 mg two tablets twice a day every 12 hours) was initiated with good tolerance and compliance. The patient was discharged with the diagnosis of bilateral pneumonia and right pleural empyema caused by *Citrobacter koseri*. In the October *follow-up* visit, the patient showed clinical improvement (residual dry cough, no fever, and decreased right chest pain) since he was discharged. The control chest X-ray showed loss of volumen of the right lung and improvement of the right alveolar basal infiltrate in comparison to the last X-ray performed during admission (Figure 4).

The patient was again admitted 2 weeks after discharge, because of swelling and pain in the area where the pigtail catheter was previously placed. An ecography of the right thoracic wall was performed. The ecography showed a fluid collection of 17×4 mm with a fistulous pleural tract with minimal pleural effusion (3.6 mm) associated with a small subcutaneous abscess in the area where the pigtail catheter was originally inserted, with the risk of producing a fistula to

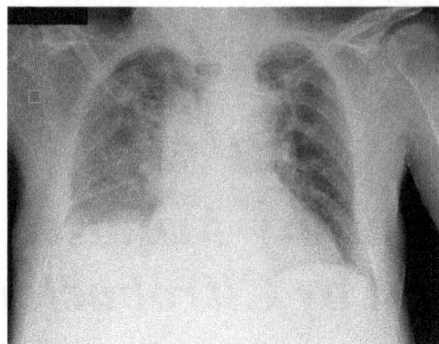

FIGURE 1: Chest X-ray on admission. Bilateral alveolar infiltrates with associated right pleural effusion.

skin (Figure 5). The abscess was drained with a small incision on the skin, and the sample was sent to the microbiology department for culture. A new pigtail drainage catheter was placed, draining 200 mL of purulent fluid. *Citrobacter koseri* was isolated again in the area of the subcutaneous abscess and in the pigtail purulent fluid. The patient was discharged with amoxicillin clavulanic acid for one more month. A control chest X-ray performed four weeks later showed radiological improvement (Figure 6). In total, the patient was treated for 12 days with piperacillin/tazobactam and levofloxacin and for three months with amoxicillin clavulanic acid. A control CT scan performed 2 months ago showed almost complete resolution of the right lower lobe consolidation (Figure 7). The patient remained well on the 3-month *follow-up* visit.

3. Discussion

Citrobacter, a Gram-negative bacterium belonging to Enterobacteriaceae, is a rare cause of lung abscess. *Citrobacter* infections usually occur in patients with underlying comorbidities or immunosuppression [10]. The infections caused by *Citrobacter* are difficult to treat with usual broad spectrum antibiotics owing to rapid generation of mutants and have been associated with high death rates in the past [10]. In our case, the patient was an immunocompetent adult with no underlying important comorbidities, making this a very unusual clinical case because this organism commonly affects neonates and immunocompromised infants. A retrospective study from Taiwan on *Citrobacter* bacteraemia reported 45 patients over a period of thirteen years [10]. Patients with malignancies (48.9% mostly intra-abdominal) or hepatobiliary stones (22.2%) were found to have high predilection for *Citrobacter* bacteraemia. Abdominal cavity (51.1%) was the most common site for initial infection, with other sites being urinary tract (20%) and lung (11.1%) [10]. Intra-abdominal infections included hepatobiliary tree infection (including three patients who had liver abscesses), peritonitis, and perianal abscess [10]. Another report of three cases noted two patients one with *Citrobacter*-related iliopsoas abscess and another patient with renal and liver abscess in a patient with diabetes owing to *C. koseri* [11].

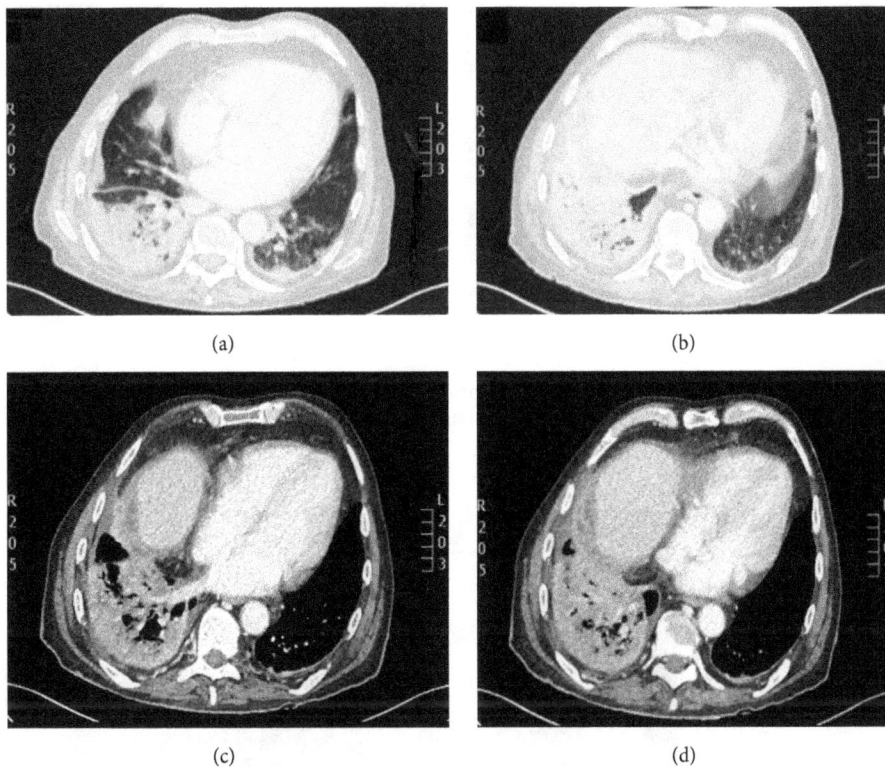

FIGURE 2: Computed tomography of the chest on admission. Right lower lobe alveolar consolidation with air bronchogram and in the left lower lobe and posterior segment of the left upper lobe similar lesions were identified in relation to a bilateral pneumonic process with associated loculated right pleural effusion and diffuse pleural thickening related to empyema.

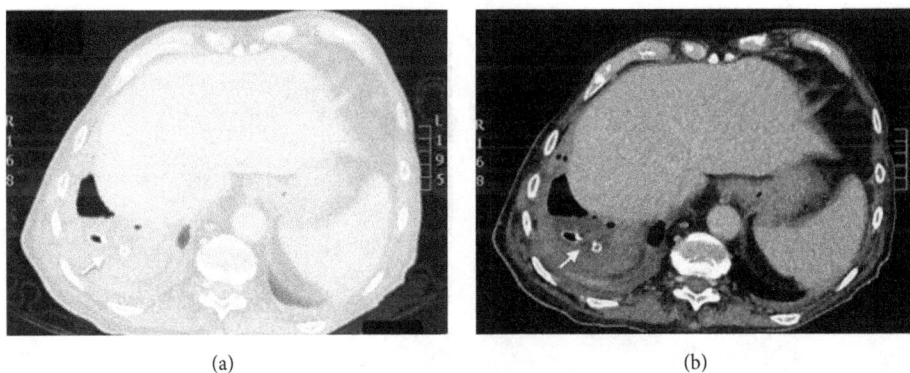

FIGURE 3: Computed tomography. Pigtail catheter correctly placed in the right lower lobe.

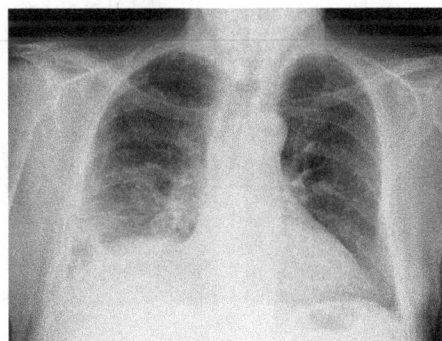

FIGURE 4: Control chest X-ray. Loss of volumen of the right lung and improvement of the right alveolar basal infiltrate.

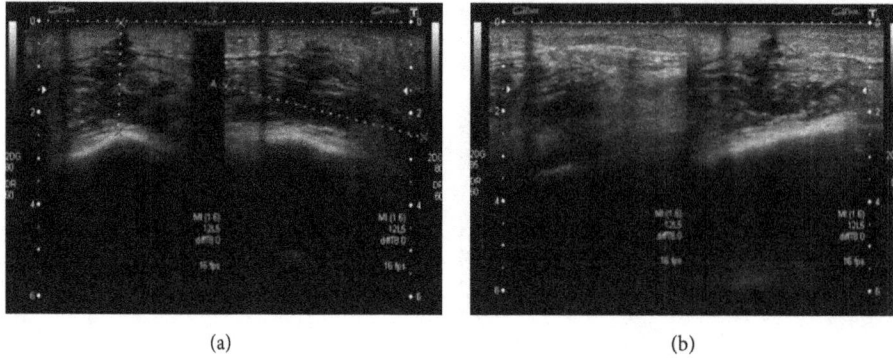

(a)

(b)

FIGURE 5: Right thoracic wall ecography. Fluid collection of 17×4 mm with a fistulous pleural tract with minimal pleural effusion (3.6 mm) associated with a small subcutaneous abscess in the area where the pigtail catheter was originally inserted, with the risk of producing a fistula to skin.

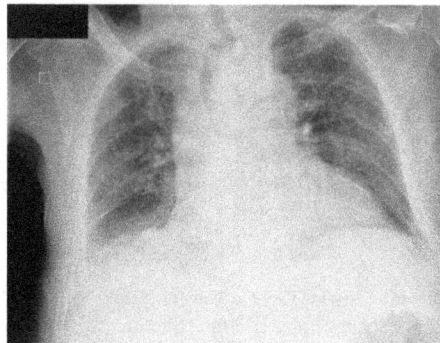

FIGURE 6: Control chest X-ray on the follow-up visit. Radiological improvement of the right lower lobe alveolar infiltrate.

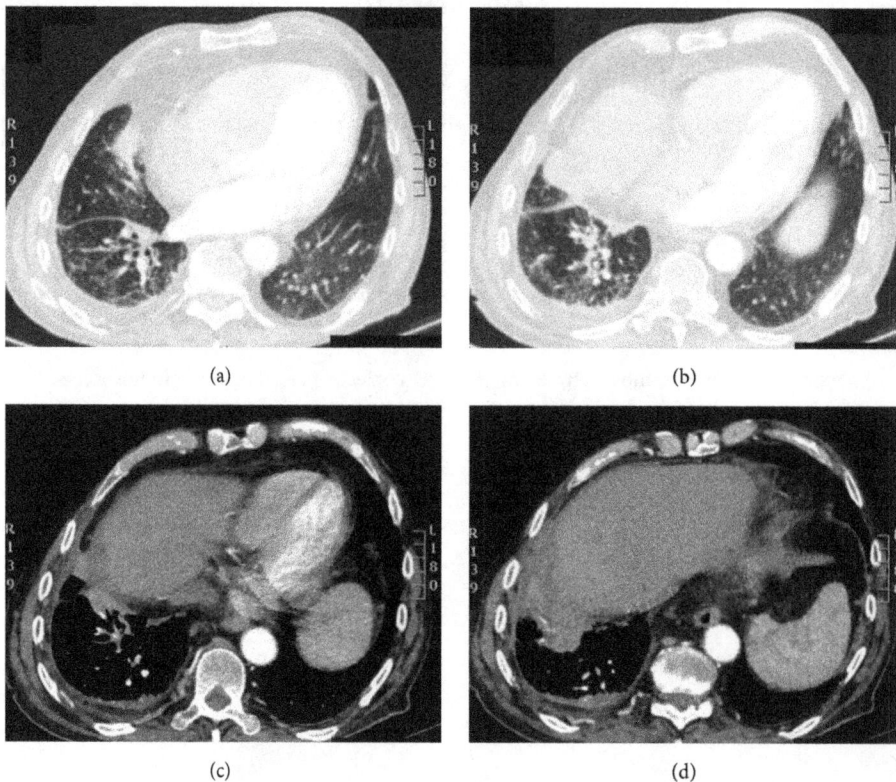

(a)

(b)

(c)

(d)

FIGURE 7: Control computed tomography of the chest. Almost complete resolution of the right lower lobe consolidation.

The literature on *Citrobacter* abscess in adults is scant [12]. We performed a PubMed search with the terms "*Citrobacter koseri*", "*Citrobacter koseri* pneumonia", and "*Citrobacter koseri* empyema". Nine cases of abscess secondary to *C. koseri* infection in adults were found in this search. None of these cases were associated with lung abscess, pneumonia, or empyema. This is the first described case in the literature of community-acquired pneumonia and empyema caused by *Citrobacter koseri* in an immunocompetent adult patient. Regarding treatment, it was observed in the study on *Citrobacter*-related bacteraemia that use of a cephalosporin within 14 days promoted the emergence of cefotaxime-resistant strains and multidrug-resistant strains [10]. Another study at a north Indian tertiary institute depicted a high degree of resistance to the third-generation and the fourth-generation cephalosporins, as well as piperacillin, gentamicin, and ciprofloxacin [13]. In our case, the isolate was sensitive to piperacillin and all third and fourth generation cephalosporins. In spite of broad spectrum antibiotic treatment according to the sensitivity reports, patient's condition showed a very slow improvement; *Citrobacter koseri* was still isolated from the pigtail catheter drainage and subcutaneous abscess after 30 days of antibiotic treatment. Imipenem has been consistently found to be active against *Citrobacter* spp. [14, 15]. As for gentamicin, despite earlier reports showing the susceptibility of *Citrobacter* spp. to this agent [14], the rates of resistance appear to be rising [15]. Rising resistance to ciprofloxacin is also of concern [15]. We could speculate that a beta-lactamase inhibitor may become the first choice for complicated *Citrobacter* infection that requires prolonged courses of antibiotics.

4. Conclusion

The present case highlights *Citrobacter koseri* as a rare cause of empyema. Although *Citrobacter* infections occur more often in immunocompromised neonates and young infants predominantly causing meningitis and liver abscess, pneumonia and empyema should be added to the spectrum of disease in immunocompetent adult patients, where a combined and prolonged treatment (invasive intervention/drainage and medication) is probably the faster and more efficient solution.

Abbreviations

HTN: Hypertension
CRP: C-reactive protein
PCT: Procalcitonin
NT-proBNP: N-terminal probrain natriuretic peptide
HIV: Human immunodeficiency virus
CT: Computed tomography.

Authors' Contribution

Miguel Angel Ariza-Prota, Ana Pando-Sandoval, Marta García-Clemente, and Ramón Fernández performed research and collected data; Miguel Angel Ariza-Prota wrote paper; Pere Casan performed the case report design and review of paper and helped to draft the paper. All authors read and approved the final paper.

References

[1] J. M. Janda, S. L. Abbott, W. K. W. Cheung, and D. F. Hanson, "Biochemical identification of citrobacteria in the clinical laboratory," *Journal of Clinical Microbiology*, vol. 32, no. 8, pp. 1850–1854, 1994.

[2] D. A. Schwartz, "Citrobacter infections," in *Pathology of Infectious Diseases. Stanford, Connecticut: Appleton and Lange*, D. H. Connor, F. W. Chandler, D. A. Schwartz, H. J. Manz, and E. E. Lack, Eds., pp. 513–516, 1997.

[3] N. Holmes and H. M. Aucken, "Citrobacter, Enterobacter, Klebsiella, Serratia and other members of the Enterobacteriaceae," in *Topley and Wilson's Microbiology and Microbial Infections*, L. Collier, A. Balows, and M. Sussman, Eds., vol. 2, pp. 999–1033, Oxford University Press, New York, NY, USA, 9th edition, 1998.

[4] S. Arens and L. Verbist, "Differentiation and susceptibility of Citrobacter isolates from patients in a university hospital," *Clinical Microbiology and Infection*, vol. 3, no. 1, pp. 53–57, 1997.

[5] C. Pepperell, J. V. Kus, M. A. Gardam, A. Humar, and L. L. Burrows, "Low-virulence Citrobacter species encode resistance to multiple antimicrobials," *Antimicrobial Agents and Chemotherapy*, vol. 46, no. 11, pp. 3555–3560, 2002.

[6] G. Altmann, I. Sechter, D. Cahan, and C. B. Gerichter, "Citrobacter diversus isolated from clinical material," *Journal of Clinical Microbiology*, vol. 3, no. 4, pp. 390–392, 1976.

[7] G. R. Hodges, C. E. Degener, and W. G. Barnes, "Clinical significance of citrobacter isolates," *American Journal of Clinical Pathology*, vol. 70, no. 1, pp. 37–40, 1978.

[8] B. A. Lipsky, E. W. Hook III, A. A. Smith, and J. J. Plorde, "Citrobacter infections in humans: experience at the Seattle Veterans Administration Medical Center and a review of the literature," *Reviews of Infectious Diseases*, vol. 2, no. 5, pp. 746–760, 1980.

[9] S. Mohanty, R. Singhal, S. Sood, B. Dhawan, A. Kapil, and B. K. Das, "Citrobacter infections in a tertiary care hospital in Northern India," *Journal of Infection*, vol. 54, no. 1, pp. 58–64, 2007.

[10] C.-C. Shih, Y.-C. Chen, S.-C. Chang, K.-T. Luh, and W.-C. Hsieh, "Bacteremia due to Citrobacter species: significance of primary intraabdominal infection," *Clinical Infectious Diseases*, vol. 23, no. 3, pp. 543–549, 1996.

[11] S.-Y. Lin, M.-W. Ho, Y.-F. Yang et al., "Abscess caused by Citrobacter koseri infection: three case reports and a literature review," *Internal Medicine*, vol. 50, no. 12, pp. 1333–1337, 2011.

[12] U. Kariholu, J. Rawal, and S. Namnyak, "Neonatal citrobacter koseri meningitis and brain abscess," *The Internet Journal of Pediatrics and Neonatology*, vol. 10, no. 1, 2008.

[13] M. Shahid, "*Citrobacter* spp. Simultaneously harboring bla-CTX-M, blaTEM, blaSHV, blaampC, and insertion sequences IS26 and orf513: an evolutionary phenomenon of recent concern for antibiotic resistance," *Journal of Clinical Microbiology*, vol. 48, no. 5, pp. 1833–1838, 2010.

[14] G. Samonis, D. H. Ho, G. F. Gooch, K. V. Rolston, and G. P. Bodey, "In vitro susceptibility of *Citrobacter* species to various antimicrobial agents," *Antimicrobial Agents and Chemotherapy*, vol. 31, no. 5, pp. 829–830, 1987.

[15] J.-T. Wang, S.-C. Chang, Y.-C. Chen, and K.-T. Luh, "Comparison of antimicrobial susceptibility of *Citrobacter freundii* isolates in two different time periods," *Journal of Microbiology, Immunology and Infection*, vol. 33, no. 4, pp. 258–262, 2000.

18

Clinical Management of Acute Interstitial Pneumonia

Yang Xia,[1,2] Zhenyu Liang,[1] Zhenzhen Fu,[2] Laiyu Liu,[1] Omkar Paudel,[2] and Shaoxi Cai[1]

[1] *Chronic Airways Diseases Laboratory, Department of Respiration, Nanfang Hospital, Southern Medical University, Guangzhou 510515, China*
[2] *Division of Pulmonary and Critical Care Medicine, Department of Medicine, Johns Hopkins University School of Medicine, Baltimore, MD, USA*

Correspondence should be addressed to Shaoxi Cai, caishaox@fimmu.com

Academic Editors: M. Berman and W. Gao

We describe a 51-year-old woman who was admitted to hospital because of cough and expectoration accompanied with general fatigue and progressive dyspnea. Chest HRCT scan showed areas of ground glass attenuation, consolidation, and traction bronchiectasis in bilateral bases of lungs. BAL fluid test and transbronchial lung biopsy failed to offer insightful evidence for diagnosis. She was clinically diagnosed with acute interstitial pneumonia (AIP). Treatment with mechanical ventilation and intravenous application of methylprednisolone (80 mg/day) showed poor clinical response and thus was followed by steroid pulse therapy (500 mg/day, 3 days). However, she died of respiratory dysfunction eventually. Autopsy showed diffuse alveolar damage associated with hyaline membrane formation, pulmonary interstitial, immature collagen edema, and focal type II pneumocyte hyperplasia.

1. Introduction

The idiopathic interstitial pneumonias (IIP) is defined as a group of chronic, progressive diffuse parenchymal lung diseases with unclear cause, characterized by expansion of the interstitial compartment of inflammatory cells, and is potential to develop pulmonary fibrosis in many cases. By and large, IIP team is divided into seven distinct groups—idiopathic pulmonary fibrosis (IPF), nonspecific interstitial pneumonia (NSIP), respiratory bronchiolitis interstitial lung disease (RBILD), desquamative interstitial pneumonia (DIP), acute interstitial pneumonia (AIP), cryptogenic organizing pneumonia (COP), and lymphoid interstitial pneumonia (LIP) [1, 2], among which IPF usually occurs primarily in older adults, and limits to the lungs is the most common form [3]. However, AIP, also known as Hamman-Rich syndrome, though displaying a very poor prognosis, with its rare morbidity, remains unfamiliar to physicians. In this report, we present a case of a mid-age female with AIPwho, though treated with intensive physical and pharmacologic care, still displayed a rapid progressive pathophysiologic process, and eventually died of respiratory failure.

2. Case Presentation

A 51-year-old woman, nonsmoker, without underlying diseases, no suspicious case history was admitted to the hospital for further workup of symptoms of cough, expectoration, and progressive dyspnea. Chest radiograph and HRCT thorax a month ago revealed increased lung markings associated with areas of bilateral and patchy ground glass shadowing. A poor response to short-term broad-spectrum antibiotic was manifested. Only one month leading up to her hospital admission again, she became virtually incapacitated by shortness of breath and exercise tolerance decreased to several feet walk at one time.

Blood pressure was 113/69 mmHg, heart rate 119 beats/min, respiration rate >30 breaths/min, oxygen saturation of 93% with high flow oxygen (10 L/min) via nasal cannula at rest, and she was about to desaturate to 88% after minimal exertion. Temperature was normal. Physical examination findings revealed a distinct respiratory distress, positive three depressions sign, and cyanopathy. Pulmonary examination findings showed remarkably decreased breath sounds and diffused velcro rale. No crackles or wheezing

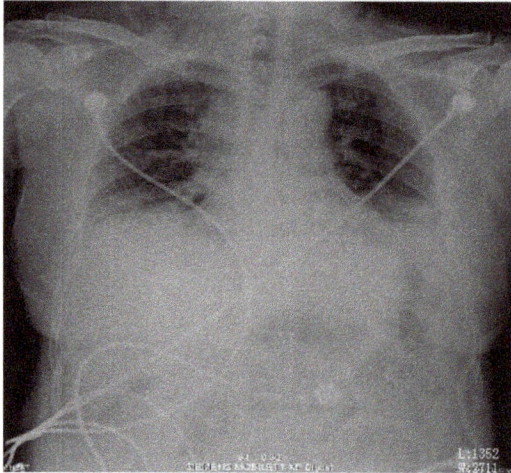

FIGURE 1: Chest radiograph with remarkable reduction of lung volume as well as increased lung markings.

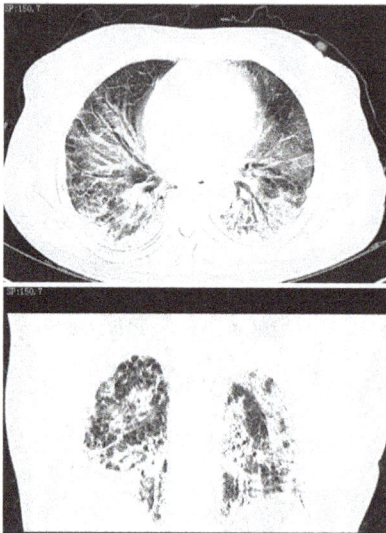

FIGURE 2: HRCT depicting diffuse areas of pulmonary infiltration, a bilateral geographic distribution of ground glass opacity and consolidation in the more dependent lung with associated traction bronchiectasis.

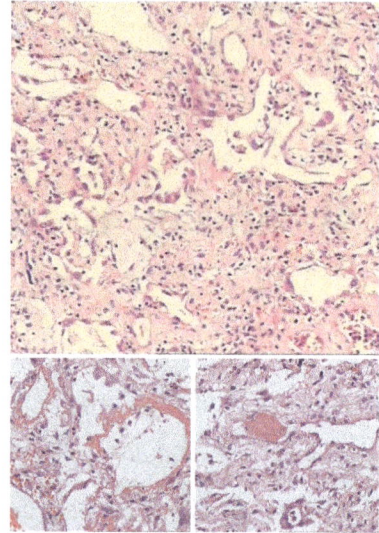

FIGURE 3: Lung biopsy reveals scattered hyaline membranes lining alveolar septa that are thickened by interstitial edema and inflammatory cell infiltration besides hyperplasia of type II pneumocytes.

were appreciated. Cardiac examination revealed regular rhythm, no gallop, or edema. There was no skin rash, joint deformity, hepatosplenomegaly, or lymphadenopathy.

Blood gas analysis revealed Po_2 8.54 KPa, Pco_2 4.9 KPa, pH 7.421, $FiO_2/PaO_2 = 120$. WBCs and HGB were within normal limits. NEU% of 74.1% was slightly increased. Serologic examinations including ANA, Sm, UI-NRnp, Jo-1, Scl-70, SSA, SSB, P-ANCA, RF, C-ANCA, and HIV were all negative. ECG demonstrated sinus tachycardia. Chest radiography was performed which is shown in Figure 1. Her chest CT scan (Figure 2) revealed areas of ground glass attenuation and consolidation in bilateral bases of her lungs accompanied with traction bronchiectasis.

Bronchoscopy was performed and the results suggested absence of microorganism infection or tumor cell and eosinophil count was normal. Cytology and culture results for mycobacterium, fungus, and bacteria were all negative. BAL fluid test results for cytomegalovirus, chlamydia, Legionella, herpes simplex virus, and respiratory syncytial virus were negative too. Transbronchial lung biopsy (TBLB) showed slight proliferation of inflammatory and fibrous tissue.

The patient was treated with high-concentration oxygen therapy, broad-spectrum antibiotics therapy, intravenous application of methylprednisolone (80 mg/day) in conjunction with noninvasive ventilation (Bi-PAP) which was terminated after 2 hours for man-machine counteraction. But all of the treatments were unremarkable. Dyspnea was increasingly aggravated since the 4th day after admittance to the hospital. Oxygenation index slumped to 99.9 mmHg. Based on the clinical and radiologic features she was diagnosed with AIP. Tracheotomy associated mechanical ventilation was required and methylprednisolone pulse therapy (500 mg/day, three consecutive days) was administrated. However, irreversible exacerbation of postoperative oxygenation index dropped further to 32.5 mmHg and blood pressure deteriorated as it fell to 90/60 mmHg. She eventually expired due to respiratory failure on the 7th day of admission. Percutaneous lung biopsy was performed and the slides (Figure 3) showed diffuse alveolar damage (DAD) associated with hyaline membrane formation, pulmonary interstitial edema, and immature collagen edema, and focal type II pneumocyte hyperplasia were also visible.

3. Discussion

Acute interstitial pneumonia, which occurs over a wide range of ages, with an approximate mean age of 50, [4] early characterized by a viral upper respiratory infection with constitutional symptoms, soon develops respiratory failure over a couple of days and within weeks. It is synonymous with

Hamman-Rich syndrome, demonstrating no sex predominance or correlation with smoking and tending to occur in patients without preexisting lung disease. Pulmonary function tests show a restrictive pattern with reduced diffusing capacity [1, 2]. Bronchoalveolar lavage fluid contains increased numbers of red blood cells, neutrophils, and occasionally lymphocytes. It has a grave prognosis with >50% mortality in 2 months, despite being under intensive medical care.

Due to the lack of well-accepted accuracy of diagnostic method, diagnosis should be accomplished with a multidisciplinary discussion among pulmonologists, radiologists, and pathologists experienced in the diagnosis of IIPs [5]. Generally, the suggested criteria for AIP include an unexplained worsening of dyspnea within 2 months; evidence of HRCT showing diffuse bilateral radiographic infiltrates; clean history of chest radiograph; organized or proliferative diffuse alveolar damage on lung biopsy; absence of any known inciting event or predisposing condition, such as, but may beyond, infection, systemic inflammatory response syndrome, environmental or toxic exposures, connective tissue disease, and prior interstitial lung disease [6].

Historically, the classic pattern of AIP shows diffuse alveolar damage. DAD, however, can also be found in some other diseases, such as acute hypersensitivity pneumonitis, acute respiratory distress syndrome (ARDS), connective tissue disease, drug-induced lung disease, infection, inhalants, toxins, and acute exacerbation of interstitial pneumonia fibrosis (AE-IPF) [7]. Therefore, diagnosis of AIP based on histology alone is obviously too arbitrary and careful evaluation of alternative etiologies containing comorbidities, medication use, occupational/environmental health, and family history is essential. And on top, physical examination, physiological testing, and laboratory evaluation such as serologic autoimmune antibody have to be performed in order to distinguish AIP from connective tissue disease (especially in young woman) and infection.

It is of particular importance to evaluate patients thoroughly for possible ARDS and AE-IPF, since such patients may mimic AIP. Although not only the clinical manifestation, but DAD features in histology of ARDS is similar to AIP, in contrast to the idiopathy of AIP, [4] the indispensable cause must be present in ARDS. Also, the fibrosis in AIP has its peculiarity which is active and proliferative with minimal deposition of collagen. However, some researchers propose AIP as a possible cause or subtype of ARDS for their high similarities that is still controversial [8, 9]. Whilst, AE-IPF, characterized by rapid deterioration at any point in the course of the disease, which is not secondary to infection, pulmonary embolism, or heart failure [10, 11], is an acute insult to the lung over and above the underlying UIP. In short, the different etiology and HRCT feature are the critical points for antidiastole AIP from AE-IPF.

Regarding the significant role of histology in AIP diagnosis, the obtainment of lung biopsy comes to be a combined problem. Although transbronchial biopsy specimens, to some degree, may contribute to the diagnosis of IIP [12], the sensitivity, specificity, biopsy quality, quantity, and position of this approach for the diagnosis is far from satisfactory [13, 14]. Furthermore, in patients with AIP, the risks of surgical lung biopsy may outweigh the benefits of establishing a secure diagnosis in terms of a severe physiologic impairment. In our case, the lack of direct evidence via transbronchial biopsy specimens supporting the diagnosis of AIP led to the delay of steroid pulse therapy possibly inducing the final consequence of death. However, in contrast, the severe disease itself in our patient also deprived her of the tolerance to any surgical lung biopsy. Thus, the final decision regarding whether or not to pursue a surgical lung biopsy must be tailored to the individuals.

The features of chest radiography from our patient are consistent with typical AIP appearances: progressive, patchy-distributed but not limited to, airspace consolidation and ground-glass attenuation in bilateral lung often diffusely involves the mid and lower zones on X-ray, with the decreased lung volumes. HRCT scan shows bilateral and patchy ground glass attenuation located distinctly at either subpleural or central, leading to a geographic appearance of preserved areas of lung lobules [1, 2]. Consolidation, most common in the dependent area of lung which is seen in the absence of traction bronchiectasis, provides an early radiographic clue to underlying fibrosis [15]. Intralobar linear opacities and subpleural honeycombing may be seen in a minority of cases after the duration of the process continues for more than a month. Later, traction bronchiectasis and architectural distortion which may increase with the duration of the disease [16] are common findings in patients imaged at an organizing stage of disease. Also, cysts and other lucent areas of lung become more common in the late stages of AIP. In reported case, HRCT showed diffused pulmonary infiltration and ground glass attenuation in a geographic appearance, consolidation with associated traction bronchiectasis which confidently fitted into the feature of later phase AIP. The later stage should be another factor to make the pathologic process irreversible even when treated with a steroid pulse therapy.

Besides the supportive care including supplemental oxygen and mechanical ventilation, the use of intravenous glucocorticoids in treatment of AIP is considered to be beneficial, [6] though lacking in convincing support [17]. Let alone the immunosuppressive therapy and lung transplant. In general, the pulmonologists have reached the consensus that the earlier intervention is associated with higher survival rates.

Although we could not do much to help in survival of patients with AIP, we still had some encouraging progress: the use of evidence-based medicine in formulating recommendations for disease management, the booming development of lung transplant in curing severe AIP patients, the well establishment of lung rehabilitation, the various molecular biomarkers of IIP used to identify the diagnosis, predict the susceptibility, prognosis, and drug efficiency [18]. However, these significant efforts in AIP field are beyond sufficient and it is obviously beyond the capability of any single center. Thus, an AIP consortium consisting of clinicians, industry, patient advocacy organizations, and the scientific community should be organized aimed to win the war against the AIP. Finally, for the clinician, they should update the information timely. Understand more, survive more.

References

[1] C. Agusti, "American Thoracic Society/European Respiratory Society International Multidisciplinary Consensus Classification of the Idiopathic Interstitial Pneumonias," *American Journal of Respiratory and Critical Care Medicine*, vol. 165, pp. 277–305, 2002.

[2] C. Agustí, "Erratum: American Thoracic Society/European Respiratory Society International Multidisciplinary Consensus Classification of the Idiopathic Interstitial Pneumonias (American Journal of Respiratory and Critical Care Medicine (2000) 165 (277–304))," *American Journal of Respiratory and Critical Care Medicine*, vol. 166, no. 3, p. 426, 2002.

[3] G. Raghu, H. R. Collard, J. J. Egan et al., "An official ATS/ERS/JRS/ALAT statement: idiopathic pulmonary fibrosis: evidence-based guidelines for diagnosis and management," *American Journal of Respiratory and Critical Care Medicine*, vol. 183, no. 6, pp. 788–824, 2011.

[4] D. Bouros, A. C. Nicholson, V. Polychronopoulos, and R. M. Du Bois, "Acute interstitial pneumonia," *European Respiratory Journal*, vol. 15, no. 2, pp. 412–418, 2000.

[5] K. R. Flaherty, T. E. King Jr., G. Raghu et al., "Idiopathic interstitial pneumonia: what is the effect of a multidisciplinary approach to diagnosis?" *American Journal of Respiratory and Critical Care Medicine*, vol. 170, no. 8, pp. 904–910, 2004.

[6] J. S. Vourlekis, "Acute interstitial pneumonia," *Clinics in Chest Medicine*, vol. 25, no. 4, pp. 739–747, 2004.

[7] A. Churg, N. L. Müller, C. I. S. Silva, and J. L. Wright, "Acute exacerbation (acute lung injury of unknown cause) in UIP and other forms of fibrotic interstitial pneumonias," *American Journal of Surgical Pathology*, vol. 31, no. 2, pp. 277–284, 2007.

[8] L. B. Ware, "The acute respiratory distress syndrome (vol 342, pg 1334, 2000)," *The New England Journal of Medicine*, vol. 343, no. 7, p. 520, 2000.

[9] J. Bruminhent, S. Yassir, and J. Pippim, "Acute interstitial pneumonia (hamman-rich syndrome) as a cause of idiopathic acute respiratory distress syndrome," *Case Reports in Medicine*, vol. 2011, Article ID 628743, 4 pages, 2011.

[10] F. J. Martinez, S. Safrin, D. Weycker et al., "The clinical course of patients with idiopathic pulmonary fibrosis," *Annals of Internal Medicine*, vol. 142, no. 12, pp. 963–967, 2005.

[11] K. Konishi, K. F. Gibson, K. O. Lindell et al., "Gene expression profiles of acute exacerbations of idiopathic pulmonary fibrosis," *American Journal of Respiratory and Critical Care Medicine*, vol. 180, no. 2, pp. 167–175, 2009.

[12] E. A. Berbescu, A. L. A. Katzenstein, J. L. Snow, and D. A. Zisman, "Transbronchial biopsy in usual interstitial pneumonia," *Chest*, vol. 129, no. 5, pp. 1126–1131, 2006.

[13] G. W. Hunninghake, M. B. Zimmerman, D. A. Schwartz et al., "Utility of a lung biopsy for the diagnosis of idiopathic pulmonary fibrosis," *American Journal of Respiratory and Critical Care Medicine*, vol. 164, no. 2, pp. 193–196, 2001.

[14] K. R. Flaherty, E. L. Thwaite, E. A. Kazerooni et al., "Radiological versus histological diagnosis in UIP and NSIP: survival implications," *Thorax*, vol. 58, no. 2, pp. 143–148, 2003.

[15] D. A. Lynch, W. D. Travis, N. L. Müller et al., "Idiopathic interstitial pneumonias: CT features," *Radiology*, vol. 236, no. 1, pp. 10–21, 2005.

[16] T. Johkoh, N. L. Müller, H. Taniguchi et al., "Acute interstitial pneumonia: thin-section CT findings in 36 patients," *Radiology*, vol. 211, no. 3, pp. 859–863, 1999.

[17] L. S. Avnon, O. Pikovsky, N. Sion-Vardy, and Y. Almog, "Acute interstitial pneumonia-hamman-rich syndrome: clinical characteristics and diagnostic and therapeutic considerations," *Anesthesia and Analgesia*, vol. 108, no. 1, pp. 232–237, 2009.

[18] Y. Zhang and N. Kaminski, "Biomarkers in idiopathic pulmonary fibrosis," *Current Opinion in Pulmonary Medicine*, vol. 18, no. 5, pp. 441–446, 2012.

19

Multicentric Spinal Tuberculosis with Sternoclavicular Joint Involvement: A Rare Presentation

Balaji Saibaba,[1] Umesh Kumar Meena,[2] Prateek Behera,[1] and Ramesh Chand Meena[2]

[1] Department of Orthopaedics, SMS Medical College, Jaipur, Rajasthan 302004, India
[2] Department of Orthopaedics, SMS Medical College and Hospital, Jaipur 302004, India

Correspondence should be addressed to Umesh Kumar Meena; drumesh_meena@yahoo.co.in

Academic Editor: Tun-Chieh Chen

Background. Tuberculosis is a chronic disease which may have varied presentations. Though pulmonary tuberculosis is the commonest, extrapulmonary tuberculosis involving skeletal system is often seen. Individuals with poor nourishment and immunological status are especially susceptible for disseminated and multicentric tuberculosis. *Case Report.* We here present a case of tuberculosis involving multiple anatomical locations in an immune-competent patient which was diagnosed with radiological studies and confirmed with histological examination. Patient was put on multidrug antitubercular therapy and responded well to the treatment with improvement in clinical and radiological picture. *Clinical Relevance.* This report of a rare case makes us aware of the varied presentations which tuberculosis can present with. It should be kept as a differential diagnosis in patients with cough and fever but not responding to conventional treatment. This is even more important in countries with poor socioeconomic conditions.

1. Introduction

Tuberculosis (TB) is still a very common disease in developing countries [1]. Pulmonary tuberculosis is the commonest form of tuberculosis but patients may present with lesions in location not involving the lungs. Skeletal tuberculosis constitutes around 10% of the extrapulmonary cases. Spinal tuberculosis is most common and a dangerous form of skeletal tuberculosis in adults. The lower thoracic and upper lumbar vertebrae are the most common sites of involvement. The cervical spine is rarely affected; cervical spine involvement occurs in approximately 0.03% of all tuberculosis cases [1, 2]. Isolated cervical spine [1] or sternoclavicular joint involvement [2, 3] also has been reported in literature but multicentric involvement is extremely rare [4–6]. Involvement of sternoclavicular joint along with spinal tuberculosis has never been reported previously in English literature. This case report describes a rare type of tuberculosis involving multiple anatomical structures (i.e., atlantoaxial junction, dorsal spine, and sternoclavicular joint with concomitant pulmonary tuberculosis) which we can hence label as multicentric tuberculosis. It was treated successfully with multidrug antitubercular therapy.

2. Case Report

A 24-year-old unmarried female presented to the outpatient clinic with painful swelling of the right sternoclavicular joint of 2-month duration without any discharging sinus (Figure 1). The swelling was gradually increasing in size and was accompanied with mild pain. The pain was dull, continuous, and limited to the site of the lesion. She also complained of neck stiffness and pain on neck movements. There was no history of any injury. History of cough, weight loss, night cries (severe pain at night), and low grade fever was present for the past 4 months. There was no history of previous tuberculosis or contact with an open case of tuberculosis. She had been prescribed several antibiotics and analgesics at another centre but had no symptomatic improvement. On physical examination the swelling (2×3 cm) was present over right sternoclavicular joint and was associated with presence of mild tenderness, erythema, and local rise of temperature. Laboratory tests revealed haemoglobin of 10.4 gm%; total leukocyte count was 10.300/mm^3. Her ESR was 34 mm in first hour. She was negative for HIV based on ELISA method. On radiographic evaluation there was destruction with sclerosis on the medial end of the right clavicle along with features of

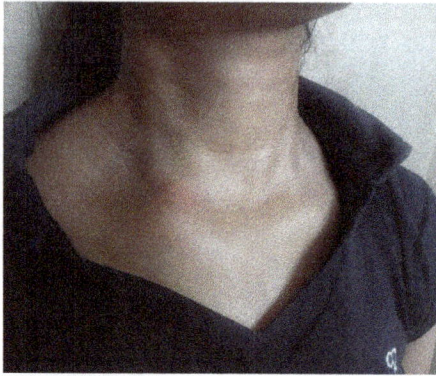

Figure 1: Clinical picture showing erythematous swelling over right sternoclavicular joint region.

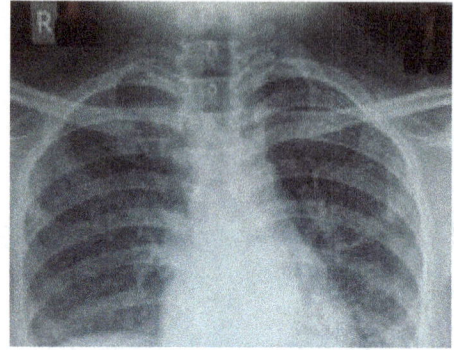

Figure 2: Radiology of patient showing diffuse pulmonary infiltrate along with destruction with sclerosis on the medial end of the right clavicle.

diffuse pulmonary infiltrate (Figure 2). MRI revealed bilateral upper lung lobe infiltrate with arthritis of right sternoclavicular joint, with regional fluid collection. A destruction of the atlanto-axial junction, D7-8 intervertebral disc space along with a pus collection from D5 to D8 region could also be appreciated (Figures 3(a), 3(b), and 3(c)). An early morning sputum sample was sent for Ziehl-Neelsen (ZN) staining and it came out positive suggesting the diagnosis of pulmonary tuberculosis. Fine needle aspiration of the right sternoclavicular lesion was done using a 22-gauge needle and sent for Gram staining, staining for acid-fast bacilli (AFB), histopathology, and cultures including a tubercular culture. The histologic picture was that of chronic inflammation with a caseating granuloma compatible with tuberculosis. The Ziehl-Neelsen stained smear also showed the presence of acid-fast bacilli (AFB), confirming the diagnosis of tuberculosis. The culture for *Mycobacterium tuberculosis* came out as negative. Antitubercular chemotherapy with four first line antitubercular drugs (rifampicin, isoniazid, ethambutol, and pyrazinamide) was started. The patient had a good clinical response within 6 weeks and was switched to three drugs (rifampicin, isoniazid, and ethambutol) after 3 months of therapy with four drugs. The clinical, haematological, and radiological parameters showed complete healing of the lesion after 1 year of treatment with ATT, which was further continued for a total duration of 18 months. After successfully completing the therapy for 18 months, the patient was followed up for 2 years and showed no recurrence of symptoms.

3. Discussion

Tuberculosis is a communicable disease caused by *M. tuberculosis*. It primarily affects the lungs and spreads by droplets and aerosols produced by coughing and sneezing by patients who are active cases of pulmonary tuberculosis. Extrapulmonary tuberculosis involving the skeletal system is not uncommon with skeletal tuberculosis accounting for 10% of extrapulmonary tuberculosis cases. Weight bearing joints involved in extrapulmonary tuberculosis are the spine, hip, and knees in the order of decreasing frequency. Involvement

of the spine constitutes 60% of skeletal tuberculosis and the lower thoracic and upper lumbar vertebrae are more often affected; an involvement of the cervical spine is rare [1]. The usual pattern of spinal tuberculosis is of contiguous or continuous vertebral involvement but multicentric involvement is extremely rare [4–6]. Considering that the patients with skeletal tuberculosis may not present with the classical constitutional symptoms of tuberculosis, these patients may not be diagnosed early in the course of disease. Common predisposing factors for multicentric tuberculosis are immunocompromised status, intravenous drug use, diabetes mellitus, alcohol abuse, and hepatic cirrhosis [4, 7], but none of these risk factors was present in our case. The mode of involvement is most likely hematogenous, as suggested by its multicentric nature. Other routes of multicentric tuberculous involvement are direct inoculation, extension from adjacent bones or joints, and lymphogenous spread [4].

Cervical pain is common in young patients with or without history of trauma but a diagnosis of tuberculosis should be kept in mind in patients with atraumatic cervical pain of long duration and should be evaluated thoroughly if not relieved with initial therapy to prevent neurological complications. Our patient was also initially treated with this form of treatment without any improvement. Most patients with cervical lesions heal with adequate local support and antitubercular therapy, but surgical decompressio may required in presence of neurological impairment, instability, large cold abscess causing mechanical compressions or in refractory cases [1].

The occurrence of sternoclavicular tuberculosis is extremely rare and is difficult to diagnose on conventional radiographs. To prevent complications early diagnosis and treatment is essential. The differential diagnosis of sternoclavicular tuberculosis includes low grade pyogenic infection, rheumatoid disease, myeloma, or secondary metastatic deposits [1]. Poor response to ordinary antibiotic therapy should lead to suspicion of underlying tuberculosis especially in underdeveloped nations with poor living conditions and relevant investigations should be carried out. It has been suggested that all radiological and imaging modalities are complementary but MRI is probably the best imaging modality for early detection and diagnosis of

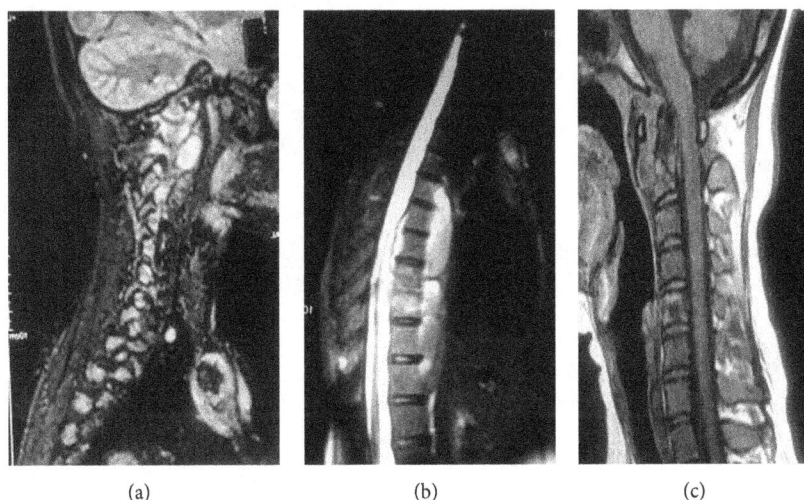

(a)   (b)   (c)

FIGURE 3: MRI images showing involvement of sternoclavicular joint along with dorsal and upper cervical involvement.

sternoclavicular joint tuberculosis [8], and final diagnosis should be made only after confirmation with bacteriological or histological examination, as image findings are not fully reliable for differentiating spinal TB from other infections or neoplasms [9]. In our case, the MRI confirmed a lytic lesion on the medial end of the clavicle along with sclerosis and a collection of fluid around right sternoclavicular joint and could also suggest the possibility of concomitant pulmonary and spinal tuberculosis. Presence of pulmonary tuberculosis was confirmed by examination of the sputum of the patient. The final histological and microbiological confirmation of skeletal tuberculosis is by fine needle aspiration or open biopsy [3]. Diagnosis in our case too was confirmed by demonstration of AFB on ZN stain and by histological examination. In countries where tuberculosis is a common condition, a physician tends to attend to multiple cases of pulmonary tuberculosis. Some patients have skeletal tuberculosis with or without presence of concomitant pulmonary tuberculosis [6, 10–12]. It is very important that the treating physician picks up these cases early in the course of the disease. A physician needs to be aware that patients with pulmonary tuberculosis need to be investigated or screened for presence of skeletal involvement if they have any swelling in the neck or neck and back pain and should not be passed off as malaise.

Usual pulmonary TB treatment lasts from 9 to 12 months but in pulmonary TB if there is skeletal involvement prolonged antibiotic treatment is to be given as per majority consensus [13]. A 14–18-month duration of antitubercular therapy is required in spinal and sternoclavicular tuberculosis [3, 13]. Total duration of antitubercular therapy in our case was also of 18 months.

To conclude, a diagnosis of multicentric tuberculosis should be kept in mind in case of patients with atypical presentations in unusual locations with constitutional symptoms in endemic areas especially among undernourished and among those living in poor conditions. Examination of sputum should be performed in each case of suspected pulmonary tuberculosis. Imaging modalities should be supplemented with fine needle aspiration cytology or open biopsy to confirm the diagnosis. Timely diagnosis and treatment of multicentric tuberculosis will prevent further complications including paraplegia or deformity because of spinal tuberculosis or compression or erosion of the large blood vessels at the base of the neck and migration of the tuberculous abscess to the mediastinum in case of tuberculosis of sternoclavicular joint. Also the role of proper multidrug antitubercular therapy needs to be emphasized as tuberculosis can be very well managed with medications.

References

[1] S. M. Tuli, *Tuberculosis of the Skeletal System: Bones, Joints, Spine and Bursal Sheaths*, Jaypee, New Delhi, India, 1993.

[2] A. Shrivastav, J. Pal, P. S. Karmakar, and N. B. Debnath, "Tuberculosis of sternoclavicular joint-uncommon manifestation of a common disease," *Journal of Medicine*, vol. 11, no. 1, pp. 102–104, 2010.

[3] M. S. Dhillon, R. K. Gupta, R. Bahadur, and O. N. Nagi, "Tuberculosis of the sternoclavicular joints," *Acta Orthopaedica Scandinavica*, vol. 72, no. 5, pp. 514–517, 2001.

[4] S. Singh, C. Nagaraj, G. N. Khare, and V. Kumaraswamy, "Multicentric tuberculosis at two rare sites in an immunocompetent adult," *Journal of Orthopaedics and Traumatology*, vol. 12, no. 4, pp. 223–225, 2011.

[5] S. Nachimuthu, L. N. Gopal, S. Alrawi, V. Natesan, T. Seenivasan, and S. K. Raju, "Multicentric spinal tuberculosis with a possible concomitant bacterial infection," *Hospital Physician*, vol. 36, pp. 61–66, 2000.

[6] B. K. Adams, E. Ahmed, and Z. Y. Al-Haider, "Multicentric skeletal tuberculosis in the absence of pulmonary disease," *Clinical Nuclear Medicine*, vol. 29, no. 8, pp. 507–508, 2004.

[7] A. Mofredj, J.-M. Guerin, F. Leibinger, and R. Masmoudi, "Primary sternal osteomyelitis and septicaemia due to *Staphylococcus aureus*," *Scandinavian Journal of Infectious Diseases*, vol. 31, no. 1, pp. 98–100, 1999.

[8] P. Khare, V. Sharma, and S. Khare, "Tuberculosis of the Sternoclavicular Joint," *Journal of Orthopaedics, Trauma and Rehabilitation*, vol. 17, no. 2, pp. 96–98, 2013.

[9] I. M. Francis, D. K. Das, U. K. Luthra, Z. Sheikh, M. Sheikh, and M. Bashir, "Value of radiologically guided fine needle aspiration cytology (FNAC) in the diagnosis of spinal tuberculosis: a study of 29 cases," *Cytopathology*, vol. 10, no. 6, pp. 390–401, 1999.

[10] A. Kaya, Z. Topu, S. Fitoz, and N. Numanoglu, "Pulmonary tuberculosis with multifocal skeletal involvement," *Monaldi Archives for Chest Disease*, vol. 61, no. 2, pp. 133–135, 2004.

[11] D. K. Sen, "Skeletal tuberculosis associated with pulmonary tuberculosis. A review of 24 cases," *Journal of the Indian Medical Association*, vol. 36, pp. 146–149, 1961.

[12] S. Blaustein and M. Wysell, "Pulmonary and skeletal tuberculosis," *The Mount Sinai Journal of Medicine*, vol. 64, no. 6, p. 419, 1997.

[13] A. Hazra and B. Laha, "Chemotherapy of osteoarticular tuberculosis," *Indian Journal of Pharmacology*, vol. 37, no. 1, pp. 5–12, 2005.

20

Congenital Pulmonary Airway Malformation in an Adult Male: A Case Report with Literature Review

Dipti Baral,[1] Bindu Adhikari,[2] Daniel Zaccarini,[1] Raj Man Dongol,[2] and Birendra Sah[1]

[1]SUNY Upstate Medical University, East Adams Street, Syracuse, NY 13210, USA
[2]College of Medical Sciences, Bharatpur 44207, Nepal

Correspondence should be addressed to Dipti Baral; diptibaral@gmail.com

Academic Editor: Manel Luján

Congenital pulmonary airway malformation (CPAM) is a rare cystic lung lesion formed as a result of anomalous development of airways in fetal life. Majority of the cases are recognized in neonates and infants with respiratory distress with very few presenting later in adult life. A 24-year-old male with history of three separate episodes of pneumonia in the last 6 months presented with left sided pleuritic chest pain for 4 days. He was tachycardic and tachypneic at presentation. White blood count was 14×10^9/L. Chest X-ray showed left lower lobe opacity. CT angiogram of thorax showed a well-defined area of low attenuation in the left lower lobe with dedicated pulmonary arterial and venous drainage and resolving infection, suggesting CPAM. He underwent left lower lobe lobectomy. Histopathology confirmed type 2 CPAM. CPAM is a rare congenital anatomic abnormality that can present with recurrent infections in adults. As a number of cases remain asymptomatic and symptomatic cases are often missed, prevalence of CPAM might be higher than currently reported.

1. Background

Congenital pulmonary airway malformation (CPAM), previously known as congenital cystic adenomatoid malformation (CCAM), is a developmental lesion of the lung comprising single or multiple cysts of uniform or varying sizes arising from anomalous growth of airways. Most of the cases are identified in infants and neonates with respiratory distress. CPAM can be a cause of pulmonary hypoplasia, severe nonimmune fetal hydrops, and fetal death [1]. On rare occasions, CPAM can present in adulthood with recurrent chest infections, pneumothorax, hemoptysis, or dyspnea [2]. CPAM has been found to be associated malignancies. Ignorance about the existence of this lung condition can lead to missed and delayed diagnosis. We report a rare case of a 24-year-old male who was diagnosed with CPAM during the work-up of recurrent pneumonia.

2. Case Summary

A 24-year-old male presented to the hospital with four-day history of moderate left sided chest pain radiating to the back.

The chest pain got worse with deep inspiration. He denied fever, chills, cough, hemoptysis, night sweats, weight loss, and recent travel. Past medical history was significant for three episodes of left lower lobe pneumonia in the past 6 months. He was treated initially with ceftibuten and azithromycin and then with a course of oral levofloxacin and most recently with amoxicillin-clavulanic acid for recurring symptoms of cough, pleuritic chest pain, and subjective fever. Currently, he was taking meloxicam as needed for chest pain. Past surgical history included right inguinal hernia repair five years ago. There was no family history of cancer, early death, or cardiac disease. He had immigrated from Guatemala four years ago and was single and unemployed. He denied any high-risk sexual behaviors or drug abuse in the present or past. He drank two beers about once or twice per week and denied smoking history. His differential diagnoses at this point include lung abscess, tuberculosis infection, foreign body aspiration, HIV with opportunistic infection, congenital immunodeficiency states, and congenital developmental anomaly of the lung.

On examination, he was tachycardic with a pulse rate of 101/min and was tachypneic at 22/min. Rest of the physical examination including respiratory examination was normal.

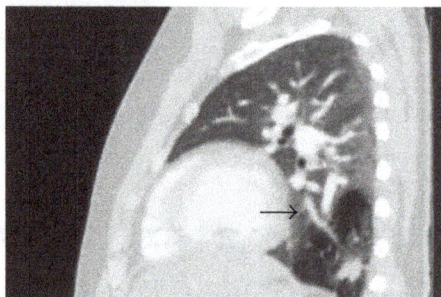

FIGURE 1: CT thorax sagittal image showing hypodense lesion in the left lower lobe posteriorly with resolving infiltrates within. Arrow: pulmonary vein branch.

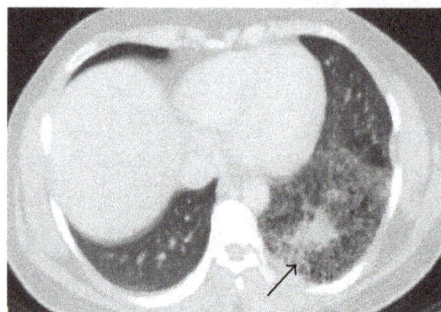

FIGURE 3: CT scan 4 months ago showing infiltrates in the left lower lung.

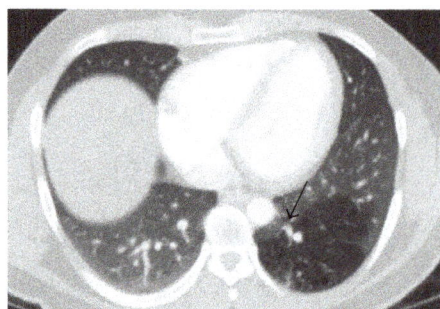

FIGURE 2: CT angiography shows dedicated pulmonary artery and vein supplying the hypolucent area. Small cysts can be appreciated within the hypolucent area.

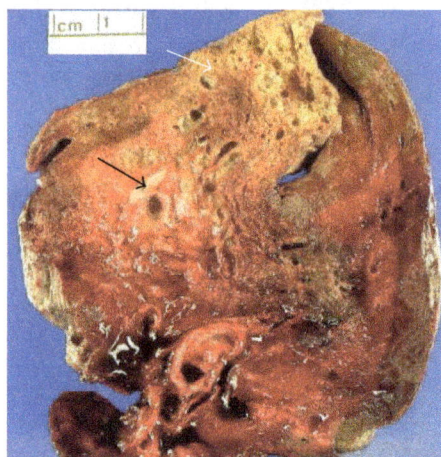

FIGURE 4: Gross photograph showing multiple air filled microcysts at periphery of lung (white arrow) and a larger cyst (black arrow).

Labs revealed complete blood counts of 14×10^9/L with 75% neutrophils. Basic metabolic panel and liver function tests were normal. Urine legionella antigen was negative, as well as antibodies to human immunodeficiency virus. His chest X-ray showed left lower lobe opacity. He was started on ceftriaxone and azithromycin for community acquired pneumonia and was admitted to the floor. Tuberculin skin test was positive with 18 mm induration at 72 hours. Interferon gamma release assay was negative. Blood cultures demonstrated no growth for 5 days.

CT angiogram of thorax showed 9 cm well-defined area of low attenuation in the left lower lobe (Figure 1) with infiltrates inside. This lesion demonstrated a dedicated pulmonary artery and pulmonary vein (Figure 2); these vessels were emerging from the hilar region. No systemic arteries or anomalous arterial supply was identified within the lesion. There was no pleural involvement or abnormal lymphadenopathy. A radiologic diagnosis of congenital pulmonary airway malformation (CPAM) was made. Review of previous chest X-rays and computed tomography (CT) of the thorax from the time of his previous episodes of pneumonia revealed various degrees of consolidation in left lower base in this particular area (Figure 3). CT abdomen pelvis did not show any abnormal intra-abdominal masses or pathology but showed some hepatic steatosis.

As his CT images were highly suggestive of congenital cystic lung lesion, surgical excision was planned to prevent further episodes of pneumonias. Bronchoscopy prior to

the surgery revealed normal segmental airways in the left lower lobe. Initially left thoracoscopy was tried; however posterolateral thoracotomy was required for better visualization of the involved anatomy. Upon direct visualization, the complete lobe was involved in chronic inflammation. The lesion had no abnormal arterial supply from aorta or below the diaphragm and was connected through air passages. Left lower lobectomy was done. On gross examination, a relatively well-demarcated lesion with a 1.5 × 1.5 cm thin walled cyst with inspissated mucus within and multiple air filled microcysts at the peripheral aspect of the cyst was noted (Figure 4). Microscopic examination revealed larger cyst with columnar ciliated epithelium (Figure 5) and dispersed bronchiole-like structures within the alveolated parenchyma (Figure 6). The pathologic diagnosis was consistent with type 2 CPAM. There was no major surgical complication. He developed a small hydro pneumothorax postoperatively, which resolved on its own. Patient has been doing well 12 months after the diagnosis.

3. Discussion

Congenital pulmonary airway malformation involves increased proliferation and cystic dilatation of different parts of the airways. CPAM comprises around 25% of all congenital

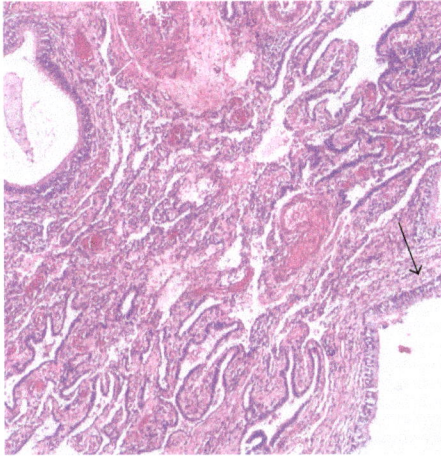

FIGURE 5: Higher power view of largest cyst (black arrow) showing columnar ciliated epithelium and adjacent smaller cyst (white arrow) with similar lining.

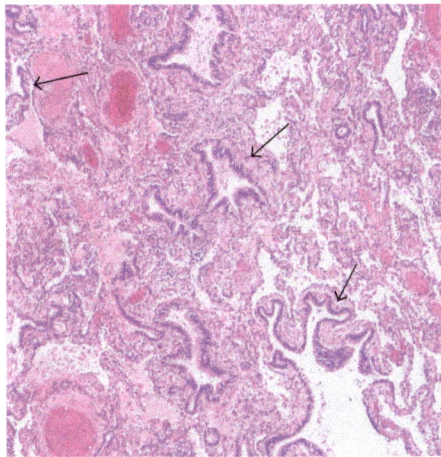

FIGURE 6: Numerous bronchiole-like structures (black arrows).

lung lesions [3] with an estimated incidence of 1 in 25,000–35,000 pregnancies [4]. CCAM was first described in 1949 by Chin and Tank [5]. Stocker et al. [6] initially classified CCAM into three types in 1977 based on the size and number of the cysts. In 1994, Stocker further expanded the CCAM classification into five categories (Table 1). There are five stages of fetal lung development-embryonic phase, pseudoglandular phase, canalicular phase, saccular phase, and alveolar phase. Types 0–3 originate during the pseudoglandular stage of lung development and type 4 originates during the saccular stage of lung development. This expanded reclassification of CCAM, now renamed CPAM, demonstrates that, as you progress from type 0 to type 4, the main pathologic origin moves from the bronchus, to bronchiole, and then to alveolar tissue. Accordingly, the epithelium varies from pseudostratified to cuboidal to low-cuboidal and simple squamous [7]. It is important to note that frequently there is an overlap between the different types [8]. Type 1 and type 4 CPAM, which have larger cysts, are difficult to differentiate from

cystic pleuropulmonary blastoma because of its cystic nature [9].

Histologically the different types of CCAM can usually be distinguished. Type 1 is the commonest type comprising 50–65% of all cases and is characterized by single or multiple larger cysts more than 2 or 3 cm in diameter lined by pseudostratified ciliated columnar epithelium and, sometimes, mucinous type epithelium [2, 7, 10, 11]. Type 2 lesions are characterized by multiple, uniform small (<2–2.5 cm) terminal bronchiole-like cysts lined by cuboidal to columnar epithelium [10]. Our case demonstrated these features and was diagnosed as type 2 CPAM. Type 2 is frequently associated with other congenital lesions [8]. Type 3 CPAM consists of bronchiole-like structures lined by ciliated cuboidal epithelium separated by alveolus-sized structures. Cysts in type 3 CPAM are small and not grossly visible [8]. This type usually involves an entire lung and has spongy appearance with bulk gland-like structures [6].

The exact mechanism of the formation of CPAM is still unknown. No clear hereditary association has been derived so far. However, it has been related to chromosomal abnormalities like trisomy 18 and hereditary renal dysplasia [8]. Some authors believe these lesions develop during the sixth and seventh week of fetal development from arrested growth of localized portions of bronchial tree while others have a concept that they are hamartomatous growth of the bronchial tree [12, 13]. Mutation disrupting TTF-1 (thyroid transcription factor-1), a factor expressed in bronchial and alveolar epithelium that regulates lung epithelial differentiation, has also been considered for the development of CPAMs [2]. Abnormal airways in CPAM have been shown to express high levels of HoxB5 (Homeobox protein) compared to normal lung tissues. Normally HoxB5 gene encodes a protein that regulates normal lung development by working as a sequence-specific transcription factor. This is a part of the developmental regulatory system that provides cells with specific positional identities on the anterior-posterior axis. So it has been postulated that this abnormal expression of HoxB5 gene could also be responsible for the development of CPAM by causing aberrant airway branching patterns [3].

For the most part, CPAM presents with acute respiratory distress in neonates and infants, but occasionally it can remain unnoticed until adolescence or later life [14]. McDonough et al. identified 42 cases of CPAM in the literature up until February 2012 presenting at an age greater than 17 years with equal prevalence in males and females [2]. We found five more cases of CPAM recognized in that age group in the English literature review from February 2012 to February 2015 [15–19]. Almost 44% of CPAM patients are found to have lower lobe lung lesions, primarily unilateral [3]. The most common clinical presentation in adults is recurrent pulmonary infection, pneumothorax, hemoptysis, fever, and dyspnea [2]. Our patient presented with recurrent pneumonia and persistent chest pain in the same location of the lung. 24% of all 42 CPAM cases identified by McDonough were asymptomatic with only radiologic abnormalities. Morelli et al. in their literature review found 9 asymptomatic cases among 45 cases (20%); their review included CPAM cases between ages 6 months and 65 years [20]. Hence, it is

TABLE 1

	Type 0	Type 1	Type 2	Type 3	Type 4
Also called	Acinar dysplasia		Intermediate	Solid	
Frequency	1–3%	50–65%,	20–25%,	8%	10%
Relative frequency	Fifth	Most common	Second most common	Fourth	Third
Presumed site of development	Tracheobronchial	Bronchial or bronchiolar	Bronchiolar	Bronchiolar/alveolar	Distal acinar
Clinical presentation as adult	No reports	If smaller, may present later in life with recurrent infections (36 reported cases) [2, 15–19]	10 previously reported cases [2, 15]	No reports	One case [18]
Cyst size	0.5 cm	2 to 10 cm	<2–2.5 cm	<0.2 cm	Varying, up to 7 cm
Cyst lining	Ciliated pseudostratified	Cuboidal to pseudostratified columnar	Cuboidal to columnar, ciliated, may resemble ectatic bronchiole-like structures	Ciliated cuboidal, resembling fetal lung in canalicular stage	Types 1 and 2 alveolar, resembling bullous emphysema
Cyst wall	Connective tissue and vasculature	Broad fibromuscular connective tissue	Small amount of fibrovascular connective tissue	Usually solid	Thin, uniform, central loose vascular tissue
Other histologic findings	Bronchial-like structures, cartilaginous airways, smooth muscle	Cartilage islands, one-third showing mucous cells, sometimes in clusters	Entrapped bronchovascular bundles near edge of lesion; occasionally mature skeletal muscle	Solid, curved channels	Large cysts usually in peripheral lung
Risk of malignancy	Not identified	Bronchioloalveolar Carcinoma	Not identified	Not identified	Must rule out pleuropulmonary blastoma

Adapted from [2, 7, 10, 11].

difficult to estimate the prevalence of CPAM in general adult population. Other congenital lesions like bronchopulmonary sequestrations, lobar emphysema, renal dysgenesis, intestinal atresia, esophageal cysts, congenital cardiac disease, and so forth have been associated with CPAM [21] and can cause various presenting symptoms depending on the involved organ system. Among the 5 types, type 2 has been found to frequently coexist with these congenital lesions [20].

CPAM is diagnosed by CT scans or MRI of chest. CPAM can be diagnosed prenatally by ultrasonography and is categorized into two groups based on the size of the cysts. Echogenic and solid cysts with diameter <5 mm are microcystic lesions and those with one or more cysts with diameter >5 mm are macrocystic lesions [22, 23]. However ultrasonography can misdiagnose other pathologies like congenital diaphragmatic hernia, bronchopulmonary sequestration, lung atresia, tracheal atresia, and bronchial stenosis as CPAM. Therefore MRI should be the diagnostic imaging choice during prenatal life [24, 25]. Incidence of prenatal diagnosis has increased with the increased use of ultrasound; however it is important to remember that up to 56% of these lesions regress later [8]. The recommended diagnostic test for CPAM in postnatal life is CT scan of the chest [9, 24, 26, 27]. CPAM appears as a large cyst or a cluster of cysts filled with gas or liquid resembling a solid mass in CT scans [28]. CT scan findings vary depending upon the type of CPAM and clinical presentation.

The differential diagnosis of CPAM in adults includes pulmonary sequestration, bronchogenic cysts, and acquired cystic lesions. Bronchogenic cysts arise as an abnormal budding from the primitive tracheobronchial tube. One-fourth of bronchogenic cysts are intrapulmonary, while the rest occur in the mediastinum. Intrapulmonary cysts are usually located in the lower lobes [1]. They are usually unilocular and contain bronchial cartilage, smooth muscle, and mucous gland histologically. Bronchogenic cysts usually do not communicate with alveoli, while adenomatoid malformations do [11]. Pulmonary sequestration is seen as a mass of pulmonary tissue that does not connect with the bronchial passages and has an anomalous blood supply [10]. If the mass is outside the pleura it is defined as extralobar pulmonary sequestration (ELPS). It is called intralobar if it shares pleura with the lung. ELPS is usually detected in the prenatal and neonatal period while late childhood and adulthood diagnosis is common with ILPS [1]. Pulmonary sequestrations can be ruled out radiologically as they have anomalous systemic arterial supply arising from thoracic or abdominal aorta unlike CPAM. It is also wise to be aware that acquired cystic lesions can occur in Ehlers-Danlos syndrome and should be included in the differential diagnosis [29].

It is estimated that approximately 1% of CPAMs, particularly types I and IV, transform into malignancy although the exact incidence is unknown [30]. Mucous cells in type 1 CPAM have tendency to undergo malignant changes

[31]. The most common malignancy associated in adults is bronchioloalveolar carcinoma; however, other malignancies like rhabdomyosarcoma, pleuropulmonary blastoma, and adenocarcinoma of lung have been recognized as well [32]. Malignant transformation might start during uterine life with the transformation of epithelial cells in CPAM tissues to atypical epithelial cells via the EGFR pathway. The atypical cells can then progress to papillary predominant adenocarcinoma. The detection of these atypical epithelial cells in the pathological examination of resected tissue emphasizes the importance of complete surgical resection [16].

Due to the risk of malignant transformation and recurrent respiratory infections, most suggest surgical resection at the time of diagnosis for the definitive treatment of symptomatic CPAM cases. In the pediatric population, surgical resection of all cystic lung lesions is generally recommended to prevent complications that may lead to more complex operation later on and also to pick up occult malignancies that are not identified preoperatively [33, 34]. For any age, the type and extent of surgical resection remain a debate. Traditionally lobectomy has been preferred because of the fear of incomplete removal of the pulmonary malformation [35] and complications like air leak associated with lung sparing surgeries [34]. Fascetti-Leon et al. in their retrospective review of 81 patients found lung sparing resection to be safe and effective with no increased risk of residual disease and recurrence if accurately planned in selected patients [36]. Bagrodia et al. came up with similar conclusion, while they suggested thoracotomy and possible lobectomy may still be necessary in cases with limited pulmonary reserve and larger malformations [35]. The resected specimen should always be carefully examined to look for occult malignancy [33]. Patients with bilateral CPAM with extensive lung involvement are mostly managed with conservative treatments, as surgery is risky and difficult [15]. Diagnosis in these cases can be confirmed by lung biopsy.

The treatment of asymptomatic CPAM is not well defined as the true incidence of complications in asymptomatic CPAM is unknown. Some authors argue against prophylactic surgeries stating that the risk of malignancy is overemphasized [2, 32]. They suggest close observation if the patient is agreeable after understanding the possible complications [32]. Also, prophylactic resection of CPAM lesions might not always be fully protective. Papagiannopoulos et al. state that prophylactic resection of lesions in CPAM patients does not protect them from later development of pleuropulmonary blastoma [34]. Even after resection of the lesion, it is recommended to closely observe patients for malignancy. Balkanli et al. described a case of bronchioloalveolar carcinoma in 19-year-old patient after undergoing resection of CPAM in infancy [32]. EGFR tyrosine kinase inhibitors can be beneficial in treating adenocarcinoma arising from type 1 CPAM with EGFR-mutation [16].

Survival rate at 6 months of age seems to have improved [14] probably because of the increased number of identified CPAM from the more common use of prenatal ultrasound. Prognoses among adult CPAM cases vary. Enuh et al. reported CPAM with aspergillosis in a 59-year-old male who died secondary to massive hemoptysis and development of disseminated intravascular coagulation during lobectomy [14]. Morelli et al. described CPAM in a 38-year-old male with persistent cough and hemoptysis who did well after lobectomy [20]. Because of the higher percentage of asymptomatic cases of CPAM and various degrees of lung involvement, it might be difficult to determine the prognosis in adults.

4. Conclusion

In otherwise healthy individuals presenting with recurrent pneumonias, causes for repeated infections need to be sought. If the same location is involved repeatedly, then any anatomic abnormality in the area needs to be considered. Careful review of history and images can reveal congenital lesions like CPAM. Though CPAM is extremely rare in adult patients, it should still be considered in the differential diagnosis of cystic lung disease. The prevalence of CPAM in adults might be higher than currently reported. CT scans are the initial diagnostic choices. Surgical resection prevents further episodes of infections and malignant transformation. Because of a small but definite risk of malignancy, it is also recommended to closely observe the individuals with CPAM for malignancy even after resection of the lesion.

References

[1] A. Turkyilmaz, Y. Aydin, A. Erdem, A. Eroglu, and N. Karaoglanoglu, "Congenital cystic pulmonary malformations in children: our experience with 19 patients," *The Eurasian Journal of Medicine*, vol. 41, no. 1, pp. 15–21, 2009.

[2] R. J. McDonough, A. S. Niven, and K. A. Havenstrite, "Congenital pulmonary airway malformation: a case report and review of the literature," *Respiratory Care*, vol. 57, no. 2, pp. 302–306, 2012.

[3] E. Taştekin, U. Usta, A. Kaynar et al., "Congenital pulmonary airway malformation type 2: a case report with review of the literature," *Japanese Journal of Clinical Oncology*, vol. 44, no. 3, pp. 278–281, 2014.

[4] J. M. Laberge, H. Flageole, D. Pugash et al., "Outcome of the prenatally diagnosed congenital cystic adenomatoid lung malformation: a Canadian experience," *Fetal Diagnosis and Therapy*, vol. 16, no. 3, pp. 178–186, 2001.

[5] K. T. Chin and M. Y. Tank, "Congenital adenomatoid malformation of one lobe of lung with general anasarca," *Archives of Pathology & Laboratory Medicine*, vol. 48, no. 3, pp. 221–229, 1949.

[6] J. T. Stocker, J. E. Madewell, and R. M. Drake, "Congenital cystic adenomatoid malformation of the lung. Classification and morphologic spectrum," *Human Pathology*, vol. 8, no. 2, pp. 155–171, 1977.

[7] J. T. Stocker, "Cystic lung disease in infants and children," *Fetal and Pediatric Pathology*, vol. 28, no. 4, pp. 155–184, 2009.

[8] A. M. Collins, P. F. Ridgway, R. P. Killeen, J. D. Dodd, and M. Tolan, "Congenital cystic adenomatoid malformation of the

lung: hazards of delayed diagnosis," *Respirology*, vol. 14, no. 7, pp. 1058–1060, 2009.

[9] M. Shimohira, M. Hara, M. Kitase et al., "Congenital pulmonary airway malformation: CT-pathologic correlation," *Journal of Thoracic Imaging*, vol. 22, no. 2, pp. 149–153, 2007.

[10] A.-L. A. Katzenstein, F. B. Askin, and V. A. Livolsi, *Katzenstein and Askin's Surgical Pathology of Non-Neoplastic Lung Disease*, vol. 13, Saunders, 1997.

[11] K. O. Leslie and M. R. Wick, *Practical Pulmonary Pathology: A Diagnostic Approach*, Elsevier Health Sciences, 2005.

[12] J. T. Stocker, "The respiratory tract," in *Pediatric Pathology*, J. T. Stocker and L. P. Dehner, Eds., pp. 445–517, Lippincott Williams & Wilkins, Philadelphia, Pa, USA, 2nd edition, 2001.

[13] J. A. Whitsett, "Genetic disorders influencing lung formation and function at birth," *Human Molecular Genetics*, vol. 13, no. 2, pp. R207–R215, 2004.

[14] H. A. Enuh, E. L. Arsura, Z. Cohen et al., "A fatal case of congenital pulmonary airway malformation with aspergillosis in an adult," *International Medical Case Reports Journal*, vol. 7, no. 1, pp. 53–56, 2014.

[15] A. Feng, H. Cai, Q. Sun, Y. Zhang, L. Chen, and F. Meng, "Congenital cystic adenomatoid malformation of lung in adults: 2 rare cases report and review of the literature," *Diagnostic Pathology*, vol. 7, no. 1, article 37, 2012.

[16] M. Hasegawa, F. Sakai, K. Arimura et al., "EGFR mutation of adenocarcinoma in congenital cystic adenomatoid malformation/congenital pulmonary airway malformation: a case report," *Japanese Journal of Clinical Oncology*, vol. 44, no. 3, pp. 278–281, 2014.

[17] S. Tetsumoto, T. Kijima, E. Morii et al., "Echinoderm microtubule-associated protein-like 4 (EML4)-anaplastic lymphoma kinase (ALK) rearrangement in congenital pulmonary airway malformation," *Clinical Lung Cancer*, vol. 14, no. 4, pp. 457–460, 2013.

[18] E. D. McLoney, P. T. Diaz, J. Tran, K. Shilo, and S. Ghosh, "Congenital pulmonary airway malformation presenting as unilateral cystic lung disease," *The American Journal of Respiratory and Critical Care Medicine*, vol. 188, no. 8, pp. 1030–1031, 2013.

[19] N. Harini, R. Chakravarthy, and L. Archana, "Congenital pulmonary airway malformation with mucoepidermoid carcinoma: a case report and review of literature," *Indian Journal of Pathology and Microbiology*, vol. 55, no. 4, pp. 540–542, 2012.

[20] L. Morelli, I. Piscioli, S. Liccill, S. Donato, A. Catalucci, and F. Del Nonno, "Pulmonary congenital cystic adenomatoid malformation, type I, presenting as a single cyst of the middle lobe in an adult: case report," *Diagnostic Pathology*, vol. 2, no. 1, article 17, 2007.

[21] D. Ankers, N. Sajjad, P. Green, and J. L. McPartland, "Antenatal management of pulmonary hyperplasia (congenital cystic adenomatoid malformation)," *BMJ Case Reports*, vol. 2010, 2010.

[22] N. Scott Adzick, M. R. Harrison, P. L. Glick et al., "Fetal cystic adenomatoid malformation: prenatal diagnosis and natural history," *Journal of Pediatric Surgery*, vol. 20, no. 5, pp. 483–488, 1985.

[23] N. S. Adzick, M. R. Harrison, T. M. Crombleholme, A. W. Flake, and L. J. Howell, "Fetal lung lesions: management and outcome," *The American Journal of Obstetrics and Gynecology*, vol. 179, no. 4, pp. 884–889, 1998.

[24] A. M. Hubbard, N. S. Adzick, T. M. Crombleholme et al., "Congenital chest lesions: diagnosis and characterization with prenatal MR imaging," *Radiology*, vol. 212, no. 1, pp. 43–48, 1999.

[25] Á. Harmath, Á. Csaba, E. Hauzman, J. Hajdú, B. Pete, and Z. Papp, "Congenital lung malformations in the second trimester: prenatal ultrasound diagnosis and pathologic findings," *Journal of Clinical Ultrasound*, vol. 35, no. 5, pp. 250–255, 2007.

[26] M. De Santis, L. Masini, G. Noia, A. F. Cavaliere, N. Oliva, and A. Caruso, "Congenital cystic adenomatoid malformation of the lung: antenatal ultrasound findings and fetal-neonatal outcome. Fifteen years of experience," *Fetal Diagnosis and Therapy*, vol. 15, no. 4, pp. 246–250, 2000.

[27] M. Hernanz-Schulman, "Cysts and cyst like lesions of the lung," *Radiologic Clinics of North America*, vol. 31, no. 3, pp. 631–649, 1993.

[28] E. F. Patz Jr., N. L. Müller, S. J. Swensen, and L. G. Dodd, "Congenital cystic adenomatoid malformation in adults: CT findings," *Journal of Computer Assisted Tomography*, vol. 19, no. 3, pp. 361–364, 1995.

[29] J. Rosai, *Rosai and Ackerman's Surgical Pathology*, Elsevier Health Sciences, Philadelphia, Pa, USA, 10th edition, 2011.

[30] S. Lantuejoul, A. G. Nicholson, G. Sartori et al., "Mucinous cells in type 1 pulmonary congenital cystic adenomatoid malformation as mucinous bronchioloalveolar carcinoma precursors," *The American Journal of Surgical Pathology*, vol. 31, no. 6, pp. 961–969, 2007.

[31] V. Benouaich, B. Marcheix, H. Begueret, L. Brouchet, J. F. Velly, and J. Jougon, "Malignancy of congenital cystic adenomatoid malformation of lung in aged," *Asian Cardiovascular and Thoracic Annals*, vol. 17, no. 6, pp. 634–636, 2009.

[32] S. Balkanli, MA. Özturk, M. Köse et al., "A report of adenocarcinoma in situ and congenital pulmonary airway malformation in a three-day-old infant with a review of the literature," *The Turkish Journal of Pediatrics*, vol. 56, no. 3, pp. 299–302, 2014.

[33] K. Papagiannopoulos, S. Hughes, A. G. Nicholson, and P. Goldstraw, "Cystic lung lesions in the pediatric and adult population: surgical experience at the Brompton hospital," *The Annals of Thoracic Surgery*, vol. 73, no. 5, pp. 1594–1598, 2002.

[34] K. A. Papagiannopoulos, M. Sheppard, A. P. Bush, and P. Goldstraw, "Pleuropulmonary blastoma: is prophylactic resection of congenital lung cysts effective?" *Annals of Thoracic Surgery*, vol. 72, no. 2, pp. 604–605, 2001.

[35] N. Bagrodia, S. Cassel, J. Liao, G. Pitcher, and J. Shilyansky, "Segmental resection for the treatment of congenital pulmonary malformations," *Journal of Pediatric Surgery*, vol. 49, no. 6, pp. 905–909, 2014.

[36] F. Fascetti-Leon, D. Gobbi, S. V. Pavia et al., "Sparing-lung surgery for the treatment of congenital lung malformations," *Journal of Pediatric Surgery*, vol. 48, no. 7, pp. 1476–1480, 2013.

21

Delayed Presentation of Traumatic Diaphragmatic Rupture with Herniation of the Left Kidney and Bowel Loops

Amiya Kumar Dwari,[1] Abhijit Mandal,[1] Sibes Kumar Das,[2] and Sudhansu Sarkar[3]

[1] *Department of Pulmonary Medicine, Bankura Sammilani Medical College, Bankura, West Bengal 722101, India*
[2] *Department of Pulmonary Medicine, Medical College, 88 College Street, Kolkata, West Bengal 700073, India*
[3] *Departtment of Surgery, Bankura Sammilani Medical College, Bankura 722101, India*

Correspondence should be addressed to Sibes Kumar Das; sibesdas67@gmail.com

Academic Editors: J. Murchison and K. Watanabe

Rupture of the diaphragm mostly occurs following major trauma. We report a case of delayed presentation of traumatic diaphragmatic hernia on the left side in a 44-year-old male who presented two weeks after a minor blunt trauma. Left kidney and intestinals coils were found to herniate through the diaphragmatic tear. This case demonstrates the importance of considering the diagnosis in all cases of blunt trauma of the trunk. It also illustrates the rare possibility of herniation of kidney through the diaphragmatic tear.

1. Introduction

Traumatic diaphragmatic hernias (DH) represents only small percentage of all diaphragmatic hernias but it is no longer an uncommon entity. Injury is mostly caused by severe blunt or penetrating trauma [1]. DH may be recognized during the period of hospitalization immediately following trauma. If the diaphragmatic injury is not recognized during the immediate posttraumatic period, the patient may recover and remain symptom free or present either with chronic thoracoabdominal symptoms or with acute emergency due to intestinal strangulation [2]. During the delayed presentation with chronic thoracoabdominal symptoms, the trauma responsible for the injury is often forgotten and the diagnosis is not suspected. A careful history, physical examination, and awareness of the possibility are the prerequisite for timely diagnosis.

Abdominal organs that commonly herniate are stomach, spleen, liver, mesentery, and small and large bowels. Kidney is rarely found to herniate through the diaphragmatic tear [3]. The case is unique due to occurrence of the DH with minor trauma, its delayed presentation, and herniation of the left kidney into the thorax.

2. Case Report

A 44-year-old male patient was kicked in his left lower chest and upper abdomen by a neighbour during a family quarrel. Considering it to be a minor trauma, he continued his daily activities for the next two weeks. He presented to pulmonary medicine outpatient department with left sided dull aching chest pain and nonproductive cough for ten days. There was no history of abdominal pain or haematuria. On examination, he was afebrile but dyspneic (MMRC grade 2) with respiratory rate of 22 breaths/min, oxygen saturation of 96% with room air, pulse rate of 90/min, and blood pressure of 138/84 mm of Hg. On examination of the chest, there was dull note over left infraclavicular area and bowel sounds were audible over the left side of the chest. Examination of other systems was within normal limits.

His chest X-ray PA view revealed a heterogeneous opacity in left lower zone but no evidence of any fracture of rib (Figure 1). He was admitted in the chest indoor. Barium meal examination of stomach and intestine revealed presence of loops of intestine within the left hemithorax (Figure 2). USG of abdomen revealed empty left renal fossa and no free fluid in abdomen. Computed tomography scan of thorax

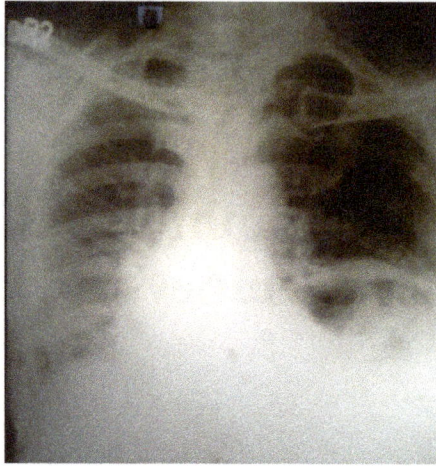

FIGURE 1: Chest X-ray PA view showing a heterogeneous opacity in the left lower zone.

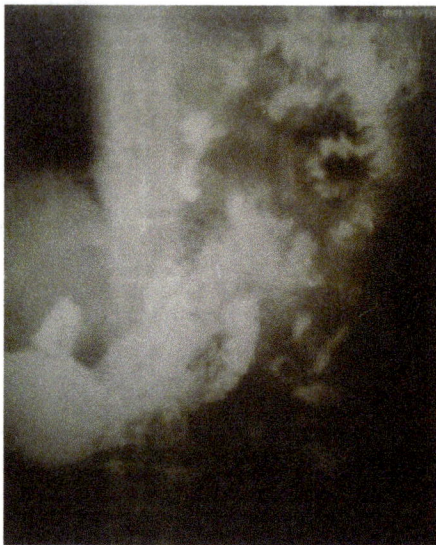

FIGURE 2: Barium meal examination of stomach and intestine showing presence of loops of intestine within the left hemithorax.

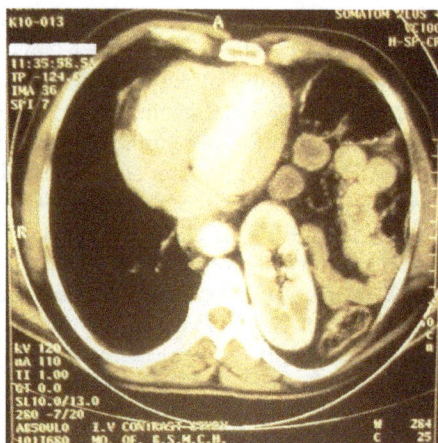

FIGURE 3: Computed tomography scan of thorax showing presence of bowel loops and kidney in the left hemithorax.

showed presence of bowel loops and kidney in the left hemithorax (Figure 3). He was diagnosed to have traumatic left diaphragmatic rupture (DR) with herniation of the intestine and left kidney.

He was shifted to the surgery ward and an emergency thoracoabdominal exploration was performed in the operation theatre. At operation, a rent of 8 cm length with irregular margin was detected in the posterolateral part of the left dome of the diaphragm with herniation of parts of small and large intestine and left kidney into the left thoracic cavity. Intestinal coils and kidney were mobilized from thoracic cavity to abdomen without difficulty. Then the rent was repaired with single layer nonabsorbable suture. His postoperative recovery was uneventful and he was keeping well on followup.

3. Discussion

The traumatic DH was apparently reported by Sennertus in 1541 [4]. Ambroise Pare described the first case of DH at autopsy in 1579. Antemortem diagnosis of traumatic DH was first made by Bowditch in 1853 and the first successful repair was done by Riolfi in 1886 [5].

The reported incidence of diaphragmatic rupture is between 0.8 and 1.6 percent of the patients admitted to the hospital with blunt trauma. The incidence rises upto 15% among patients with penetrating trauma [4]. Male to female ratio of traumatic DH is 4 : 1 and most of them present in the third decade of life.

A 75% of rupture is from blunt abdominothoracic trauma of severe grade (mainly motor vehicle accidents) and 25% from penetrating trauma (from gunshot and stab injury) [6]. Rare causes of rupture include vomiting, coughing, exercise, pregnancy, and iatrogenic injury. Mechanisms of rupture of diaphragm include (a) sudden increase in intrathoracic/intra-abdominal pressure against a fixed diaphragm, (b) shearing stress on a stretched diaphragm, and (c) avulsion of the diaphragm from its point of attachment [7]. Commonest site of rupture is the posterolateral surface along the embryonic fusion line because it is the weakest part of the diaphragm. Left sided rupture occurs in 70%–80% cases, right sided rupture in 15%–24% cases, and bilateral in 5%–8% cases [8]. The greater prevalence of left sided rupture is due to buffer effect of the liver, embryonic weakness of left hemidiaphragm, and underdiagnosis of right diaphragmatic rupture [9–11]. Intrathoracic kidney is very rare and can occur in three possible situations like congenital DH, traumatic DH, or a congenital ectopic kidney. Herniation of left kidney sometimes occurs in Bochdalek hernia which is more common in new born [12].

Grimes has appropriately described the presentation into three phases—the acute phase, latent phase, and obstructive phase [13]. Acute phase is dominated in 95%–100% cases by associated injuries like rib fracture, pelvic fracture, splenic rupture, closed head injury, liver laceration, haemothorax, pneumothorax, and pulmonary contusion. The diagnosis is frequently missed in the acute phase because of the presence of shock, respiratory failure, concomitant visceral injury, and coma which dominate the clinical picture. Delayed presentation of the DH in the latent phase is with upper gastrointestinal symptoms, chest pain, and dyspnea or an abnormal chest radiograph without symptoms. Patients with obstructive phase often present months to years later with incarceration, obstruction, strangulation, or perforation.

Delayed presentation may be due to delayed detection or delayed rupture [14], the former being more likely. Detection may be delayed if diaphragmatic tear remains asymptomatic at the time of injury and manifests only when hernia occurs. Delayed rupture is possible if diaphragmatic tissue is devitalized at the time of injury but maintains a tenuous barrier until several days later when superadded inflammation weakens it.

Diagnosis of traumatic DH is done preoperatively in 43.5% cases, incidentally at laparotomy or thoracotomy or autopsy in 41.3% cases, and a delayed diagnosis in 14.6% cases [6]. Although chest radiograph is the initial diagnostic modality [15], it is diagnostic only in 33% cases of left sided rupture and 18% cases of right sided rupture [16]. Pathognomonic signs include visualization of herniated stomach or bowel in the chest and extension of intragastric tube above the level of diaphragm [16–18]. Suggestive signs are irregularity of the diaphragmatic contour, elevated diaphragm in the absence of atelectasis, contralateral mediastinal shift in the absence of pulmonary or pleural cause, and persistent basal opacity mimicking collapse or supra-phrenic mass [16–18]. Immediate intubation or presence of concomitant pleural effusion or haemothorax may reduce the diagnostic accuracy of chest X-ray. CT scan of the thorax is a useful aid in the diagnosis in urgent or uncertain cases. The important signs are sharp discontinuation of the diaphragm, intrathoracic visceral herniation, lack of visualization of the diaphragm (absent diaphragm sign), and constriction of bowel or stomach at the site of herniation (collar sign) [19–22]. Thoracoscopy in the acute phase within 24 hours of injury or laparoscopy in delayed cases is advised as alternative diagnostic tool [6].

In the acute presentation, operation is mandatory as soon as proper resuscitation is made. Laparotomy is advocated in this stage to look for concomitant abdominal injury, though some advocates thoracotomy in acute DR of right side for better access and repair [23]. Thoracotomy (if required, extended into a thoracoabdominal incision) is advised in the patients with delayed presentation since the adhesions within the chest can be freed easily and reduction and repair of hernia will be easily accomplished. Laparoscopy and video-assisted thorascopic surgery are newer options in patients with delayed presentations as they require hemodynamically stable state. Preoperative examination of the border of the rent in the diaphragm will help in the differentiation between traumatic and congenital DH. If the border is smooth, it is likely a congenital hernia whereas irregular border suggests traumatic rupture. The latter was the finding in this case.

In conclusion, traumatic DH is often missed if it occurs after seemingly innocuous injury or has a delayed presentation. Diagnosis should be reached as early as possible to reduce mortality. To make radiological diagnosis, radiologists should be familiar with a variety of imaging presentation of injury and maintain a high index of suspicion. In a clinically suspected case, if the chest X-ray is noncontributory, further imaging should be advised. Open surgery or endoscopic surgery should be performed immediately to diagnose and treat the injury.

References

[1] M. M. Hegarty, J. V. Bryer, I. B. Angorn, and L. W. Baker, "Delayed presentation of traumatic diaphragmatic hernia," *Annals of Surgery*, vol. 188, no. 2, pp. 229–233, 1978.

[2] B. N. Carter, J. Giuseffi, and B. Felson, "Traumatic diaphragmatic hernia," *The American Journal of Roentgenology, Radium Therapy, and Nuclear Medicine*, vol. 65, no. 1, pp. 56–72, 1951.

[3] Z. Cohen, A. Gabriel, S. Mizrachi, V. Kapuler, and A. J. Mares, "Traumatic avulsion of kidney into the chest through a ruptured diaphragm in a boy," *Pediatric Emergency Care*, vol. 16, no. 3, pp. 180–181, 2000.

[4] D. Bosanquet, A. Farboud, and H. Luckraz, "A review diaphragmatic injury," *Respiratory Medicine CME*, vol. 2, no. 1, pp. 1–6, 2009.

[5] A. Rekha and A. Vikram, "Traumatic diaphragmatic hernia," *Sri Ramachandra Journal of Medicine*, vol. 3, pp. 23–25, 2010.

[6] R. Shah, S. Sabanathan, A. J. Mearns, and A. K. Choudhury, "Traumatic rupture of diaphragm," *Annals of Thoracic Surgery*, vol. 60, no. 5, pp. 1444–1449, 1995.

[7] J. L. Cameron, "Diaphragmatic injury," in *Current Surgical Therapy*, pp. 1095–1100, Mosby, Louis, Mo, USA, 7th edition, 2001.

[8] S. Eren, M. Kantarci, and A. Okur, "Imaging of diaphragmatic rupture after trauma," *Clinical Radiology*, vol. 61, no. 6, pp. 467–477, 2006.

[9] K. Ala-Kulju, K. Verkkala, P. Ketonen, and P.-T. Harjola, "Traumatic rupture of the right hemidiaphragm," *Scandinavian Journal of Thoracic and Cardiovascular Surgery*, vol. 20, no. 2, pp. 109–114, 1986.

[10] B. R. Boulanger, D. P. Milzman, C. Rosati, and A. Rodriguez, "A comparison of right and left blunt traumatic diaphragmatic rupture," *Journal of Trauma*, vol. 35, no. 2, pp. 255–260, 1993.

[11] C. H. Andrus and J. H. Morton, "Rupture of the diaphragm after blunt trauma," *The American Journal of Surgery*, vol. 119, no. 6, pp. 686–693, 1970.

[12] M. Obatake, T. Nakata, M. Nomura et al., "Congenital intrathoracic kidney with right Bochdalek defect," *Pediatric Surgery International*, vol. 22, no. 10, pp. 861–863, 2006.

[13] O. F. Grimes, "Traumatic injuries of the diaphragm. Diaphragmatic hernia," *The American Journal of Surgery*, vol. 128, no. 2, pp. 175–181, 1974.

[14] C. D. Johnson, "Blunt injuries of the diaphragm," *British Journal of Surgery*, vol. 7, pp. 226–230, 1988.

[15] B. K. P. Goh, A. S. Y. Wong, K.-H. Tay, and M. N. Y. Hoe, "Delayed presentation of a patient with a ruptured diaphragm complicated by gastric incarceration and perforation after apparently minor blunt trauma," *Canadian Journal of Emergency Medicine*, vol. 6, no. 4, pp. 277–280, 2004.

[16] R. Gelman, S. E. Mirvis, and D. Gens, "Diaphragmatic rupture due to blunt trauma: sensitivity of plain chest radiographs," *American Journal of Roentgenology*, vol. 156, no. 1, pp. 51–57, 1991.

[17] A. B. van Vugt and F. J. Schoots, "Acute diaphragmatic rupture due to blunt trauma: a retrospective analysis," *Journal of Trauma*, vol. 29, no. 5, pp. 683–686, 1989.

[18] S. A. Groskin, "Selected topics in chest trauma," *Radiology*, vol. 183, no. 3, pp. 605–617, 1992.

[19] E.-Y. Kang and N. L. Müller, "CT in blunt chest trauma: pulmonary, tracheobronchial, and diaphragmatic injuries," *Seminars in Ultrasound CT and MRI*, vol. 17, no. 2, pp. 114–118, 1996.

[20] M. L. van Hise, S. L. Primack, R. S. Israel, and N. L. Müller, "CT in blunt chest trauma: indications and limitations," *Radiographics*, vol. 18, no. 5, pp. 1071–1084, 1998.

[21] S. A. Worthy, E. Y. Kang, T. E. Hartman, J. S. Kwong, J. R. Mayo, and N. L. Müller, "Diaphragmatic rupture: CT findings in 11 patients," *Radiology*, vol. 194, no. 3, pp. 885–888, 1995.

[22] J. G. Murray, E. Caoili, J. F. Gruden, S. J. J. Evans, R. A. Halvorsen Jr., and R. C. Mackersie, "Acute rupture of the diaphragm due to blunt trauma: diagnostic sensitivity and specificity of CT," *American Journal of Roentgenology*, vol. 166, no. 5, pp. 1035–1039, 1996.

[23] O. Kozak, O. Mentes, A. Harlak et al., "Late presentation of blunt right diaphragmatic rupture (hepatic hernia)," *American Journal of Emergency Medicine*, vol. 26, no. 5, pp. 638.e3–638.e5, 2008.

22

High-Flow Nasal Cannula Therapy in a Patient with Reperfusion Pulmonary Edema following Percutaneous Transluminal Pulmonary Angioplasty

Kiyoshi Moriyama,[1] **Toru Satoh,**[2] **Akira Motoyasu,**[1] **Tomoki Kohyama,**[1] **Mariko Kotani,**[1] **Riichiro Kanai,**[1] **Tadao Ando,**[1] **and Tomoko Yorozu**[1]

[1] *Department of Anesthesiology, Kyorin University School of Medicine, 6-20-2 Shinkawa, Mitaka, Tokyo 181-8611, Japan*
[2] *Second Department of Internal Medicine, Kyorin University School of Medicine, 6-20-2 Shinkawa, Mitaka, Tokyo 181-8611, Japan*

Correspondence should be addressed to Kiyoshi Moriyama; mokiyokeio@gmail.com

Academic Editor: Reda E. Girgis

A 62-year-old woman with Wolff-Parkinson-White syndrome was with recent worsening of dyspnea to New York Heart Association functional status Class III. The patient was diagnosed as having central type chronic thromboembolic pulmonary hypertension. By cardiac catheterization, her mean pulmonary artery pressure was 53 mmHg with total pulmonary resistance 2238 dynes·sec·cm^{-5}. After medical therapies with tadalafil, furosemide, ambrisentan, beraprost, and warfarin were initiated, percutaneous transluminal pulmonary angioplasty (PTPA) was performed. Following PTPA, life-threating hypoxemia resulting from postoperative reperfusion pulmonary edema developed. High-flow nasal cannula therapy (HFNC) was applied, and 100% oxygen at 50 L/min of flow was required to keep oxygenation. HFNC was continued for 3 days, and the patient was discharged on 8th postoperative day with SpO$_2$ of 97% on 3 L/min of oxygen inhalation. Because of the simplicity of the technique, the lower cost of equipment, and remarkable patient tolerance to the treatment, we speculate that HFNC can take over the post of noninvasive ventilation as first-line therapy for patients with acute respiratory failure.

1. Introduction

For patients with chronic thromboembolic pulmonary hypertension (CTEPH), percutaneous transluminal pulmonary angioplasty (PTPA) was originally reported in 2001 in USA [1] and now developing in Japan [2, 3]. A troublesome complication associated with PTPA is reperfusion pulmonary edema, which almost always occurs within 48 h after vessel dilation [4]. We experienced a patient suffering from postoperative reperfusion pulmonary edema that was successfully managed with high-flow nasal cannula therapy (HFNC).

2. Case Presentation

A woman with Wolff-Parkinson-White syndrome noticed exercise intolerance and dyspnea at 61 years old. Her symptoms developed from New York Heart Association (NYHA) functional status Class II to III in 3 months. She was diagnosed to have CTEPH by lung perfusion scintigraphy and contrast CT image. Cardiac catheterization was performed and her mean pulmonary arterial pressure (mPAP) was 53 mmHg with total pulmonary resistance 2238 dynes·sec·cm^{-5}. Her brain natriuretic peptide (BNP) level was 306.5 pg/dL, and she started to take tadalafil, furosemide, ambrisentan, beraprost, and warfarin. Because her symptoms worsened on supine position, ambulatory oxygen inhalation therapy while sleeping was started, and PTPA was scheduled.

On admission to our hospital, the patient's NYHA functional status was Class III. Preoperative cardiac catheterization showed that medical therapies decreased her mPAP from 53 to 42 mmHg, total pulmonary resistance from 2238 to 1223 dynes·sec·cm^{-5}, and BNP level from 306.5 to 48.0 pg/dL. Her SaO$_2$ was 93.7% and cardiothoracic ratio on chest X-ray was 56% (Figure 1(a)).

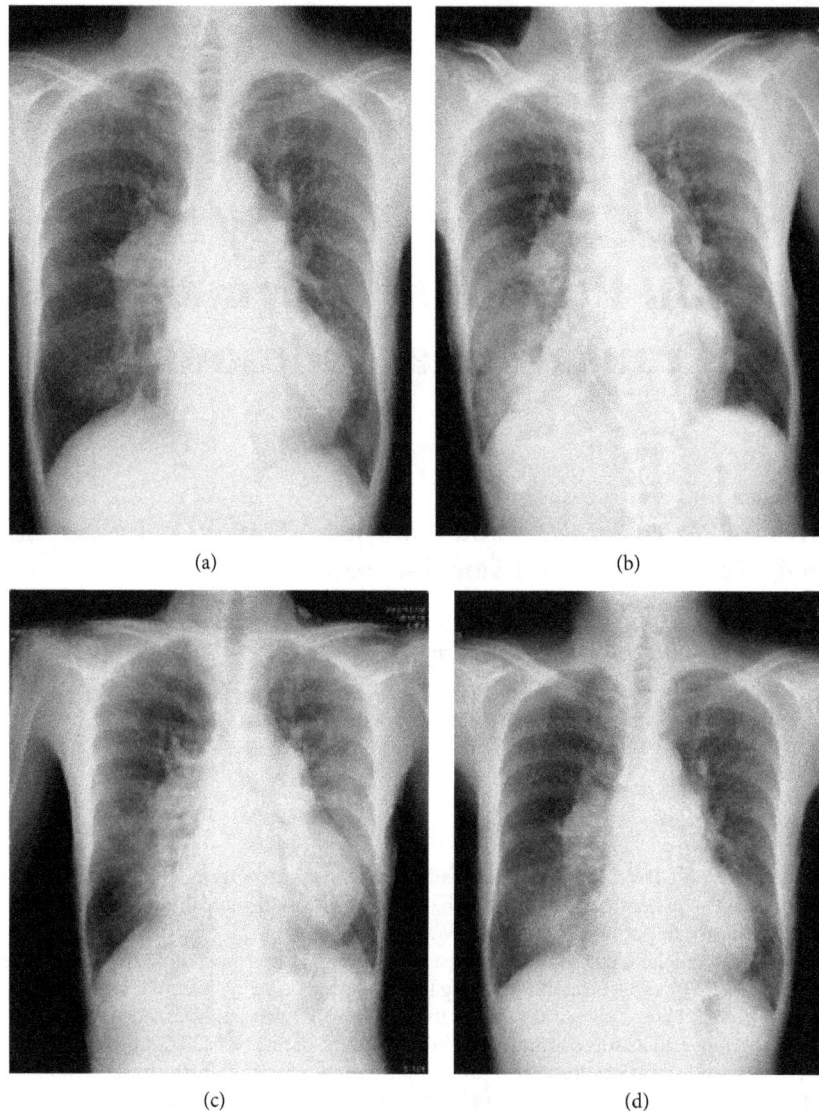

FIGURE 1: Chest X-ray obtained before percutaneous transluminal pulmonary angioplasty (a), on the first postoperative day (POD1) (b), POD4 (c), and POD8 (d). The patient had localized consolidation and atelectasis on her right lower lobe on POD1, 4, and 8, designating postsurgical pulmonary edema in the dilated segment.

Initial PTPA was performed for her right pulmonary artery. The A8 region of her right pulmonary artery was dilated by the balloon (Figure 2). On admission to the ICU (day 0), her mPAP was 37 mmHg and her SpO$_2$ was 99% with 3 L/min of oxygen inhalation through a nasal cannula with no complaint of dyspnea. Twelve hours after admission to the ICU, her SpO$_2$ decreased to 77% with 5 L/min of oxygen inhalation, and pink frothy sputum was noticed with increases in mPAP up to 49 mmHg. To avoid hypoxemia and increases in PAP, HFNC was applied simultaneously with the administration of methylprednisolone (1000 mg/day) and furosemide (10 mg/day).

The initial setting of HFNC was 90% oxygen at 35 L/min of flow. Immediately after applying HFNC, her SpO$_2$ rose up to 93% and her mPAP decreased to 30 mmHg. On day 1, her chest X-ray revealed localized consolidation on her right lower lobe with atelectasis (Figure 1(b)). To avoid the development of pulmonary edema, the flow of HFNC was arisen up to 50 L/min. Figure 3 shows CT scan images obtained on day 3. On day 3, with 50 L/min of flow unchanged, oxygen concentration was decreased to 50%. HFNC was finally discontinued on day 4 with her mPAP 34 mmHg (Figure 1(c)). The patient was discharged on the 8th postoperative day with SpO$_2$ of 97% on 3 L/min of oxygen inhalation (Figure 1(d)).

3. Discussion

PTPA is a catheterization-based interventional management strategy for patients compromised with CTEPH, who are deemed nonsurgical or high-risk surgical candidates of pulmonary thromboendarterectomy [5]. Sugimura et al.

(a)

(b)

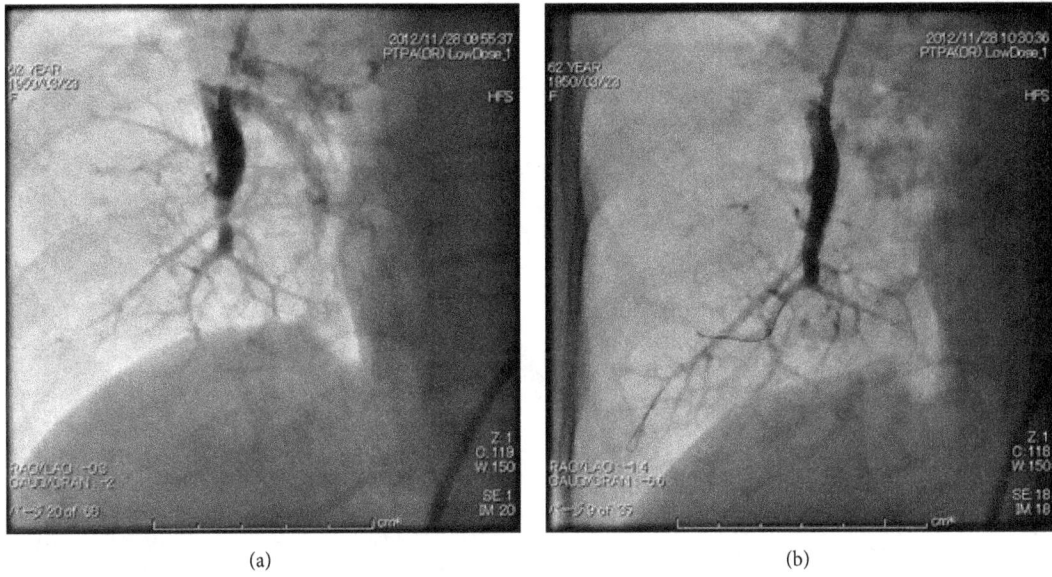

FIGURE 2: Initial percutaneous transluminal pulmonary angioplasty was performed for the right pulmonary artery (a). The A8 region of her right pulmonary artery was dilated by the balloon (plain old balloon atherectomy, b).

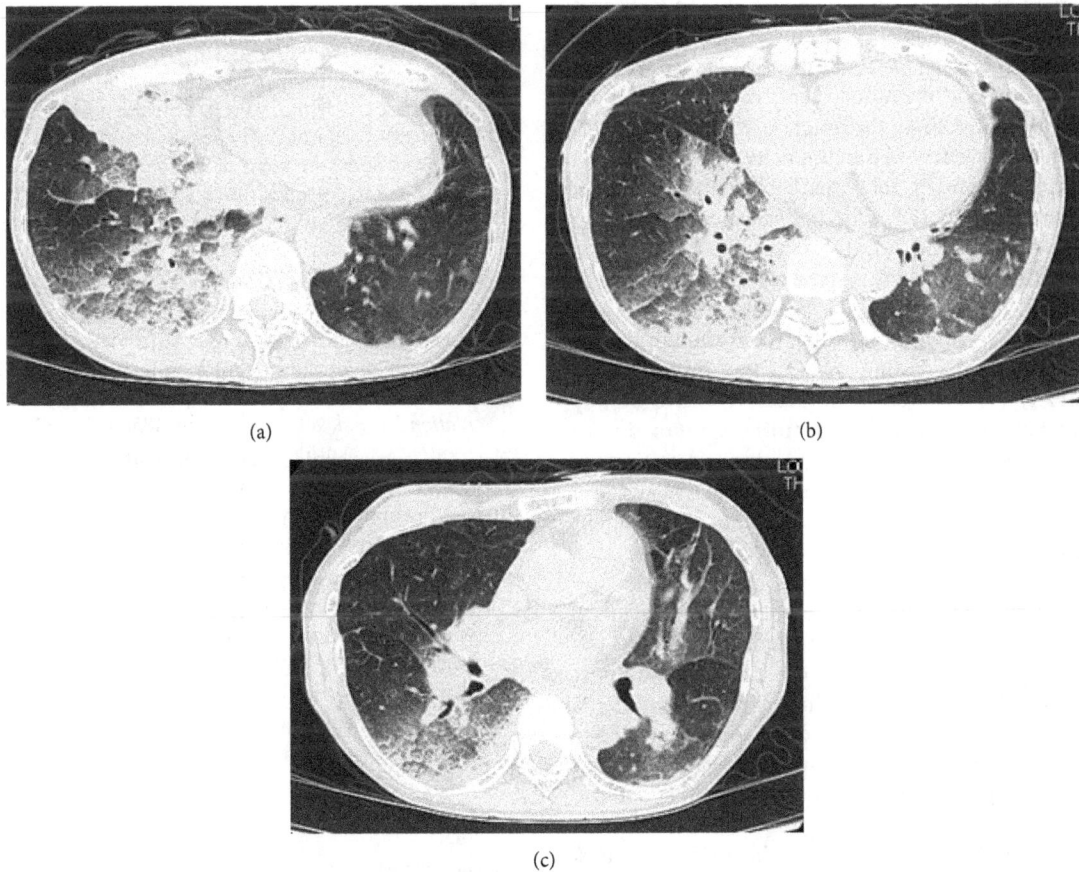

(a)

(b)

(c)

FIGURE 3: CT scan images obtained on the third postoperative day (POD3). The patient had localized consolidation on her right lower lobe with atelectasis, designating postsurgical pulmonary edema in the dilated segment.

reported that PTPA combined with conventional vasodilator treatment was effective in improving pulmonary hemodynamics in patients with distal-type CTEPH [6]. Feinstein et al. reported [1] that the reperfusion pulmonary edema was the most life-threatening postoperative complication following PTPA, and 3/18 patients required mechanical ventilation and 1 patient died 1 week after PTPA.

Typical management of reperfusion pulmonary edema includes diuretics and oxygen. In cases with worsening hypoxemia, noninvasive ventilation has been a first-line intervention to avoid endotracheal intubation [7]. Noninvasive ventilation is a technique to augment alveolar ventilation delivered by face mask, without endotracheal intubation. We previously reported a patient with postsurgical reperfusion pulmonary edema following PTPA [8]. This patient accepted a long duration of 16 days of noninvasive ventilation. However, because of mask tolerance, a long duration of noninvasive ventilation with an almost full-day dependence on ventilatory support is not applicable to all patients, even with slight sedative administration. Díaz-Lobato et al. reported a patient with acute respiratory failure of neuromuscular origin, who did not tolerate noninvasive ventilation but was treated successfully with HFNC [9].

HFNC oxygen therapy is a new alternative to conventional oxygen therapy [10]. HFNC delivers consistent and accurate oxygen concentrations and generates flows up to 60 L/min with optimal heat and humidity (37°C and 44 mg H_2O/L) through a nasal cannula. The therapeutic advantages of HFNC are (1) preventing air dilution, (2) minimizing CO_2 rebreathing, (3) generating moderate positive airway pressure [11], (4) increasing end-expiratory lung volumes and tidal volumes, and (5) maintaining the function of the mucociliary transport system, as well as (6) the simplicity of the technique, the lower cost of equipment, and remarkable patient tolerance to the treatment compared with endotracheal intubation or noninvasive ventilation [9]. These advantages benefited critical care patients with acute respiratory failure [12].

In this case, (1) preventing air dilution was necessary as the patient was severely hypoxemic. (2) Although hypercapnia was absent, decreasing $PaCO_2$ was preferable to decrease mPAP, (3) generating moderate positive airway pressure was helpful to reduce pink frothy sputum due to reperfusion pulmonary edema. (4) Increasing end-expiratory lung volumes and tidal volumes was also helpful because the patient was also compromised with atelectasis. The patient was able to take medications and meals without hypoxemia and had no complaint of HFNC during 4 days.

Because of the simplicity of the technique, the lower cost of equipment, and remarkable patient tolerance to the treatment, we speculate that HFNC can take over the post of noninvasive ventilation as first-line therapy for patients with acute respiratory failure. Parke et al. compared HFNC with conventional high-flow face mask (HFFM) oxygen therapy [13] in 60 patients with hypoxic respiratory failure. They showed that HFNC significantly reduced desaturations and the rate of noninvasive ventilation. In their study, 10% of patients on HFNC required noninvasive ventilation due to worsening respiratory failure. When applying HFNC to patients with respiratory failure, we always need to consider noninvasive ventilation or endotracheal intubation in cases when increased dyspnea, respiratory fatigue, worsening gas exchange, or intolerance of allocated therapy continues.

In summary, we experienced a patient with postsurgical, reperfusion pulmonary edema following PTPA. Severe hypoxemia was successfully treated with HFNC. We speculate that HFNC can take over the post of noninvasive ventilation as first-line therapy for patients with acute respiratory failure.

References

[1] J. A. Feinstein, S. Z. Goldhaber, J. E. Lock, S. M. Ferndandes, and M. J. Landzberg, "Balloon pulmonary angioplasty for treatment of chronic thromboembolic pulmonary hypertension," Circulation, vol. 103, no. 1, pp. 10–13, 2001.

[2] H. Mizoguchi, A. Ogawa, M. Munemasa, H. Mikouchi, H. Ito, and H. Matsubara, "Refined balloon pulmonary angioplasty for inoperable patients with chronic thromb oembolic pulmonary hypertension," Circulation: Cardiovascular Interventions, vol. 5, no. 6, pp. 748–755, 2012.

[3] M. Kataoka, T. Inami, K. Hayashida et al., "Percutaneous transluminal pulmonary angioplasty for the treatment of chronic thromboembolic pulmonary hypertension," Circulation: Cardiovascular Interventions, vol. 5, no. 6, pp. 756–762, 2012.

[4] N. Yamada, "Percutaneous transluminal pulmonary angioplasty for distal-type chronic thromboembolic pulmonary hypertension," Circulation Journal, vol. 76, no. 2, pp. 307–308, 2012.

[5] N. Galiè, M. M. Hoeper, M. Humbert et al., "ESC Committee for Practice Guidelines (CPG). Guidelines for the diagnosis and treatment of pulmonary hypertension: the Task Force for the Diagnosis and Treatment of Pulmonary Hypertension of the European Society of Cardiology (ESC) and the European Respiratory Society (ERS), endorsed by the International Society of Heart and Lung Transplantation (ISHLT)," European Heart Journal, vol. 30, pp. 2493–2537, 2009.

[6] K. Sugimura, Y. Fukumoto, K. Satoh et al., "Percutaneous transluminal pulmonary angioplasty markedly improves pulmonary hemodynamics and long-term prognosis in patients with chronic thromboembolic pulmonary hypertension," Circulation Journal, vol. 76, no. 2, pp. 485–488, 2012.

[7] C. C. Koutsogiannidis, F. C. Ampatzidou, O. G. Ananiadou, T. E. Karaiskos, and G. E. Drossos, "Noninvasive ventilation for post-pneumonectomy severe hypoxemia," Respiratory Care, vol. 57, no. 9, pp. 1514–1516, 2012.

[8] K. Moriyama, S. Sugiyama, K. Uzawa, M. Kotani, T. Satoh, and T. Yorozu, "Noninvasive positive pressure ventilation against reperfusion pulmonary edema following percutaneous transluminal pulmonary angioplasty," Case Reports in Anesthesiology, vol. 2011, Article ID 204538, 3 pages, 2011.

[9] S. Díaz-Lobato, M. A. Folgado, A. Chapa, and S. Mayoralas Alises, "Efficacy of high-flow oxygen by nasal cannula with active humidification in a patient with acute respiratory failure of neuromuscular origin," Respir Care, vol. 58, pp. e164–e167, 2013.

[10] M. F. El-Khatib, "High-flow nasal cannula oxygen therapy during hypoxemic respiratory failure," Respiratory Care, vol. 57, no. 10, pp. 1696–1698, 2012.

[11] R. Parke, S. McGuinness, and M. Eccleston, "Nasal high-flow therapy delivers low level positive airway pressure," *British Journal of Anaesthesia*, vol. 103, no. 6, pp. 886–890, 2009.

[12] B. Sztrymf, J. Messika, F. Bertrand et al., "Beneficial effects of humidified high flow nasal oxygen in critical care patients: a prospective pilot study," *Intensive Care Medicine*, vol. 37, no. 11, pp. 1780–1786, 2011.

[13] R. L. Parke, S. P. McGuinness, and M. L. Eccleston, "A preliminary randomized controlled trial to assess effectiveness of nasal high-flow oxygen in intensive care patients," *Respiratory Care*, vol. 56, no. 3, pp. 265–270, 2011.

23

Undiagnosed Chronic Granulomatous Disease, *Burkholderia cepacia complex* Pneumonia, and Acquired Hemophagocytic Lymphohistiocytosis: A Deadly Association

Maxime Maignan,[1] Colin Verdant,[2,3] Guillaume F. Bouvet,[1] Michael Van Spall,[4] and Yves Berthiaume[1,2,5]

[1] *Institut de Recherches Cliniques de Montréal, Université de Montréal, Montréal, QC, Canada H2W 1R7*
[2] *Département de Médecine, Université de Montréal, Montréal, QC, Canada H3T 1J4*
[3] *Département de Médecine, Hôpital Sacré Cœur, Université de Montréal, Montréal, QC, Canada H4J 1C5*
[4] *Centre de Recherche du Centre hospitalier de l'Université de Montréal, Montréal, QC, Canada H2W 1T8*
[5] *Service de Pneumologie, Centre Hospitalier de l'Université de Montréal, Montréal, QC, Canada H2W 1T8*

Correspondence should be addressed to Yves Berthiaume; yves.berthiaume@ircm.qc.ca

Academic Editors: T. Peros-Golubicic and R. Vender

Background. Chronic granulomatous disease is a rare inherited disorder of the phagocyte nicotinamide adenine dinucleotide phosphate (NADPH) oxidase. The clinical course of the disease is marked by recurrent infections, including *Burkholderia cepacia complex* infection. *Case Report.* Here we report the case of a 21-year-old male hospitalized for a *Burkholderia cepacia complex* pneumonia. Despite the broad spectrum antibiotic treatment, fever continued and patient's condition worsened. Anemia and thrombocytopenia developed together with hypofibrinogenemia. The patient died of multiple organ dysfunction 17 days after his admission. Autopsy revealed hemophagocytosis, suggesting the diagnosis of acquired hemophagocytic lymphohistiocytosis. DNA analysis showed a deletion in the p47phox gene, confirming the diagnosis of autosomal recessive chronic granulomatous disease. *Discussion.* In addition to chronic granulomatous disease, recent findings have demonstrated that *Burkholderia cepacia complex* can decrease activity of the NADPH oxidase. Interestingly, hemophagocytic lymphohistiocytosis is characterized by an impaired function of the T-cell mediated inflammation which is partly regulated by the NADPH oxidase. Physicians should therefore pay particular attention to this deadly association.

1. Introduction

Chronic granulomatous disease (CGD) is an inherited disorder of the phagocyte nicotinamide adenine dinucleotide phosphate (NADPH) oxidase, which results in impaired production of reactive oxygen species and subsequent compromised antimicrobial defenses [1, 2]. CGD accounts for 1.1% of cases of primary immunodeficiency and the prevalence has been estimated to be close to 1/300000 [3].

There are different forms of CGD caused by different mutations in the genes coding for the NADPH oxidase protein complex. However, the majority of cases encountered in clinical practice followed an X-linked pattern of inheritance [3] and originated from a defect of gp1-phox gene, either the gene expression or the protein function. This type of CGD is more severe, and diagnosis is usually made within the first year of life because of recurrent infections [3]. The autosomic recessive form of CGD involves genes that encode p22-phox, p67-phox, and p47-phox. This form is less severe, and consequently, the diagnosis is usually made during the second decade of life.

One of the most frequent germs encountered in CGD patients is *Burkholderia cepacia complex* (Bcc). This motile Gram negative bacillus is involved in at least 3% to 7% of pneumonia and in 18% of deaths in CGD [3, 4]. The treatment of Bcc infection is challenging due to antibiotic multiresistant Bcc strains [5, 6]. Bcc is also known to produce several virulence factors such as catalases, hemolysins, proteases, lipases, and some respiratory mucin-binding adhesins [7–9]. Understanding the complex interplay of these mechanisms of adaptation is of great importance to improve the treatment of Bcc infection [10].

We present a patient with undiagnosed CGD suffering from a Bcc pneumonia whose clinical course is marked by the occurrence of hemophagocytic lymphohistiocytosis (HLH), a syndrome characterized by an uncontrolled immune response. This case report describes the deadly potential of this association as well as a potential common pathophysiological pathway between CGD, Bcc, and HLH.

2. Case Presentation

A 21-year-old Caucasian male was admitted to our ICU for severe pneumonia. His past medical and family history was unremarkable with no serious or recurrent infections. He was vaccinated properly and never had any adverse reactions. He had been working in a greenhouse but had become unemployed a few months before being admitted. He smoked half a pack a day and drank alcohol only socially. He had no allergies and was not taking any medication. He had not travelled recently and had not been in contact with an ill person.

The patient initially had flu-like symptoms and diarrhea. Two weeks after the onset of symptoms, he was admitted to the medical ward for a left lower lobe pneumonia with moderate pleural effusion. Basic laboratory studies showed a white blood cell count of $11,900/mm^3$, with 92% neutrophils, 3% lymphocytes, and no eosinophils. Hemoglobin was 11.5 g/dL and platelet count was $398/mm^3$. Biochemical tests only revealed elevated levels of serum GOT (60UI/L) and GPT (30UI/L). Oxygen and intravenous erythromycin and cefotaxime were started, but cefotaxime was replaced by ciprofloxacin on the 5th day because of a rash. The chest X-ray performed on the 5th day is presented in Figure 1. Blood culture was sterile and a tuberculin shin test was not reactive at 48 hours. Sputum culture revealed Bcc.

On the 7th day, the patient became severely hypoxemic and was transferred to our ICU. Medical examination and tests showed extensive bilateral pneumonia with increased pleural effusion (Figure 2), splenomegaly, and hepatic cytolysis. The arterial blood gases at 100% oxygen by mask were pH 7.51, PO_2 93 mmHg, PCO_2 32 mmHg, and HCO_3 25 mmol/L. Blood count revealed white-cell count of $4,300/mm^3$, hemoglobin of 88 g/L, and platelet count of $225/mm^3$. Biochemical tests were unchanged. A chest tube was inserted, and piperacillin-tazobactam, netilmicin, and vancomycin were added to ciprofloxacin therapy. Analysis of the effusion yielded pH 7.41, glucose 4.5 mmol/L, LDH 751 UI/L, and protein 33 g/L with cytology negative for tumoral cells.

On the 11th day, the patient was placed on mechanical ventilation because of respiratory failure. The antibiogram showed imipenem and aminoglycoside resistance (Table 1),

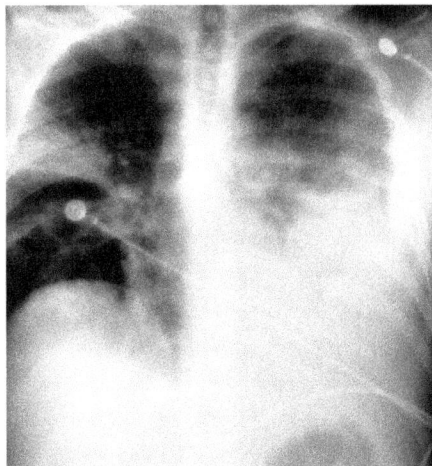

FIGURE 1: Chest X-ray on the 5th day.

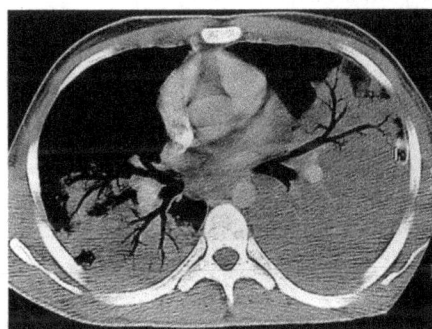

FIGURE 2: Thoracic CT scan on the 7th day after hospitalization showing a bilateral pneumonia with pleural effusion.

and antibiotic therapy was switched to ceftazidime and ongoing ciprofloxacin. On the 15th day, hypofibrinogenemia (1.1 g/L), thrombocytopenia ($80/mm^3$), and deep anemia (64 g/L) were observed; two units of packed red blood cells were administered. The patient became hypotensive on the 17th day, and despite intensive vasopressor therapy, he died from multiple organ failure, twenty days after hospital admission. An autopsy revealed severe bilateral bronchopneumonia and left empyema associated with hemophagocytosis, prompting the diagnosis of acquired HLH (Table 2). A culture of crushed lung tissues from the autopsy revealed three different species of Bcc. A postmortem DNA analysis showed a deletion (delta GT) in the p47-phox gene, confirming the diagnosis of autosomal recessive CGD.

3. Discussion

Although the association of CGD with Bcc infection is well known, only few case reports have described the presence of HLH [11–14] (Table 3) during the course of Bcc infection in CGD patients. Furthermore, although other medical conditions could lead to infection with Bcc [7], we are not aware of any report of HLH during Bcc infection in absence of CGD. These reports raise the question of a specific

TABLE 1: *In vitro* sensitivity of the 3 types of *Burkholderia cepacia complex* (Bcc) isolated from sputum cultures.

	Minimal inhibitory concentrations (ug/mL) and interpretation		
	Bcc 1	Bcc 2	Bcc 3
Amikacin	>64 R	>64 R	>64 R
Aztreonam	>32 R	>32 R	>32 R
Cefoxitin	>32 R	>32 R	>32 R
Ceftazidime	<8 S	>32 R	>32 R
Ceftizoxime	16 I	128 R	>256 R
Ciprofloxacin	<0.5 S	>4 R	>4 R
Gentamicin	>16 R	>16 R	>16 R
Imipenem	>16 R	>16 R	>16 R
Piperacillin	128 R	>256 R	>256 R
Ticarcillin/clavulanate	>256 R	>256 R	>256 R
Tobramycin	>16 R	>16 R	>16 R
Trimethoprim/sulfamethoxazole	<16 S	<16 S	160 R

S: susceptible; I: intermediate; R: resistant.

TABLE 2: Clinical, laboratory, and autopsy findings corresponding to acquired hemophagocytic lymphohistiocytosis diagnostic criteria.

Hemophagocytic lymphohistiocytosis diagnostic criteria (diagnosis is established by fulfilling 5 out of 8 of the following)	Patient's findings
Fever	Yes
Splenomegaly	Yes
Cytopenia (affecting ≥ 2 cell lineages, hemoglobin < 9 g/dL; platelets < 100 G/L; neutrophils < 1.0 G/L)	Hemoglobin 6.4 g/dL Platelets 80 G/L
Hypertriglyceridemia (≥265 mg/dL) and/or hypofibrinogemia (≤1.5 g/L)	yes
Low or absent natural killer cell cytotoxicity	NI
Hyperferritinemia (>500 ng/mL)	NI
Elevated sCD25 (>2.400 U/mL)	NI
Hemophagocytosis in the bone marrow, spleen, or lymph nodes without malignancy	Bone marrow and spleen

NI: not investigated.
Note: adapted from the 2nd International HLH study, http://www.histio.org/page.aspx?pid=389.

TABLE 3: Chronic granulomatous patients with *Burkholderia cepacia complex* infection and acquired hemophagocytic lymphohistiocytosis.

Sex	Age	Mutation	Site of infection	Outcome	Reference
M	36 months	X-linked	Abdomen	Survived	[11]
F	19 years	p22-phox	Vagina	Survived	[12]
M	17 months	NS	Spleen	Survived	[13]
M	40 months	X-linked	Lung	Deceased	[14]
M	21 years	p47-phox	Lung	Deceased	Present case

NS: non specified.

interplay between CGD, Bcc, and HLH. Bcc exhibits multiple mechanisms of adaptation, including interference with the phagosome maturation [15, 16]. Moreover, Bcc is able to lessen phagocyte NADPH-oxidase activity, which enables it to survive in phagocyte vacuoles [17]. Thus, in CGD patients, Bcc could further decrease the production of reactive oxidant species by the NADPH oxidase and contribute to the dysregulation of the immune response.

HLH is characterized by an uncontrolled immune response with severe hyperinflammation [18]. There are two forms of HLH: a familial or genetic one and an acquired one triggered by infections and autoimmune and/or malignant diseases. The clinical course of HLH is mainly characterized by a prolonged fever unresponsive to antibiotics. Patients often present a hepatosplenomegaly and a moderate cytolytic hepatitis. Neurological symptoms as meningism, seizures, and ataxia may be present [19–21]. Adenopathy, edema, or rash may also be encountered, especially in acquired HLH. The diagnosis of HLH has to be made early in the course of the disease in order to initiate potential life-saving treatments with immune modulator treatments such as corticosteroids, cyclosporine A, and methotrexate [22]. This diagnosis is often tricky because of the initial similarity between sepsis and HLH [22]. An eight-criteria panel (Table 2) has been proposed, but diagnosis pitfalls remain [18]. In this case report, the patient fulfilled five of the criteria, which is the threshold for a clinical diagnosis. However, HLH was not diagnosed and the patient did not receive immunosuppressive drugs.

The pathophysiology of HLH remains controversial, but the common feature of both forms of HLH is an impaired function of natural killer and cytotoxic T cells and their regulatory mechanisms [18]. The secretion of proinflammatory cytokines is increased, while the clearance of pathogens is reduced. Interestingly, recent findings demonstrated that NADPH oxidase plays a crucial role in T-cell mediated inflammation [23]. Human macrophages with the p47-phox mutation exhibit reduced regulatory T-cell induction and T-cell suppression [24]. In CGD patients, the decreased NADPH oxidase activity not only reduced the production of reactive oxidant species and the subsequent pathogens clearance but also impaired the ability of the host to regulate the inflammatory response [1]. Our hypothesis is that the presence of a Bcc infection could further impair the NADPH oxidase activity and, as a consequence, the inflammatory response. Finally, these cooperating mechanisms could explain the association of HLH in CGD patients especially when infected by Bcc.

This pathophysiological cooperation may account for an increased severity. However, there is no cohort study available to investigate the mortality of the CGD, Bcc, and HLH association. We can only state from the published case reports that 2 patients out of 5 died (Table 3). Bcc infection is a recognized severity factor in CGD patients and mortality of infection-associated HLH is close to 20% [3, 25]. The association of these three diseases is likely to have a worse outcome especially in the light of the shared pathophysiological pathways. These considerations may have a strong clinical impact on the general management of CGD patients and on the care of autosomic recessive CGD patients in particular. Autosomic recessive CGD is known to be less severe and to be diagnosed later than the X-linked CGD [4]. Nonetheless, this case report shows that in some autosomic recessive CGD patients, the disease can be revealed by a very severe form of sepsis. The occurrence of HLH in such infected CGD patients may worsen their prognosis especially if CGD and/or HLH are not suspected.

In conclusion, HLH, CGD, and Bcc infections share pathophysiological pathways, and this possibly explains their relatively frequent association. In light of this case, CGD mutations should be sought out in previously healthy adult patients with Bcc infection, and particular attention should be paid to HLH occurrence during Bcc infections.

References

[1] B. H. Segal, P. Veys, H. Malech, and M. J. Cowan, "Chronic granulomatous disease: lessons from a rare disorder," *Biology of Blood and Marrow Transplantation*, vol. 17, no. 1, supplement, pp. S123–S131, 2011.

[2] N. Rieber, A. Hector, T. Kuijpers, D. Roos, and D. Hartl, "Current concepts of hyperinflammation in chronic granulomatous disease," *Clinical and Developmental Immunology*, vol. 2012, Article ID 252460, 6 pages, 2012.

[3] J. A. Winkelstein, M. C. Marino, R. B. Johnston Jr. et al., "Chronic granulomatous disease: report on a national registry of 368 patients," *Medicine*, vol. 79, no. 3, pp. 155–169, 2000.

[4] J. M. van den Berg, E. van Koppen, A. Åhlin et al., "Chronic granulomatous disease: the European experience," *PLoS ONE*, vol. 4, no. 4, Article ID e5234, 2009.

[5] P. Drevinek and E. Mahenthiralingam, "*Burkholderia cenocepacia* in cystic fibrosis: epidemiology and molecular mechanisms of virulence," *Clinical Microbiology and Infection*, vol. 16, no. 7, pp. 821–830, 2010.

[6] A. Horsley and A. M. Jones, "Antibiotic treatment for *Burkholderia cepacia complex* in people with cystic fibrosis experiencing a pulmonary exacerbation," *Cochrane Database Systematic Review*, vol. 10, Article ID CD009529, 2012.

[7] S. McClean and M. Callaghan, "*Burkholderia cepacia complex*: epithelial cell-pathogen confrontations and potential for therapeutic intervention," *Journal of Medical Microbiology*, vol. 58, no. 1, pp. 1–12, 2009.

[8] J. H. Leitão, S. A. Sousa, A. S. Ferreira, C. G. Ramos, I. N. Silva, and L. M. Moreira, "Pathogenicity, virulence factors, and strategies to fight against *Burkholderia cepacia complex* pathogens and related species," *Applied Microbiology and Biotechnology*, vol. 87, no. 1, pp. 31–40, 2010.

[9] S. Ganesan and U. S. Sajjan, "Host evasion by *Burkholderia cenocepacia*," *Frontiers in Cellular and Infection Microbiology*, vol. 1, p. 25, 2011.

[10] E. Mahenthiralingam, T. A. Urban, and J. B. Goldberg, "The multifarious, multireplicon *Burkholderia cepacia complex*," *Nature Reviews Microbiology*, vol. 3, no. 2, pp. 144–156, 2005.

[11] A. Álvarez-Cardona, A. L. Rodríguez-Lozano, L. Blancas-Galicia et al., "Intravenous immunoglobulin treatment for macrophage activation syndrome complicating chronic granulomatous disease," *Journal of Clinical Immunology*, vol. 32, no. 2, pp. 207–211, 2011.

[12] M. Hisano, K. Sugawara, O. Tatsuzawa, M. Kitagawa, A. Murashima, and K. Yamaguchi, "Bacteria-associated haemophagocytic syndrome and septic pulmonary embolism caused by *Burkholderia cepacia complex* in a woman with chronic granulomatous disease," *Journal of Medical Microbiology*, vol. 56, no. 5, pp. 702–705, 2007.

[13] S. Sirinavin, C. Techasaensiri, S. Pakakasama, M. Vorachit, R. Pornkul, and R. Wacharasin, "Hemophagocytic syndrome and *Burkholderia cepacia* splenic microabscesses in a child with chronic granulomatous disease," *Pediatric Infectious Disease Journal*, vol. 23, no. 9, pp. 882–884, 2004.

[14] J. M. Van Montfrans, E. Rudd, L. D. Van Corput et al., "Fatal hemophagocytic lymphohistiocytosis in x-linked chronic granulomatous disease associated with a perforin gene variant," *Pediatric Blood and Cancer*, vol. 52, no. 4, pp. 527–529, 2009.

[15] K. K. Huynh, J. D. Plumb, G. P. Downey, M. A. Valvano, and S. Grinstein, "Inactivation of macrophage Rab7 by *Burkholderia*

cenocepacia," *Journal of Innate Immunity,* vol. 2, no. 6, pp. 522–533, 2010.

[16] J. Lamothe, K. K. Huynh, S. Grinstein, and M. A. Valvano, "Intracellular survival of *Burkholderia cenocepacia* in macrophages is associated with a delay in the maturation of bacteria-containing vacuoles," *Cellular Microbiology,* vol. 9, no. 1, pp. 40–53, 2007.

[17] K. E. Keith, D. W. Hynes, J. E. Sholdice, and M. A. Valvano, "Delayed association of the NADPH oxidase complex with macrophage vacuoles containing the opportunistic pathogen *Burkholderia cenocepacia,*" *Microbiology,* vol. 155, no. 4, pp. 1004–1015, 2009.

[18] G. E. Janka, "Familial and acquired hemophagocytic lymphohistiocytosis," *Annual Review of Medicine,* vol. 63, pp. 233–246, 2012.

[19] P. Ruppert, E. C. Edmonds, M. Brook M et al., "Neuropsychological assessment in a case of adult-onset hemophagocytic lymphohistiocytosis (HLH)," *The Clinical Neuropsychologist,* vol. 26, no. 6, pp. 1038–1052, 2012.

[20] K. Deiva, N. Mahlaoui, F. Beaudonnet et al., "CNS involvement at the onset of primary hemophagocytic lymphohistiocytosis," *Neurology,* vol. 78, no. 15, pp. 1150–1156, 2012.

[21] L. Chiapparini, G. Uziel, C. Vallinoto et al., "Hemophagocytic lymphohistiocytosis with neurological presentation: MRI findings and a nearly miss diagnosis," *Neurological Sciences,* vol. 32, no. 3, pp. 473–477, 2011.

[22] J.-I. Henter, A. Horne, M. Aricó et al., "HLH-2004: diagnostic and therapeutic guidelines for hemophagocytic lymphohistiocytosis," *Pediatric Blood and Cancer,* vol. 48, no. 2, pp. 124–131, 2007.

[23] B. H. Segal, M. J. Grimm, A. N. H. Khan et al., "Regulation of innate immunity by NADPH oxidase," *Free Radical Biology and Medicine,* vol. 53, no. 1, pp. 72–80, 2012.

[24] M. D. Kraaij, N. D. L. Savage, S. W. Van Der Kooij et al., "Induction of regulatory T cells by macrophages is dependent on production of reactive oxygen species," *Proceedings of the National Academy of Sciences of the United States of America,* vol. 107, no. 41, pp. 17686–17691, 2010.

[25] E. Ishii, S. Ohga, S. Imashuku et al., "Nationwide survey of hemophagocytic lymphohistiocytosis in Japan," *International Journal of Hematology,* vol. 86, no. 1, pp. 58–65, 2007.

24

Severe Respiratory Distress in a Child with Pulmonary Idiopathic Hemosiderosis Initially Presenting with Iron-Deficiency Anemia

A. Potalivo, L. Finessi, F. Facondini, A. Lupo, C. Andreoni, G. Giuliani, and C. Cavicchi

Department of Emergency, Anaesthesia and Intensive Care Section, Infermi Hospital, Viale Luigi Settembrini 2, 47923 Rimini, Italy

Correspondence should be addressed to L. Finessi; lfinessi1981@gmail.com

Academic Editor: Maria Plataki

Idiopathic pulmonary hemosiderosis (IPH) is a rare cause of alveolar hemorrhage in children but should be considered in children with anemia of unknown origin who develop respiratory complications. It is commonly characterized by the triad of recurrent hemoptysis, diffuse parenchymal infiltrates, and iron-deficiency anemia. Pathogenesis is unclear and diagnosis may be difficult along with a variable clinical course. A 6-year-old boy was admitted to the hospital with a severe iron-deficiency anemia, but he later developed severe acute respiratory failure and hemoptysis requiring intubation and mechanical ventilation. The suspicion of IPH led to the use of immunosuppressive therapy with high dose of corticosteroids with rapid improvement in clinical condition and discharge from hospital.

1. Background

Idiopathic pulmonary hemosiderosis (IPH) is a rare cause of alveolar hemorrhage in children [1, 2]. It is commonly characterized by the triad of recurrent hemoptysis, diffuse parenchymal infiltrates, and iron-deficiency anemia [3–5]. Pathogenesis is unclear and diagnosis may be difficult due to a variable clinical course [5, 6]. About 500 cases of this disease have been described in medical literature [5, 7]. IPH is usually a diagnosis of exclusion as not one identifying test has been described [6]. Currently used intensive care therapies include high dose steroid and immunosuppressive treatment along with conventional and high-frequency oscillatory ventilation. In children who cannot maintain adequate oxygenation with conventional therapies extracorporeal life support has been described [6, 8, 9]. The aim of this paper is to present the diagnostic challenge and intensive care unit management of a 6-year-old boy with a severe respiratory failure due to IPH initially presenting as an iron-deficiency anemia.

2. Case Presentation

A 6-year-old boy of 20 kg weight was admitted to the hospital, with a recent history of progressive paleness and general fatigue. The patient was alert, with profound dyspnea, and unable to maintain oxygen saturation in room air (SaO_2 < 80%); his cardiac frequency was 130 bpm and BP was 90/40 mmHg. Physical examination was positive for skin and mucous membrane pallor. The chest radiograph was positive for multiple alveolar-type opacities with a background of interstitial reticular pattern (Figure 1). History was positive for previous tonsillectomy and familiar cases of celiac disease. One month before the child was again hospitalized for severe anemia requiring blood transfusions, laboratory investigations showed severe anemia with hemoglobin (Hb) 4.6 g/dL, microcytosis, and hypocromia with level of serum iron and transferritin decreased. His vital signs were normal; bleeding from gastrointestinal tract was excluded and bone marrow biopsy showed nonspecific findings of dyserythropoiesis. Serologic studies were negative. He was discharged from hospital but subsequent follow-up showed persistent anemia despite iron therapy and several blood transfusion with packet red blood cell units.

When he was readmitted to emergency department he was febrile (37.9°C) with severe respiratory distress; laboratory confirmed persistent anemia and elevated inflammatory indices (white blood cells 18.830 × 10^3/μL and C-reactive protein of 21.9 mg/L).

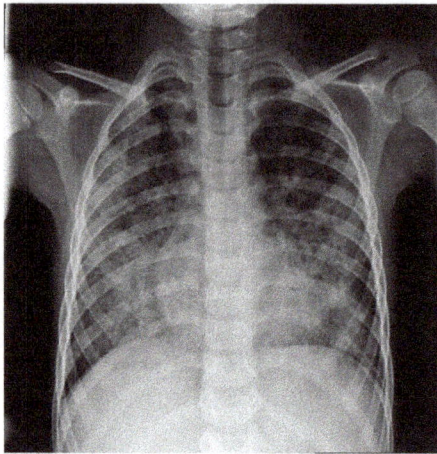

FIGURE 1: Posteroanterior chest radiography showing diffuse bilateral pulmonary infiltrations.

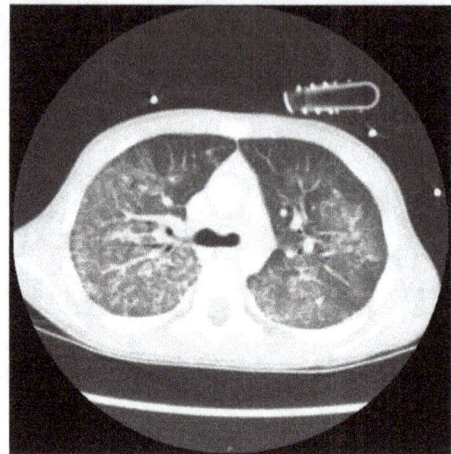

FIGURE 2: Chest computed tomography shows areas of ground-glass attenuation and a reticular micronodular appearance in both lung fields.

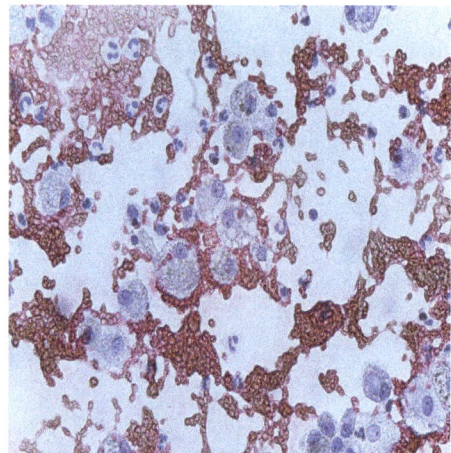

FIGURE 3: BAL specimen showing hemosiderin-laden macrophages. Staining for iron (Perls' Prussian blue). Magnification ×400.

He was transferred to the ICU after starting broad spectrum antibiotics with suspicion of severe sepsis or transfusion related acute lung injury. Few hours later severe hemoptysis occurred and a diagnosis of IPH was supposed. The patient was treated with bolus infusion of methilprednisolone 10 mg/kg and subsequentially 20 mg prednisone four times daily, but worsening respiratory failure required endotracheal intubation and mechanical ventilation. He was sedated with infusion of Propofol 6 mg/kg/h and Remifentanyl 0.05 μg/kg/min and he was ventilated with protective strategy using low tidal volume values and positive end-expiratory pressure of 5 cmH$_2$O due to severe respiratory distress (PaO$_2$/FiO$_2$ ratio of 90). Rapid clinical improvement was noted and the following day a CT scan showed diffuse alveolar consolidation compatible with a recent bleeding (Figure 2). A bronchoscopy was performed and microscopic examination of the bronchoalveolar lavage fluid revealed the presence of many hemosiderin-laden macrophages (Figure 3) with no evidence of infection. Laboratory work-up including antinuclear antibodies (ANA), anti-neutrophil cytoplasmic antibodies (ANCA), extractable nuclear antigens (ENA) antibodies, rheumatoid factor, antigliadin, tissue transglutaminase antibody IgA class, antiglomerular basement membrane (antiGBM), and specific cow's milk IgE and complement was negative. Cyclic citrullinated peptide antibodies (anti-CCP) were also negative. Improvement in gas exchanges led to extubation four days later. Noninvasive ventilation support was started due to persistence of mild respiratory distress. The child was transferred to medical ward after eight days of ICU stay and then discharged from hospital after other nine days. Prolonged follow-up showed good clinical recovery with methilprednisolone pulses of 30 mg/kg for three days and repeated monthly. During progressive tapering off of corticosteroids the child suffered of another self-limiting episode of hemoptysis without sequelae. For this reason current daily maintaining dose of oral prednisone is 1 mg/kg/day and methilprednisolone pulses were resumed. Despite negative serologic findings, the child followed a gluten-free diet without any apparently long term benefit. There was not any adverse effect of corticosteroid treatment. Outcome is satisfactory, but patient's quality of life got worse due to exertional dyspnea.

3. Discussion

Idiopathic pulmonary hemosiderosis is a rare and life threatening type of diffuse alveolar hemorrhage (DAH) that preferentially affects children and young adults [1, 4, 5]. Pathophysiology of the disease is complex and elusive and its etiology remains unknown. Allergic, environmental, genetic, and/or autoimmune hypotheses have been proposed to explain the structural lesions of alveolar-endothelial membrane seen in IPH [1]. While there is no definitive etiology of IPH, an underlying immune process is likely, given its typical responsiveness to immunosuppressive therapy [10, 11].

Estimated pediatric IPH incidence is 0.24 and 1.23 cases per million, with a mortality rate as high as 50% in previous reports [11, 12]. It commonly occurs in the ages of 1–7 years

[13], but 20% of cases are adult-onset patients [4]. It is classically characterized by a triad of hemoptysis, iron-deficiency anemia, and pulmonary infiltrates [4, 5, 14]. However, any of these features may be the first presenting manifestation, so the diagnosis of IPH can be difficult [11]. In previous reports the classic triad was found only in 15% to 26% of patients diagnosed with IPH [15, 16]. Anemia and dyspnea are the most frequent clinical features and hemoptysis occurs in about 50% of patients [3], but its incidence could be underestimated in young children, who frequently swallow their sputum [4].

In our case iron-deficiency anemia preceded other symptoms and signs, so the diagnosis of IPH was delayed. Pulmonary hemorrhages and hemoptysis are rare in children and the absence of respiratory symptoms led us to look for other causes of iron-deficiency anemia like cystic fibrosis, congenital heart diseases, malignancies, and gastrointestinal or laryngeal pathologies [5, 17]. It should be stressed to consider the diagnosis of a rare pathology like IPH when there is no response to iron therapy and blood transfusions and no clear site of bleeding [4, 18]. Dyspnea and hemoptysis along with severe respiratory distress that occurred with second clinical presentation drew our attention to a possible DAH.

DAH syndromes are heterogeneous pathologies taking place as a result of injury to the small lung vessels (capillaries, but also arterioles and venules) and they can occur with or without pulmonary capillaritis [19]. IPH is a disorder where there is no cardiovascular cause and no evidence of capillaritis. Renal and systemic manifestations are absent. There are reports of patients, initially diagnosed with IPH, who are later found to have Goodpasture's syndrome, systemic lupus erythematosus, or microscopic polyangiitis. IPH should be considered a diagnosis of exclusion [19, 20] as in our case where all serologic findings were negative.

The lung biopsy still remains the gold standard for definite diagnosis, but IPH can also be confirmed by bronchoscopy with bronchoalveolar lavage showing hemosiderin-laden macrophages [1–5].

We decided not to perform lung biopsy, due to severe respiratory distress and given the fact that the bronchoalveolar lavage was highly suggestive.

Interestingly there was a positive familiar history of celiac disease in our patient. IPH has frequently been associated with celiac disease. This association is well-known as the Lane-Hamilton syndrome and there are reports of positive respiratory outcome with a gluten-free diet [21, 22]. Some authors suggest to systematically perform gastrointestinal endoscopies and biopsies in IPH patients, even in the absence of gastrointestinal symptoms, when the severity of anemia is disproportionate to radiologic findings [21, 23]. We screened for specific antibodies of celiac disease (antigliadin and anti-tranglutaminase antibodies), but they were negative so we did not request HLA types. However the child did not apparently benefit of a gluten-free diet.

It is essential to make a prompt diagnosis in order to avoid complications of recurrent alveolar hemorrhages like interstitial fibrosis [4, 10, 11]. High resolution CT scan is useful for early detection of pulmonary fibrosis [10, 24], and it helped us to exclude this complication.

Pulmonary function testing techniques are well established in children and adolescents. However children aged 2–6 years represent a real challenge in pulmonary function assessment due to lack in cooperation. Lung diffusing capacity of carbon monoxide (DLCO) is often markedly reduced and may be abnormal before any radiologic abnormalities [2].

There are no evidence-based recommendations regarding treatment for acute onset DAH and in particular for IPH [1, 3–5, 10]. Corticosteroids have long been used for treatment of IPH [3, 11]. Their use is associated with a decrease of the frequency of hemorrhages, although it is not known if they have any effect on the course of the disease and progression to pulmonary fibrosis [4]. Immunosoppressive therapy has also been used, especially in cases of steroid-dependence or steroid-resistance diseases [1, 11, 14]. Among immunosuppressant agents, azathioprine in combination with corticosteroids might be the best therapeutic regimen, especially in preventing IPH exacerbations [1, 4]. In our cases corticosteroids therapy was effective and clinical outcome was satisfactory. Only few cases of single-lung transplantation have been reported as a therapy of end stage IPH, with failure of this therapeutic option due to reoccurrence of the disease [25, 26]. Long term follow-up should take into account the numbers and severity of hemorrhagic episodes and the progression of interstitial disease (as expressed by the decline of DLCO) [1]. Fortunately the prognosis of IPH seems to improve over time. Two decades ago the mean survival was 3 years, but recent data indicate a 5-year survival of 86% of cases possibly due to the long term use of immunosuppressant therapy [4, 5, 11].

Respiratory distress in our patient was particularly severe leading to intubation and mechanical ventilation. Little is known about need for ventilatory support in pediatric patients with severe IPH. Rabe and coworkers report a series of 37 adult patients with DAH admitted to ICU for severe respiratory distress. Eighty-six percent of them (32 patients) were mechanically ventilated [27]. Sun and coworkers described a 11-year-old case of pediatric IPH leading to ARDS and ventilatory support [9]. In their case conventional ventilatory support failed to maintain adequate respiratory gas exchanges so extracorporeal membrane oxygenation (ECMO) was started. Another case of extracorporeal life support in a 5-week-old infant with IPH has been described with good clinical outcome [6]. Our case did not require ECMO given the fact that respiratory gas exchanges rapidly ameliorated after starting corticosteroid therapy.

Although mechanical ventilation could be life-saving in these situations, it is essential to limit the possibility of ventilation induced lung injury (VILI) [28]. Artificial lung ventilation can further damage the alveolar-endothelial membrane, so it is recommended to limit tidal volume to 4–6 mL/kg and give positive end-expiratory alveolar pressure (PEEP) in order to limit cyclic collapse and opening of terminal airways during tidal ventilation [29]. Increasing the PEEP during mechanical ventilation may otherwise produce a tamponade effect to limit capillary bleeding from disrupted alveolar-capillary membranes [19].

Our case emphasizes the importance for the respiratory physician to consider IPH as a possible diagnosis when a child with idiopathic anaemia develops severe respiratory failure, in order to avoid the possible long term sequelae of untreated disease.

Abbreviations

DAH: Diffuse alveolar hemorrhage
IPH: Idiopathic pulmonary hemosiderosis
Hb: Haemoglobin
ICU: Intensive care unit
ANA: Antinuclear antibodies
ANCA: Anti-neutrophil cytoplasmic antibodies
ENA: Extractable nuclear antigens
GBM: Glomerular basement membrane
ARDS: Acute respiratory distress syndrome
VILI: Ventilation induced lung injury
DLCO: Diffusing capacity for carbon monoxide
PEEP: Positive end-expiratory pressure.

Authors' Contribution

A. Potalivo and C. Cavicchi collected the patient data. All authors were involved in the treatment of patient. L. Finessi drafted the paper. A. Potalivo, F. Facondini, and C. Andreoni revised and edited the paper. A. Potalivo obtained approval from the institutional review board.

Acknowledgment

The authors would like to thank the Department of Pathology and Radiology of "Infermi Hospital" of Rimini for their collaboration in acquisition of data.

References

[1] O. C. Ioachimescu, S. Sieber, and A. Kotch, "Idiopathic pulmonary haemosiderosis revisited," *European Respiratory Journal*, vol. 24, no. 1, pp. 162–170, 2004.

[2] A. Clement, N. Nathan, R. Epaud, B. Fauroux, and H. Corvol, "Interstitial lung diseases in children," *Orphanet Journal of Rare Diseases*, vol. 5, no. 1, article 22, 2010.

[3] J. Taytard, N. Nathan, J. de Blic et al., "New insights into pediatric idiopathic pulmonary hemosiderosis: the French RespiRare cohort," *Orphanet Journal of Rare Diseases*, vol. 8, article 161, 2013.

[4] I. Bakalli, L. Kota, D. Sala et al., "Idiopathic pulmonary hemosiderosis—a diagnostic challenge," *Italian Journal of Pediatrics*, vol. 40, article 35, 2014.

[5] E. Kamienska, T. Urasinski, A. Gawlikowska-Sroka, B. Glura, and A. Pogorzelski, "Idiopathic pulmonary hemosiderosis in a 9-year-old girl," *European Journal of Medical Research*, vol. 14, supplement 4, pp. 112–115, 2009.

[6] S. Gutierrez, S. Shaw, S. Huseni et al., "Extracorporeal life support for a 5-week-old infant with idiopathic pulmonary hemosiderosis," *European Journal of Pediatrics*, vol. 173, no. 12, pp. 1573–1576, 2014.

[7] K. Sawielajc, J. Krus, and A. Balcar-Boron, "Spontaneous pulmonary hemosiderosis in a four-year-old boy," *Wiad Lek*, vol. 47, pp. 210–212, 1994.

[8] N. S. Kolovos, D. J. E. Schuerer, F. W. Moler et al., "Extracorporal life support for pulmonary hemorrhage in children: a case series," *Critical Care Medicine*, vol. 30, no. 3, pp. 577–580, 2002.

[9] L.-C. Sun, Y.-R. Tseng, S.-C. Huang et al., "Extracorporeal membrane oxygenation to rescue profound pulmonary hemorrhage due to idiopathic pulmonary hemosiderosis in a child," *Pediatric Pulmonology*, vol. 41, no. 9, pp. 900–903, 2006.

[10] N. Milman and F. M. Pedersen, "Idiopathic pulmonary haemosiderosis. Epidemiology, pathogenic aspects and diagnosis," *Respiratory Medicine*, vol. 92, no. 7, pp. 902–907, 1998.

[11] M. M. Saeed, M. S. Woo, E. F. MacLaughlin, M. F. Margetis, and T. G. Keens, "Prognosis in pediatric idiopathic pulmonary hemosiderosis," *Chest*, vol. 116, no. 3, pp. 721–725, 1999.

[12] K. H. Soergel and S. C. Sommers, "Idiopathic pulmonary hemosiderosis and related syndromes," *The American Journal of Medicine*, vol. 32, no. 4, pp. 499–511, 1962.

[13] D. C. Heiner, "Pulmonary hemosiderosis," in *Disorders of the Respiratory Tract in Children*, V. Chernick and E. L. Kendig Jr., Eds., pp. 498–509, WB Saunders, Philadelphia, Pa, USA, 1990.

[14] H. Willms, K. Gutjahr, U. R. Juergens et al., "Diagnostics and therapy of idiopathic pulmonary hemosiderosis," *Medizinische Klinik*, vol. 102, no. 6, pp. 445–450, 2007.

[15] C. Bulucea and D. Sorin, "Idiopathic pulmonary hemosiderosis in children: a Romanian experience," *Pediatrics*, vol. 121, supplement, pp. S158–S159, 2008.

[16] S. K. Kabra, S. Bhargava, R. Lodha, A. Satyavani, and M. Walia, "Idiopathic pulmonary hemosiderosis: clinical profile and follow up of 26 children," *Indian Pediatrics*, vol. 44, no. 5, pp. 333–338, 2007.

[17] S. Godfrey, "Pulmonary hemorrhage/hemoptysis in children," *Pediatric Pulmonology*, vol. 37, no. 6, pp. 476–484, 2004.

[18] S. Sankararaman, K. Shah, K. Maddox, S. Velayuthan, and L. K. Scott, "Clinical case of the month. Idiopathic pulmonary hemosiderosis presenting as a rare cause of iron deficiency anemia in a toddler—a diagnostic challenge," *The Journal of the Louisiana State Medical Society*, vol. 164, no. 5, pp. 293–296, 2012.

[19] S. C. Susarla and L. L. Fan, "Diffuse alveolar hemorrhage syndromes in children," *Current Opinion in Pediatrics*, vol. 19, no. 3, pp. 314–320, 2007.

[20] D. J. Serisier, R. C. W. Wong, and J. G. Armstrong, "Alveolar haemorrhage in anti-glomerular basement membrane disease without detectable antibodies by conventional assays," *Thorax*, vol. 61, no. 7, pp. 636–639, 2006.

[21] D. H. Mayes and M. L. Guerrero, "A few good men: a marine with hemoptysis and diarrhea," *Chest*, vol. 134, no. 3, pp. 644–647, 2008.

[22] G. R. Sethi, K. K. Singhal, A. S. Puri, and M. Mantan, "Benefit of gluten-free diet in idiopathic pulmonary hemosiderosis in association with celiac disease," *Pediatric Pulmonology*, vol. 46, no. 3, pp. 302–305, 2011.

[23] O. Keskin, M. Keskin, E. Guler et al., "Unusual presentation: pulmonary hemosiderosis with celiac disease and retinitis pigmentosa in a child," *Pediatric Pulmonology*, vol. 46, no. 8, pp. 820–823, 2011.

[24] D. L. Buschman and R. Ballard, "Progressive massive fibrosis associated with idiopathic pulmonary hemosiderosis," *Chest*, vol. 104, no. 1, pp. 293–295, 1993.

[25] F. Calabrese, C. Giacometti, F. Rea et al., "Recurrence of idiopathic pulmonary hemosiderosis in a young adult patient after bilateral single-lung transplantation," *Transplantation*, vol. 74, no. 11, pp. 1643–1645, 2002.

[26] B. M. Wroblewski, C. R. Stefanovic, V. M. McDonough, and P. J. Kidik, "The challenges of idiopathic pulmonary hemosiderosis and lung transplantation," *Critical Care Nurse*, vol. 17, no. 3, pp. 39–44, 1997.

[27] C. Rabe, B. Appenrodt, C. Hoff et al., "Severe respiratory failure due to diffuse alveolar hemorrhage: clinical characteristics and outcome of intensive care," *Journal of Critical Care*, vol. 25, no. 2, pp. 230–235, 2010.

[28] D. Dreyfuss and G. Saumon, "Ventilator-induced lung injury lessons from experimental studies," *American Journal of Respiratory and Critical Care Medicine*, vol. 157, no. 1, pp. 294–323, 1998.

[29] D. R. Hess, "Approaches to conventional mechanical ventilation of the patient with acute respiratory distress syndrome," *Respiratory care*, vol. 56, no. 10, pp. 1555–1572, 2011.

25

Successful Treatment of Bulla with Endobronchial Valves

Erdoğan Çetinkaya,[1] Mehmet Akif Özgül,[1] Şule Gül,[1] Hilal Boyacı,[2] Ertan Cam,[1] Emine Kamiloglu,[3] and Mustafa Çörtük[4]

[1]*Department of Chest Diseases, Yedikule Chest Disease and Chest Surgery Education and Research Hospital, İstanbul, Turkey*
[2]*Amasya Merzifon Kara Mustafa Pasa State Hospital, Amasya, Turkey*
[3]*Dr. Burhan Nalbantoğlu State Hospital, Lefkose, Northern Cyprus, Turkey*
[4]*Karabük University Education and Research Hospital, Karabuk, Turkey*

Correspondence should be addressed to Erdoğan Çetinkaya; ecetinkaya34@yahoo.com

Academic Editor: Tomonobu Koizumi

Emphysematous bullae are a complication of end-stage COPD. Patients with large bullae and poor respiratory function have limited treatment options. Surgical resection is a recognized treatment, but functional improvement after bullectomy is not satisfactory in patients with forced expiratory volume in 1 s (FEV1) < 35% predicted. When this 59-year-old male end-stage COPD patient was assessed, he was cachectic and lung function tests showed a FEV1 of 0.56 L (19% predicted) and a RV of 7 L (314% predicted), while 6MWT was 315 m and MRC dyspnea score was 4. Chest X-ray revealed a massive bulla of 10 cm in diameter in the right middle lobe. A fibrobronchoscopy was performed under local anesthesia and 2 Zephyr 4.0 valves were placed in the right middle lobe. Chest X-ray and CT scan performed 36 days later showed the complete resolution of the bulla. Seven months later, the patient demonstrated an improvement in FEV1 (+30%) and a decrease in RV from 314 to 262% predicted. This case report shows that the Zephyr valves may be successfully used to treat a large bulla in the right middle lobe in a patient with diffuse emphysema and severely impaired lung function.

1. Introduction

Emphysema is characterized by parenchymal lung destruction and loss of elastic recoil which results in hyperinflation. Bullae are thought to develop from a parenchymal weakness which, once it exceeds a certain size, will result in a space within the lung which will fill preferentially. The bulla does not participate in ventilation to any great extent because of the large volume. Similarly gas exchange is reduced because of the relatively reduced, avascular surface area [1]. Either due to compression of the surrounding lung tissue or simply due to loss of elastic recoil in adjacent airways, there will be occlusion and atelectasis of lung tissue adjacent to the bulla.

Whilst surgical resection of the bulla is a recognized treatment, it has been shown that functional improvement after bullectomy is unsatisfactory in patients with poor respiratory reserve [2].

We report here a case of successful treatment of a large bulla in a patient with poor pulmonary function who had limited treatment options.

2. Case Report

A 59-year-old male patient was referred to our center for the assessment of his end-stage chronic obstructive airways disease.

He was an ex-smoker having smoked one pack per day for 40 years until two and a half years prior to the consultation. He had a long history of cough and shortness of breath and was diagnosed with COPD two years earlier. He had worked as a farmer but his worsening COPD had caused him to discontinue his occupation. He was unable to dress or wash himself without assistance, had shortness of breath on minimal exertion, and as a result had become bedridden. Despite

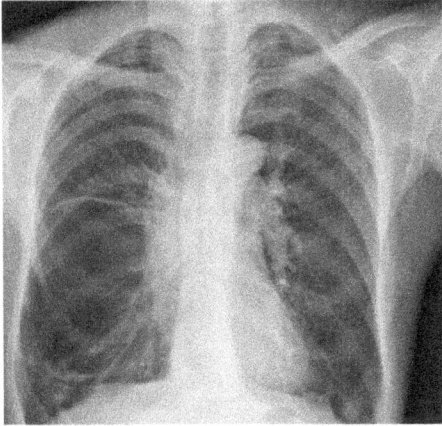

FIGURE 1: Pretreatment chest X-ray.

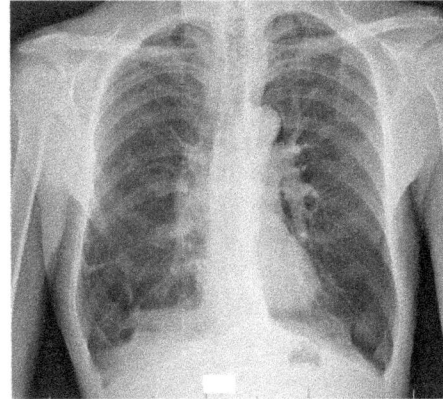

FIGURE 2: Pretreatment CT scan.

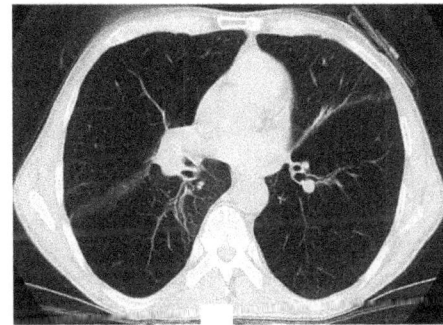

FIGURE 3: Posttreatment chest X-ray.

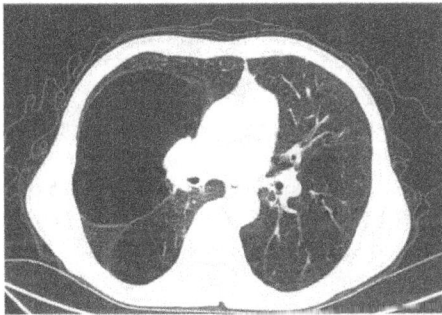

FIGURE 4: Posttreatment CT scan.

maximum use of bronchodilators, inhaled steroids, and long-term oxygen therapy he suffered frequent exacerbations of his COPD requiring hospital admissions. He had no other associated comorbidities and no family history of note.

When assessed in our unit for the first time, he was cachectic with a BMI of 17.9. Blood gases on air revealed a PaO2 of 54.9 torr and PaCO2 of 34 torr. Pulmonary function tests showed a forced expiratory volume in 1 s (FEV1) of 0.56 liters (19% predicted normal value). He had severe hyperinflation with a residual volume (RV) of 7 liters (314% predicted). His 6-minute walk test (6MWT) was 315 meters. His MRC dyspnea score was 4 and lowest oxygen saturation was 76% at rest.

Chest X-ray revealed a bilateral flattening of the diaphragm and bilateral hyperinflation. There was a massive bulla of approximately 10 cm in diameter occupying the right middle lobe (Figure 1). The CT scan confirmed bilateral emphysema and the giant bulla (166 × 85 mm diameter) in the right middle lobe causing compression atelectasis of the right middle and lower lobes (Figure 2). SPECT/CT showed a gross defect in ventilation and perfusion in the area of the right upper and middle lobes.

The patient was assessed for surgical bullectomy. However, it was considered that he would not be a good candidate for surgery in view of the severity of his COPD with the associated poor pulmonary function. Additionally, surgical bullectomy is associated with a significant risk of prolonged postoperative air leak which the patient would not be able to

tolerate. After discussion with the patient, it was decided to place one-way endobronchial valves in an attempt to collapse the bulla and allow surrounding lung tissue to expand again.

A fiber-optic bronchoscopy was performed under local anesthesia using lidocaine with the patient under conscious sedation with midazolam. Two Zephyr 4.0 valves were placed in the right middle lobe at B4 and B5. Postoperative chest X-ray did not show any evidence of pneumothorax. The patient made an uneventful recovery and was discharged after a two-day hospital stay.

Chest X-ray and CT scan performed 36 days after the procedure showed complete resolution of the right middle lobe bulla (Figures 3 and 4).

Seven months later, the patient demonstrated an improvement in 6MWT of 39% (437 meters). His FEV1 had improved by 30% to 0.73 liters (24% predicted). His RV has reduced from 314% predicted to 262% predicted. He was able to dress himself without help and to travel independently. At this time, he required oxygen supplementation only during exercise. His lowest oxygen saturation has increased 90% at rest.

Additional follow-up data are given in Table 1.

3. Discussion

Patients with large bullae and poor respiratory function have limited treatment options. Medical management is limited and whilst surgical resection of the bulla is a recognized

TABLE 1: Investigation results before treatment and at 7 months and 17 months after treatment.

	Before treatment (% predicted)	7 months after treatment (% predicted)	17 months after treatment (% predicted)
6MWT (m)	315	437	378
Pulmonary function tests			
FVC (L)	2.05 (54)	2.76 (73)	2.43 (65)
FEV1 (L)	0.56 (19)	0.73 (24)	0.61 (20)
IC (L)	0.83 (29)	1.42 (49)	1.20 (41)
TLC (L)	9.14 (146)	8.79 (140)	8.70 (139)
RV (L)	7.00 (314)	5.86 (262)	6.02 (267)
MRC dyspnea score	4	3	Not available

treatment, it has been shown that functional improvement after bullectomy is unsatisfactory in patients who have an FEV1 < 35% predicted, severe hypercapnia, and hypoxia [2]. Mortality in patients with diffuse emphysema who had underwent surgical resection of the bulla is higher than in those who did not have diffuse emphysema [3].

Less invasive approaches for patients with poor respiratory cell reserve have been considered. Takizawa et al. used CT guided drainage but prolonged air leak was a significant problem [4]. Bhattacharyya et al. decompressed an emphysematous bulla via a transbronchial aspiration needle and instilled autologous blood into the bulla to induce fibrosis. However, the risk of pneumothorax and bronchopleural fistula makes this procedure unsuitable for peripheral bullae [5].

The Zephyr Endobronchial Valve (Zephyr EBV) is designed to create volume reduction in patients with hyperinflation associated with emphysema. The device consists of a one-way, silicone, duckbill valve attached to a nickel-titanium (Nitinol), self-expanding retainer that is covered with a silicone membrane. It is implanted in the target bronchus using a flexible delivery catheter that is guided to the targeted bronchus by inserting it through a 2.8 mm working channel of a bronchoscope. It allows air and secretions to escape from the occluded lobe on expiration but prevents air from entering on inspiration [6].

For the treatment of a bulla, by placing EBV in the airways communicating with the bulla, air is able to escape from the bulla on expiration but no air enters on inspiration and, as a result, the bulla deflates. Respiratory function should improve either as a result of less compression of the surrounding tissue or simply as a result of the elimination of dead space allowing better ventilation and breathing mechanics. The EBVs are designed to be a permanent implant. However, in the event that there is no positive benefit or an adverse effect, the EBVs can easily be removed via a bronchoscope.

Santini et al. have reported a series of nine patients who benefited from EBV placement for the treatment of giant bullae. Mean FEV1 was 1.0 (35% predicted) and mean RV was 5.5 liters (231% predicted) [7]. In the case reported here, the patient was severely compromised with a FEV1 of 0.56 liters (19% predicted) and a RV of 7 liters (314%

predicted), but treatment was successful with resolution of the bulla, improved pulmonary function tests, and improved performance with an increase in 6MWT and the ability to recommence daily life activities.

In the Santini's series, the bullae were situated in the left upper lobe in five patients, right upper lobe in two patients, left lower lobe in one patient, and bilateral upper lobes in one patient [7]. Fiorelli et al. have published 15 patients with emphysema and 10 patients have isolated giant bullous. They found improvement in FEV1 for patient who has giant bullous higher than who has emphysema (11.7% versus 7%) [8]. In this study, occupation of the giant bulla in the chest, as well as compression of surrounding tissue and diaphragm, therefore after EBV applying that reported improvement in lung function. In our case, the bulla was situated in the right middle lobe and was successfully treated. It is not certain what role collateral ventilation has in maintaining the structure of bullae. However, when EBVs are used to create lung volume reduction in emphysema, superior results are obtained in the absence of collateral ventilation. Raasch et al. found that the fissures between the right middle lobe and adjacent lobes were incomplete in a high proportion of cases (94% minor fissure, 70% right upper major, and 47% right lower major), suggesting a high likelihood of collateral ventilation between right middle and adjacent lobes [9]. Success in this case may be explained because the placement of EBV blocked all airways feeding the bulla or, if additional channels were present, the resistance may have been sufficiently high that air preferentially escaped via the EBV, thus reducing the size of the bulla and increasing the resistance of collateral channels further.

4. Conclusion

In this case, the Zephyr Endobronchial Valves were successfully used to treat a large bulla in the right middle lobe in a patient with diffuse emphysema and severely impaired pulmonary function. Although a single case report, this case provides additional evidence to the case series of Santini et al. that EBV can be used to offer a safe treatment option for patients with emphysematous bullae who are not good candidates for surgery.

References

[1] M. D. L. Morgan, C. W. Edwards, J. Morris, and H. R. Matthews, "Origin and behaviour of emphysematous bullae," *Thorax*, vol. 44, no. 7, pp. 533–538, 1989.

[2] K. Nakahara, K. Nakaoka, K. Ohno et al., "Functional indications for bullectomy of giant bulla," *Annals of Thoracic Surgery*, vol. 35, no. 5, pp. 480–487, 1983.

[3] A. Palla, M. Desideri, G. Rossi et al., "Elective surgery for giant bullous emphysema: a 5-year clinical and functional follow-up," *Chest*, vol. 128, no. 4, pp. 2043–2050, 2005.

[4] H. Takizawa, K. Kondo, S. Sakiyama, and Y. Monden, "Computed tomography-guided drainage for large pulmonary bullae," *Interactive Cardiovascular and Thoracic Surgery*, vol. 3, no. 2, pp. 283–285, 2004.

[5] P. Bhattacharyya, D. Sarkar, S. Nag, S. Ghosh, and S. Roychoudhury, "Transbronchial decompression of emphysematous bullae: a new therapeutic approach," *European Respiratory Journal*, vol. 29, no. 5, pp. 1003–1006, 2007.

[6] ZEPHYR Endobronchial Valve System Instructions for Use, Pulmonx.

[7] M. Santini, A. Fiorelli, G. Vicidomini, V. G. Di Crescenzo, G. Messina, and P. Laperuta, "Endobronchial treatment of giant emphysematous bullae with one-way valves: a new approach for surgically unfit patients," *European Journal of Cardio-thoracic Surgery*, vol. 40, no. 6, pp. 1425–1431, 2011.

[8] A. Fiorelli, M. Petrillo, G. Vicidomini et al., "Quantitative assessment of emphysematous parenchyma using multidetector-row computed tomography in patients scheduled for endobronchial treatment with one-way valves," *Interactive Cardiovascular and Thoracic Surgery*, vol. 19, no. 2, pp. 246–255, 2014.

[9] B. N. Raasch, E. W. Carsky, E. J. Lane, J. P. O'Callaghan, and E. R. Heitzman, "Radiographic anatomy of the interlobar fissures: a study of 100 specimens," *American Journal of Roentgenology*, vol. 138, no. 6, pp. 1043–1049, 1982.

26

Perioperative Identification of an Accessory Fissure of the Right Lung

Yannick Taverne,[1,2] **Gert-Jan Kleinrensink,**[2] **and Peter de Rooij**[3]

[1]*Department of Cardiothoracic Surgery, Erasmus Medical Center, 's-Gravendijkwal 230, 3015 CE Rotterdam, Netherlands*
[2]*Department of Anatomy (ERCATHAN), Erasmus Medical Center, 's-Gravendijkwal 230, 3015 CE Rotterdam, Netherlands*
[3]*Department of General Surgery, Maasstad Hospital, Olympiaweg 350, 3078 RT Rotterdam, Netherlands*

Correspondence should be addressed to Yannick Taverne; y.j.h.j.taverne@erasmusmc.nl

Academic Editor: Fabio Midulla

Anatomical variations of lungs are common in clinical practice; however, they are sometimes overlooked in routine imaging. Surgical anatomy of the lung is complex and many variations are known to occur. A defective pulmonary development gives rise to variations in lobes and fissures. Morphological presentation is of clinical importance and profound knowledge of the organogenesis and functional anatomy is imperative for the interpretation and evaluation of lung pathophysiology and subsequent surgical intervention. However, appreciating them on radiographs and CT scans is difficult and they are therefore often either not identified or completely misinterpreted. As presented in this case report, an accessory fissure separating the superior segment of the right lower lobe from its native lobe was seen perioperatively and could only retrospectively be defined on X-rays and CT scan. It is imperative to keep in mind that accessory fissures can be missed on imaging studies and thus can make the surgical procedure more challenging.

1. Introduction

Anatomical variations of lungs are common in clinical practice and have been reported up to 40% in anatomical specimens [1, 2]. However, appreciating them on radiographs and CT scans is difficult and they are therefore either not identified or completely misinterpreted [1, 3]. Defective pulmonary development gives rise to variations in lobes and fissures which can only be comprehended from knowledge of embryology and developmental anatomy.

2. Case Report

We present a 33-year-old male admitted with progressive dyspnea and a nonproductive cough. Medical history includes an earlier admission with an atypical pneumonia (CURB 0: CURB-score is a clinical prediction rule that has been validated for predicting mortality in community-acquired pneumonia and infection of any site. In this case, CURB 0 represents a 30-day risk of death of 0.6%).

CT scan showed a pneumomediastinum with an interstitial lung disease without significant lymphadenopathy. Bronchoalveolar lavage and serology were negative. Therefore, video-assisted thoracoscopic (VATS) approach was used to obtain pulmonary biopsies. During VATS, we discovered an interesting anatomical variation of the lower lobe of the right lung; that is, the superior segment of the right lower lobe appeared separated from its native lobe through an extra fissure (Figures 1(a)–1(d)), thus giving this lung the image of a four-lobed organ. This finding was not visible on the plain X-ray (Figures 2(a)-2(b)) or detected during routine examination of the preoperative CT scan (Figures 3(a)–3(d)). Only after reexamination of the CT scan, the accessory fissure was detected.

3. Discussion

Fissures are defined as spaces separating individual bronchopulmonary buds or segments which get obliterated, except along two planes [4]. These planes will later be the horizontal

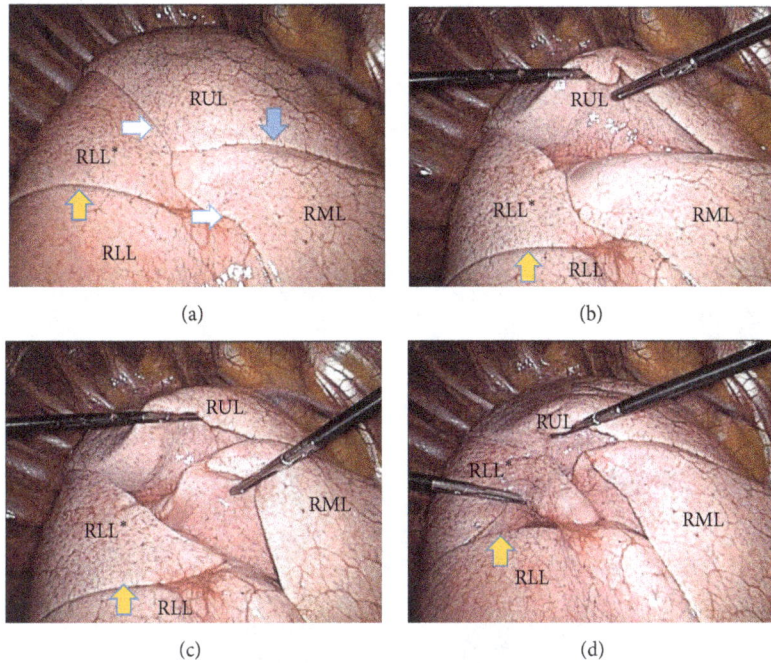

FIGURE 1: Perioperative pictures during VATS. All photographs were taken from the camera port distally with the patient lying on his left side and the arm in 90 degrees so the respective sides of these photographs concur with apical, ventral, distal, and dorsal positions, respectively. On the ventral side, the right internal mammary artery and vein running near the sternum can be seen. Pictures (a) to (d) display the different fissures as shown with long shaft instruments. RUL: right upper lobe; RML: right middle lobe; RLL: basal segments of the right lower lobe; RLL*: apical segment of the right lower lobe. Solid white arrows: horizontal fissure; blue arrow: oblique fissure; orange solid arrow: superior accessory fissure of the right lower lobe.

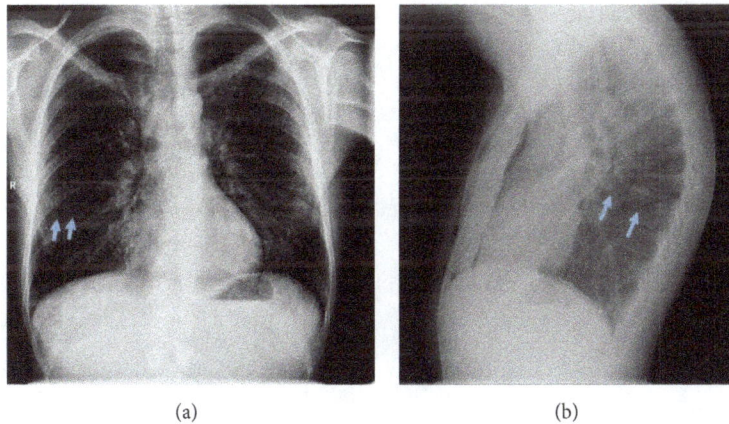

FIGURE 2: Plain X-rays. (a) anteroposterior X-ray; (b) lateral X-ray. Blue arrows show the superior accessory fissures (R = right side).

or oblique fissure. When these spaces are not obliterated, accessory fissures of the lung are created. All variations in lobulation and fissures are the result of altered pulmonary development. The presence of a variant fissure can be due to partial or complete failure of obliteration of these fissures [5–7].

The most common accessory fissures of the right lung detected on CT scans are the inferior accessory fissure, demarcating the medial basal segment, and the superior fissure which defines the superior segment [1]. As in our case, a superior accessory fissure separates the superior segment of

the lower lobe from the basal segment and is more common on the right side than on the left [8]. Superior accessory fissures have a reported incidence of 5–30% in autopsy studies as compared to the 3% incidence in high resolution CT scans [1, 5, 9]. In many cases, an accessory fissure fails to be detected on CT scan due to its incompleteness, thick CT scan sections, or orientation in relation to a particular anatomical plane [10].

From a functional and evolutionary point of view, a variant fissure separating the medial and lateral bronchopulmonary segments of the middle lobe and the basal segment from each basal segment, respectively, may be of advantage

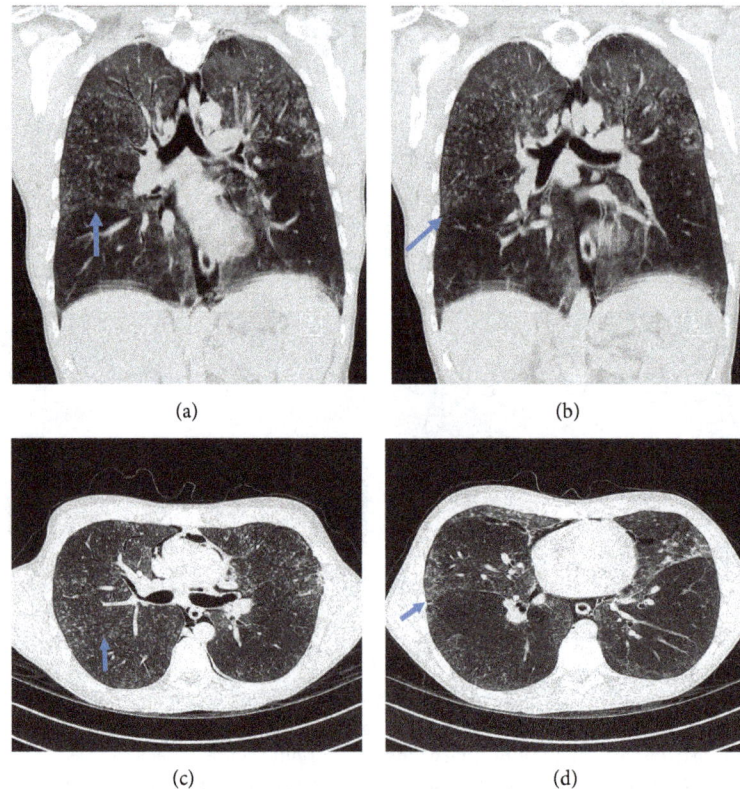

FIGURE 3: CT scan. (a)-(b) Coronal sections showing the bifurcation of the bronchus to the apical segment and the basal segments. There is no evidence of accessory branching, so no morphological extra lobe; hence there is only an accessory fissure (arrows). CT scans (a) and (b) have respiratory artifacts as seen at the level of the diaphragm. (c)-(d) Transversal sections showing the superior accessory fissure of the lower lobe of the right lung.

as it might limit the spread of infection [5]. It forms a sharp demarcated pneumonia which can be wrongly interpreted as atelectasis or consolidation [8]. Also, incomplete fissures are responsible for altering the spread of any lung disease [5].

4. Conclusion

It is imperative to keep in mind that an accessory fissure can be missed on imaging studies. Also, perioperative identification of the completeness of fissures and the presence of segmental localization is imperative before performing lobectomy. This is because individuals with an incomplete fissure are more prone to develop postoperative air leakage and thus possibly require further procedures such as a sleeve lobectomy.

References

[1] C. A. Ozmen, H. Nazaroglu, A. H. Bayrak, S. Senturk, and H. O. Akay, "Evaluation of interlobar and accessory pulmonary fissures on 64-row MDCT," *Clinical Anatomy*, vol. 23, no. 5, pp. 552–558, 2010.

[2] U. G. Esomonu, M. G. Taura, M. H. Modibbo, and A. O. Egwu, "Variation in the lobar pattern of the right and left lungs: a case report," *Australasian Medical Journal*, vol. 6, no. 10, pp. 511–514, 2013.

[3] K. Hayashi, A. Aziz, K. Ashizawa, H. Hayashi, K. Nagaoki, and H. Otsuji, "Radiographic and CT appearances of the major fissures," *Radiographics*, vol. 21, no. 4, pp. 861–874, 2001.

[4] M. Herriges and E. E. Morrisey, "Lung development: orchestrating the generation and regeneration of a complex organ," *Development*, vol. 141, no. 3, pp. 502–513, 2014.

[5] S. Meenakshi, K. Y. Manjunath, and V. Balasubramanyam, "Morphological variations of the lung fissures and lobes," *The Indian Journal of Chest Diseases & Allied Sciences*, vol. 46, no. 3, pp. 179–182, 2004.

[6] S. Joshi and S. Kotecha, "Lung growth and development," *Early Human Development*, vol. 83, no. 12, pp. 789–794, 2007.

[7] R. J. Metzger, O. D. Klein, G. R. Martin, and M. A. Krasnow, "The branching programme of mouse lung development," *Nature*, vol. 453, no. 7196, pp. 745–750, 2008.

[8] J. D. Godwin and R. D. Tarver, "Accessory fissures of the lung," *American Journal of Roentgenology*, vol. 144, no. 1, pp. 39–47, 1985.

[9] A. Yildiz, F. Gölpinar, M. Çalikoglu, M. N. Duce, C. Özer, and F. D. Apaydin, "HRCT evaluation of the accessory fissures of the lung," *European Journal of Radiology*, vol. 49, no. 3, pp. 245–249, 2004.

[10] O. M. Ariyürek, M. Gülsün, and F. B. Demirkazik, "Accessory fissures of the lung: evaluation by high-resolution computed tomography," *European Radiology*, vol. 11, no. 12, pp. 2449–2453, 2001.

27

A Cause of Bilateral Chylothorax: A Case of Mesothelioma without Pleural Involvement during Initial Diagnosis

Ercan Kurtipek,[1] Meryem İlkay Eren Karanis,[2] Nuri Düzgün,[3] Hıdır Esme,[3] and Mustafa Çaycı[4]

[1]Department of Chest Diseases, Konya Training and Research Hospital, 42090 Konya, Turkey
[2]Department of Pathology, Konya Training and Research Hospital, 42090 Konya, Turkey
[3]Department of Thoracic Surgery, Konya Training and Research Hospital, 42090 Konya, Turkey
[4]Department of Nuclear Medicine, Konya Training and Research Hospital, 42090 Konya, Turkey

Correspondence should be addressed to Ercan Kurtipek; kurtipek14@hotmail.com

Academic Editor: Gunnar Hillerdal

Chylothorax is characterized by fluid accumulation in the pleural cavity containing chylomicrons due to disruption of lymphatic drainage in the thoracic ductus and development of chylothorax. A 60-year-old male patient presented to our clinic with shortness of breath and displayed bilateral pleural effusion and diffuse mediastinal lymph nodes in his computed chest tomography images. There were no thickening and nodular formation on the pleural surfaces. PET-CT showed no pathological FDG uptake. Thoracentesis showed a chylous effusion. Drainage reduced during monitoring could not be stopped; therefore, surgical intervention was considered. The patient underwent right thoracotomy. There were no pathological findings in the parietal and visceral pleura during the surgery. Initially lymphoma was considered. Perioperative samples were collected from the mediastinal lymph node. The pathology analysis reported metastasis of malignant mesothelioma. Evaluation of a repeated chest computed tomography showed nodular formations on the pleural surfaces. Mediastinal lymph nodes compressed the ductus thoracicus, resulting with chylothorax. The present case, with malignant mesothelioma, bilateral chylothorax, and mediastinal lymph node without any pleural involvement during initial diagnosis, is rare and will hence contribute to the literature.

1. Introduction

Formation of chylous in the pleural space due to a damage or blockage of the thoracic duct is called chylothorax. It can result from tumors, lymphatic involvement, direct invasion, or tumor embolus, leading to spontaneous chylothorax. Lymphoma is the most common cause of nontraumatic chylothorax [1]. The majority of them develop secondary to obstruction of the lymphatic pathways from mediastinal lymphomas. Other malignancies with mediastinal involvement and infectious diseases may be associated with chylothorax [2]. Granulomatous diseases are also associated with chylothorax [2]. Malignant pleural mesothelioma (MPM) is a locally aggressive tumor with a very poor prognosis, where exposure to asbestos is the major etiology. Rare causes of MPM include radiotherapy, tuberculosis, and chronic empyema. Common findings of MPM from imaging studies include nodular pleural thickening, pleural plaques, and pleural effusion. We aimed to present a case whose thoracoscopy showed no pathological evidence on pleural surfaces while a computed tomography of the chest showed pleural thickening, and PET showed no pathological FDG uptake but resulted in bilateral chylothorax whose mediastinal lymph node sampling was reported as MPM.

2. Case Presentation

A 60-year-old male presented to our clinic with a complaint of shortness of breath. A computed tomography (CT) showed bilateral pleural effusion (Figure 1(a)) while CT analysis showed no thickening of pleural surfaces and nodular formation. Thoracentesis showed a chylous effusion. A biochemical analysis of the pleural fluid sample showed a triglyceride

(a)

(b)

(c)

(d)

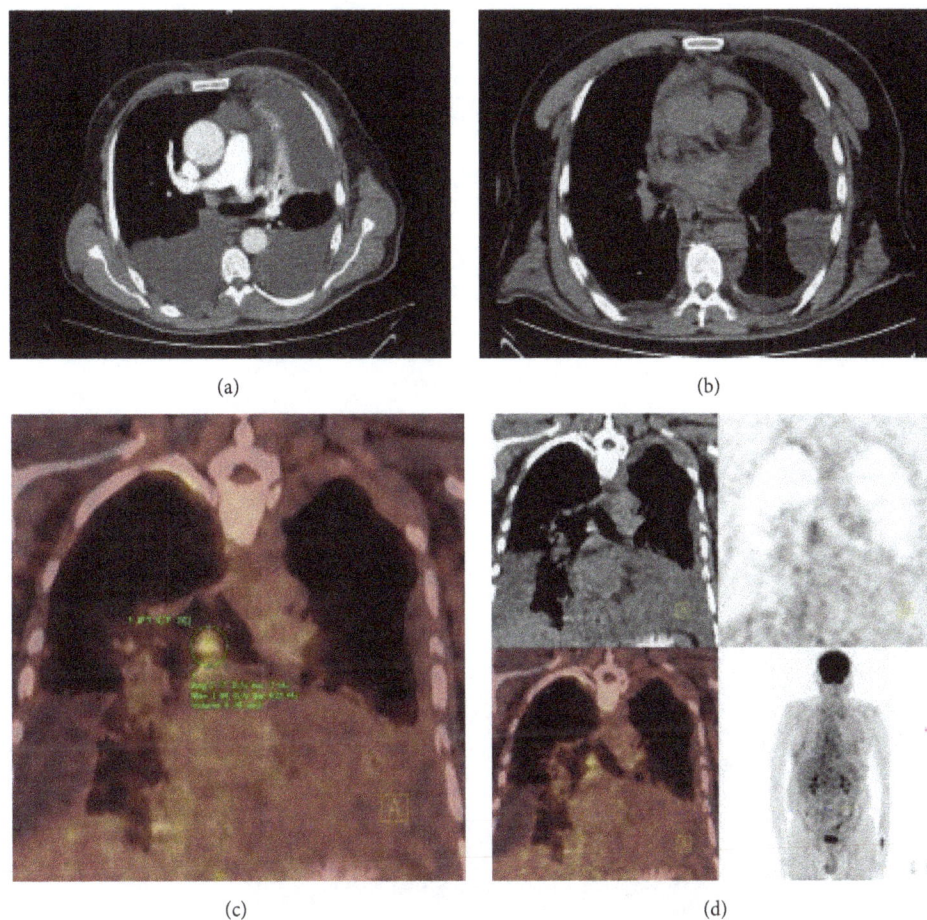

FIGURE 1: (a) A bilateral pleural effusion is noted in the CT obtained during first presentation. (b) A CT scan shows no nodular formation in the pleural surfaces following the drainage of pleural effusion. (c) A coronal PETCT image at the level of the mediastinal nodes. (d) PET-CT images are shown.

level of 1228 mg/dL and a cholesterol level of 149 mg/dL. The patient received bilateral thoracic drainage after withdrawal of oral nutrition, and he was initiated on a protein-rich and fat-poor parenteral nutrition. A new CT, which was repeated to prevent overlooking any potential lesions in the parenchyma after drainage of effusion, showed no thickening of pleural surfaces or any nodular formation (Figure 1(b)). Similarly, PET-CT showed no pathological FDG uptake (Figures 1(c)-1(d)). During monitoring, a surgery was planned at day 10 since drainage was reduced to less than 500 cc but persisted above 250 cc. The patient received 200 cc olive oil by nasogastric tube 2 hours before the surgery. He underwent right thoracotomy, and ductus thoracicus was identified between azygos vein and esophagus during the operation. It was followed by mass ligation just above the diaphragm. No pathology was observed in parietal and visceral pleura during the surgery suggesting mesothelioma. Specimens were collected from the mediastinal lymph nodes and sent to the pathology laboratory. A microscopic examination of the lymph node showed tumoral infiltration in a scattered pattern with layers under the capsule and between lymphoid follicles. Tumor cells are medium large cells with large eosinophilic cytoplasm, oval round vesicular nucleus, and

distinct nucleolus (Figure 2(a)). The immunohistochemical analysis showed diffuse and strong staining with Pan-CK (Figure 2(b)), Calretinin (Figure 2(c)), WT-1 (Figure 2(d)), vimentin, CK7, HBME-1, and D2-40 and focal staining with CK5/6 (Figure 2(e)), CEA, and EMA in tumor cells. No immune reaction was observed in tumor cells with CD68, TTF-1, Napsin-A, Melan-A, S-100, HMB45, LCA, Heppar-1, PLAP, and CK20 used for differential diagnosis. Based on these findings, the patient was diagnosed with metastasis of malignant mesothelioma. A recent CT which was performed at postoperative month 1 due to persistence of patient's complaints showed diffuse nodular formation. A pathological analysis of the lymph node reported MPM. Following a consultation with the medical oncology, a chemotherapy regimen was prescribed; however, the patient was unable to receive the treatment due to his impaired general condition.

3. Discussion

Clinically patients with chylothorax develop progressive dyspnea and tachypnea. Auscultation reveals decreased respiratory sound on the relevant side. Our patient presented to our

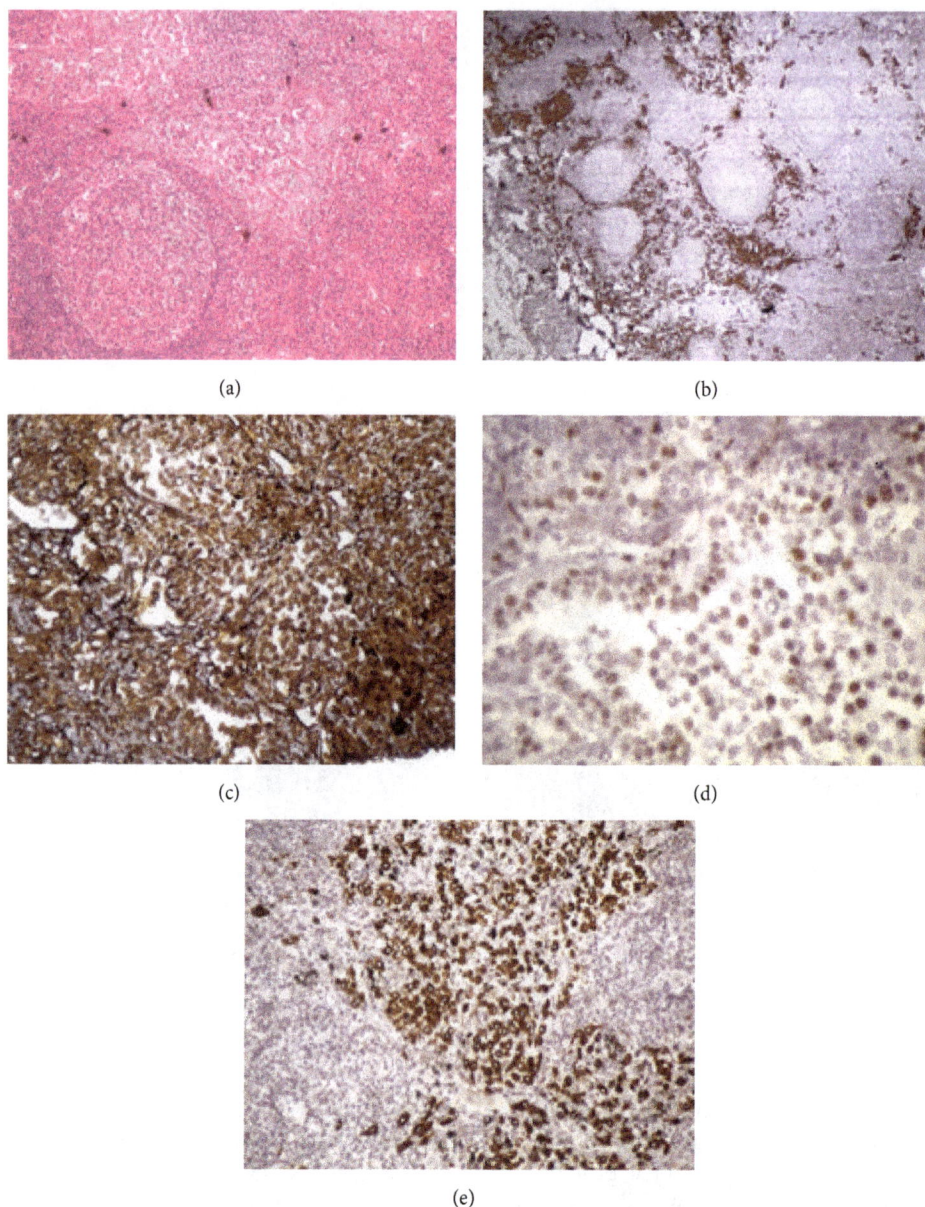

FIGURE 2: (a) Tumoral infiltration was seen between the lymphoid follicles. Tumor cells are medium large cells with large eosinophilic cytoplasm, oval round vesicular nucleus, and distinct nucleolus (HE × 200). (b) Cytoplasmic staining in tumor cells with immunohistochemical Pan-CK stain. Pan-CK × 100. (c) Cytoplasmic and nuclear staining in tumor cells with immunohistochemical Calretinin stain. Calretinin × 400. (d) Nuclear staining in tumor cells by immunohistochemical WT-1 stain. WT-1 × 400. (e) Cytoplasmic staining of tumor cells with immunohistochemical CK 5/6 stain. CK 5/6 × 200.

clinic with such complaints. Lymphoma is the most common cause of nontraumatic chylothorax [1]. Computed tomography is not efficient in locating the site of chyle leakage but is helpful in identifying the location of a mediastinal or thoracic lesion [3]. Fifty percent of patients with Hodgkin's lymphoma have lymphadenopathy in their thorax [4]. Puncture of pleural effusion common in most of the patients is the first diagnostic method for diagnosis of MPM. A cytologic examination of the pleural fluid allows establishment of diagnosis in 20% to 50% of patients. A percutaneous pleural biopsy may help in the diagnosis of one-third of the patients. Treatment

of chylothorax initially requires drainage of the chylous in the pleural space. However, surgical treatment is recommended in case of inefficient drainage and development of nutritional complications despite conservative management [1, 5]. The mortality of chylothorax was around 50% in the absence of surgery. The landmark in the treatment of chylothorax has been the initial successful treatment of a patient by ligation of ductus thoracicus in 1948 by Lampson [6].

Malignant pleural mesothelioma (MPM) is a rare condition, most commonly caused by exposure to asbestos, with increasing incidence worldwide. It generally occurs in the 5th to 7th decades of life, and 70–80% of patients are males. It is more common in men, which is mainly attributed to occupational exposure. The most common presenting complaints are shortness of breath and chest pain. One third of patients have shortness of breath without chest pain [7]. Our patient also had only a complaint of shortness of breath. Imaging has an important role in evaluating the response (especially in terms of resectability), treatment planning, monitoring, and diagnosis of patients with MPM. The imaging modalities used for diagnosis and treatment of MPM include X-ray, computed tomography (CT), magnetic resonance imaging (MRI), and positron emission tomography (PET). In BT, any evidence of unilateral pleural effusion, circumferential diffuse or pleural thickening, and shrinkage in hemithorax suggests MPM [8–10]. Our patient had no involvement of pleural surfaces during first presentation. There are some histological challenges in the diagnosis. A major challenge is the differentiation of malignant mesothelioma from reactive mesothelial cells. The same challenge exists for differentiation from lung adenocarcinomas [11].

Although several methods are available for treatment of MPM, there exists a consensus only for chemotherapy. The prognosis is usually poor in malignant mesotheliomas. A mean survival time of 4–12 months has been reported. The prognosis is better in female patients whose symptoms manifest in a period more than six months in younger ages without chest pain and involvement of visceral pleura [12].

In conclusion, MPM should be considered in patients presenting with particularly unilateral pleural effusion, pleural thickening, and chest pain. We believe that in our patient, the combination of MPM and bilateral chylothorax was associated with the rupture of the ductus thoracicus as a result of the invasion of the tumor in the mediastinal pleura into the mediastinum and ductus thoracicus.

References

[1] V. G. Valentine and T. A. Raffin, "The management of chylothorax," *Chest*, vol. 102, no. 2, pp. 586–591, 1992.

[2] F. Maldonado, R. Cartin-Ceba, F. J. Hawkins, and J. H. Ryu, "Medical and surgical management of chylothorax and associated outcomes," *American Journal of the Medical Sciences*, vol. 339, no. 4, pp. 314–318, 2010.

[3] R. A. Malthaner and R. I. Inculet, "The thoracic duct and chylothorax," in *Thoracic Surgery*, F. G. Pearson, J. D. Cooper, and J. Deslauriers, Eds., pp. 1228–1240, Churchill Livingstone, Philadelphia, Pa, USA, 2nd edition, 2002.

[4] R. Pugatch, "Thoracic neoplasms," in *Textbook of Diagnostic Imaging*, C. E. Putman and C. E. Ravin, Eds., pp. 562–580, W.B. Saunders Company, Philadelphia, Pa, USA, 1994.

[5] I. Opitz, "Management of malignant pleural mesothelioma. The European experience," *Journal of Thoracic Disease*, vol. 6, supplement 2, pp. S238–S252, 2014.

[6] R. S. Lampson, "Traumatic chylothorax. A review of the literature and report o a case treated by mediastinal ligation of the thoracic duct," *The Journal of Thoracic Surgery*, vol. 17, p. 778, 1948.

[7] I. Ahmed, S. A. Tipu, and S. Ishtiaq, "Malignant mesothelioma," *Pakistan Journal of Medical Sciences*, vol. 29, no. 6, pp. 1433–1438, 2013.

[8] E. F. Patz Jr., K. Shaffer, D. R. Piwnica-Worms et al., "Malignant pleural mesothelioma: value of CT and MR imaging in predicting resectability," *American Journal of Roentgenology*, vol. 159, no. 5, pp. 961–966, 1992.

[9] R. Eibel, S. Tuengerthal, and S. O. Schoenberg, "The role of new imaging techniques in diagnosis and staging of malignant pleural mesothelioma," *Current Opinion in Oncology*, vol. 15, no. 2, pp. 131–138, 2003.

[10] Z. J. Wang, G. P. Reddy, M. B. Gotway et al., "Malign plevral mezotelyoma: CT, MR görüntüleme, PET ile değerlendirme," *Radiographics*, vol. 24, no. 1, pp. 105–119, 2004.

[11] Ö. Üçer, A. F. Dağli, A. Kiliçarslan, and G. Artaş, "Value of Glut-1 and Koc markers in the differential diagnosis of reactive mesothelial hyperplasia, malignant mesothelioma and pulmonary adenocarcinoma," *Turkish Journal of Pathology*, vol. 29, no. 2, pp. 94–100, 2013.

[12] E. Taioli, A. S. Wolf, M. Camacho-Rivera, and R. M. Flores, "Women with malignant pleural mesothelioma have a threefold better survival rate than men," *Annals of Thoracic Surgery*, vol. 98, no. 3, pp. 1020–1024, 2014.

28

An Unusual Case of Pulmonary Nocardiosis in Immunocompetent Patient

Zehra Yaşar,[1] **Murat Acat,**[2] **Hilal Onaran,**[3] **Mehmet Akif Özgül,**[3] **Neslihan Fener,**[4]
Fahrettin Talay,[1] **and Erdoğan Çetinkaya**[3]

[1] *Department of Chest Diseases, Abant Izzet Baysal University School of Medicine, Gölköy, 14280 Bolu, Turkey*
[2] *Department of Chest Diseases, Karabuk University School of Medicine, 78000 Karabuk, Turkey*
[3] *Pulmonary Division, Yedikule Chest Diseases and Surgery Teaching and Research Hospital, 34010 Istanbul, Turkey*
[4] *Yedikule Chest Diseases and Surgery Teaching and Research Hospital, 34010 Istanbul, Turkey*

Correspondence should be addressed to Zehra Yaşar; zehraasuk@hotmail.com

Academic Editor: Akif Turna

Pulmonary nocardiosis is a subacute or chronic necrotizing pneumonia caused by aerobic actinomycetes of the genus *Nocardia* and rare in immune-competent patients. A 35-year-old male, who had treated with antituberculosis drugs, presented with cough, dyspnea, and expectoration with episodes of hemoptysis with purulent sputum. The diagnosis of nocardiosis was made by microscopic examination of the surgically resected portion of the lung and revealed filamentous Gram-positive bacteria.

1. Introduction

Nocardiosis, caused by Gram-positive, weakly acid-fast, filamentous aerobic actinomycetes, is an opportunistic infection and remains as a possible cause of pulmonary and systemic infection in immunocompromised patients [1]. But it can be isolated in otherwise immune-competent patients that consisted at least 15% of the infections in patients without a definable predisposing condition [2]. *Nocardia* species are common natural inhabitants of the soil throughout the world. Pulmonary nocardiosis is usually acquired by direct inhalation of *Nocardia* species form contaminated soil, and person-to-person transmission is rare [3]. Pulmonary nocardiosis is difficult to be diagnosed and is often mistaken for other lung diseases. We report a case of pulmonary nocardiosis that resembled tuberculosis, in a 35-year-old patient without a definable predisposing condition.

2. Case Report

A 35-year-old male presented with cough, dyspnea, and expectoration with episodes of hemoptysis with purulent sputum for 2 years. He took an antitubercular treatment for six months. With antitubercular treatment his fever had subsided but the sputum and hemoptysis had continued. Two months ago he referred to a general physician with low grade fever associated with productive cough and received some medication without any improvement. His condition became worsened. Chest X-ray showed infiltrations in right upper lobe with cavity formation (Figure 1(a)) and computed tomography (CT) revealed the presence of areas of consolidation with air bronchograms and cavitary lesions containing air and infiltration beginning from the apical segment lying to anterior segment of right lower lobe (Figure 2). The FDG PET/BT revealed a hypermetabolic lesion over the right upper lobe of the lung of the patient, with a maximum standardized uptake value (SUV) of 5.9–7.1 which favors a malignancy (Figure 2). Then, he received some antibiotics such as ceftazidime and ciprofloxacin. But he did not have any improvement in respiratory symptoms. Several sputum samples were collected and tested for the presence of acid-fast bacilli, but all smears were negative. The patient then underwent bronchoscopy and aspirated material was negative for tuberculosis, fungi (including Pneumocystis

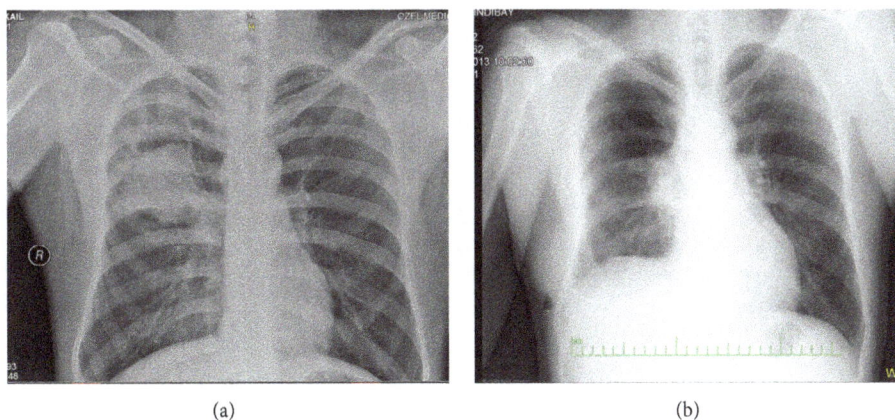

(a)　　　　　　　　　　　　　　　　(b)

FIGURE 1

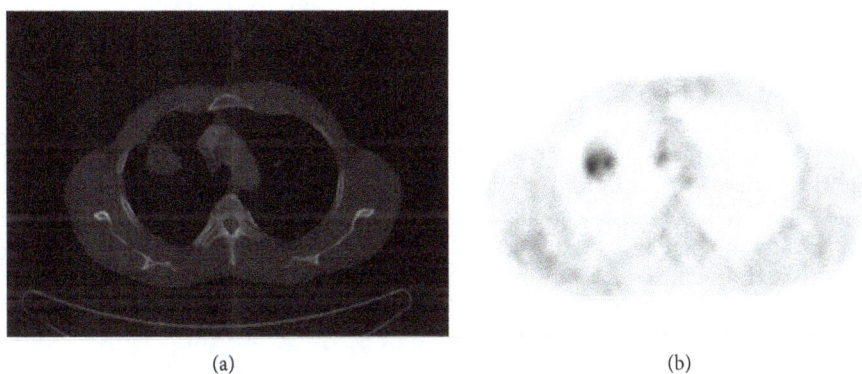

(a)　　　　　　　　　　　　　　　　(b)

FIGURE 2

jirovecii), and malignancy. FNAC was done from the right upper lung lesion. Aspirated material was negative for tuberculosis and malignancy. Because of progressive worsening of clinical status, right upper lobectomy was performed. On gram staining, the organism appeared as Gram-positive, thin branching filaments. Modified Ziehl-Neelsen staining showed many branching acid-fast bacilli, consistent with the morphology of *Nocardia* species (Figure 3). The patient was started on trimethoprim-sulfamethoxazole. The patient improved remarkably both clinically and radiographically (Figure 1(b)).

3. Discussion

Nocardia infection is a rare disorder caused by bacteria, which tends to affect the lung, brain, and skin. Pulmonary nocardiosis is a subacute or chronic pneumonia caused by a species of the family Nocardiaceae. Seven species have been associated with human disease. *N. asteroides* is responsible for about 70% of infection caused by these organisms [4], and debilitated patients have a 45% mortality rate even with appropriate therapy. The typical lesions of nocardiosis are abscesses extensively infiltrated with neutrophils. There is usually extensive necrosis; granulation tissue often surrounds the lesions.

Nocardia infections are rare among normal population. Nocardiosis typically develops in immunocompromised persons, such as those suffering from a lymphoreticular malignancy and Cushing's disease, those with acquired immune deficiency syndrome, those with transplanted organs, and those receiving high-dose corticosteroids [5]. Suppression of cellular immunity appears to play a key role in the establishment of *Nocardia* infection [6]. Bronchopulmonary or disseminated nocardiosis can occur in various rheumatologic diseases, including SLE, temporal arteritis, polyarthritis nodosa, intermittent hydrarthrosis, vasculitis, or uveitis [7]. Persons with pulmonary alveolar proteinosis are also at increased risk [8]. Nocardiosis can occur in apparently healthy population but further detailed immunologic evaluation particularly considering interleukin-12-gamma interferon pathway deficiency or other immunologic systems may help in diagnosis of these patients' underlying diseases in the future. Amatya et al. have also reported a case of immunocompetent individual with subcutaneous involvement involving *Nocardia* brasiliensis [9]. In our case any definable predisposing conditions were detected.

The clinical presentation of pulmonary nocardiosis is variable and nonspecific with a chronic course [6]. Symptoms usually have been present for days or weeks at presentation. In this case symptoms were present for two years before referring to our clinic. The usual symptoms are that of

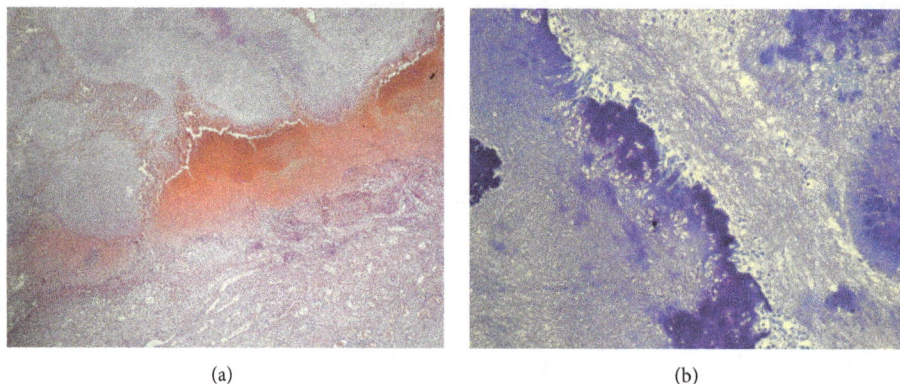

(a)   (b)

FIGURE 3

dyspnea, productive cough, and fever. In our case presenting symptoms were those of chronic cough with productive sputum, low grade fever, weakness, and failure to respond to ATT (antitubercular therapy).

The chest radiographic manifestations are pleomorphic and nonspecific. Consolidations and large irregular nodules, often cavitary, are most common; nodules, masses, and interstitial patterns also occur [10]. Upper lobes are more commonly involved [3]. Computed tomography findings include consolidation with or without cavitation, multiple discrete pulmonary nodules, pleural effusion, and chest wall extension.

Since the clinical and radiologic manifestations are non-specific, and the microbiological diagnosis is often difficult, it seems likely that, in some patients, pulmonary nocardiosis will be mistaken for other infections, such as tuberculosis, bacterial pneumonia, or malignancies. In countries where tuberculosis is very common, antituberculous drugs are started on basis of radiology and clinical symptoms like our case. A classic radiographic evidence of tuberculosis that is unresponsive to medication raises the suspicion of other diseases. Kumar et al. reported a case of pulmonary tuber-culosis; however in our case the patient was not suffering from pulmonary tuberculosis but was mimicking pulmonary tuberculosis, because of which there was failure to respond to ATT [11]. Similar cases mimicking pulmonary tuberculosis had been reported [12, 13] but invasive diagnostic procedures were not needed for diagnosis like our case.

Difficulty and slowness of culture growth, along with the lack of a serologic test for nocardiosis, necessitate its inclusion in the differential diagnosis for both immunocompromised and immunocompetent patients in whom an apparent pul-monary infection cannot be rapidly diagnosed. If sputum examinations do not yield the diagnosis in a suspected case and the diagnosis cannot be made easily from lesions elsewhere in the body, more invasive diagnostic procedures like bronchoscopy, needle aspiration, and open lung biopsy should be performed [11]. Because of progressive worsening of clinical status and a hypermetabolic lesion over the right upper lobe of the lung which favors a malignancy in our case, open lung biopsy and right upper lobectomy was performed.

The treatment of choice for this infection includes sulphonamides and, more recently, trimethoprim and sul-phamethoxazole associated with surgical drainage when required but other regimens like amikacin, imipenem, minocycline, linezolid, and cephalosporins are alternatives [14, 15]. Therapy must be prolonged to prevent relapses. The duration of treatment for nocardiosis depends on disease site. For pulmonary involvement, therapy is usually continued for 6 to 12 months or for 2 to 3 months after disease resolution [16].

This case highlights that pulmonary nocardiosis should be keep in mind in also immunocompetent patients, espe-cially in suspected cases of tuberculosis not responding to antitubercular therapy and showing no tubercle bacilli either in the direct smears or cultures.

References

[1] R. Martínez Tomás, R. Menéndez Villanueva, S. Reyes Calzada et al., "Pulmonary nocardiosis: risk factors and outcomes," *Respirology*, vol. 12, no. 3, pp. 394–400, 2007.

[2] B. L. Beaman, J. Burnside, B. Edwards, and W. Causey, "Nocar-dial infections in the United States, 1972–1974," *The Journal of Infectious Diseases*, vol. 134, no. 3, pp. 286–289, 1976.

[3] R. Menéndez, P. J. Cordero, M. Santos, M. Gobernado, and V. Marco, "Pulmonary infection with Nocardia species: a report of 10 cases and review," *European Respiratory Journal*, vol. 10, no. 7, pp. 1542–1546, 1997.

[4] J. H. Hwang, W.-J. Koh, G. Y. Suh et al., "Pulmonary nocardiosis with multiple cavitary nodules in a HIV-negative immunocom-promised patient," *Internal Medicine*, vol. 43, no. 9, pp. 852–854, 2004.

[5] R. B. Uttamchandani, G. L. Daikos, R. R. Reyes et al., "Nocar-diosis in 30 patients with advanced human immunodeficiency virus infection: clinical features and outcome," *Clinical Infec-tious Diseases*, vol. 18, no. 3, pp. 348–353, 1994.

[6] K. Hızel, K. Çağglar, H. Cabadak, and C. Külah, "Pulmonary nocardiosis in a non-Hodgkin's lymphoma patient," *Infection*, vol. 30, no. 4, pp. 243–245, 2002.

[7] P. D. Gorevic, E. I. Katler, and B. Agus, "Pulmonary nocardiosis. Occurrence in men with systemic lupus erythematosus," *Archives of Internal Medicine*, vol. 140, no. 3, pp. 361–363, 1980.

[8] M. B. Goetz and S. M. Finegold, "Nocardiosis," in *Textbook of Respiratory Medicine*, J. F. Murray and J. A. Nadel, Eds., Saunders, 3rd edition, 2000.

[9] R. Amatya, R. Koirala, B. Khanal, and S. Dhakal, "Nocardia brasiliensis primary pulmonary nocardiosis with subcutaneous involvement in an immunocompetent patient," *Indian Journal of Medical Microbiology*, vol. 29, no. 1, pp. 68–70, 2011.

[10] D. S. Feigin, "Nocardiosis of the lung: chest radiographic findings in 21 cases," *Radiology*, vol. 159, no. 1, pp. 9–14, 1986.

[11] A. Kumar, A. Mehta, G. Kavathia, and M. Madan, "Pulmonary and extra pulmonary tuberculosis along with pulmonary nocardiosis in a patient with human immuno deficiency virus infection," *Journal of Clinical and Diagnostic Research*, vol. 5, no. 1, pp. 109–111, 2011.

[12] V. Chopra, G. C. Ahir, G. Chand, and P. K. Jain, "Pulmonary nocardiosis mimicking pulmonary tuberculosis," *Indian Journal of Tuberculosis*, vol. 48, p. 211, 2001.

[13] G. Depaak and D. Gunjan, "Pulmonary nocardiosis mimicking tuberculosis—a case report," *Journal of Contemporary Medicine*, vol. 1, pp. 24–28, 2013.

[14] P. I. Lerner, "Nocardia species," in *Principles & Practice of Infectious Diseases*, G. I. Mandell, R. G. Douglas, and J. E. Benett, Eds., p. 192, John Wiley & Sons, New York, NY, USA, 2nd edition, 1985.

[15] M. A. Saubolle and D. Sussland, "Nocardiosis: review of clinical and laboratory experience," *Journal of Clinical Microbiology*, vol. 41, no. 10, pp. 4497–4501, 2003.

[16] A. R. Tunkel, J. K. Crane, and F. G. Hayden, "Pulmonary nocardiosis in AIDS," *Chest*, vol. 100, no. 1, pp. 295–296, 1991.

29

Endobronchial Enigma: A Clinically Rare Presentation of *Nocardia beijingensis* in an Immunocompetent Patient

Nader Abdel-Rahman,[1,2] **Shimon Izhakain,**[1,2] **Walter G. Wasser,**[3,4] **Oren Fruchter,**[1,2] **and Mordechai R. Kramer**[1,2]

[1] *The Pulmonary Institute, Rabin Medical Center, Beilinson Hospital, 49100 Petah Tikva, Israel*
[2] *The Sackler Faculty of Medicine, Tel Aviv University, 69978 Tel Aviv, Israel*
[3] *Mayanei HaYeshua Medical Center, 51544 Bnei Brak, Israel*
[4] *Rambam Health Care Campus, 3109601 Haifa, Israel*

Correspondence should be addressed to Shimon Izhakain; shimixyz@gmail.com

Academic Editor: Tun-Chieh Chen

Nocardiosis is an opportunistic infection caused by the Gram-positive weakly acid-fast, filamentous aerobic Actinomycetes. The lungs are the primary site of infection mainly affecting immunocompromised patients. In rare circumstances even immunocompetent hosts may also develop infection. Diagnosis of pulmonary nocardiosis is usually delayed due to nonspecific clinical and radiological presentations which mimic fungal, tuberculous, or neoplastic processes. The present report describes a rare bronchoscopic presentation of an endobronchial nocardial mass in a 55-year-old immunocompetent woman without underlying lung disease. The patient exhibited signs and symptoms of unresolving community-acquired pneumonia with a computed tomography (CT) scan that showed a space-occupying lesion and enlarged paratracheal lymph node. This patient represents the unusual presentation of pulmonary *Nocardia beijingensis* as an endobronchial mass. Pathology obtained during bronchoscopy demonstrated polymerase chain reaction (PCR) confirmation of nocardiosis. Symptoms and clinical findings improved with antibiotic treatment. This patient emphasizes the challenge in making the diagnosis of pulmonary nocardiosis, especially in a low risk host. A literature review presents the difficulties and pitfalls in the clinical assessment of such an individual.

1. Introduction

Nocardia infection was initially reported by Nocard, a French veterinarian in 1888 [1], who described an uncommon Gram-positive bacterial infection caused by aerobic Actinomycetes. Currently there are 85 identified species of *Nocardia* classified by using 16S rRNA gene sequence; approximately 25 species are associated with human infections. These include *Nocardia asteroides* complex (more than 50% human cases), *N. brasiliensis*, *N. abscessus*, *N. cyriacigeorgica*, *N. farcinica*, *N. nova*, *N. transvalensis* complex, *N. nova* complex, *N. pseudobrasiliensis*, *Nocardia veteran*, *N. cerradoensis* [2], and recently reported *N. beijingensis* [3–8]. Sputum isolation of *Nocardia* always represents an infection since *Nocardia* is not part of the human normal flora.

The clinical presentation of pulmonary nocardiosis can be acute, subacute, or chronic pneumonia. The diagnosis can be challenging, as often signs and symptoms are nonspecific including fever, night sweats, fatigue, anorexia, weight loss, dyspnea, cough, hemoptysis, and pleuritic chest pain [9, 10]. Moreover, there are a wide range of radiographic presentations such as lobar infiltrates, effusion, abscesses, cavities, lobar consolidations, subpleural plaques, and masses.

Nocardiosis has been observed to be associated with a wide range of conditions, especially those with impaired cell mediated immunity, including solid organ and hematopoietic stem cell transplantation, acquired immunodeficiency syndrome (AIDS), and hematologic and solid organ malignancies as well as chronic systemic steroid use. Nevertheless, there are a limited number of reports of nocardial infection of immunocompetent individuals described in the literature [11–20]. Structural lung abnormalities such as bronchiectasis and COPD have been shown to be associated with nocardial infection among immunocompetent individuals [11–14].

The present report describes the clinical presentation of *N. beijingensis* as an endobronchial mass in an immunocompetent middle aged woman, without evidence of lung disease.

2. Case Presentation

A 55-year-old female presented to our hospital with a low grade fever, productive cough, and hemoptysis, which had developed over the previous 6 months.

Her past medical history included breast cancer, which was operated on without complications 9 years prior to her current admission. Based on symptoms, physical examinations, and imaging studies, she was diagnosed with community-acquired pneumonia and treated with several courses of doxycillin, amoxicillin, and cefuroxime. However, symptoms of low grade fever and cough persisted despite therapy.

The patient represented with an exacerbation of the fever and cough, now accompanied by progressive weight loss, and severe malaise having lost 5 Kg during the previous 6-month period.

On physical examination her temperature was 38°C, heart rate was 82 beats per minute, and her blood pressure was 142/84 mmHg. The patient's chest was clear to auscultation and no lymphadenopathy was present.

Laboratory studies demonstrated a hemoglobin (HB) level of 11.9 gr/dL, Hematocrit (HCT) of 36.6%, White Blood Cell (WBC) count of 21,820 K/μL with 91.2% neutrophils, Erythrocyte Sedimentation Rate (ESR) of 85 mm/h, and C-Reactive Protein (CRP) of 14.2 mg/dL.

Serum liver enzymes and function tests were all within the normal limits. Evaluation of renal function revealed blood urea nitrogen (BUN) of 28 mg/dL, creatinine of 0.71 mg/dL, and normal urinalysis.

Serologic investigation for autoimmune disease revealed normal findings including anti-proteinase, anti-myeloperoxidase, anti-JO-1, anti-SCL, anti-SSA, anti-SSB, and anti-Smith antibodies, anti-nuclear antibodies, anti-double stranded DNA, and alpha-1 antitrypsin.

A computed tomography (CT) of her chest with contrast revealed an enlarged paratracheal lymph node of 15 mm, a space-occupying lesion with a diameter of 4.2 cm that externally compressed the right upper lobe, and cavitary lesion with a diameter of 3.2 cm in the right lower lobe (Figure 1).

Three bronchoscopies were performed over period of 3 months. The first bronchoscopy was performed on the 25th hospital day, a repeat bronchoscopy was performed 22 days later, and a third bronchoscopy was performed 30 days later.

The first bronchoscopy revealed white friable skipped lesions on the end bronchial surface of the right lower lobe. Multiple endobronchial and transbronchial biopsies were extracted and analyzed. A bronchoalveolar lavage (BAL) was also performed and fungal and bacterial cultures were obtained and plated on blood agar, chocolate agar, MacConkey agar, buffered charcoal yeast extract (BCYE) agar, and Lowenstein medium. Specimens were sent for

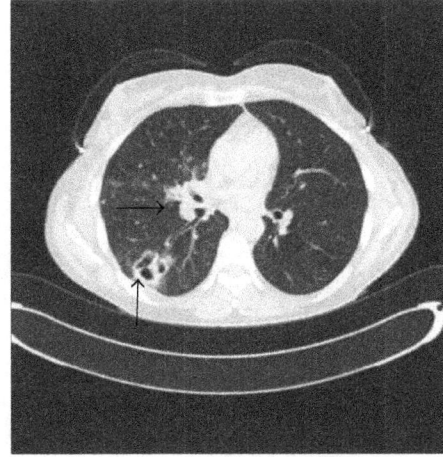

FIGURE 1: CT scan of the lung, axial view: the horizontal arrow is pointing toward nocardial mass in the right lower lob, while the longitudinal arrow is pointing toward nocardial cavitary lesion in the same lobe.

Ziehl-Neelsen stain. The biopsy results showed granulation tissues with abscesses, mixed inflammation, and no signs of malignancy or granulomas. The bronchoscopic cultures were negative for pathogens.

Steroid therapy for a presumed vasculitic lesion was begun with prednisone 30 mg daily with a tapering dose until discontinued after 21 days. This yielded a brief general improvement at the first few days.

The patient returned after worsening of her symptoms and underwent a second bronchoscopy which did not present any additional information. She was discharged with antimicrobial empirical treatment with ciprofloxacin.

In the following week, she was admitted again with high grade fever, coughing, weight loss, and general deterioration. A third bronchoscopy was performed which showed white friable material which was previously described (Figures 2(a) and 2(b)). We obtained viral (cytomegalovirus, adenovirus), bacterial (Legionella), and fungal cultures from the bronchoalveolar lavage. We also send the material for staining (PAS and silver stain) and performing PCR studies for *Pneumocystis carinii*, *Cryptococcus*, *Aspergillus*, and *Nocardia*. All of these lab examination revealed negative results. The only positive results were the encoded genes "RNA 16S" and "HSP 65" of the Actinomycetes family, consistent with *Nocardia beijingensis* which showed a 98% match.

After several days of prolonged incubation, *Nocardia* colonies were visible. Antibiotic sensitivities showed the *Nocardia* species to be sensitive to all antibiotics and resistant only to ciprofloxacin (Table 1). A review of the bronchoscopic biopsy revealed Gram-positive filamentous microorganism, also confirming the diagnosis of *Nocardia* (Figure 3).

Thus, a diagnosis of endobronchial pulmonary nocardiosis was obtained and the patient was treated for 3 months with oral trimethoprim-sulfamethoxazole (TMP-SMX) and intravenous ceftriaxone for 1 month. Antibiotic treatment was followed by complete patient recovery.

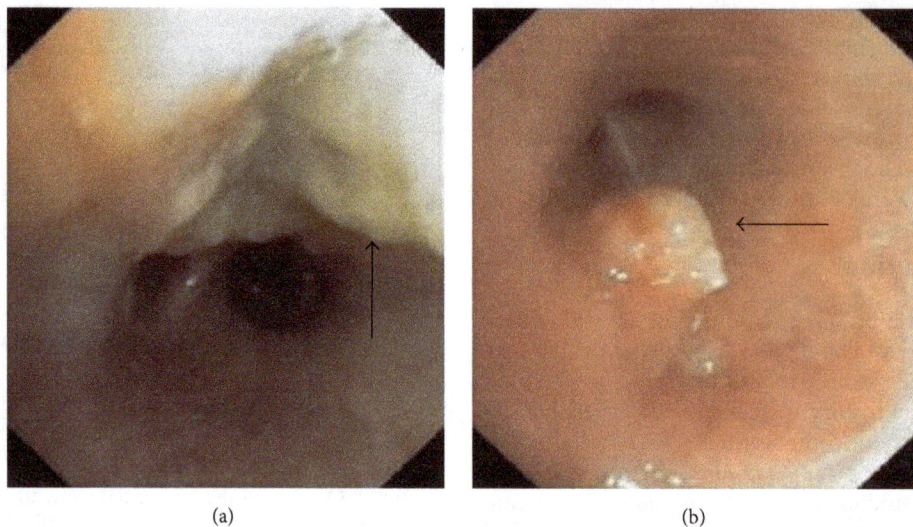

(a)   (b)

FIGURE 2: Bronchoscopic images: the arrows are pointing to different views of nocardial white friable lesions (a) and mass (b) in the right lower lobe.

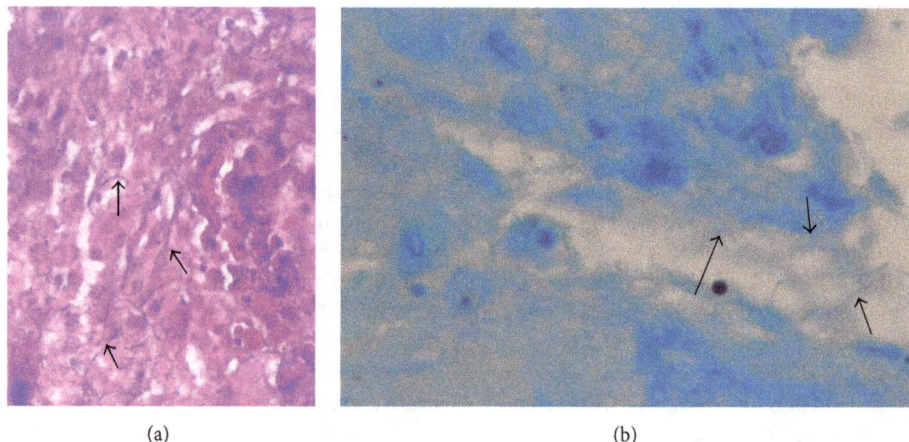

(a)   (b)

FIGURE 3: (a) Gram stain (×40). Arrows point toward Gram-positive filamentous microorganism. (b) Ziehl-Neelsen stain (×100). Arrows point toward partially acid-fast beaded branching filaments.

TABLE 1: *N. beijingensis* isolate antimicrobial susceptibility results.

Antibiotic	Susceptibility
Amikacin	Sensitive
Ciprofloxacin	Sensitive
Ceftriaxone	Sensitive
Imipenem	Sensitive
Minocycline	Sensitive
Sulfamethoxazole/trimethoprim	Sensitive
Ertapenem	Sensitive

3. Discussion

Nocardiosis is thought to be a rare, opportunistic disease. One would expect an increase in its prevalence due to immunosuppression and the increasing use of corticosteroids. In this report, we are able to demonstrate that the increased sensitivity of modern laboratory techniques enhanced our ability to detect nocardial infection even in a healthy individual.

Pulmonary nocardiosis in immunocompetent patients is the subject of a number of recent reports [11–20]. Although some of these patients had underlying lung abnormalities such as COPD or asthma, they did not receive therapy with immunosuppressives or steroids [11–14]. These sporadic reports indicate chronic air flow obstruction to be a risk factor for pulmonary nocardiosis. What makes the present description unusual is that our patient neither received immunosuppressive therapy nor had any underlying lung disease [15–20].

The diagnosis of pulmonary nocardiosis is difficult to document. Precious time may elapse, and during that time the condition of the patient might deteriorate. The median time for diagnosis of pulmonary nocardiosis was 32–42 days, which may increase to 55 days with dissemination to

TABLE 2: Summary of pulmonary nocardiosis cases presented as endobronchial mass.

Number	Age/sex	Smoking status	Clinical presentation	CXR/CT	Bronchoscopic findings	Identified species	Main treatment
1	73/male	Ex-smoker	Cough, fever, malaise, night sweats, and weight loss	Air space opacity RUL	Polypoid mass at the RUL [21]	Nocardia asteroides	TMP-SMX therapy, for 6 months
2	51/male	Ex-smoker	Malaise, low grade fever, chills, and cough	Infiltrate in the anterior segment of RUL	White exophytic lesion occluding the anterior segment RUL [22]	Nocardia asteroides	TMP-SMX therapy, for 3 months
3	28/male	Nonsmoker	Cough, fever, malaise, weight loss, night sweats, and dyspnea	Paramediastinal mass occluding RMB	Large fungating mass extending from the RMB [23]	Nocardia asteroides	Triple-sulfa therapy, for 6 months, gentamicin, for 3 months. RUL lobectomy
4	56/male	Ex-smoker	Cough, night sweats, and malaise	Left lung infiltrate	Mucosal edema and endobronchial mass [24]	Nocardia asteroides	Sulfisoxazole therapy, for 1 year
5	32/female	Unspecified	Fever, cough, and hemoptysis	RUL thick wall cavity with suspected fungal ball inside [25]	No bronchoscopy, on thoracotomy, fungal ball on RLL segments	Nocardia sp. (unspecified)	RML and RLL resection (unspecified antibiotics)
6	70/male	Smoker	Cough, dyspnea, anorexia, and weight loss	Mass in the RUL bronchus	Obstructing "tumor" of the RMB [26]	Nocardia asteroides	Minocycline, for 10 months
7	25/female	Nonsmoker	Persistent cough, pleuritic chest pain, and hemoptysis	Infiltrates RUL, RML, and RLL pleural effusion	Friable lesion "pearly white" occluding the entire segment [27]	Nocardia sp. (unspecified)	Antituberculosis medication. TMP-SMX therapy (unspecified duration)
8	55/female	Ex-smoker	Cough, weight loss, and hemoptysis	Endobronchial mass and cavitary lesion	Friable weight material, our case	Nocardia beijingensis	TMP-SMX therapy, for 3 months, ceftriaxone, for 1 month

RUL, right upper lobe; RML, right middle lobe; RLL, right lower lobe; RMB, right middle bronchus of lung; TMP-SMX, trimethoprim-sulfamethoxazole.
All patients had symptoms resolution after initiating the appropriate treatment, except in case 5 where the patient died due to late diagnosis.

the nervous system [28]. Diagnosis in our patient required a total of 51 days. Mortality due to pulmonary nocardiosis continues to be high, between 14 and 40%, and increases significantly when there is dissemination to nervous system [28–30].

Several factors contribute to difficulties of diagnosis. Firstly, fungal cultures are time-consuming process; typical colonies are usually seen after 3 to 5 days and may even take up to 4 weeks [31]. Thus, it is critical to notify the laboratory when nocardial infection is suspected so that appropriate measures may be taken to optimize recognition and recovery of the organism. Secondly, it has been reported that in up to half of pulmonary nocardiosis cases the diagnosis cannot be achieved by sputum alone, thereby requiring further assessment of bronchoalveolar lavage or other respiratory samples [32]. Thirdly, prescribing empirical antibiotics therapy can contribute to difficulties in isolating the organism, which can

cause complications when further invasive assessments are needed. Fourthly, serology is usually not useful, as no single serological technique can detect all of the clinically relevant species. Moreover, the antibody response is usually impaired in immunocompromised patients [33]. Fifthly, diagnosis is extremely difficult since nocardiosis is a rare disease, not well known by clinicians in daily practice. Finally, the clinical and radiographic findings in pulmonary and disseminated nocardiosis are nonspecific and may be mistaken for a variety of other bacterial infections, including actinomycosis and tuberculosis, as well as fungal infections, malignancies, and other diseases.

Uttamchandani et al., reporting a series of 30 cases of pulmonary nocardiosis, demonstrated infiltrates in 23 patients located in the upper lobe mimicking tuberculosis [10]. In others reports, empirical treatment for pulmonary tuberculosis was actually begun [11, 27, 34].

Nocardia beijingensis was first isolated by Wang et al. from soil in a sewage ditch in China in 2001 [3]. In 2004, the first human infections were reported in Thailand and Japan [4]. In 2008, a case of cutaneous *N. beijingensis* in an immunocompetent host was reported in France [5]. In 2011, the first pulmonary case outside Asia was reported [7]. In 2014, the first pulmonary case in the Western Hemisphere was reported [8].

No prospective randomized trials have determined the most effective therapy for nocardiosis. In addition, it is unlikely that such trials will ever be performed due to the uncommon nature and diverse clinical presentation. Thus, the choice of antimicrobials is based upon retrospective experience, animal model investigation, and *in vitro* antimicrobial activity profiles [35].

Treatment regimens effective against *Nocardia* spp. include trimethoprim-sulfamethoxazole (TMP-SMX), amikacin, imipenem, and third generation cephalosporins (ceftriaxone and cefotaxime). However, antibiotic susceptibilities vary among isolates [36].

In our patient, the pulmonary lesion was rare presentation of an endobronchial nocardial mass. This presentation mimics similar mass lesions seen in granulomatous or neoplastic diseases. *Nocardia* has been described as an endobronchial mass in 7 previous reports [21–27] presented in Table 2. In 2 previous reports, masses occluded one of the lung lobes and cause even severe atelectasis [21, 22].

In conclusion, pulmonary nocardiosis should be considered in the differential diagnosis of unresolving pneumonia or an endobronchial mass lesion in an immunocompetent individual. The diagnosis of an endobronchial mass lesion due to nocardial infection is rare and may be easily confused for tuberculosis or bronchogenic tumor. Appropriate tests need to be expeditiously obtained to document the diagnosis and beginning of therapy with an appropriately sensitive antibiotic such as trimethoprim-sulfamethoxazole. Prompt initiation of therapy is required to prevent central nervous system dissemination and increased patient morbidity and mortality.

References

[1] M. E. Nocard, "Note sur la maladie des boeufs de la Guadeloupe: connue sous le nom de farcin," *Annales de l'Institut Pasteur*, vol. 2, pp. 293–302, 1888.

[2] V. Kandi, "Human *Nocardia* infections: a review of pulmonary nocardiosis," *Cureus*, vol. 7, no. 8, article e304, 2015.

[3] L. Wang, Y. Zhang, Z. Lu et al., "Nocardia beijingensis sp. nov., a novel isolate from soil," *International Journal of Systematic and Evolutionary Microbiology*, vol. 51, part 5, pp. 1783–1788, 2001.

[4] A. Kageyama, N. Poonwan, K. Yazawa, Y. Mikami, and K. Nishimura, "Nocardia beijingensis, is a pathogenic bacterium to humans: the first infectious cases in Thailand and Japan," *Mycopathologia*, vol. 157, no. 2, pp. 155–161, 2004.

[5] C. Derancourt, R. Theodose, L. Deschamps et al., "Primary cutaneous nocardiosis caused by *Nocardia beijingensis*," *British Journal of Dermatology*, vol. 167, no. 1, pp. 216–218, 2012.

[6] C. Martinaud, C. Verdonk, A. Bousquet et al., "Isolation of *Nocardia beijingensis* from a pulmonary abscess reveals human immunodeficiency virus infection," *Journal of Clinical Microbiology*, vol. 49, no. 7, pp. 2748–2750, 2011.

[7] E. R. Lederman and N. F. Crum, "A case series and focused review of nocardiosis: clinical and microbiologic aspects," *Medicine*, vol. 83, no. 5, pp. 300–313, 2004.

[8] J. A. Crozier, S. Andhavarapu, L. M. Brumble, and T. Sher, "First report of *Nocardia beijingensis* infection in an immunocompetent host in the United States," *Journal of Clinical Microbiology*, vol. 52, no. 7, pp. 2730–2732, 2014.

[9] R. Martínez Tomás, R. Menéndez Villanueva, S. Reyes Calzada et al., "Pulmonary nocardiosis: risk factors and outcomes," *Respirology*, vol. 12, no. 3, pp. 394–400, 2007.

[10] R. B. Uttamchandani, G. L. Daikos, R. R. Reyes et al., "Nocardiosis in 30 patients with advanced human immunodeficiency virus infection: clinical features and outcome," *Clinical Infectious Diseases*, vol. 18, no. 3, pp. 348–353, 1994.

[11] F. Rivière, M. Billhot, C. Soler, F. Vaylet, and J. Margery, "Pulmonary nocardiosis in immunocompetent patients: can COPD be the only risk factor?" *European Respiratory Review*, vol. 20, no. 121, pp. 210–212, 2011.

[12] L. Verfaillie, J. De Regt, A. De Bel, and W. Vincken, "*Nocardia asiatica* visiting Belgium: nocardiosis in a immunocompetent patient," *Acta Clinica Belgica*, vol. 65, pp. 425–427, 2010.

[13] M. Nisbet, T. Eaton, S. Roberts, D. Milne, K. Rogers, and A. Woodhouse, "Pulmonary nocardiosis in an immunocompetent host: successful treatment with moxifloxacin and minocycline of multiple drug-resistant nocardia transvalensis complex," *Infectious Disease in Clinical Practice*, vol. 14, no. 1, pp. 55–58, 2006.

[14] J. M. Brechot, F. Capron, J. Prudent, and J. Rochemaure, "Unexpected pulmonary nocardiosis in a non-immunocompromised patient," *Thorax*, vol. 42, no. 6, pp. 479–480, 1987.

[15] S. De and P. Desikan, "Pulmonary nocardiosis mimicking relapse of tuberculosis," *BMJ Case Reports*, 2009.

[16] K. Wakamatsu, N. Nagata, H. Kumazoe, A. Kajiki, and Y. Kitahara, "*Nocardia transvalensis* pulmonary infection in an immunocompetent patient with radiographic findings consistent with nontuberculous mycobacterial infections," *Journal of Infection and Chemotherapy*, vol. 17, no. 5, pp. 716–719, 2011.

[17] W. O. Tam, C. F. Wong, and P. C. Wong, "Endobronchial nocardiosis associated with broncholithiasis," *Monaldi Archives for Chest Disease*, vol. 69, no. 4, pp. 183–185, 2008.

[18] S. Sud, T. B. S. Buxi, I. Anand, and A. Rohatgi, "Case series: nocardiosis of the brain and lungs," *Indian Journal of Radiology and Imaging*, vol. 18, no. 3, pp. 218–221, 2008.

[19] O. Dikensoy, A. Filiz, N. Bayram et al., "First report of pulmonary Nocardia otitidiscaviarum infection in an immunocompetent patient from Turkey," *International Journal of Clinical Practice*, vol. 58, no. 2, pp. 210–213, 2004.

[20] E. Gupta, B. Dhawan, M. M. Thabah, B. K. D. S. Sood, and A. Kapil, "*Nocardia* pyopneumothorax in an immunocompetent patient," *Indian Journal of Medical Research*, vol. 124, no. 3, pp. 363–364, 2006.

[21] M. Alanezi, S. Pugsley, D. Higgins, M. Smieja, and C. H. Lee, "An elderly man with nonresolving cough, leukocytosis and a pulmonary mass," *Canadian Medical Association Journal*, vol. 169, no. 2, pp. 134–135, 2003.

[22] F. E. Casty and M. Wencel, "Endobronchial nocardiosis," *European Respiratory Journal*, vol. 7, no. 10, pp. 1903–1905, 1994.

[23] A. Brown, S. Geyer, M. Arbitman, and B. Postic, "Pulmonary nocardiosis presenting as a bronchogenic tumor," *Southern Medical Journal*, vol. 73, no. 5, pp. 660–663, 1980.

[24] J. Q. Henkle and S. V. Nair, "Endobronchial pulmonary nocardiosis," *Journal of the American Medical Association*, vol. 256, no. 10, pp. 1331–1332, 1986.

[25] R. Tilak, D. Agarwal, T. K. Lahiri, and V. Tilak, "Pulmonary nocardiosis presenting as fungal ball—a rare entity," *Journal of Infection in Developing Countries*, vol. 2, no. 2, pp. 143–145, 2008.

[26] K. D. McNeil, D. W. Johnson, and W. A. Oliver, "Endobronchial nocardial infection," *Thorax*, vol. 48, no. 12, pp. 1281–1282, 1993.

[27] N. Kumar and R. Ayinla, "Endobronchial pulmonary nocardiosis," *Mount Sinai Journal of Medicine*, vol. 73, no. 3, pp. 617–619, 2006.

[28] M. B. Chedid, M. F. Chedid, N. S. Porto, C. B. Severo, and L. C. Severo, "Nocardial infections: report of 22 cases," *Revista do Instituto de Medicina Tropical de São Paulo*, vol. 49, pp. 239–246, 2007.

[29] M. J. Agterof, T. van der Bruggen, M. Tersmette, E. J. ter Borg, J. M. M. van den Bosch, and D. H. Biesma, "Nocardiosis: a case series and a mini review of clinical and microbiological features," *Netherlands Journal of Medicine*, vol. 65, no. 6, pp. 199–202, 2007.

[30] J. Muñoz, B. Mirelis, L. M. Aragón et al., "Clinical and microbiological features of Nocardiosis 1997–2003," *Journal of Medical Microbiology*, vol. 56, pp. 545–550, 2007.

[31] L. R. Ashdown, "An improved screening technique for isolation of *Nocardia* species from sputum specimens," *Pathology*, vol. 22, no. 3, pp. 157–161, 1990.

[32] C.-H. Hui, V. W. K. Au, K. Rowland, J. P. Slavotinek, and D. L. Gordon, "Pulmonary nocardiosis re-visited: experience of 35 patients at diagnosis," *Respiratory Medicine*, vol. 97, no. 6, pp. 709–717, 2003.

[33] B. A. Brown-Elliott, J. M. Brown, P. S. Conville, and R. J. Wallace Jr., "Clinical and laboratory features of the *Nocardia* spp. based on current molecular taxonomy," *Clinical Microbiology Reviews*, vol. 19, no. 2, pp. 259–282, 2006.

[34] M. A. John, T. E. Madiba, P. Mahabeer, K. Naidoo, and A. W. Sturm, "Disseminated nocardiosis masquerading as abdominal tuberculosis," *South African Journal of Surgery*, vol. 42, no. 1, pp. 17–19, 2004.

[35] B. A. Brown-Elliott, J. Biehle, P. S. Conville et al., "Sulfonamide resistance in isolates of *Nocardia* spp. from a US multicenter survey," *Journal of Clinical Microbiology*, vol. 50, no. 3, pp. 670–672, 2012.

[36] K. B. Uhde, S. Pathak, I. McCullum Jr. et al., "Antimicrobial-resistant *Nocardia* isolates, United States, 1995–2004," *Clinical Infectious Diseases*, vol. 51, no. 12, pp. 1445–1448, 2010.

30

Primary Pleural Angiosarcoma in a 63-Year-Old Gentleman

Ahmed Abu-Zaid[1] and Shamayel Mohammed[2]

[1] *College of Medicine, Alfaisal University, P.O. Box 50927, Riyadh 11533, Saudi Arabia*
[2] *Department of Pathology and Laboratory Medicine, King Faisal Specialist Hospital and Research Center (KFSH&RC),*
P.O. Box 3354, Riyadh 11211, Saudi Arabia

Correspondence should be addressed to Ahmed Abu-Zaid; aabuzaid@alfaisal.edu

Academic Editors: T. Koizumi and A. Turna

Primary pleural angiosarcomas are extremely rare. As of 2010, only around 50 case reports have been documented in the literature. Herein, we report the case of a 63-year-old gentleman who presented with a 3-month history of right-sided chest pain, dyspnea, and hemoptysis. Chest X-ray showed bilateral pleural effusion with partial bibasilar atelectasis. Ultrasound-guided thoracocentesis showed bloody and exudative pleural fluid. Cytologic examination was negative for malignant cells. An abdominal contrast-enhanced computed tomography (CT) scan showed two right diaphragmatic pleural masses. Whole-body positron emission tomography/computed tomography (PET/CT) scan showed two hypermetabolic fluorodeoxyglucose-(FDG-) avid lesions involving the right diaphragmatic pleura. CT-guided needle-core biopsy was performed and histopathological examination showed neoplastic cells growing mainly in sheets with focal areas suggestive of vascular spaces lined by cytologically malignant epithelioid cells. Immunohistochemical analysis showed strong positivity for vimentin, CD31, CD68, and Fli-1 markers. The overall pathological and immunohistochemical features supported the diagnosis of epithelioid angiosarcoma. The patient was scheduled for surgery in three weeks. Unfortunately, the patient died after one week after discharge secondary to pulseless ventricular tachycardia arrest followed by asystole. Moreover, we also present a brief literature review on pleural angiosarcoma.

1. Introduction

Angiosarcoma is an exceedingly uncommon malignant neoplasm derived from endothelial cells [1]. It accounts for roughly 1%-2% of all soft tissue neoplasms [2]. It most frequently occurs in skin and soft tissues [3]. Primary pleural angiosarcomas are extremely rare. As of 2010, only around 50 case reports have been documented in the literature [4]. Herein, we report a case of primary epithelioid angiosarcoma of the right pleura in a 63-year-old gentleman who presented with a 3-month history of right-sided chest pain, dyspnea, and hemoptysis. In addition, a literature review on pleural angiosarcoma is included.

2. Case Report

A 63-year-old gentleman presented to King Faisal Specialist Hospital and Research Center (KFSH&RC) with a 3-month history of right-sided chest pain, dyspnea, and hemoptysis.

Past medical history was remarkable for diabetes mellitus type 2, hypertension, ischemic heart disease, and congestive heart failure. The patient did not have previous history of tuberculous infection or asbestos exposure. Clinical respiratory examination was remarkable for bilateral reduced airway entry. All laboratory tests were normal.

A chest plain radiograph (X-ray) showed bilateral pleural effusion, partial bibasilar atelectasis, and linear pleural calcifications involving the right lung (Figure 1). Ultrasound-guided thoracocentesis showed bloody and exudative pleural fluid. Cytologic examination was negative for malignant cells. A chest, abdominal, and pelvic contrast-enhanced computed tomography (CT) scan showed bilateral pleural effusion, partial bibasilar atelectasis, and peripheral linear dense calcifications and thickening of the right lung. In addition, two pleural masses touching the right hemidiaphragm were identified and measured 3.2 × 2.1 cm and 4.3 × 4.8 cm. The masses were suspicious for neoplastic lesions. No axillary or mediastinal lymphadenopathy was identified. Furthermore, no evidence

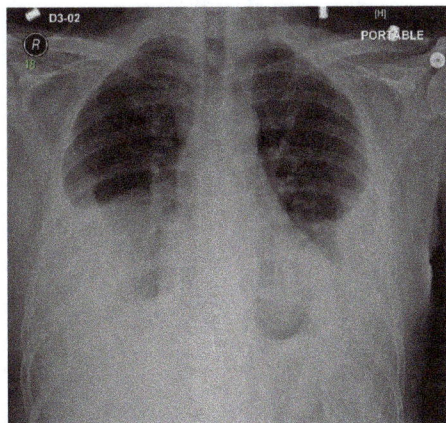

FIGURE 1: A chest plain radiograph (X-ray) showing bilateral pleural effusion, partial bibasilar atelectasis, and linear pleural calcifications involving the right lung.

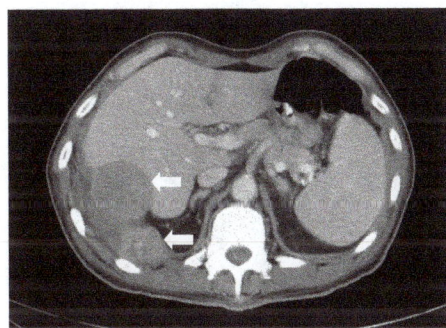

FIGURE 2: An axial chest, abdominal, and pelvic contrast-enhanced computed tomography (CT) scan showing bilateral pleural effusion, partial bibasilar atelectasis, and peripheral dense calcifications of the right lung. In addition, two pleural masses touching the right hemidiaphragm were identified and measured 3.2 × 2.1 cm and 4.3 × 4.8 cm (white arrows). The masses were suspicious for neoplastic lesions. No axillary or mediastinal lymphadenopathy was identified. Furthermore, no evidence of distant metastasis was identified.

of distant metastasis was identified (Figure 2). CT-guided needle-core biopsy was performed, and the histopathological and immunohistochemical examinations revealed epithelioid angiosarcoma. Whole-body positron emission tomography/computed tomography (PET/CT) scan showed two hypermetabolic fluorodeoxyglucose- (FDG-) avid lesions involving the right diaphragmatic pleura, suggesting neoplastic lesions and supporting the earlier pathological CT scan and CT-guided needle-core biopsy findings (Figure 3). Accordingly, the patient was scheduled for surgery in three weeks.

Histopathological examination showed neoplastic proliferation consisting of highly atypical large epithelioid cells with abundant eosinophilic cytoplasm, round to oval nuclei with marked pleomorphism, vesicular chromatin, and prominent single nucleoli. The neoplastic cells grew mainly in sheets with focal areas suggestive of vascular spaces lined by cytologically malignant epithelioid cells (Figure 4(a)).

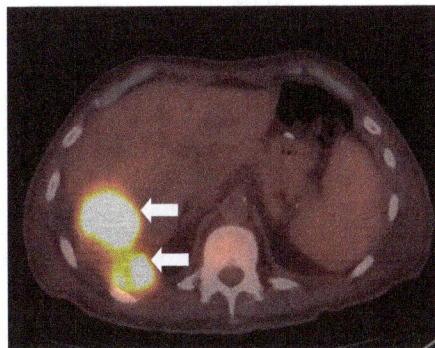

FIGURE 3: An axial chest positron emission tomography/computed tomography (PET/CT) scan showing two hypermetabolic fluorodeoxyglucose- (FDG-) avid mass lesions involving the right diaphragmatic pleura, suggestive of neoplastic lesions (white arrows).

In addition, focal hemorrhagic areas were also identified (Figure 4(b)).

Immunohistochemical analysis showed strong positivity for mesenchymal (vimentin) and endothelial (CD31, CD68, and Fli-1) markers (Figures 5(a)–5(d)). The tumor cells were negative for cytokeratin, cytokeratin 7, cytokeratin 20, cytokeratin 5/6, cytokeratin 8/18, calretinin, WT-1, HMB45, Mclan A, MITF, P63, S100, TTF 1, PLAP, PSA, AFP, EMA, HSA, CD10, CD20, CD30, CD38, and CD45. The overall pathological and immunohistochemical features supported diagnosis of a malignant epithelioid vascular tumor, consistent with epithelioid angiosarcoma.

The patient was discharged on the second day after the CT-guided needle-core biopsy in a stable condition. Unfortunately, the patient died after one week secondary to pulseless ventricular tachycardia arrest followed by asystole.

3. Discussion

Angiosarcoma is an exceedingly uncommon malignant neoplasm derived from uncontrolled proliferation of anaplastic vascular endothelial cells that line abnormal blood-filled sacs [1]. It accounts for approximately 1%-2% of all soft tissue neoplasms [2]. Skin and soft tissues (such as breast, heart, liver, spleen, and skeletal muscle) are the most frequent sites of involvement [3]. Pleural angiosarcomas are almost always secondary (metastatic) neoplasms from other primary sites [5]. Primary pleural angiosarcomas are exceptionally rare. As of 2010, only around 50 case reports of primary pleural angiosarcomas have been documented in the English literature so far [4]. Average age at presentation is 57 years, and males are affected more frequently than females (male-female ratio is 9 : 1) [6]. Etiology remains unknown. However, reported predisposing etiological factors are many and include exposure to chronic tuberculous pyothorax, chronic lymphedema, viral infections, radiation therapy, asbestos, and thorium [1, 2, 7]. When etiology is unrelated to predisposing factors, the term "de novo neoplasm" is applied [3, 7].

Clinical signs and symptoms are nonspecific. The most frequently presenting clinical signs and symptoms include

(a)

(b)

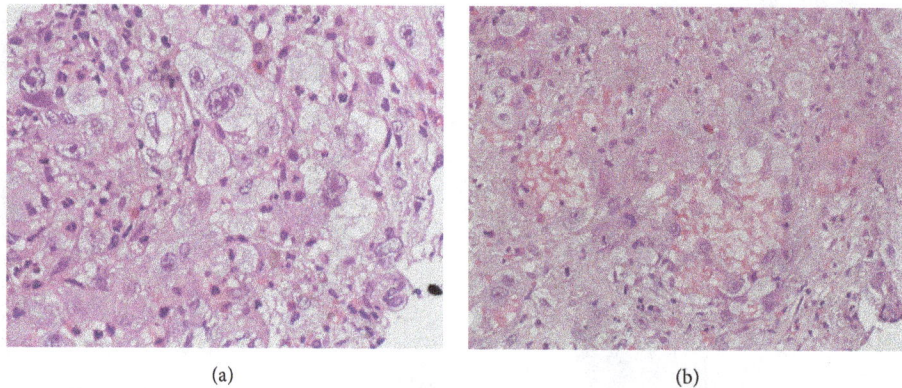

FIGURE 4: (a) Histopathological examination of the right diaphragmatic pleural masses (magnification power, 40x) showing the neoplastic cells that grew mainly in sheets with focal areas suggestive of vascular spaces lined by cytologically malignant epithelioid cells. The neoplastic proliferation consisted of highly atypical large epithelioid cells with abundant eosinophilic cytoplasm, round to oval nuclei with marked pleomorphism, vesicular chromatin, and prominent single nucleoli. (b) Focal hemorrhagic areas were identified.

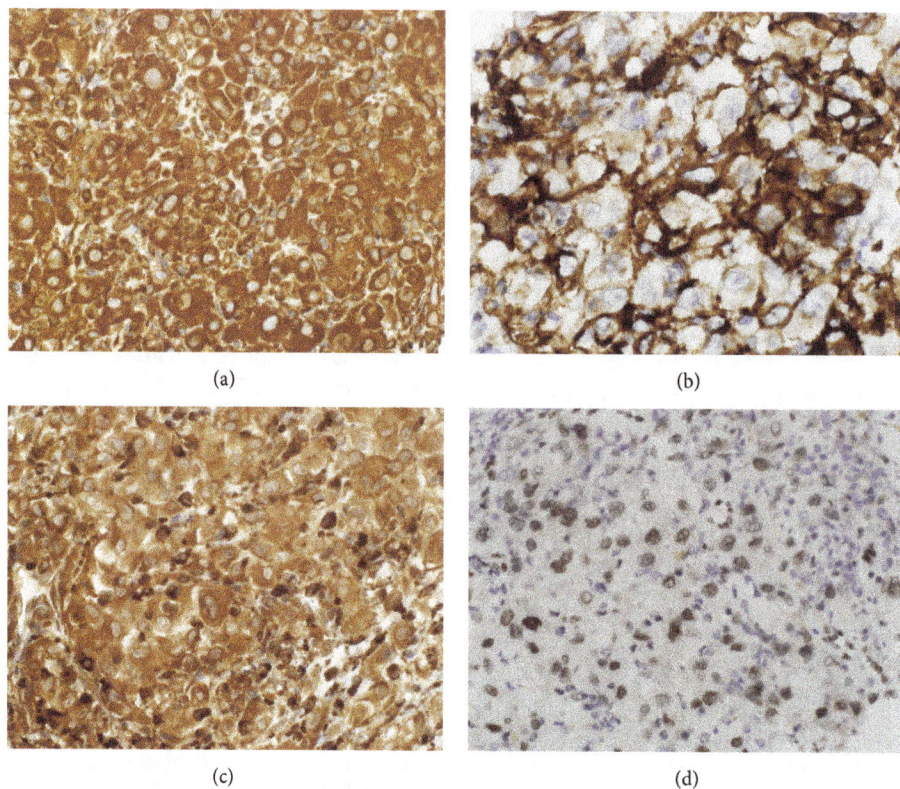

(a)

(b)

(c)

(d)

FIGURE 5: Immunohistochemical examination of the resected right diaphragmatic pleural masses. (a) Tumor cells stained positive for vimentin (magnification power, 40x). (b) Tumor cells stained positive for CD31 (magnification power, 40x). (c) Tumor cells stained positive for CD68 (magnification power, 40x). (d) Tumor cells stained positive for Fli-1 (magnification power, 40x).

chest pain, pleuritic chest pain, shortness of breath, cough, hemoptysis, anemia, and massive recurrent hemothorax [3, 5, 8]. Radiological findings are also nonspecific and cannot differentiate pleural angiosarcomas from other primary or metastatic pleural neoplastic lesions. Chest plain radiographs (X-rays) usually demonstrate pleural mass lesions, diffused pleural thickening, and unilateral or bilateral pleural effusions [3, 5, 8]. Computed tomography (CT) scans typically exhibit pleural heterogeneous contrast-enhanced lobulated masses (blood-filled cysts) with ill-defined margins [8]. Positron emission tomography (PET) scans generally illustrate homogenous or diffused fluorodeoxyglucose- (FDG-) avid lesions, and are often utilized in delineating the extent of disease [8]. Collectively, clinical signs and symptoms as well as radiological findings are nonspecific and similar to the other closely related pleural neoplasms that will be considered in the differential diagnosis, such as mesotheliomas and adenocarcinomas.

Cytological examination of thoracocentesis (pleural effusion tap) specimens is frequently negative for malignancy, hence unhelpful in making the diagnosis [7]. Definitive diagnosis of pleural angiosarcoma is established by surgical biopsy specimens for histopathological and immunohistochemical examinations [1, 9].

Microscopically, there are two histological variants of pulmonary/pleural angiosarcoma: classical and epithelioid [10, 11]. Classical angiosarcomas exhibit vasoformative patterns such as irregularly and variably sized anastomosing vascular channels lined by atypical and pleomorphic malignant endothelial cells. Conversely, vasoformative patterns are minimal in epithelioid angiosarcomas. Furthermore, epithelioid angiosarcomas are characterized by solid-sheeted nodular growth patterns, large round to polygonal epithelioid neoplastic cells with plentiful eosinophilic cytoplasm, large pleomorphic nuclei and prominent nucleoli. Nemours mitotic figures and variable proportions of necrosis and hemorrhage can be present [10, 11]. Extravasations of red blood cells (intracytoplasmic lumen containing red blood cells) can be visualized [10, 11]. Although not routinely performed due to availability of specific immunohistochemical markers, electron microscopic recognition of several Weibel-Palade bodies and pinocytic vesicles highly confirms neoplasms of endothelial-derived origins [12]. Epithelioid histological variant is deemed to be an element of higher malignant potential when compared to the classical histological variant [13]. Pleural angiosarcomas are commonly epithelioid variants in about 75% of the cases [1, 7, 14] and are often misdiagnosed as mesotheliomas or adenocarcinomas [15, 16].

Immunohistochemical examination is essential for distinguishing pleural angiosarcomas from the other histologically related mesotheliomas or adenocarcinomas [17]. Epithelial markers (e.g., cytokeratin) always stain strongly positive in mesotheliomas and adenocarcinomas whereas they occasionally stain positive in pleural angiosarcomas, particularly the epithelioid histological variants of pleural angiosarcomas [11]. Interestingly, our case report stained negative for epithelial markers. Endothelial (vascular) markers are necessary for warranting definitive diagnosis of angiosarcoma such as CD31, CD34, and factor VIII-related antigens [7]. By far, CD31 is the most sensitive and specific marker for vascular neoplasms and has been shown to hardly ever stain positive with nonvascular neoplasms (such as mesotheliomas and adenocarcinomas) [7, 18, 19]. Coexpression of mesenchymal (vimentin) and endothelial (particularly CD31 and Fli-1) markers along with epithelioid histopathological features confirms diagnosis of epithelioid angiosarcoma.

Management modalities of pleural angiosarcoma include surgery, radiotherapy, and chemotherapy [3, 7, 18, 20]. Surgery must be performed whenever possible and is indicated in conditions of complete surgical resection, debulking with pneumonectomy and rib excision, as well as cauterization of bleeding sources [2, 3]. Radiotherapy may have a beneficial role in postoperative settings in the absence of diffuse or metastatic disease [3]. Chemotherapy generally has minimal effect and is merely utilized for purposes of symptom palliation, and is rarely used in patients with poor performance status [2]. Preoperative vascular embolization can be used to reduce tumor vascularity and accordingly intraoperative pleural bleeding [2, 7].

In conclusion, pleural angiosarcoma remains a highly aggressive malignant neoplasm with a rapidly fetal clinical course, despite the varying treatment modalities (surgery, radiotherapy, and chemotherapy) [20]. Prognosis is extremely poor and death often occurs soon within 24 months from the time of diagnosis (mostly by the 7th month) [20].

Acknowledgment

The authors sincerely acknowledge the editorial assistance of Ms. Ranim Chamseddin, College of Medicine, Alfaisal University, Riyadh, Saudi Arabia.

References

[1] D. E. Maziak, F. M. Shamji, R. Peterson, and D. G. Perkins, "Angiosarcoma of the chest wall," *Annals of Thoracic Surgery*, vol. 67, no. 3, pp. 839–841, 1999.

[2] C. Alexiou, C. A. Clelland, D. Robinson, and W. E. Morgan, "Primary angiosarcomas of the chest wall and pleura," *The European Journal of Cardio-thoracic Surgery*, vol. 14, no. 5, pp. 523–526, 1998.

[3] M. Lorentziadis and A. Sourlas, "Primary de novo angiosarcoma of the pleura," *Annals of Thoracic Surgery*, vol. 93, no. 3, pp. 996–998, 2012.

[4] M. S. Roh, J. Y. Seo, and S. H. Hong, "Epithelioid angiosarcoma of the pleura : a case report," *Journal of Korean Medical Science*, vol. 16, no. 6, pp. 792–795, 2001.

[5] J.-E. Kurtz, S. Serra, B. Duclos, F. Brolly, P. Dufour, and J.-P. Bergerat, "Diffuse primary angiosarcoma of the pleura: a case report and review of the literature," *Sarcoma*, vol. 8, no. 4, pp. 103–106, 2004.

[6] P. J. Zhang, V. A. Livolsi, and J. J. Brooks, "Malignant epithelioid vascular tumors of the pleura: report of a series and literature review," *Human Pathology*, vol. 31, no. 1, pp. 29–34, 2000.

[7] C. del Frate, K. Mortele, R. Zanardi et al., "Pseudomesotheliomatous angiosarcoma of the chest wall and pleura," *Journal of Thoracic Imaging*, vol. 18, no. 3, pp. 200–203, 2003.

[8] C. S. Pramesh, B. P. Madur, S. Raina, S. B. Desai, and R. C. Mistry, "Angiosarcoma of the pleura," *Annals of Thoracic and Cardiovascular Surgery*, vol. 10, no. 3, pp. 187–190, 2004.

[9] A. Baisi, F. Raveglia, M. de Simone, and U. Cioffi, "Primary multifocal angiosarcoma of the pleura," *Interactive Cardiovascular and Thoracic Surgery*, vol. 12, no. 6, pp. 1069–1070, 2011.

[10] K. D. Branch and M. T. Smith, "Epithelioid angiosarcoma: a case review," *Pathology Case Reviews*, vol. 13, no. 6, pp. 264–268, 2008.

[11] J. Hart and S. Mandavilli, "Epithelioid angiosarcoma: a brief diagnostic review and differential diagnosis," *Archives of Pathology and Laboratory Medicine*, vol. 135, no. 2, pp. 268–272, 2011.

[12] L. Lund and R. Amre, "Epithelioid angiosarcoma involving the lungs," *Archives of pathology & laboratory medicine*, vol. 129, no. 1, pp. e7–e10, 2005.

[13] C.-F. Yang, T.-W. Chen, G.-C. Tseng, and I.-P. Chiang, "Primary pulmonary epithelioid angiosarcoma presenting as a solitary pulmonary nodule on image," *Pathology International*, vol. 62, no. 6, pp. 424–428, 2012.

[14] G. C. Maglaras, S. Katsenos, J. Kakadelis et al., "Primary angio-sarcoma of the lung and pleura," *Monaldi Archives for Chest Disease*, vol. 61, no. 4, pp. 234–236, 2004.

[15] B. T.-Y. Lin, T. Colby, A. M. Gown et al., "Malignant vascular tumors of the serous membranes mimicking mesothelioma: a report of 14 cases," *The American Journal of Surgical Pathology*, vol. 20, no. 12, pp. 1431–1439, 1996.

[16] G. Falconieri, R. Bussani, M. Mirra, and M. Zanella, "Pseudo-mesotheliomatous angiosarcoma: a pleuropulmonary lesion simulating malignant pleural mesothelioma," *Histopathology*, vol. 30, no. 5, pp. 419–424, 1997.

[17] M. Kimura, H. Ito, T. Furuta, T. Tsumoto, and S. Hayashi, "Pyo-thorax-associated angiosarcoma of the pleura with metastasis to the brain," *Pathology International*, vol. 53, no. 8, pp. 547–551, 2003.

[18] E. Dainese, B. Pozzi, M. Milani et al., "Primary pleural epithe-lioid angiosarcoma. A case report and review of the literature," *Pathology Research and Practice*, vol. 206, no. 6, pp. 415–419, 2010.

[19] B. R. de Young, M. R. Wick, J. F. Fitzgibbon, K. E. Sirgi, and P. E. Swanson, "CD31: an immunospecific marker for endothelial differentiation in human neoplasm," *Applied Immunohisto-chemistry & Molecular Morphology*, vol. 1, pp. 97–100, 1993.

[20] Y. C. Kao, J. M. Chow, K. M. Wang, C. L. Fang, J. S. Chu, and C. L. Chen, "Primary pleural angiosarcoma as a mimicker of mesothelioma: a case report ∗∗VS∗∗," *Diagnostic Pathology*, vol. 6, article 130, 2011.

31

A Case of Chronic Granulomatous Disease with a Necrotic Mass in the Bronchus: A Case Report and a Review of Literature

Ali Cheraghvandi,[1] **Majid Marjani,**[2] **Saeid Fallah Tafti,**[3]
Logman Cheraghvandi,[1] **and Davoud Mansouri**[4]

[1] *Chronic Respiratory Diseases Research Center, National Research Institute of Tuberculosis and Lung Diseases (NRITLD),*
Shahid Beheshti University of Medical Sciences, Tehran 19558 41452, Iran
[2] *Clinical Tuberculosis and Epidemiology Research Center, National Research Institute of Tuberculosis and Lung Disease (NRITLD),*
Masih Daneshvari Hospital, Shahid Beheshti University of Medical Sciences, Tehran 19558 41452, Iran
[3] *Nursing and Respiratory Health Management Research Center, National Research Institute of Tuberculosis and Lung Diseases*
(NRITLD), Shahid Beheshti University of Medical Sciences, Tehran 19558 41452, Iran
[4] *Lung Transplantation Research Center, National Research Institute of Tuberculosis and Lung Diseases (NRITLD), Shahid Beheshti*
University of Medical Sciences, Tehran 19558 41452, Iran

Correspondence should be addressed to Majid Marjani, marjani@nritld.ac.ir

Academic Editors: T. A. Chiang, I. Lang, K. M. Nugent, and K. Watanabe

Chronic granulomatous disease is a rare phagocytic disorder with recurrent, severe bacterial and fungal infections. We describe an unusual case of chronic granulomatous disease manifesting as an invasive pulmonary aspergillosis with an obstructive necrotic mass at the right middle bronchus. The patient was successfully treated with a bronchoscopic intervention for the removal of the obstructive mass and a medical therapy.

1. Introduction

Chronic granulomatous disease (CGD) is a rare primary immunodeficiency state. Affected cases are susceptible to special infections including particular fungal and bacterial disease [1, 2], most of them are diagnosed in early childhood [3]. Pneumonia is the most common infection and the most common organism is *Aspergillus* spp. [4]. CGD is a life-threatening disease so early diagnosis of an infection is very important.

2. Case Report

A 19-year-old woman was referred to our hospital with complaints of productive cough and massive hemoptysis. One month earlier she had been admitted to a hospital in the northern province of the country with symptoms of fever, weight loss, and bloody sputum. A computed tomography (CT) scan was performed and showed cavitary lesions with nodules in both lungs. Medical therapy for pulmonary infection consisting clindamycin and ceftriaxone was started, but did not respond well to the treatment after 3 weeks. So bronchoscopy was performed which reported an acute severe bronchitis. Culture of bronchoalveolar lavage specimen was negative after a 7-day inoculation and the transbronchial lung biopsy (TBLB) showed pulmonary angiitis granulomatosis compatible with Wegener's granulomatosis. Also antinuclear antibody test (ANA) was positive (1/640) but anti-dsDNA was negative. She was referred to our hospital for a complementary workup.

The patient was a young housewife originally from north Iran. Her illness started 30 days ago with fever, night sweats, weakness, and weight loss of four Kg, that followed with productive cough and hemoptysis, about 20 cc of blood in her sputum for 3 times. She had a normal delivery 5 months ago with a normal infant. She is a nonsmoker, without any history of recent travel or drug abuse. She had no significant medical history except an episode of pyelonephritis when she was 6 years old, recurrent oral aphthous ulcers, and multiple episodes of common cold in the last two years. She had four healthy, living siblings and her parents were not related. Her aunt had pulmonary tuberculosis twenty years ago.

On admission she was dyspneic and febrile with oral temperature of 39°C. Her blood pressure was 110/60 mm Hg, heart rate was 120/min, and respiratory rate was 20/min. Physical examination was unremarkable except pectus excavatum and bilateral course crackles along with rhonchi in right hemithorax. Peripheral blood leukocyte count was 16300/μL with 65% neutrophil, 10% lymphocyte, 11% monocyte, and 14% eosinophil (total eosinophil count: 2282/μL); hemoglobin and platelet counts were 8.6 mg/dL and 552×10^9 per liter. The erythrocyte sedimentation rate was 125 mm/h. All results of biochemical tests were normal. Also c-ANCA, p-ANCA, anti-PR3 IgG, and anti-MPO IgG were negative.

A chest X-ray was done and showed cavitary lesions and nodules in both lungs. Direct smear of sputum for acid fast bacilli was negative three times. Ciprofloxacin and meropenem were started but no improvement was seen in her condition.

The thorax CT scan was performed and showed biapical cavitary lesions and intracavitary soft tissue projection in the left lung. Also scattered nodular infiltration with a large mass-like consolidation was seen in the right lower lobe. Right hilar and subcarinal adenopathy there also reported (Figure 1).

Bronchoscopy was done which showed a necrotic obstructive mass at the right middle bronchus. No bacterial or fungal agents were isolated from sputum and bronchoalveolar lavage (BAL) fluid. Histopathological study showed filamentous septated hyphae with acute angle branching, without any evidence of granuloma or necrotizing vasculitis. Galactomannan assay index of serum was highly positive (10 ng/mL). Voriconazole was added to her treatment.

Aspergillus fumigatus was isolated from the culture of tissue specimen. Bronchoscopy was repeated for the removal of obstructive mass. Distal to it, a lot of necrotic material was discovered (Figure 2). Voriconazole was changed to Itraconazole 200 mg t.i.d after seven days of treatment. Brain CT scan was performed and was normal.

The patient's immune system was assessed. Ranges of the immunoglobulins were normal. The nitroblue-tetrazolium (NBT) test was 0%. Also the dihydrorhodamine 123 (DHR) assay confirmed the diagnosis of chronic granulomatous disease (CGD).

Patient's symptoms improved gradually, fever stopped, and she did not have any episodes of hemoptysis at all. Therapeutic dose of Itraconazole was continued for four months, after that it was prescribed as 100 mg once daily concomitant with Trimethoprim-sulfamethoxazole as prophylaxis up to now. Also at the follow-up visits there was no sign of recurrent infection. Screening of the other members of the family was negative for CGD.

3. Discussion

CGD was for the first time described half a century ago. It is a primary immunodeficiency state of phagocytic cells. CGD now consists of five genetic defects, related to every subunit of the five essential subunits of the phagocyte nicotinamide adenine dinucleotide phosphate (NADPH) oxidase. This enzyme generates reactive oxygen essential for the killing of some bacteria and fungi. Susceptibility to a particular spectrum of infectious agents associated with hyperinflammation and tissue granuloma formation are the characteristics of CGD [1].

Overall prevalence of CGD is about 1 in 200000 to 250000 persons. Approximately 70% of them are X-linked variant of disease (gp 91 deficient), and the remainder are autosomal recessive [2].

The majority of patients are diagnosed in early childhood [3], 76% before five years of age but 15% of patients are diagnosed in the second decade of the life [4] and on rare occasions (4%), even later [5, 6].

The X-linked form of disease presents earlier and more severe and rates of infection and death are higher [1]. In contrast, autosomal recessive forms are diagnosed in the older age and have a better outcome [2, 4, 7]. At present, about 50% of CGD cases survive until the third or fourth decades of life [8, 9].

Pneumonia is the most common complication [4], after that skin, lymph nodes, and liver infections are common. Among CGD patients five main groups of pathogens are more frequent: *Aspergillus, Staphylococcus aureus, Burkholderia, Serratia marcescens,* and *Nocardia* [1]. The most common organism is *Aspergillus* spp. [4]. Among them, *Aspergillus nidulans* is a highly likely pathogen, in contrast to infrequency among other immune deficient states [3, 10]. Consequently, the microbiological investigation for infectious agents should be performed and can be highly suggestive of CGD as the underlying condition [3].

One-third of CGD patients present a variety of inflammatory diseases, such as obstructive lesions of gastrointestinal tract and urinary systems. Also inflammatory bowel disease similar to Crohn's disease has been described among them [1, 11].

In this setting, an invasive fungal pneumonia is insidious in onset, although mortality is very high. Patients usually report chronic cough and malaise. Invasive aspergillosis is characterized by impaired ability to damage hyphae, dysregulated inflammation, and local extension to the pleura and the chest wall among one-third of the patients [12, 13].

The first element in the care of CGD patients is the early diagnosis of the infection; concerning that the classic signs of infection such as fever and leukocytosis may be absent. An elevated ESR rate may be the only indicator [2]. On the other hand, some specific opportunistic infections including invasive mold diseases and infections by *B. cepacia, S. marcescens,* and *Nocardia* species should prompt a diagnostic approach for CGD [2].

Dihydrorhodamine 1,2,3 (DHR) assay is a flow cytometry technique for the diagnosis of CGD. It is easy and more sensitive than the nitroblue-tetrazolium method (NBT) test

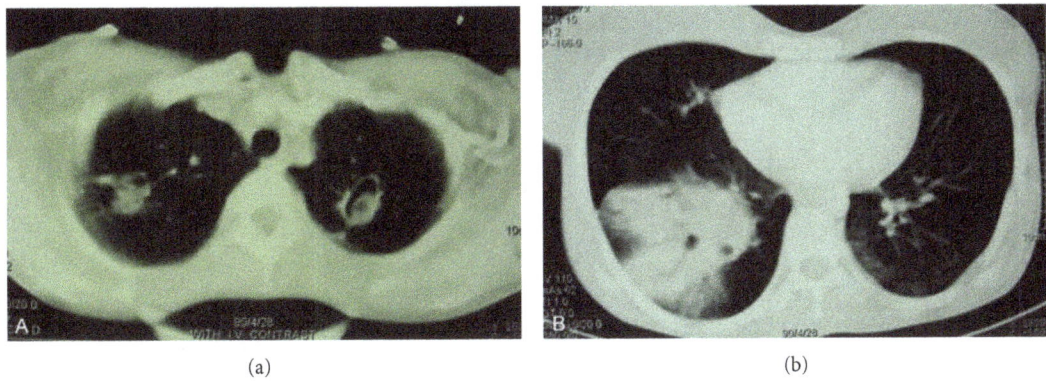

(a)   (b)

FIGURE 1: Spiral lung CT scan; (a) biapical cavitary lesions and intracavitary soft tissue projection in the left lung; (b) scattered nodular infiltration with a large mass-like consolidation was seen in the right lower lobe.

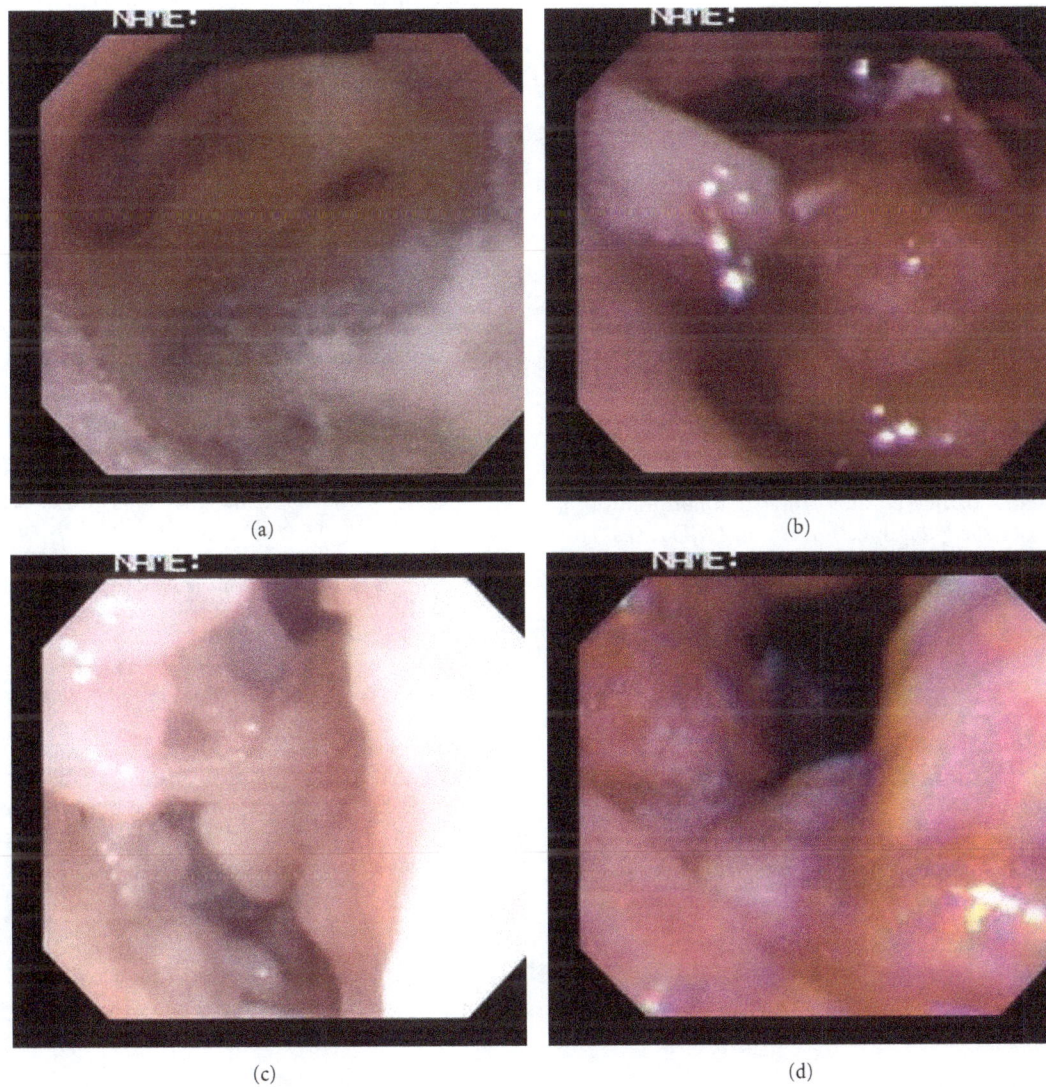

(a)   (b)

(c)   (d)

FIGURE 2: Bronchoscopic view of the right middle bronchus; (a) obstructed bronchus; (b) mass lesion; (c) necrotic material behind mass; (d) after the removal of necrotic material.

[3]. Also in some cases of autosomal recessive and variant X-linked forms of disease, low levels of NADPH oxidase activity may lead to incorrect results with NBT [2]. So DHR is preferred. DHR (dihydrorhodamine 1,2,3) enters phagocytes freely and is oxidized in the cells to rhodamine 1,2,3 by diffusible H_2O_2 after phagocytes are stimulated, which is detectible by flow cytometry [1].

During any episode of infection, every attempt should be performed for a microbiological diagnosis. Exclusion of disseminated infection, especially the involvement of central nervous system, is necessary in the cases of pneumonia caused by *Aspergillus* or *Nocardia* spp. that can be performed best by an imaging study [12]. Serum galactomannan (an *Aspergillus* antigen and a diagnostic marker for an invasive disease) appears to be insensitive among CGD patients [2].

All episodes of infection should be treated as soon as possible. Due to slow response, prolonged treatment may be necessary particularly for fungal infections (e.g., for 4–6 months). Antibiotic and antifungal prophylaxis is recommended indefinitely to prevent the recurrence or reactivation of infection. Trimethoprim-sulfamethoxazole and Itraconazole are preferred agents [12]. Cure can be achieved by haematopoietic stem cell transplantation and gene therapy [1].

The above case has some interesting characteristics. She was a 19-year-old woman, without any history of serious infections compatible with the autosomal recessive form of CGD. Typically after the detection of the *Aspergillus* as the cause of infection, CGD was introduced. Although, for the diagnosis of CGD, DHR assay is better, in our setting NBT test is more accessible. She had a history of recurrent aphthous ulcers; this may be related to CGD or not. Aphtus lesions have been reported in gp91 carriers (X-linked form of disease) [14].

A necrotic obstructive mass was observed at right middle bronchus. It may be due to hyper inflammation, a characteristic of *Aspergillus* infection among CGD cases. This mass was removed by interventional bronchoscopy as part of treatment. Although necrotizing aspergillosis of the large airways (necrotizing *Aspergillus* bronchitis) is a known entity [15], to our knowledge, until now, this form of aspergillosis has not been reported among CGD cases in the literature.

4. Conclusion

CGD can be a lethal disease. Early diagnosis of the underlying disorder of immune system is very important. We have to consider CGD in any patient with recurrent episodes of severe infections. On the other hand, the isolation of particular opportunistic infections such as *Aspergillus*, *Serratia*, *Nocardia*, and *Burkholderia* should prompt a diagnostic approach for CGD.

Acknowledgments

The authors would like to thank all colleagues at Masih Daneshvari Hospital that helped with the preparation of this paper.

References

[1] R. A. Seger, "Chronic granulomatous disease: recent advances in pathophysiology and treatment," *Netherlands Journal of Medicine*, vol. 68, no. 11, pp. 334–340, 2010.

[2] B. H. Segal, P. Veys, H. Malech, and M. J. Cowan, "Chronic granulomatous disease: lessons from a rare disorder," *Biology of Blood and Marrow Transplantation*, vol. 17, no. 1, supplement, pp. S123–S131, 2011.

[3] S. M. Holland, "Chronic granulomatous disease," *Clinical Reviews in Allergy and Immunology*, vol. 38, no. 1, pp. 3–10, 2010.

[4] J. A. Winkelstein, M. C. Marino, R. B. Johnston Jr. et al., "Chronic granulomatous disease: report on a national registry of 368 patients," *Medicine*, vol. 79, no. 3, pp. 155–169, 2000.

[5] J. S. Ma, P. Y. Chen, L. S. Fu et al., "Chronic granulomatous disease: a case report," *Journal of Microbiology, Immunology and Infection*, vol. 33, no. 2, pp. 118–122, 2000.

[6] A. Lun, J. Roesler, and H. Renz, "Unusual late onset of X-linked chronic granulomatous disease in an adult woman after unsuspicious childhood," *Clinical Chemistry*, vol. 48, no. 5, pp. 780–781, 2002.

[7] B. H. Segal, T. L. Leto, J. I. Gallin, H. L. Malech, and S. M. Holland, "Genetic, biochemical, and clinical features of chronic granulomatous disease," *Medicine*, vol. 79, no. 3, pp. 170–200, 2000.

[8] J. Liese, S. Kloos, V. Jendrossek et al., "Long-term follow-up and outcome of 39 patients with chronic granulomatous disease," *Journal of Pediatrics*, vol. 137, no. 5, pp. 687–693, 2000.

[9] A. Finn, N. Hadzić, G. Morgan, S. Strobel, and R. J. Levinsky, "Prognosis of chronic granulomatous disease," *Archives of Disease in Childhood*, vol. 65, no. 9, pp. 942–945, 1990.

[10] R. B. Johnston Jr., "Clinical aspects of chronic granulomatous disease," *Current Opinion in Hematology*, vol. 8, no. 1, pp. 17–22, 2001.

[11] M. C. B. Godoy, P. M. Vos, P. L. Cooperberg, C. P. Lydell, P. Phillips, and N. L. Müller, "Chest radiographic and CT manifestations of chronic granulomatous disease in adults," *American Journal of Roentgenology*, vol. 191, no. 5, pp. 1570–1575, 2008.

[12] R. A. Seger, "Modern management of chronic granulomatous disease," *British Journal of Haematology*, vol. 140, no. 3, pp. 255–266, 2008.

[13] B. H. Segal, L. Romani, and P. Puccetti, "Chronic granulomatous disease," *Cellular and Molecular Life Sciences*, vol. 66, no. 4, pp. 553–558, 2009.

[14] K. Kragballe, N. Borregaard, and F. Brandrup, "Relation of monocyte and neutrophil oxidative metabolism to skin and oral lesions in carriers of chronic granulomatous disease," *Clinical and Experimental Immunology*, vol. 43, no. 2, pp. 390–398, 1981.

[15] T. Franquet, F. Serrano, A. Giménez, J. M. Rodríguez-Arias, and C. Puzo, "Necrotizing aspergillosis of large airways: CT findings in eight patients," *Journal of Computer Assisted Tomography*, vol. 26, no. 3, pp. 342–345, 2002.

32

Robot-Assisted Thoracoscopic Resection of a Posterior Mediastinal Mullerian Cyst

Calvin Chao,[1] **Vijay Vanguri,**[2] **and Karl Uy** ⓘ[1]

[1]*Division of Thoracic Surgery, UMass Memorial Medical Center, University of Massachusetts Medical School, Worcester, MA, USA*
[2]*Department of Pathology, UMass Memorial Medical Center, University of Massachusetts Medical School, Worcester, MA, USA*

Correspondence should be addressed to Karl Uy; karl.uy@umassmemorial.org

Academic Editor: Daniel T. Merrick

First described in 2005, the Mullerian derived cyst in the mediastinum is a rare finding with few subsequent reports. We report a case of Mullerian cyst occurring in the mediastinum of a 49-year-old female that was resected by robot-assisted thoracoscopic surgery. To our knowledge, this is the first report of robot-assisted resection of Hattori's cyst. Histopathologic analysis revealed ciliated Mullerian-type tubal epithelium positive for paired box gene 8 (PAX8), estrogen receptor (ER), and progesterone receptor (PR), confirming Mullerian differentiation. We also review the clinical presentation, pathology, and differential diagnosis of such cysts.

1. Introduction

The Mullerian mediastinal cyst was first described by Hattori in 2005 [1]. He reported a posterior mediastinal cyst in an 18-year-old woman with no anatomic abnormalities or clinical symptoms. Since then, a number of additional cases have been reported [2]. Moreover, it appears that Mullerian mediastinal cysts are more common than once thought as retrospective analyses reveal a higher than expected percentage of mediastinal cysts which are Mullerian in origin [3]. We report a case of Hattori's cyst occurring in the posterior mediastinum of a 49-year-old female patient that was resected by robot-assisted thoracoscopic surgery (RATS).

2. Case Report

A 49-year-old woman presented to our clinic for the first time in consultation because of an incidental finding of a paraspinal mediastinal cyst. She was a healthy-appearing, obese (BMI 30.6) woman who recently moved from West Virginia. She is gravida 1, para 1, with first child born when she was 18 years old. She currently has an intrauterine device and previously took oral contraceptive pills for 15 years. The patient was status post-C5-C6 anterior cervical discectomy and fusion for spinal compression. She has a strong family

history of breast cancer and is Necdin variant positive (NDN). This gene, located in the Prader-Willi syndrome deletion region, facilitates cell cycle arrest, predisposing her to development of breast cancer. The patient has denied prophylactic mastectomy. During workup for migraine headaches and cervicalgia, a magnetic resonance imaging (MRI) scan of her cervical spine was performed, leading to an MRI of the thoracic spine. In this subsequent MRI, a well-circumscribed homogeneous mass with signals compatible with a pure cyst measuring $2.0 \times 1.2 \times 2.2$ cm was found along the right anterolateral aspect of the T5 vertebral body (Figure 1).

Though we recommended continued monitoring of the cyst, the patient, given her genetic predisposition and family history of cancer, opted for surgical intervention. The patient underwent robot-assisted thoracoscopic surgery for resection of the cyst for diagnostic and therapeutic purposes.

After induction of general anesthesia utilizing a double-lumen endotracheal tube, the patient was placed on the left lateral decubitus position and the da Vinci Si robot was docked. We utilized 4 ports placed along the 7th intercostal space with CO2 insufflation and a 0-degree 10 mm camera. After retracting the lung anteriorly, we located the cyst at the paraspinal T5 level, where it was encompassed by veins draining to the azygos system. Though the cyst was mostly adherent to the body of the spine, we were able to find

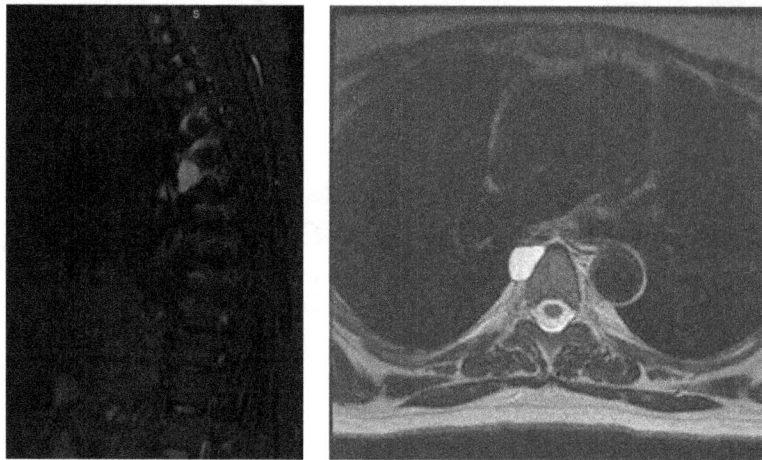

(a) Sagittal magnetic resonance imaging of Mullerian cyst at level T5

(b) Axial magnetic resonance imaging of Mullerian cyst at level T5

FIGURE 1

a distinct plane for complete excision. The cyst wall was inadvertently ruptured during the dissection and drained serous fluid but was excised completely. The patient had a severe migraine postoperatively but otherwise had a good recovery and was discharged on the second postoperative day.

Gross pathological examination revealed the paraspinal cyst to be a 1.3 × 1.0 × 0.3 cm previously disrupted pink-red cystic structure which was bisected to reveal a smooth inner and outer lining. Histopathologic analysis revealed a cyst lined by ciliated Mullerian-type tubal epithelium with no evidence of malignancy. Immunohistochemical staining with paired box gene 8 (PAX8), estrogen receptor (ER), and progesterone receptor (PR) was done to confirm a Mullerian origin as was also described by Hattori [4] (Figure 2).

3. Discussion

To our knowledge, this is the 19th documented case in the English literature of a Mullerian cyst in the mediastinum and the first reported case of such a cyst resected by robot-assisted thoracoscopic surgery [2]. Of the three mediastinal compartments, the posterior mediastinum is the least likely to contain malignant masses and is amenable for thoracoscopic approach. Important anatomic considerations in the posterior mediastinum include the descending thoracic aorta, trachea, esophagus, azygous venous system, and potential spinal involvement. Given the paraspinal location, low likelihood of malignancy, and proximity to important structures, a robotic approach was preferred. The precise manipulation of the machine arms enabled complete excision of the cyst from the spine without damage to the encompassing veins.

We considered other differential diagnoses in assessing this posterior mediastinal mass. Neoplasms such as schwannomas, neuroblastomas, ganglioneuroblastoma, gangliomas, and spinal cord lesions often appear in the posterior mediastinum but are not cystic and can be ruled out preoperatively by imaging and lack of clinical manifestation. An

anterior spinal meningocele may also present in the posterior mediastinum and will appear cyst-like on imaging due to filling of cerebrospinal fluid. However, the meningocele will communicate with the vertebral column unlike a true cyst.

The most common mediastinal cysts include bronchogenic cysts, enteric duplication cysts, pericardial cysts, and thymic cysts, though most of these cysts appear in the middle mediastinum with the exception of thymic cysts in the anterior mediastinum. Bronchogenic cysts can be ciliated and may stain positive cytokeratin (CK7) positive but rarely stain PAX8, WT-1, and ER positive [5]. Enteric duplication cysts may be ciliated and have been reported to stain PAX8 positive or CK7 positive but rarely stain PR and ER positive [6]. Pericardial cysts are quite rare (1/100,000) and typically present in the right cardiophrenic angle. They may stain cytokeratin positive but again rarely stain PAX8, ER, and PR positive. Thymic cysts are similarly quite rare and are typically a single cyst associated with a soft tissue component and connection to thymic tissue. Mesothelial cysts are another consideration but are typically sequelae of previous surgery. Therefore, having ruled out the likelihood of the above presentations, we may reasonably conclude that our cyst, having stained for CK7, WT-1, PAX8, ER, and PR, is Hattori's cyst.

The pathogenesis of a posterior mediastinal Mullerian cyst is still not yet completely understood. Previous reported cases of Hattori's cysts have posited that such cysts are the result of remnant Mullerian tissue during embryogenesis as proposed by Ludwig et al. in his study of Mayer-Rokitansky-Kuster syndrome [7, 8]. The first Mullerian duct anlage arises in the 3rd to 5th thoracic vertebral blastema in stage 16 embryos. At stage 17, the Mullerian duct appears via a deep invagination at the level of the 3rd thoracic somite and proceeds to grow caudally towards the Wolffian ducts until fusion in stage 18. The two Mullerian ducts will continue caudally until reaching the dorsal wall of the urogenital sinus at stage 23, forming the cervicovaginal canal. The cervicovaginal canal and nearby anlages will later form the

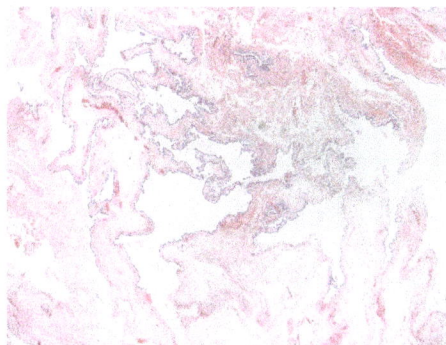

(a) 4-micron, H&E-stained, formalin-fixed, paraffin-embedded sections at 20x demonstrate a simple cystic lining with no epithelial complexity, bland fibrous tissue, and no significant associated inflammation or hemorrhage

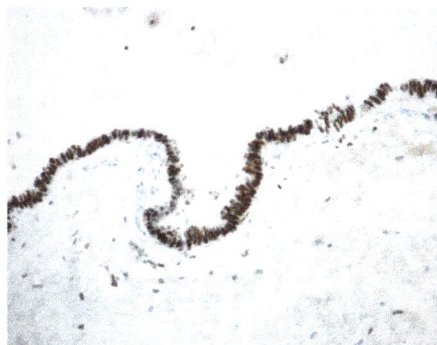

(b) Immunohistochemical stain for estrogen receptor reveals diffuse nuclear positivity of most lining epithelial cells (immunoperoxidase, 200x)

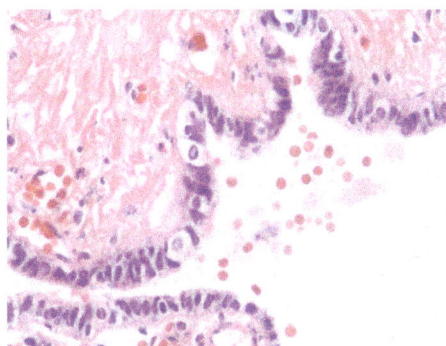

(c) 600x H&E shows simple Mullerian tubal-type columnar epithelium with mostly secretory cells and some ciliated cells

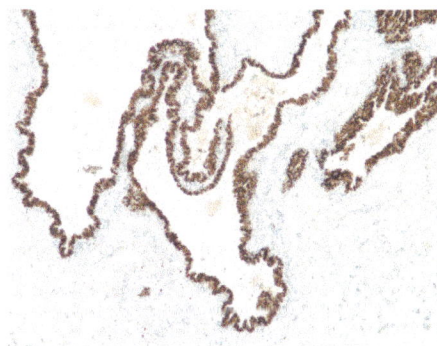

(d) 100x 4-micron formalin-fixed paraffin-embedded sections stained with PAX8 immunoperoxidase preparation highlights diffuse epithelial nuclear reactivity with the PAX8 antibody, confirming Mullerian differentiation

FIGURE 2

location between the fallopian tube and uterine horn [7]. An aberration of this process is the root cause of Mullerian agenesis and remnant structures during this migration are perhaps also the pathogenesis of Hattori's cysts [9].

In conclusion, we present a patient with a posterior mediastinal mass identified to be a cyst of Mullerian origin. At her one-month postoperative clinic visit she denied any postoperative complications and endorsed only continued migraines and cervicalgia for which she will follow with her neurologist. While rare in presentation we review the diagnosis of Hattori's cysts and present the first documented RATS approach for resection with considerations for such a robotic approach. Lastly, we overview the likely pathogenesis of such cysts as a remnant of Mullerian duct migration.

References

[1] H. Hattori, "Ciliated cyst of probable mullerian origin arising in the posterior mediastinum [1]," *Virchows Archiv*, vol. 446, no. 1, pp. 82–84, 2005.

[2] M. Simmons, L. V. Duckworth, K. Scherer, P. Drew, and D. Rush, "Mullerian cysts of the posterior mediastinum: Report of two cases and review of the literature," *Journal of Thoracic Disease*, vol. 5, no. 1, pp. E8–E10, 2013.

[3] V. Thomas-de-Montpréville and E. Dulmet, "Cysts of the posterior mediastinum showing müllerian differentiation (Hattori's cysts)," *Annals of Diagnostic Pathology*, vol. 11, no. 6, pp. 417–420, 2007.

[4] H. Hattori, "High prevalence of estrogen and progesterone receptor expression in mediastinal cysts situated in the posterior mediastinum," *CHEST*, vol. 128, no. 5, pp. 3388–3390, 2005.

[5] A. Roma, M. Varsegi, C. Magi-Galluzzi, T. Ulbright, and M. Zhou, "The distinction of bronchogenic cyst from metastatic testicular teratoma: A light microscopic and immunohistochemical study," *American Journal of Clinical Pathology*, vol. 130, no. 2, pp. 265–273, 2008.

[6] K. Faraj, L. Edwards, A. Gupta, and B. Seifman, "Completely isolated retroperitoneal enteric duplication cyst with adenocarcinoma transformation managed with robotic radical nephrectomy," *Journal of Endourology Case Reports*, vol. 3, no. 1, pp. 31–33, 2017.

[7] K. S. Ludwig, "The Mayer-Rokitansky-Kuster syndrome. An analysis of its morphology and embryology. Part II: Embryology," *Archives of Gynecology and Obstetrics*, vol. 262, no. 1-2, pp. 27–42, 1998.

33

Coexistent Non–Small Cell Carcinoma and Small Cell Carcinoma in a Patient Presenting with Hyponatremia

Mitchell D. Ross,[1] Sreeja Biswas Roy,[1] Pradnya D. Patil,[2] Jasmine L. Huang,[3] Nitika Thawani,[4] Ralph Drosten,[5] and Tanmay S. Panchabhai ⓘ [3]

[1]*Department of Internal Medicine, St. Joseph's Hospital and Medical Center, Phoenix, AZ, USA*
[2]*Department of Hematology and Oncology, Taussig Cancer Institute, Cleveland Clinic, Cleveland, OH, USA*
[3]*Norton Thoracic Institute, St. Joseph's Hospital and Medical Center, Phoenix, AZ, USA*
[4]*Department of Radiation Oncology, University of Arizona Cancer Center, St. Joseph's Hospital and Medical Center, Phoenix, AZ, USA*
[5]*Department of Radiology, St. Joseph's Hospital and Medical Center, Phoenix, AZ, USA*

Correspondence should be addressed to Tanmay S. Panchabhai; tanmay.panchabhai@dignityhealth.org

Academic Editor: Akif Turna

Despite recent advances in screening methods, lung cancer remains the leading cause of cancer-related deaths worldwide. By the time lung cancer becomes symptomatic and patients seek treatment, it is often too advanced for curative measures. Low-dose computed tomography (CT) screening has been shown to reduce mortality in patients at high risk of lung cancer. We present a 66-year-old man with a 50-pack-year smoking history who had a right upper lobe (RUL) pulmonary nodule and left lower lobe (LLL) consolidation on a screening CT. He reported a weight loss of 45 pounds over 3 months, had recently been hospitalized for hyponatremia, and was notably cachectic. A CT of the chest showed a stable LLL mass-like consolidation and a 9 × 21 mm subsolid lesion in the RUL. Navigational bronchoscopy biopsy of the RUL lesion revealed squamous non–small cell lung cancer (NSCLC). Endobronchial ultrasound-guided transbronchial needle aspiration of the LLL lesion revealed small cell lung cancer (SCLC). The final diagnosis was a right-sided Stage I NSCLC (squamous) and a left-sided limited SCLC. The RUL NSCLC was treated with stereotactic radiation; the LLL SCLC was treated with concurrent chemotherapy and radiation. In patients with multiple lung nodules, a diagnosis of synchronous multiple primary lung cancers (MPLCs) is crucial, as inadvertent upstaging of patients with MPLC (to T3 and/or T4 tumors) can lead to erroneous staging, inaccurate prognosis, and improper treatment. Recent advances in the diagnosis of small pulmonary nodules via navigational bronchoscopy and management of these lesions dramatically affect a patient's overall prognosis.

1. Introduction

Lung cancer is by far the leading cause of cancer deaths in both men and women, with roughly 222,500 new cases of lung cancer expected to be diagnosed in 2017 alone [1]. The National Lung Screening Trial (NLST) [2], published in 2011, demonstrated that lung cancer screening can detect early-stage lung cancer, thereby decreasing mortality [2]. In addition to detection of early-stage lung cancer, screening programs may incidentally reveal other findings, such as nonmalignant lung nodules and coronary artery disease (based on coronary calcium scoring) [2]. Pulmonary nodules detected during lung cancer screening are managed using the Fleischner Society recommendations [3] or the Lung-RADS™ guidelines [4].

The most common incidental finding is a single primary malignancy, but synchronous multiple primary lung cancers in varied stages are occasionally diagnosed based on lung cancer screening results [5]. However, the approach to such distinct lung nodules is not always straightforward, and appropriate staging based on tissue diagnosis is of paramount importance. In Western societies, the incidence of synchronous primary lung cancers has been reported to be anywhere from 0.2% to 20% [6–10]. Here we report the unique presentation, challenging diagnosis, and successful management of non–small cell lung cancer (NSCLC)

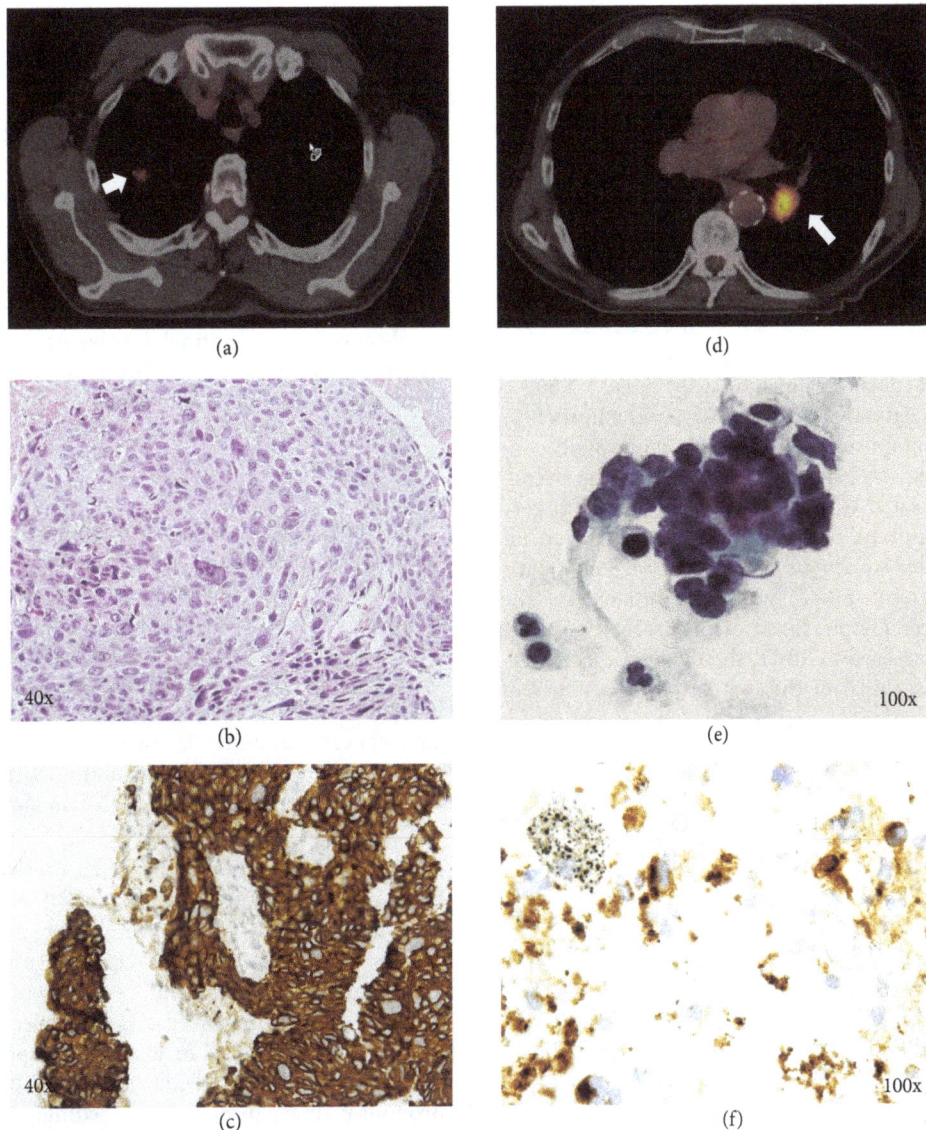

FIGURE 1: Positron emission tomogram showing mild [11F]-2-fluoro-2-deoxy-D-glucose (FDG) uptake in the right upper lobe lesion (a) (short white arrow), diagnosed as squamous cell carcinoma on biopsy ((b) hematoxylin and eosin, 40x; (c) CK5 immunostain, 40x). (d) A highly FDG-avid left infrahilar mass (long white arrow) that was diagnosed as small cell carcinoma after biopsy analysis ((e) hematoxylin and eosin, 100x; (f) synaptophysin, 100x).

and small cell lung cancer (SCLC) coexisting in the same patient.

2. Case Presentation

A 66-year-old man with a 50-pack-year smoking history and severe chronic obstructive pulmonary disease (COPD) presented to our clinic with a new right upper lobe (RUL) pulmonary nodule and a chronic left lower lobe (LLL) consolidation on screening computed tomography (CT). His pulmonary function tests (PFTs) showed airflow obstruction with an FEV_1 of 2.58 L (81% predicted). The LLL consolidation was evident on a chest radiograph 6 months before his current presentation, and the lesion had been biopsied by his local pulmonologist via conventional bronchoscopy with no evidence of malignancy.

The patient reported a 45-pound weight loss over the course of three months, as well as a recent hospitalization for severe hyponatremia (109 mEq/L). Upon physical examination, the patient was noted to be cachectic, with bilateral decreased air entry. CT of the chest showed a stable LLL consolidation along with a 9 × 21 mm subsolid lesion in the RUL. Navigational bronchoscopy and biopsy of the RUL lesion revealed squamous NSCLC with positive CK5, p63, and TTF-1 markers (Figures 1(a)–1(c)). The LLL consolidation was not sampled during this procedure, as it was located on the contralateral lung, was noted to be stable for 6 months based on a prior chest radiograph, and had been analyzed after a previous bronchoscopy with cytology and transbronchial lung biopsies without evidence of malignancy. A staging positron emission tomogram (PET) done after the navigational bronchoscopy once a malignant diagnosis was confirmed showed FDG avidity in the RUL lesion (SUV 2), along with an FDG-avid left infrahilar mass (SUV 11) within the LLL consolidation (Figure 1(d)). The absence of enlarged or FDG-avid mediastinal adenopathy made the diagnosis of a second primary cancer very likely. Endobronchial ultrasound-guided transbronchial needle aspiration (EBUS-TBNA) of the left infrahilar mass revealed a cluster of cells with minimal cytoplasm and small nuclei with nuclear cytoplasmic molding (Figures 1(d)–1(f)).

Immunohistochemical markers were consistent with an undifferentiated SCLC that was positive for CAM 5.2, TTF-1, CD56, and synaptophysin and negative for p63 and CK5 (Figure 1). The final diagnosis was a right-sided Stage I NSCLC (squamous) and a left-sided limited SCLC. Chemotherapy was initiated with etoposide and cisplatin, along with concurrent radiation for the left-sided SCLC. Given the overall poor survival associated with small cell carcinoma, surgery including segmentectomy was not a therapeutic option for the Stage I right-sided squamous cell carcinoma. Stereotactic body radiation therapy (SBRT) was then initiated for the squamous cell cancer. Despite lower rates of recurrence after segmentectomy compared to SBRT, the likelihood of recurrent SCC driving survival in this patient with concurrent SCLC was low. The patient's hyponatremia has since resolved, and his surveillance PET scan showed him to be recurrence-free at 1 year.

3. Discussion

Lung cancer screening has been shown to decrease mortality associated with lung cancer by detecting early-stage lung cancer in high-risk patients [2]. Patients at increased risk for lung cancer include those who are between the ages of 55 and 74 years and who have at least a 30-pack-year smoking history. Lung nodules detected on screening CT can then be risk-stratified based on either Fleischner Society recommendations [3] or the Lung-RADS guidelines [4]. Diagnosis of synchronous multiple primary lung cancers becomes especially important when a satellite lung nodule in the same lobe is staged as a T3 tumor whereas one in an ipsilateral lung lobe is classified as a T4 tumor. Upstaging patients with multiple primary lung cancers (MPLCs) can lead to erroneous staging, inaccurate prognosis, and, ultimately, improper treatment.

Recent advances in the diagnosis of small pulmonary nodules via navigational bronchoscopy and the management of these nodules (either surgically or with SBRT) can significantly affect patients' prognosis, survival, and treatment. To diagnose synchronous MPLCs, physicians must adhere to strict criteria and obtain tissue samples of both lesions. These samples must each be malignant and must arise independently in the lung. Benign nodules, infectious processes, or metastases from extrapulmonary sources must be excluded. Further complicating the diagnostic process is the fact that up to 50% of synchronous MPLCs are composed of multiple adenocarcinomas [11].

The accepted criteria for distinguishing a second primary malignancy from metastasis are

(1) different histology from a separate focus,

(2) same histology but anatomically distinct lesions without involvement of the mediastinum (N2/N3) and without systemic metastases,

(3) same histology but clearly different lesions (so designated based on predominant subtype, cytological features, or different biomarker patterns) [12].

Our patient met the criteria of different histology, anatomically distinct lesions, and different biomarkers. Before biopsy, the absence of mediastinal involvement on his PET scan triggered suspicion for synchronous MPLCs. Any patient with multiple lung nodules without mediastinal involvement should undergo tissue sampling of all lung lesions for definitive diagnosis.

Current recommendations suggest that clinicians initiate a discussion about lung cancer screening with patients who meet certain criteria. Patients aged 55 to 74 years who have at least a 30-pack-year smoking history, who currently smoke, or who have quit within the past 15 years and those who are in relatively good health qualify for screening [13]. The recommended screening modality is annual low-density CT. Lung cancer screening is associated with a 20% relative decrease in lung cancer deaths and a 7% relative reduction in all-cause mortality in these high-risk patients [2].

Our case depicts the insidious development of synchronous primary lung cancer with both NSCLC and SCLC, and with this case come several crucial teaching points. Patients diagnosed with one cancer are at increased risk of a second malignancy, and patients with one pulmonary neoplasm are at increased risk of a second lung tumor [8]. MPLCs are present in just 0.5% of patients diagnosed with lung cancer, and NSCLC and SCLC presenting as synchronous primary tumors are exceedingly rare. Our patient's severe hyponatremia tipped us off to these MPLCs, as severe hyponatremia is a common paraneoplastic syndrome associated with SCLC. Tissue diagnosis for such lesions (without mediastinal involvement) may have a significant impact on an individual's therapy and prognosis. Innovative modalities, including surgical resection of one primary tumor and SBRT for the other, are increasingly common for synchronous early-stage cancers (when both tumors are NSCLC). Therefore, proper diagnosis and staging of all suspicious pulmonary nodules are of paramount importance in the ever-changing, high-stakes field of lung cancer.

References

[1] R. L. Siegel, K. D. Miller, and A. Jemal, "Cancer statistics, 2017," CA: A Cancer Journal for Clinicians, vol. 67, no. 1, pp. 7–30, 2017.

[2] D. R. Aberle, A. M. Adams, and C. D. Berg, "Reduced lung-cancer mortality with low-dose computed tomographic screening," The New England Journal of Medicine, vol. 365, no. 5, pp. 395–409, 2011.

[3] H. MacMahon, D. P. Naidich, J. M. Goo et al., "Guidelines for management of incidental pulmonary nodules detected on CT images: from the Fleischner Society 2017," *Radiology*, vol. 284, no. 1, pp. 228–243, 2017.

[4] P. F. Pinsky, D. S. Gierada, W. Black et al., "Performance of lung-RADS in the national lung screening trial: A retrospective assessment," *Annals of Internal Medicine*, vol. 162, no. 7, pp. 485–491, 2015.

[5] T. M. Aziz, R. A. Saad, J. Glasser, A. N. Jilaihawi, and D. Prakash, "The management of second primary lung cancers. A single centre experience in 15 years," *European Journal of Cardio-Thoracic Surgery*, vol. 21, no. 3, pp. 527–533, 2002.

[6] F. Rea, A. Zuin, D. Callegaro, L. Bortolotti, G. Guanella, and F. Sartori, "Surgical results for multiple primary lung cancers," *European Journal of Cardio-Thoracic Surgery*, vol. 20, no. 3, pp. 489–495, 2001.

[7] H. Rostad, T.-E. Strand, A. Naalsund, and J. Norstein, "Resected synchronous primary malignant lung tumors: a population-based study," *The Annals of Thoracic Surgery*, vol. 85, no. 1, pp. 204–209, 2008.

[8] B. M. Stiles, M. Schulster, A. Nasar et al., "Characteristics and outcomes of secondary nodules identified on initial computed tomography scan for patients undergoing resection for primary non-small cell lung cancer," *The Journal of Thoracic and Cardio-vascular Surgery*, vol. 149, no. 1, pp. 19–24, 2015.

[9] T. Tanvetyanon, L. Robinson, K. E. Sommers et al., "Relation-ship between tumor size and survival among patients with resection of multiple synchronous lung cancers," *Journal of Thoracic Oncology*, vol. 5, no. 7, pp. 1018–1024, 2010.

[10] D. Trousse, F. Barlesi, A. Loundou et al., "Synchronous multiple primary lung cancer: An increasing clinical occurrence requir-ing multidisciplinary management," *The Journal of Thoracic and Cardiovascular Surgery*, vol. 133, no. 5, pp. 1193–1200, 2007.

[11] A. Bhaskarla, P. C. Tang, T. Mashtare et al., "Analysis of second primary lung cancers in the SEER database," *Journal of Surgical Research*, vol. 162, no. 1, pp. 1–6, 2010.

[12] F. C. Detterbeck, W. A. Franklin, A. G. Nicholson et al., "The IASLC lung cancer staging project: background data and proposed criteria to distinguish separate primary lung cancers from metastatic foci in patients with two lung tumors in the forthcoming eighth edition of the TNM classification for lung cancer," *Journal of Thoracic Oncology*, vol. 11, no. 5, pp. 651–665, 2016.

[13] D. E. Wood, "National Comprehensive Cancer Network (NCCN) clinical practice guidelines for lung cancer screening," *Thoracic Surgery Clinics*, vol. 25, no. 2, pp. 185–197, 2015.

34

Extracorporeal Lung Support as a Bridge to Diagnosis of Pulmonary Tumor Embolism

Vishnu Vasanthan,[1,2] Kieran Halloran,[3,4] Lakshmi Puttagunta,[3,4] and Jayan Nagendran[1,2]

[1]*Department of Surgery, University of Alberta, Edmonton, AB, Canada*
[2]*Mazankowski Alberta Heart Institute, Edmonton, AB, Canada*
[3]*Department of Medicine, University of Alberta, Edmonton, AB, Canada*
[4]*University of Alberta Hospital, Edmonton, AB, Canada*

Correspondence should be addressed to Jayan Nagendran; jayan@ualberta.ca

Academic Editor: Samer Al-Saad

Bridging to diagnosis is an emerging technique used in end-stage cardiorespiratory failure that prolongs a patient's life using various modalities of extracorporeal lung support (ECLS) to achieve antemortem diagnosis. Pulmonary tumor embolism occurs when cell clusters travel from primary malignancies through venous circulation to the lungs, causing respiratory failure through inflammatory and venoocclusive pathways. Due to its nonspecific symptomatology, pulmonary tumor embolism remains an elusive diagnosis antemortem. Herein, we bridge a patient who presented in acute respiratory failure to the diagnosis of pulmonary tumor embolism from a gastric signet-ring cell carcinoma using ECLS modalities including venoarterial extracorporeal membrane oxygenation and centrally cannulated Novalung pumpless extracorporeal lung assist. We demonstrate the utility of this approach in diagnostically uncertain cases in unstable patients who are potentially acceptable ECLS and transplant candidates.

1. Introduction

In end-stage cardiorespiratory failure, patients can be placed on various modalities of extracorporeal lung support (ECLS) as a bridge to recovery [1], transplantation [2], or diagnosis [3]. While bridging to recovery or transplantation is employed after achieving diagnosis, bridging to a diagnosis is a strategy of prolonging a patient's life to identify the cause of cardiorespiratory failure. As a patient is bridged to diagnosis, there is opportunity to assess and evaluate suitability for potential recovery, transplantation, or appropriate withdrawal of support.

Pulmonary tumor embolism occurs when clusters of cells from a primary malignant tumor invade venous circulation and travel to the lungs. This can result in pulmonary hypertension by mechanical obstruction, production of microthrombi from coagulation cascades, and induction of concentric hypertrophy via inflammatory pathways [4–6]. Pulmonary hypertension in the context of lung carcinomatosis was first described by Bristowe in 1868 [7]. Pulmonary

tumor embolism was first documented by Schmidt [8], and Kane et al. [9] used autopsy studies to report multiple tumor emboli as a cause of dyspnea. Despite previous reports, the nonspecific symptomatology makes pulmonary tumor embolism an elusive diagnosis antemortem [6].

Herein, we report the use of venoarterial extracorporeal membrane oxygenation (VA-ECMO) and Novalung pumpless extracorporeal lung assist (pECLA) as a bridge to diagnosis of pulmonary tumor embolization secondary to gastric signet-ring cell carcinoma.

2. Case Presentation

A 38-year-old previously healthy male (Table 1) presented with 2 months of MRC grade 3 dyspnea and 9 kg weight loss with no fever or night sweats. On arrival to the emergency room, he was requiring 6 L/min oxygen via nasal prongs to maintain saturations greater than 90%. Chest X-ray and chest computed tomography (CT) (Figure 1) suggested possible pneumonia overlying interstitial lung disease and pulmonary

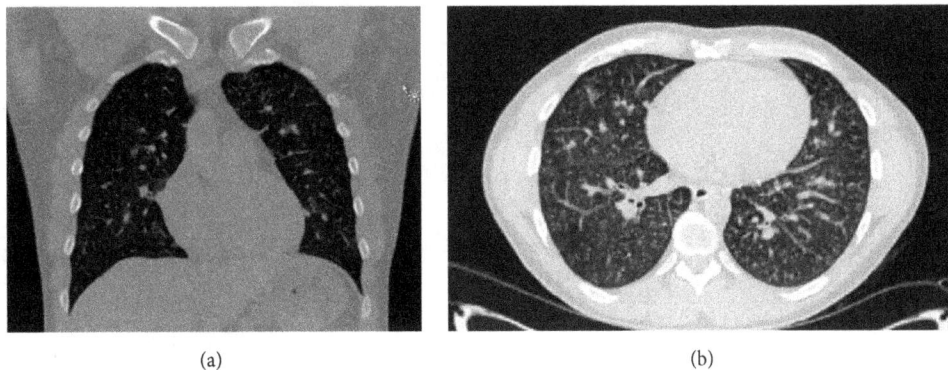

(a)   (b)

FIGURE 1: Coronal (a) and transverse (b) computed tomography views of the chest on first presentation. Images show ground-glass centrilobular micronodularities with perihilar ground-glass opacities. There is mild septal thickening and clear airways. Pulmonary artery is 3.3 cm, suggesting pulmonary hypertension.

TABLE 1: Patient characteristics.

Parameter	Characteristic
Age (y)	38
Gender	Male
Weight (kg)	86.9
Height (m)	1.8
BMI (kg/m^2)	26.8
Presentation	Respiratory failure
Procedure	Central cannulation ECLS Open lung biopsy

hypertension. CT and ultrasound showed small left axillary lymph nodes unamenable to biopsy. Abdominal ultrasound was grossly normal. Thus, the patient was diagnosed with presumed pneumonia and started on antibiotics, antiviral agents, inhaled corticosteroid, and bronchodilator therapy, with enoxaparin for venous thromboembolism prophylaxis.

Over the next 5 days, the patient's oxygen saturation was kept above 90% with 8–10 L/min oxygen via nonrebreather mask. Barriers to diagnosis included inability to produce sputum despite induction, high oxygen demands contraindicating bronchoscopy, small lymph nodes unamenable to biopsy, and intolerance of supine position needed for perfusion scans. The patient was transferred to the Thoracic Surgery service for a surgical lung biopsy on day 6. However, the patient experienced right-sided chest pain, diaphoresis, and tachycardia of 160 beats per minute, followed by a convulsive episode with no postictal symptoms. After transfer to the intensive care unit, mean systemic arterial pressures were found to be low, with transient reduction to as low as 40 mmHg when the patient coughed or spoke. Transthoracic echocardiography (Table 2) showed a dilated right ventricle with globally reduced systolic function. Right ventricular systolic pressures were shown to be 170 mmHg. Milrinone and epinephrine were started for hemodynamic support.

Due to progressive symptomatic and hemodynamic deterioration, he was transferred to the Cardiovascular Intensive Care Unit under the cardiac surgery service at another hospital to facilitate Novalung insertion via central cannulation.

The goal was to decompress the right ventricle in order to stabilize the patient's hemodynamics, as well as bridge to diagnosis and possibly lung transplant assessment.

In the operating room, the patient arrested when anesthetic induction was attempted. Thus, he was bridged to cardiopulmonary bypass via cardiac massage. Venous and arterial cannulation of the Novalung were, respectively, achieved via the pulmonary artery and left atrium through Sondergaard's groove, with simultaneous surgical lung biopsy. Novalung was started on 2 L sweep gas at 2 L flow. After sternal closure, the patient became increasingly hypotensive with transesophageal echocardiography showing right ventricular dysfunction. Thus, the patient was reopened and cardiopulmonary bypass was reinitiated. With extensive vasoplegia and increased demand for vasoconstrictors, cardiopulmonary bypass was converted to venoarterial ECMO to maintain mechanical support. At the end of the procedure, the sternum was left open with slight retraction provided by a converted 20 mL syringe, and the skin was closed.

Postoperatively, the patient was maintained on VA-ECMO and Novalung for 110 h (Table 2). Flows were maintained at 2.5–3 L/min and 2.5–3.5 L/min for VA-ECMO and Novalung, respectively. On postoperative day 2, the surgical lung biopsy demonstrated signet-ring cell pulmonary tumor embolism and lymphangitic carcinomatosis. Figures 2 and 3 depict histological sections demonstrating lymphangitic carcinomatosis of the lung and tumor thrombus in both arterial and venous pulmonary vasculatures. Figure 4 demonstrates a thrombosed pulmonary artery, explaining the subacute pulmonary hypertension. Given the extent of metastatic infiltration and the need for mechanical support, palliative chemotherapy was contraindicated. After discussion with the family, all modes of support were withdrawn in appropriate order and the patient passed away.

Autopsy results supported the diagnosis of lymphangitic carcinomatosis with signet-ring cell morphology. Vascular features suggested grades 3 and 4 pulmonary hypertension and multiple tumor thrombi. Right ventricle of the heart was moderately dilated. Examination of the stomach revealed a nonperforated 3.3 × 2 cm ulcer with involvement of poorly differentiated signet-ring cell adenocarcinoma. All sampled

TABLE 2: Surgical data.

Parameter	Value
Preoperative echocardiography	
Right ventricular dimensions (mm)	
Annulus	52
Mid-cavity	60
Longitudinal	75
Free wall thickness	8
Tricuspid annular plane systolic excursion (mm)	<10 mm
Right ventricular systolic pressure (mmHg)	170
Mean pulmonary artery pressure (mmHg)	100
Perioperative	
Total cardiopulmonary bypass time (min)	164
Postoperative	
Total ECLS time	110
VA-ECMO flow (L/min)	2.5–3
Novalung flow (L/min)	2.5–3.5
Final diagnosis	Pulmonary tumor embolism Signet-ring cell morphology
Status	Deceased

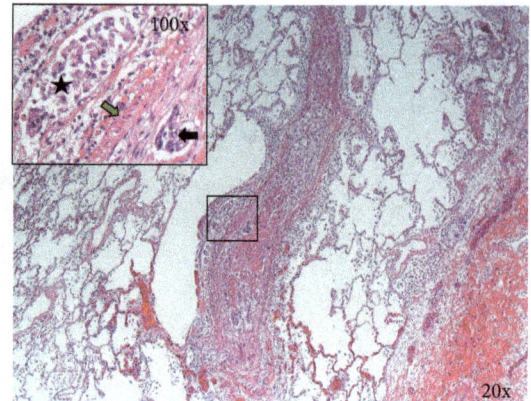

FIGURE 3: Section of lung showing diffusely thrombosed artery with recanalization and small focus of intra-arterial malignant cells (arrow). Inset also shows adjacent lymphatic channel with malignant cells (star). Green arrow points to the muscular wall of the artery. Hematoxylin and eosin.

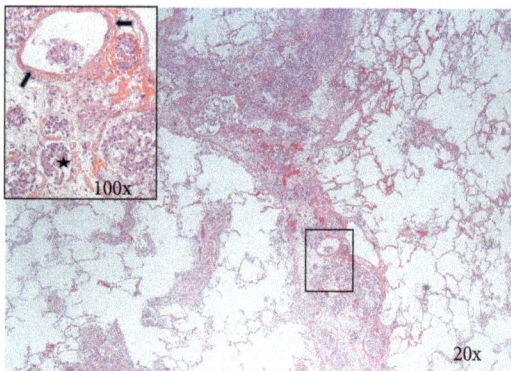

FIGURE 2: Section of postmortem lung tissue demonstrating thickened edematous interlobular septum with numerous dilated lymphatic channels filled with malignant glandular cells (starred in inset). Inset also shows tumor cells in venous channels with thicker walls (arrows). Hematoxylin and eosin.

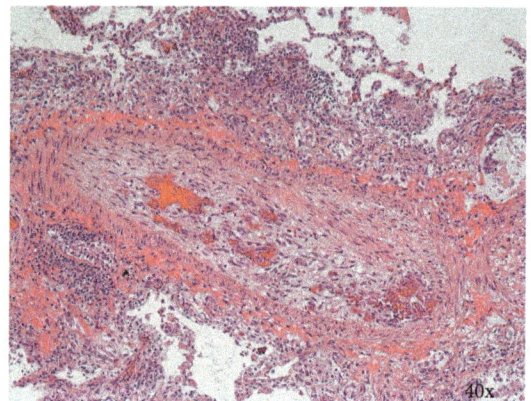

FIGURE 4: Section showing thrombosed medium-sized pulmonary artery with recanalization. Various stages of thrombosis were observed in many arteries throughout all lobes. Hematoxylin and eosin.

perigastric, peripancreatic, mesenteric, and omental nodules were positive for metastatic adenocarcinoma.

3. Discussion

Extracorporeal membrane oxygenation was first reported as a long-term bridge to recovery in 1972 [1], to transplant in 1991 [2], and to left ventricular assist devices in 1999 [10]. The use of centrally cannulated Novalung pECLA was first reported in pulmonary arterial hypertension and bridge to transplant in 2009 [11]. These modalities of ECLS are indicated in respiratory or right ventricular failure refractory to medical management, both in potentially reversible conditions and in irreversible conditions in transplant candidates [12].

Signet-ring cell gastric carcinoma is a rare tumor that is increasing in incidence in an era of risk modification for other forms of gastric adenocarcinoma. In advanced stages, this tumor is highly infiltrative and is less chemosensitive compared to other gastric adenocarcinomas. The rarity of the tumor and the nonspecific presentation of pulmonary tumor embolism were both factors in the difficulty of clinical diagnosis [13].

In this case, the rapid progression of disease and the etiology and reversibility of the patient's respiratory failure were uncertain. The acuity of respiratory and hemodynamic failure prevented our team from employing crucial diagnostic investigations, including ventilation-perfusion scans and CT angiography, both previously shown to aid in the diagnosis of PTE [14–16]. Most importantly, a tissue diagnosis from a surgical lung biopsy was not feasible due to the deteriorating clinical state. ECLS bridging facilitated these investigations, allowing for informed decision-making by both the clinical team and the patients family.

4. Conclusion

Our experience adds to the growing body of knowledge regarding the use of ECLS modalities including VA-ECMO and centrally cannulated Novalung pECLA as a bridge to diagnosis in unstable patients [1, 17, 18]. This approach facilitates good decision-making regarding withdrawal of support, bridge to recovery, or bridge to transplantation. We advocate this approach in diagnostically uncertain cases in unstable patients who are otherwise good ECLS and transplant candidates.

Competing Interests

All authors have no competing interests to disclose.

Authors' Contributions

Vishnu Vasanthan (medical student) conducted chart and literature review and composed the manuscript. Kieran Halloran (pulmonologist) and Jayan Nagendran (cardiac surgeon) performed medical/surgical patient management and edited the manuscript. Lakshmi Puttagunta provided histology images and edited the manuscript.

References

[1] J. D. Hill, T. G. O'Brien, J. J. Murray et al., "Prolonged extracorporeal oxygenation for acute post-traumatic respiratory failure (shock-lung syndrome). Use of the Bramson membrane lung," *The New England Journal of Medicine*, vol. 286, no. 12, pp. 629–634, 1972.

[2] M. J. Jurmann, A. Haverich, S. Demertzis, H.-J. Schaefers, T. O. F. Wagner, and H. G. Borst, "Extracorporeal membrane oxygenation as a bridge to lung transplantation," *European Journal of Cardio-Thoracic Surgery*, vol. 5, no. 2, pp. 94–98, 1991.

[3] L. J. Schlapbach, M. Grips, R. Justo, and T. Karl, "Extracorporeal membrane oxygenation as a bridge to diagnosis in a 20-month old girl with pulmonary hypertension and right ventricular failure," *Interactive CardioVascular and Thoracic Surgery*, vol. 15, no. 6, pp. 1088–1089, 2012.

[4] S. Z. Goldhaber, E. Dricker, J. E. Buring et al., "Clinical suspicion of autopsy-proven thrombotic and tumor pulmonary embolism in cancer patients," *American Heart Journal*, vol. 114, no. 6, pp. 1432–1435, 1987.

[5] D. J. Shields and W. D. Edwards, "Pulmonary hypertension attributable to neoplastic emboli: an autopsy study of 20 cases and a review of literature," *Cardiovascular Pathology*, vol. 1, no. 4, pp. 279–287, 1992.

[6] K. E. Roberts, D. Hamele-Bena, A. Saqi, C. A. Stein, and R. P. Cole, "Pulmonary tumor embolism: a review of the literature," *The American Journal of Medicine*, vol. 115, no. 3, pp. 228–232, 2003.

[7] J. S. Bristowe, "Colloid cancer of esophagus, stomach, lungs, and adjoining lymphatic glands," *Transactions of the Pathological Society of London*, vol. 19, pp. 228–236, 1868.

[8] M. B. Schmidt, *Die Verbreitungswege der Karzinome und die Beziehung Generalisierter Sarcome zu den Leukaemischen Neubildungen*, G. Fischer, Vienna, Austria, 1903.

[9] R. D. Kane, H. K. Hawkins, J. A. Miller, and P. S. Noce, "Microscopic pulmonary tumor emboli associated with dyspnea," *Cancer*, vol. 36, no. 4, pp. 1473–1482, 1975.

[10] F. D. Pagani, W. Lynch, F. Swaniker et al., "Extracorporeal life support to left ventricular assist device bridge to heart transplant: a strategy to optimize survival and resource utilization," *Circulation*, vol. 100, no. 19, supplement, pp. II206–II210, 1999.

[11] M. Strueber, M. M. Hoeper, S. Fischer et al., "Bridge to thoracic organ transplantation in patients with pulmonary arterial hypertension using a pumpless lung assist device," *American Journal of Transplantation*, vol. 9, no. 4, pp. 853–857, 2009.

[12] A. Beckmann, C. Benk, F. Beyersdorf et al., "Position article for the use of extracorporeal life support in adult patients," *European Journal of Cardio-Thoracic Surgery*, vol. 40, no. 3, pp. 676–680, 2011.

[13] S. Pernot, T. Voron, G. Perkins, C. Lagorce-Pages, A. Berger, and J. Taieb, "Signet-ring cell carcinoma of the stomach: impact on prognosis and specific therapeutic challenge," *World Journal of Gastroenterology*, vol. 21, no. 40, pp. 11428–11438, 2015.

[14] W. L. Chen, S. C. Cherng, W. S. Hwang, D. J. Wang, and J. Wei, "Perfusion scan in pulmonary tumor microembolism: report of a case," *Journal of the Formosan Medical Association*, vol. 90, no. 9, pp. 863–866, 1991.

[15] H. D. Sostman, M. Brown, A. Toole, S. Bobrow, and A. Gottschalk, "Perfusion scan in pulmonary vascular/lymphangitic carcinomatosis: the segmental contour pattern," *The American Journal of Roentgenology*, vol. 137, no. 5, pp. 1072–1074, 1981.

[16] R. Crane, T. G. Rudd, and D. Dail, "Tumor microembolism: pulmonary perfusion pattern," *Journal of Nuclear Medicine*, vol. 25, no. 8, pp. 877–880, 1984.

[17] Y. Hsieh, F. Siao, C. Chiu, H. Yen, and Y. Chen, "Massive Pulmonary Embolism Mimicking Acute Myocardial Infarction: successful use of extracorporeal membrane oxygenation support as bridge to diagnosis," *Heart, Lung and Circulation*, vol. 25, no. 7, pp. e78–e80, 2016.

[18] J. Mancio Silva, R. Fontes-Carvalho, and D. Valente, "Extracorporeal membrane oxygenation as bridge-to-decision in acute heart failure due to systemic light-chain amyloidosis," *American Journal of Case Reports*, vol. 16, pp. 174–181, 2015.

35

Left Functional Pneumonectomy Caused by a Very Rare Giant Intrathoracic Cystic Lesion in a Patient with Gorham–Stout Syndrome: Case Report and Review of the Literature

Nikolaos Tasis ⓘ,[1] Ioannis Tsouknidas,[1] Argyrios Ioannidis ⓘ,[1] Konstantinos Nassiopoulos,[2] and Dimitrios Filippou ⓘ [1,3]

[1]Department of Anatomy and Surgical Anatomy, Medical School, National and Kapodistrian University of Athens, Athens, Greece
[2]Hopital Daler, Fribourg, Switzerland
[3]Department of Surgical Oncology, Laparoscopic Surgery and Laser Surgery, N Athinaio Hospital, Athens, Greece

Correspondence should be addressed to Nikolaos Tasis; tasisnikolaos@gmail.com

Academic Editor: Tun-Chieh Chen

Gorham–Stout syndrome is an uncommon entity, with few cases reported in bibliography. It consists of osteolytic manifestations affecting various bones and replacing them with lymphangiomatous tissue. With pathophysiology unknown, Gorham–Stout disease affects also cardiorespiratory system usually causing lytic lesions to the bones of the thoracic cage or directly invading the thoracic duct. This is a case report of a unique respiratory manifestation of the disease and a review of its cardiorespiratory complications.

1. Introduction

Gorham–Stout syndrome or vanishing bone disease is a rare entity with very few cases reported in global bibliography. Gorham et al. in 1954 [1] and Gorham and Stout in 1955 [2] firstly described this uncommon form of massive osteolysis. Till today, etiology and pathophysiology of the disease are unknown. The syndrome consists of replacement of normal bone by nonneoplastic vascular tissue, via overgrowth of lymphatic vessels, resulting in an "invisible" hypervascular fibrous bone [3]. The prognosis varies, with some patients achieving stabilization, while others, especially if complicated with pleural effusion, showing high mortality rates [4]. We present a case report of a unique thoracic presentation of Gorham–Stout syndrome and a detailed review of the literature concerning respiratory manifestations and complications of the disease.

2. Case Presentation

In 1997, female patient, 24 years old, presented intense lower back pain. Lumbar spine CT revealed multiple osteolytic lesions in lumbar vertebrae. Further investigation by attending physicians ruled out neoplastic infiltration. Clinical and laboratory exams were normal, except for slightly decreased calcium levels of unknown origin, with normal levels of PTH, so the patient was treated conservatively with NSAIDs and careful medical advice.

In May of 2004, the patient discovered a nodule in left thyroid lobe, which gradually increased in size. Biopsy revealed follicular thyroid cancer, and a total thyroidectomy was performed. Histological exam showed papillary and follicular thyroid cancer. Histological preparation did not consist of any parathyroid gland, although patient suffered from severe hypocalcaemia for many years postoperatively until utterly controlled by attending endocrinologist with administration of calcium and salmon calcitonin. In September of 2004, a large cystic mass was detected in anterior cervical surface, left of the clavicle. Ultrasound revealed a cyst with 4 cm diameter which was surgically removed. Histological exam suggested lymphatic cyst.

In 2007, a relapse was observed and was US monitored for the next months. In 2008, the patient was referred to our department for further investigation. Clinical examination showed the palpable mass in the lower anterior section of the cervix, with 3 cm diameter, increasing in size. Lab tests were normal apart from CPK (250 IU/L), serum phosphorus (5,6 mg/dl), and serum calcium (7,8 mg/dl). Thoracic and Cervical MRI reveal a substantial cystic mass (12,5 × 2,2 × 2,3 cm) in anterior mesothorax. Two similar masses were detected one paratracheal (2,6 × 4 cm) and one in the lower cervix (2,4 × 2 cm), all communicating. Lower and upper abdomen CT showed multiple cystic lesions of the spleen, while full MRI check revealed no change in cystic lesions of lumbar vertebrae, with several similar lesions in whole vertebrae column, the clavicle and both femurs. FNA procedure took place and the sample proved to be lymph. FNA in combination with CT and MRI results indicated Gorham–Stout disease.

Patient continued receiving conservative therapy with calcium and salmon calcitonin and after six months calcium levels became normal and bone density reached normal range, improving by far patient's quality of life. Mesothorax and spinal cystic lesions were reevaluated regularly and no change in size was noted.

The next two years patient underwent two incidents which were impossible to properly diagnose. The first consisted of an intense headache, which lasted for 15 days during patient's vacation, with following improvement and the second involved a vision disorder which was examined by an ophthalmologist with no pathology defined.

However, in 2010, the patient was admitted due to intense headache, gradually increasing, affecting patient's quality of life. Although examination revealed no abnormal findings, the patient was deteriorating. A lumbar puncture took place and showed low cerebrospinal fluid (CSF) pressure (<6). Intravenous fluids were administrated and, later, patient improved and was discharged, only to come two days later with severe temporal and cervical cephalalgia and vertigo. Otorhinolaryngological examination was not pathological and patient was treated conservatively with Sibellium, Lonarid-N, and Tramal tablets. Patient improved but further examination took place. Full-body 3D CT scan with intrathecal radioactive polymer infusion revealed the following: (1) incomplete herniation of the brain stem probably due to low CSF pressure; (2) dilation of endothoracic cyst, with more than 20 cm diameter, fully compressing left lung causing functional left pneumonectomy; and (3) possible communication of CSF with mesothoracic cystic mass (Figures 1(a), 1(b), and 2).

Surgical excision was undertaken. Patient underwent thoracoscopic excision of the gargantuan cystic mass, with ligation of major lymph vessels, conserving major thoracic duct. No connection between the cyst and spinal cavity was detected, possibly because during the excision procedure the connection was ligated or shut. Patient had a smooth postoperative course and recovery.

3. Discussion

Gorham–Stout syndrome (GSS), also known as Gorham's syndrome, idiopathic massive osteolysis, disappearing bone, disease or phantom bone disease, is a rare skeletal disorder, characterized by osteolysis of various bones accompanied by proliferative angiomatosis. Almost 180 years have passed since Jackson first presented, in 1838, the case of an 18-year-old boy with idiopathic osteolysis of his right humerus [62]. In 1955, Gorham and Stout, after concentrating and studying all previous similar cases, described "a syndrome of progressive osteolysis associated with an angiomatosis proliferation of blood or lymphatic vessels" [2]. Although over 200 cases have been reported to date [63], there is still a lot to learn about this syndrome.

Gorham–Stout syndrome provokes osteolytic damage to one or multiple bones. It can affect any age, but most commonly children and young adults. Special correlation with specific race, sex, geography, or hereditary pattern has not been identified yet [64]. The shoulder and the pelvis are the most common sites to be affected according to Patel [3]. Femur as more possible first presentation is described by Ruggieri et al. [65] and Hu et al. [66]. Cases of phantom bone disease to the skull, mandible, maxillofacial skeleton, spine, scapula, clavicle, ribs, sternum, humerus, hand, and foot have also been described [3]. In our case lumbar osteolytic lesions may be considered the first sign of Gorham–Stout syndrome. Our patient experienced intense low back pain at the age of 22. The symptom was treated as common back pain and although lesions of lumbar spine were detected, no further investigation was required since neoplastic etiology was ruled out and laboratory tests were normal. Pain was relieved with NSAIDs and the patient continued everyday activity without symptoms for years. Pain is considered to be a frequent atypical symptom of GSS [64], mainly because of lymphangiomatous infiltration of bones. Maillot et al. [67] state that vertebral primary involvement is rare (10%) and associated with a poor prognosis. However, patients tend to be undiagnosed until pathological fracture takes place even if localized pain is present [65]. The fact that Gorham–Stout progression may be asymptomatic reinforces our belief of lumbar spine involvement in our case.

In the course of the case, two years after thyroidectomy, a cystic mass was spotted in lower anterior cervix of the patient. It was identified as a lymphangiomatous cyst and was surgically excised. Six months later, a relapse caused the referral of the patient to our department only to diagnose one large mesothoracic cyst (12,5 × 2,2 × 2,3 cm) with two smaller and one paratracheal (2,6 × 4 cm) cysts and one in the lower cervix (2,4 × 2 cm). In addition, osteolytic lymphangiomatous lesions, common Gorham–Stout syndrome's manifestations [64], were located in whole vertebrae column, the clavicle, and both femurs as well as in spleen. Patient was treated conservatively with calcitonin and regularly checked. Cysts were monitored and there was no change in size until patient had a thorough investigation for intense cephalalgia. Only then did we come across a unique finding. CT revealed dilation of endothoracic cyst, more than 20 cm in diameter, fully compressing left lung causing functional left pneumonectomy. Also, there was incomplete herniation of the brain stem due to low CSF pressure, probably because of possible communication of CSF with mesothoracic cystic mass, which could not be verified thoracoscopically.

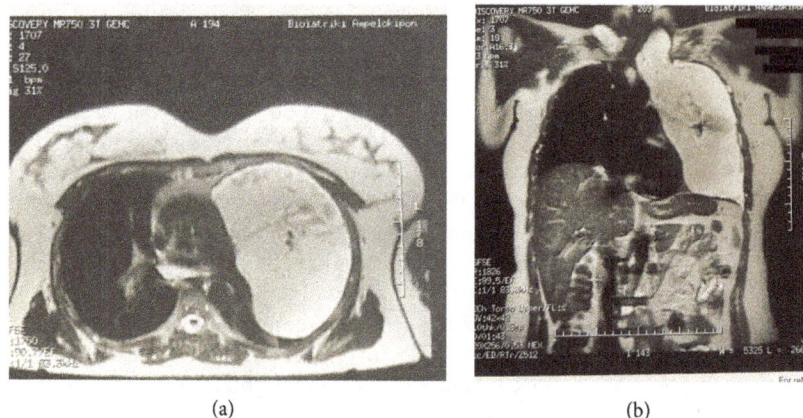

(a)   (b)

FIGURE 1: A giant cystic lesion occupying almost completely the left side of thorax causing functional pneumonectomy.

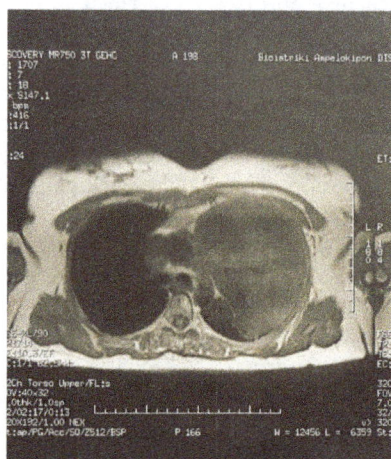

FIGURE 2: MRI of the intrathoracic cystic lesion. Osteolytic lesion in the thoracic vertebrae also obvious.

Disease of the bones of the thoracic cage often presents with pleural effusion and/or chylothorax. Chylothorax is present up to 17% of the patients [50] and increases the rate of mortality and morbidity, especially if patients do not undergo surgical intervention [68]. There are 67 confirmed cases of Gorham–Stout syndrome with cardiorespiratory invasion found in the literature (Table 1). Chylothorax was present in 60 of them (89,55%) and was the major presenting symptom in the thorax. In literature we found, also, two cases of nondescript pleural effusion [4, 56], one case of hemothorax [29], one case with hematoma [29], and three cases with bloody pleural effusion [32, 34, 47]. One unusual case of duropleural fistula [47] was noted as well. Concerning more rare cardiac presentations, there were two cases with chylotamponade [41, 52], one with hemochylopericardium [46], and two cases of nondescript pericardial effusion [4, 44] reported in literature. In these 67 cases we only encountered 2 cases of lymphangiomatous cysts [37, 61], one in the mediastinum and one located in right anterior chest wall. Our case is the third with cystic presentation of Gorham–Stout syndrome. However, the fact that the massive lymphangiomatous cyst provoked a functional left pneumonectomy due to its size and

position in the mesothorax has not been described previously in Gorham–Stout disease. Usually, the cysts are found and dealt with at early stages or erupt into the pleural cavity causing chylothorax. In this case the cyst reached 20 cm in diameter, caused left functional pneumonectomy, and was identified randomly after CT scan. Our patient underwent surgery and had an uncomplicated recovery. Mortality in Gorham–Stout disease with thoracic cage presentation as reported in the literature is high. Out of 67 cases, 22 did not survive (32,8%). Surgical ligation, pleurodesis, and other surgical or radiological treatments seem to improve survival for patients with these complications [68].

4. Conclusion

Gorham–Stout syndrome is an uncommon condition. With etiology unknown, diagnosis and treatment remain a challenge. Osteolytic lesions and/or pathological fractures should raise clinical suspicion for GSS. Attention is needed, especially when respiratory complications are present. This case offers a new presentation of the disease and along with past and future cases may contribute to a deeper understanding

TABLE 1: Presentation of all cases of patients with respiratory manifestations of Gorham–Stout syndrome reported in the literature.

Number	Author	Year	Age/sex	Hemithorax involved	Pathology	Outcome
(1)	Gorham et al. [1]	1954	16/M	R	Chylothorax	Died
(2)	De seze and Hubault [5]	1956	29/F	Bilateral	Chylothorax	N/A
(3)	Jones et al. [6]	1958	28/M	Bilateral	Chylothorax	Died
(4)	Koblenzer and Bukowski [7]	1961	4/F	R	Chylothorax	Died
(5)	Tucker [8]	1967	11/M	Bilateral	Chylothorax	Survived
(6)	Kolpakova and Iaroshevskaia [9]	1967	12/F	Bilateral	Chylothorax	Died
(7)	Vanetti et al. [10]	1968	5/F	L	Chylothorax	Survived
(8)	Morphis et al. [11]	1970	9 mo/M	Bilateral	Chylothorax	Died
(9)	Touraine et al. [12]	1970	49/M	L	Chylothorax	Survived
(10)	Takamoto et al. [13]	1971	21/M	R	Chylothorax	Survived
(11)	Gutierrez and Spjut [14]	1972	4/M	Bilateral	Chylothorax	Died
(12)	Berberich et al. [15]	1975	3.5/M	Bilateral	Chylothorax	Survived
(13)	Noziska et al. [16]	1974	14/M	Bilateral	Chylothorax	Died
(14)	Fessard et al. [17]	1974	2/F	R	Chylothorax	Died
(15)			3/F	Bilateral	Chylothorax	Died
(16)	Patrick [18]	1976	30/M	L	Chylothorax	Survived
(17)	Rousselin et al. [19]	1977	30/F	L	Chylothorax	Died
(18)	Feigl et al. [20]	1981	26/F	Bilateral	Chylothorax	Survived
(19)	Young et al. [21]	1983	2/M	R	Chylothorax	Survived
(20)	Pedicelli et al. [22]	1984	18/F	L	Chylothorax	Survived
(21)	Brown et al. [23]	1986	30/M	Bilateral	Chylothorax	Died
(22)	Choma et al. [24]	1987	23/M	R	Chylothorax	Survived
(23)	Hejgaard and Olsen [25]	1987	9/M	R	Chylothorax	Survived

TABLE 1: Continued.

Number	Author	Year	Age/sex	Hemithorax involved	Pathology	Outcome
(24)	Joseph and Bartal [26]	1987	7/F	R	Chylothorax	Died
(25)	Marymont [27]	1987	7/F	R	Chylothorax	Died
(26)	Romero et al. [28]	1989	61/M	R	Chylothorax	Survived
(27)	Meller et al. [29]	1993	7 mo/M	R	Hemothorax	Survived
(28)			14/M	R	Hematoma	Survived
(29)	Tie et al. [30]	1994	18/M	L	Chylothorax	Survived
(30)	Drewry et al. [31]	1994	13/M	L	Chylothorax	Survived
(31)	Ng and Wang [32]	1995	63/F	R	Pleural effusion (Blood stained serous fluid)	Died
(32)	Riantawan et al. [33]	1996	27/M	Bilateral	Chylothorax	Died
(33)	McNeil et al. [34]	1996	21/M	R	Pleural effusion (Bloodstained fluid)	Survived
(34)	Aoki et al. [35]	1996	19/F	R	Chylothorax	Survived
(35)	Chavanis et al. [36]	2001	45/F	L	Chylothorax	Survived
(36)	Yoo et al. [37]	2002	38/M	Bilateral	Chylothorax, Mediastinal cystic mass (with turbid pinkish fluid)	Survived
(37)	Fujiu et al. [38]	2002	15/M	Bilateral	Chylothorax	Died
(38)	Miller [39]	2002	2/M	R	Chylothorax	Died
(39)	Lee et al. [40]	2002	25/F	R	Chylothorax	Survived
(40)	Swelstad et al. [41]	2003	31/F	R	Chylothorax, chylotamponade	Survived

TABLE 1: Continued.

Number	Author	Year	Age/sex	Hemithorax involved	Pathology	Outcome
(41)	Lee et al. [42]	2003	6/F	N/A	Chylothorax	Died
(42)	Lee et al. [42]	2003	9/F	N/A	Chylothorax	Died
(43)	Fontanesi [43]	2003	M	R	Chylothorax	Survived
(44)	Takahashi et al. [44]	2005	2/F	L	Chylothorax, Pericardial effusion	Survived
(45)	Kren et al. [45]	2005	7/M	L	Chylothorax	Survived
(46)	Duffy et al. [46]	2005	31/F	Bilateral	Chylothorax, hemochylopericardium	Survived
(47)	Agrawal et al. [47]	2006	25/F	L	Bloody pleural effusion, DPF	Survived
(48)	Pfleger et al. [48]	2006	18/M	R	Chylothorax	Survived
(49)	Yildiz et al. [49]	2009	6/M	Bilateral	Chylothorax	Survived
(50)	Kose et al. [50]	2009	9/F	R	Chylothorax	Survived
(51)	De Smet et al. [51]	2010	8/M	L	Chylothorax	Survived
(52)	Wijesinghe et al. [52]	2010	50/F	L	Chylothorax, Chylotamponade	Survived
(53)	Kuriyama et al. [53]	2010	16/F	L	Chylothorax	Survived
(54)	Deveci et al. [54]	2011	6/M	Bilateral	Chylothorax	Died
(55)	Brodszki et al. [55]	2011	2.5/M	R	Chylothorax	Survived
(56)			4/F	Bilateral	Chylothorax	Survived
(57)	Min-Wen et al. [56]	2012	5/F	L	Pleural effusion	Survived
(58)	Hopman et al. [57]	2012	12 mo/M	R	Chylothorax	Died
(59)	Noda et al. [58]	2013	15/M	R	Chylothorax	Survived
(60)	Jayaprakash et al. [59]	2013	9/F	Bilateral	Chylothorax	Died
(61)	Maillot et al. [60]	2014	30/F	L	Chylothorax	Survived
(62)			32/F	Bilateral	Pleural effusion, Pericardial effusion	Survived
(63)			15/M	Bilateral	Chylothorax	Survived
(64)	Liu et al. [4]	2014	32/M	Bilateral	Chylothorax	Survived
(65)			22/F	L	Chylothorax	Survived
(66)			23/M	R	Chylothorax	Survived
(67)	Davalos et al. [61]	2015	9/F	R	Large cystic mass, chylothorax	Survived

of this extraordinary clinical entity, the Gorham–Stout Syndrome.

References

[1] L. W. Gorham, A. W. Wright, H. H. Shultz, and F. C. Maxon Jr., "Disappearing bones: A rare form of massive osteolysis. Report of two cases, one with autopsy findings," *American Journal of Medicine*, vol. 17, no. 5, pp. 674–682, 1954.

[2] L. W. Gorham and A. P. Stout, "Massive osteolysis (Acute spontaneous absorption of bone, phantom bone, disappearing bone)," *The Journal of Bone & Joint Surgery*, vol. 37, no. 5, pp. 985–1004, 1955.

[3] D. V. Patel, "Gorham's Disease or Massive Osteolysis," *Clinical Medicine & Research*, vol. 3, no. 2, pp. 65–74, 2005.

[4] Y. Liu, D.-R. Zhong, P.-R. Zhou et al., "Gorham-Stout disease: radiological, histological, and clinical features of 12 cases and review of literature," *Clinical Rheumatology*, vol. 35, no. 3, pp. 813–823, 2016.

[5] S. De seze and A. Hubault, "Essential osteolysis scapulo-thoraco-brachial," *Revue du Rhumatisme et des Maladies Osteo-Articulaires*, vol. 23, no. 6, pp. 517–523, 1956.

[6] G. B. Jones, R. L. Midgley, G. S. Smith et al., "Massive osteolysis-disappearing bones," *The Journal of Bone and Joint Surgery*, pp. 40B–494, 1958.

[7] P. G. Koblenzer and M. J. Bukowski, "Angiomatosis (Hamarto-matosis—Hem-Lymphangiomatosis). Report of a case with diffuse involvement," *Pediatrics*, vol. 28, p. 65, 1961.

[8] S. M. Tucker, "Bilateral chylothorax with multiple osteolytic lesions? Generalized abnormality of lymphatic system," *Proceedings of the Royal Society of Medicine*, vol. 60, no. 1, pp. 17–19, 1967.

[9] L. V. Kolpakova and E. N. Iaroshevskaia, "A case of massive regional osteolysis," *Arkh Patol*, vol. 29, no. 5, pp. 75–77, 1967.

[10] A. Vanetti, J. D. Picard, M. Fandre et al., "A case of apparently spontaneous chylothorax in children associated with osseous lesions of the osteolytic type," *Annales de chirurgie thoracique et cardio-vasculaire*, vol. 7, no. 1, pp. 99–104, 1968.

[11] L. G. Morphis, E. L. Arcinue, and J. R. Krause, "Generalized lymphangioma in infancy with chylothorax," *Pediatrics*, vol. 46, no. 4, pp. 566–575, 1970.

[12] R. Touraine, J. P. Trouillier, and A. M. Balander, "Chylothorax et maladie de Gorham," *Lyon Med*, vol. 224, pp. 445–466, 1970.

[13] R. M. Takamoto, R. G. Armstrong, W. Stanford, L. J. Fontenelle, and G. Troxler, "Chylothorax with multiple lymphangiomata of the bone.," *CHEST*, vol. 59, no. 6, pp. 687–689, 1971.

[14] R. M. Gutierrez and H. J. Spjut, "Skeletal angiomatosis: report of three cases and review of the literature.," *Clinical Orthopaedics and Related Research*, vol. 85, pp. 82–97, 1972.

[15] F. R. Berberich, I. D. Bernstein, H. D. Ochs, and R. T. Schaller, "Lymphangiomatosis with chylothorax," *Journal of Pediatrics* vol. 87, no. 6, pp. 941–943, 1975.

[16] Z. Nozicka, V. Herout, and Fingerland A., "Gorhauv-Stoutuv syndrome zpusobeny hemangio-lymfangiomen," *Czech Patol*, vol. 10, pp. 56–62, 1974.

[17] C. I. Fessard, C. Boulesteix, C. H. Roudil, N. Grynblat, A. Fondimare, R. Dumas et al., "ascite chyleuse, chylothorax et ectasiescapillares intra-osseuses," *Arch Fr Pediatr*, vol. 31, pp. 489–506, 1974.

[18] J. H. Patrick, "Massive osteolysis complicated by chylothorax successfully treated by pleurodesis," *The Journal of Bone & Joint Surgery (British Volume)*, vol. 58, no. 3, pp. 347–349, 1976.

[19] L. Rousselin, G. Roche, and M. F. Carette, "Les epanchements pleuraux (chyleux ou non) avec osteolyse regionale," *Le Poumon et le Coeur*, vol. 3, pp. 203–207, 1977.

[20] D. Feigl, L. Seidel, and A. Marmor, "Gorham's disease of the clavicle with bilateral pleural effusions," *CHEST*, vol. 79, no. 2, pp. 242–244, 1981.

[21] J. W. R. Young, M. Galbraith, J. Cunningham et al., "Case report: Progressive vertebral collapse in diffuse angiomatosis," *Metabolic Bone Disease and Related Research*, vol. 5, no. 2, pp. 53–60, 1983.

[22] G. Pedicelli, P. Mattia, A. A. Zorzoli, A. Sorrone, F. De Martino, and V. Sciotto, "Gorham syndrome," *Journal of the American Medical Association*, vol. 252, no. 11, pp. 1449–1451, 1984.

[23] L. R. Brown, H. M. Reiman, E. C. Rosenow III, P. M. Gloviczki, and M. B. Divertie, "Intrathoracic lymphangioma," *Mayo Clinic Proceedings*, vol. 61, no. 11, pp. 882–892, 1986.

[24] N. D. Choma, C. V. Biscotti, T. W. Bauer, A. C. Mehta, and A. A. Licata, "Gorham's syndrome: A case report and review of the literature," *American Journal of Medicine*, vol. 83, no. 6, pp. 1151–1156, 1987.

[25] N. Hejgaard and P. R. Olsen, "Massive gorham osteolysis of the right hemipelvis complicated by chylothorax: Report of a case in a 9-year-old boy successfully treated by pleurodesis," *Journal of Pediatric Orthopaedics*, vol. 7, no. 1, pp. 96–99, 1987.

[26] J. Joseph and E. Bartal, "Disappearing bone disease: A case report and review of the literature," *Journal of Pediatric Orthopaedics*, vol. 7, no. 5, pp. 584–588, 1987.

[27] J. V. Marymont, "Comparative imaging. Massive osteolysis (Gorham's syndrome, disappearing bone disease)," *Clinical Nuclear Medicine*, vol. 12, no. 2, pp. 153-154, 1987.

[28] J. Romero, R. Kunz, U. Münch, and U. Neff, "Successful treatment of a chylothorax in lymphangiomatosis of the ribs (Gorham-Stout syndrome)," *Schweiz Med Wochenschr*, vol. 119, no. 20, pp. 671–677, 1989.

[29] J. L. Meller, M. Curet-Scott, P. Dawson, A. S. Besser, and D. W. Shermeta, "Massive osteolysis of the chest in children: An unusual cause of respiratory distress," *Journal of Pediatric Surgery*, vol. 28, no. 12, pp. 1539–1542, 1993.

[30] M. L. H. Tie, G. A. Poland, and E. C. Rosenow III, "Chylothorax in Gorham's syndrome: A common complication of a rare disease," *CHEST*, vol. 105, no. 1, pp. 208–213, 1994.

[31] G. R. Drewry, C. R. Martinez, and S. G. Brantley, "Gorham disease of the spine," *The Spine Journal*, vol. 19, no. 19, pp. 2213-2222, 1994.

[32] S. E. S. Ng and Y. T. Wang, "Gorhams syndrome with pleural effusion and colonic carcinoma," *Singapore Medical Journal*, vol. 36, pp. 102–104, 1995.

[33] P. Riantawan, S. Tansupasawasdikul, and P. Subhannachart, "Bilateral chylothorax complicating massive osteolysis (Gorham's syndrome)," *Thorax*, vol. 51, no. 12, pp. 1277-1278, 1996.

[34] K. D. McNeil, K. M. Fong, Q. J. Walker, P. Jessup, and P. V. Zimmerman, "Gorham's syndrome: A usually fatal cause of pleural effusion treated successfully with radiotherapy," *Thorax*, vol. 51, no. 12, pp. 1275-1276, 1996.

[35] M. Aoki, F. Kato, H. Saito, K. Mimatsu, and H. Iwata, "Successful treatment of chylothorax by bleomycin for Gorham's disease," *Clinical Orthopaedics and Related Research*, no. 330, pp. 193–197, 1996.

[36] N. Chavanis, P. Chaffanjon, G. Frey, G. Vottero, and P.-Y. Brichon, "Chylothorax complicating Gorham's disease," *The Annals of Thoracic Surgery*, vol. 72, no. 3, pp. 937–939, 2001.

[37] S. Y. Yoo, J. M. Goo, and J.-G. Im, "Mediastinal Lymphangioma and Chylothorax: Thoracic Involvement of Gorham's Disease," *Korean Journal of Radiology*, vol. 3, no. 2, pp. 130–132, 2002.

[38] K. Fujiu, R. Kanno, H. Suzuki, N. Nakamura, and M. Gotoh, "Chyothorax associated with massive osteolysis (Gorham's syndrome)," *The Annals of Thoracic Surgery*, vol. 73, no. 6, pp. 1956-1957, 2002.

[39] G. Miller, "Treatment of chylothorax in Gorhams disease: case report and literature review," *Canadian Journal of Surgery*, vol. 45, no. 4, 2002.

[40] W. S. Lee, S. H. Kim, I. Kim et al., "Chylothorax in Gorham's disease," *Journal of Korean Medical Science*, vol. 17, no. 6, pp. 826–829, 2002.

[41] M. R. Swelstad, C. Frumiento, A. Garry-McCoy, R. Agni, and T. L. Weigel, "Chylotamponade: An unusual presentation of Gorham's Syndrome," *The Annals of Thoracic Surgery*, vol. 75, no. 5, pp. 1650–1652, 2003.

[42] S. Lee, L. Finn, R. W. Sze, J. A. Perkins, and K. C. Sie, "Gorham Stout Syndrome (Disappearing Bone Disease): Two Additional Case Reports and a Review of the Literature," *Archives of Otolaryngology—Head and Neck Surgery*, vol. 129, no. 12, pp. 1340–1343, 2003.

[43] J. Fontanesi, "Radiation therapy in the treatment of Gorham disease," *Journal of Pediatric Hematology/Oncology*, vol. 25, no. 10, pp. 816-817, 2003.

[44] A. Takahashi, C. Ogawa, T. Kanazawa et al., "Remission induced by interferon alfa in a patient with massive osteolysis and extension of lymph-hemangiomatosis: A severe case of Gorham-Stout syndrome," *Journal of Pediatric Surgery*, vol. 40, no. 3, pp. E47–E50, 2005.

[45] L. Kren, P. Rotterova, M. Hermanova et al., "Chylothorax as a possible diagnostic pitfall: A report of 2 cases with cytologic findings," *Acta Cytologica*, vol. 49, no. 4, pp. 441–444, 2005.

[46] B. Duffy, R. Manon, R. Patel, and J. Welsh, "A Case of gorhams disease with chylothorax treated curatively with radiation therapy," *CM & R*, vol. 3, no. 2, pp. 83–86, 2005.

[47] R. Agrawal, I. Mohammed, and P. G. Reilly, "Duropleural fistula as a consequence of Gorham-Stout syndrome: A combination of 2 rare conditions," *The Journal of Thoracic and Cardiovascular Surgery*, vol. 131, no. 5, pp. 1205-1206, 2006.

[48] A. Pfleger, W. Schwinger, A. Maier, J. Tauss, H. H. Popper, and M. S. Zach, "Gorham-Stout syndrome in a male adolescent - Case report and review of the literature," *Journal of Pediatric Hematology/Oncology*, vol. 28, no. 4, pp. 231–233, 2006.

[49] T. S. Yildiz, A. Kus, M. Solak, and K. Toker, "The Gorham-Stout syndrome: One lung ventilation with a bronchial blocker. A case of Gorham's disease with chylothorax," *Pediatric Anesthesia*, vol. 19, no. 2, pp. 190-191, 2009.

[50] M. Kose, S. Pekcan, D. Dogru et al., "Gorham-Stout syndrome with chylothorax: Successful remission by interferon alpha-2b," *Pediatric Pulmonology*, vol. 44, no. 6, pp. 613–615, 2009.

[51] K. De Smet, M. De Maeseneer, E. Huijssen-Huisman, V. Van Gorp, S. Hachimi-Idrissi, and C. Ernst, "A rare cause of dyspnea due to chylothorax," *Emergency Radiology*, vol. 17, no. 6, pp. 503–505, 2010.

[52] N. Wijesinghe, Z. Lin, M. J. Swarbrick, and D. M. Jogia, "Chylotamponade an unusual manifestation of gorham-stout syndrome," *Circulation: Cardiovascular Imaging*, vol. 3, no. 2, pp. 223-224, 2010.

[53] D. K. Kuriyama, S. C. McElligott, D. W. Glaser, and K. S. Thompson, "Treatment of gorham-stout disease with zoledronic acid and interferon-α: A case report and literature review," *Journal of Pediatric Hematology/Oncology*, vol. 32, no. 8, pp. 579–584, 2010.

[54] M. Deveci, N. Inan, F. Çorapçioğlu, and G. Ekingen, "Gorham-Stout syndrome with chylothorax in a six-year-old boy," *The Indian Journal of Pediatrics*, vol. 78, no. 6, pp. 737–739, 2011.

[55] N. Brodszki, J.-K. Länsberg, M. Dictor et al., "A novel treatment approach for paediatric Gorham-Stout syndrome with chylothorax," *Acta Paediatrica*, vol. 100, no. 11, pp. 1448–1453, 2011.

[56] Z. Min-Wen, M. Yang, Q. Jian-Xin et al., "Gorham-stout syndrome presenting in a 5-year-old girl with a successful bisphosphonate therapeutic effect," *Experimental and Therapeutic Medicine*, vol. 4, no. 3, pp. 449–451, 2012.

[57] S. M. J. Hopman, R. R. Van Rijn, C. Eng et al., "PTEN hamartoma tumor syndrome and Gorham-Stout phenomenon," *American Journal of Medical Genetics Part A*, vol. 158, no. 7, pp. 1719–1723, 2012.

[58] M. Noda, C. Endo, Y. Hoshikawa et al., "Successful management of intractable chylothorax in Gorham-Stout disease by awake thoracoscopic surgery," *General Thoracic and Cardiovascular Surgery*, vol. 61, no. 6, pp. 356–358, 2013.

[59] B. Jayaprakash, B. Prajeesh, and D. S. Nair, "Gorham's Disease," *The Journal of the Association of Physicians of India*, vol. 61, 2013.

[60] C. Maillot, T. Cloche, and J. C. Le Huec, "Thoracic osteotomy for Gorham-Stout disease of the spine: a case report and literature review," *European Spine Journal*, 2014.

[61] E. A. Davalos, N. M. Gandhi, D. Barank, and R. K. Varma, "Gorham-stout disease presenting with dyspnea and bone pain in a 9-year-old girl," *Radiology Case Reports*, vol. 10, no. 2, p. 1110, 2015.

[62] J. B. S. Jackson, "A Boneless Arm," *The Boston Medical and Surgical Journal*, vol. 18, pp. 368-369, 1838.

[63] U. Brunner, K. Rückl, C. Konrads, M. Rudert, and P. Plumhoff, "Gorham-Stout syndrome of the shoulder," *SICOT-J from Société Internationale de Chirurgie Orthopédique et de Traumatologie*, vol. 2, no. 25, pp. 1–7, 2016.

[64] V. S. Nikolaou, D. Chytas, D. Korres, and N. Efstathopoulos, "Vanishing bone disease (gorham-stout syndrome): A review of a rare entity," *World Journal of Orthopedics*, vol. 5, no. 5, pp. 694–698, 2014.

[65] P. Ruggieri, M. Montalti, A. Angelini, M. Alberghini, and M. Mercuri, "Gorham-Stout disease: The experience of the Rizzoli Institute and review of the literature," *Skeletal Radiology*, vol. 40, no. 11, pp. 1391–1397, 2011.

[66] P. Hu, X. Yua, X. Hu, F. Shen, and J. Wang, "Gorham-Stout syndrome in mainland China: a case series of 67 patients and review of the literature," *J Zhejiang Univ-Sci B (Biomed & Biotechnol)*, vol. 14, no. 8, pp. 729–735, 2013.

36

Airway Complications from an Esophageal Foreign Body

Ismael Garcia,[1] Joseph Varon,[2,3,4] and Salim Surani[5]

[1]*Facultad de Medicina Tampico, Universidad Autónoma de Tamaulipas, Tampico, TAMPS, Mexico*
[2]*Dorrington Medical Associates, Houston, TX, USA*
[3]*Foundation Surgical Hospital, Houston, TX, USA*
[4]*The University of Texas Health Science Center at Houston, Houston, TX 77030, USA*
[5]*Texas A&M University, Corpus Christi, TX 78413, USA*

Correspondence should be addressed to Salim Surani; srsurani@hotmail.com

Academic Editor: Fabio Midulla

Introduction. Foreign body impaction (FBI) in the esophagus can be a serious condition, which can have a high mortality among children and adults, if appropriate diagnosis and treatment are not instituted urgently. 80–90% of all foreign bodies trapped in the esophagus usually pass spontaneously through the digestive tract, without any medical or surgical intervention. 10–20% of them will need an endoscopic intervention. *Case Report.* We hereby present a case of a large chicken piece foreign body impaction in the esophagus in a 25-year-old male with mental retardation. Patient developed hypoxemic respiratory failure requiring intubation. The removal required endoscopic intervention. *Conclusions.* Foreign bodies trapped in the upper gastrointestinal tract are a serious condition that can be fatal if they are not managed correctly. A correct diagnosis and treatment decrease the chances of complications. Endoscopic treatment remains the gold standard for extracting foreign body impaction.

1. Introduction

A foreign body impaction (FBI) in the esophagus can be a serious condition with high mortality rate among children and adults. A foreign body can be defined as the presence of any object, food, or material in the upper gastrointestinal tract, swallowed by accident or intentionally [1]. Children are more commonly affected by these conditions than adults. In the adult population, certain special conditions, such as mental retardation, psychiatric disorders, alcohol intake, and demented or edentulous patients, put them in a higher risk for developing an FBI [2].

Studies have shown that 80–90% of all foreign bodies trapped in the esophagus pass spontaneously whereas the remaining 10–20% of cases will require an endoscopic intervention to remove the FBI [3].

Radiological imaging of the neck and abdomen can allow the clinician to identify the radiopaque object and complications as esophageal perforation [4]. There are various ways to achieve removal of a FBI; these include nonendoscopic methods and endoscopic methods, which include flexible endoscopy versus rigid endoscopy. The rigid endoscopy is considered the gold standard for the treatment of FBI [5]. In cases when the airway of the patients seems compromised the use of a rigid endoscopy and intubation are the best treatment option [6, 7]. The choice by the clinician relies on the patient condition, the characteristics of the object, and the location, type, form, size of material, object or food that got impacted, and the anatomical portion of the esophagus which gets affected, and the duration of FBI episode [8].

We hereby present a case of a foreign body in the esophagus caused by a food bolus impaction with a piece of chicken in a 25-year-old male with mental retardation; patient developed hypoxemic complications which were resolved. This was managed endoscopically via using flexible video endoscope by Olympus.

2. Case Report

25-year-old gentlemen presented to the emergency department (ED) due to acute shortness of breath and bronchospasms after ingesting the chicken piece. Patient past

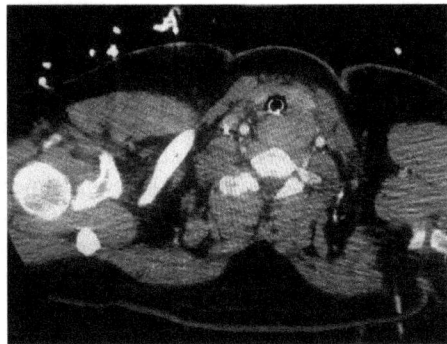

FIGURE 1: Computerized tomography of chest demonstrating foreign body impaction versus mass in esophagus.

medical history was significant for mental retardation, bipolar disorder, seizure disorder, and hypertension.

Patient was eating a chicken piece for meal, according to the witness he started to have a choking episode, Heimlich maneuver was performed, and a piece of the chicken was expelled. He started having severe respiratory distress after the incident and was transferred to the ED via ambulance. On arrival in ED, the patient was in significant respiratory distress. Patient was placed on oxygen supplementation with nonrebreather mask at 15 L/min. On auscultation stridor was heard in upper airway and rhonchi were heard in all lung fields. Patient blood pressure was 162/97 mmhg, heart rate was 103 beats/min, respiratory rate was 30/min, and pulse oximetry showed an oxygen saturation of 100%. Patient temperature was 99.3°F. An X-ray with lateral view of the neck was performed, showing no radiopaque foreign body within the pharyngeal or laryngeal region. Cervical spine X-ray to the level of C5 was within normal limits. Patient WBC count was 18.5 mm^3. Electrolytes and electrocardiogram were within normal limits. Patient underwent an emergent bronchoscopy in the ED revealing no foreign body and normal airway. Patient continued to have respiratory distress and bronchospasms, which failed to improve postracemic epinephrine and steroid. Patient was intubated with excellent arterial blood gas (ABG) with no significant A-a gradient. Patient was also placed on empiric broad-spectrum antibiotic with piperacillin and tazobactam. In the following day, patient had an excellent oxygenation on arterial blood gas. Patient was extubated. Immediately after extubation patient went into severe respiratory distress and bronchospasm, requiring immediate reintubation.

CT scan of the chest was performed which showed a large soft tissue mass 8 × 6 cm posterior to the trachea, extending to the left of midline posterior to the left thyroid lobe (Figure 1). The mass displaces the trachea anteriorly and slightly to the right. Differential diagnosis included esophageal mass versus large left thyroid versus possible nonopaque foreign body. Other findings reported were posterior right upper lobe and bilateral lower lobe consolidations.

In the view of the patient history of possible foreign body ingestion, patient underwent esophagogastroduodenoscopy (EGD). The flexible video endoscope was inserted and passed without difficulty up to the upper esophageal sphincter, where a very large piece of chicken was identified occluding the proximal esophagus and causing significant pressure on the posterior tracheal wall. A tunnel in the middle of the chicken piece was made and grabbed in pieces with a snare and eventually removed as much as possible, weakening the center piece so the rest of the piece could pass easily into the stomach. The scope was advanced into the duodenum, which was in the normal limits without any acute findings.

Following the EGD, the patient was able to be successfully extubated. Patient initially received intravenous antibiotics, which was switched to oral antibiotics, and was discharged home on oral antibiotics in 3 days.

3. Discussion

The foreign body impaction (FBI) is considering an emergent situation. FBI is defined as the presence of any object, material, or food that gets trapped in the upper gastrointestinal tract, usually swallowed by accident or in some cases, intentionally. Some data reports that around 100,000 of FBI occur each year in the United States of America [9]. This event can lead to high morbidity and mortality [10]. It is estimated that between 1,500 and 1,600 patients die yearly due to FBI and esophageal perforation being the most dreaded complication [11].

We presented a case of a FBI in a 25-year-old adult. Although children's are the ones most commonly affected (specially between 6 and 72 months of age), [6, 10–12], our patient with history of mental retardation made him a high-risk person for FBI. In addition, other factors for adults include gastrointestinal alterations [9, 12, 13], psychiatric disorders, alcohol/drug intoxication, being edentulous elderly, baseline dementia, or altered mental status [8, 11].

Numerous objects and food can get impacted in the upper gastrointestinal tract [6, 10, 11, 14]. In our case a piece of chicken was swallowed. The literature reveals that in adults FBI with food occurs more frequently, especially meat products, fish, or chicken bones [15]. Among the pediatric population, coins and small batteries are the most common objects [6, 14].

Majority of the FBIs do not need any kind of intervention or treatment, data reports that around 80 and 90% of the FBIs will pass from the esophagus to the stomach without any intervention, the remaining 10–20% will need endoscopic intervention, and 1% of the FBIs cases will require surgical intervention [6, 8, 10, 14, 15]. In our case the need of endoscopic intervention was needed as it compromised the airway by extrinsic pressure on the membranous wall of the trachea, leading to the tracheal collapse. The clinical presentation as seen in our patient causing airway compromise is seen in 10% of the cases [16]. In some cases, patients with FBI may be asymptomatic, to be diagnosed later on during imaging studies or examination as an incidental finding. In other circumstances, patient presents with array of symptoms (see Table 1) [11, 14, 16].

In most cases making an accurate diagnosis is simple, as patient presents with the history or has been witnessed, and other times it can be complex, especially in case of very

TABLE 1: Clinical manifestation of foreign body impaction.

System	Symptoms
Gastrointestinal	(i) Abdominal pain
	(ii) Dysphagia
	(iii) Halitosis
	(iv) Hematemesis
	(v) Nausea
	(vi) Odynophagia
	(vii) Regurgitation
	(viii) Vomiting
Respiratory	(i) Cough
	(ii) Drooling
	(iii) Dyspnea
	(iv) Stridor
	(v) Wheezing

small children or adult with dementia or mental retardation that may not be able to provide adequate history. In our case, the information presented was provided by the family members of our patient and a choking episode with the chicken piece was witnessed. When ingestion of a foreign body is suspected, either by symptoms, when present, or by clinical history imaging studies with X-ray of neck, chest, and abdomen may help in diagnosis [17]. We performed an X-ray with lateral view of the neck and no radiopaque foreign body was seen in the pharyngeal or laryngeal region, as literature suggests [18, 19]. In the event of the negative X-ray and patient with a high index of suspicion for FBI, we performed a chest computerized tomography as our next step for diagnosis, which reported the presence of a mass posterior to the trachea, as mentioned above.

In any case of FBI the first line of treatment is to protect the airway [8]. Our patient presented with symptoms of respiratory distress and was intubated. The management used in our case was the flexible video endoscopic removal of the foreign body. The flexible endoscopy which is readily available and can be done at the bedside was the first choice. Though rigid scope can be used instead or in the cases when flexible scope fails to remove the FBI [14]. Minor complications have been reported in literature when endoscopic methods are performed [19]. The chicken piece in our patient was successfully removed with a flexible endoscope and patient then was successfully extubated and discharged home. Regardless of the methodology used after removal of the foreign body, follow-up imaging studies need to be done to ensure complete removal and rule out any complication.

FBI, though having a low complication rate, error in diagnosis or the delay in the management of these situations can lead to very critical and life treating situations. The most severe of them is perforation of the esophageal wall, which can lead to mediastinitis, abscess, fistula formation, empyema, sepsis, and death [11, 13, 15, 20–22]. Other life treating complications are airway compromise as occurred in our patient, which was treated initially by endotracheal intubation and later endoscopic removal of the FBI. Other complications from FBI are direct damage to the esophageal wall and migration of foreign body to trachea or mediastinum [6, 18].

4. Conclusions

Foreign bodies trapped in the upper gastrointestinal tract are a serious condition that can be fatal if not managed correctly. Accurate diagnosis and urgent treatment decrease the complications risk. Although majority of these events resolve spontaneously by themselves, some do require intervention. Endoscopic treatment remains as the standard for extracting foreign body impaction. Physicians need to perform adequate history and if unavailable or in doubt imaging studies need to be done to identify the FBI and site of impaction.

Competing Interests

The authors declare that there are no competing interests.

References

[1] K. H. Hong, Y. J. Kim, J. H. Kim, S. W. Chun, H. M. Kim, and J. H. Cho, "Risk factors for complications associated with upper gastrointestinal foreign bodies," *World Journal of Gastroenterology*, vol. 21, no. 26, pp. 8125–8131, 2015.

[2] M. H. Emara, E. M. Darwiesh, M. M. Refaey, and S. M. Galal, "Endoscopic removal of foreign bodies from the upper gastrointestinal tract: 5-year experience," *Clinical and Experimental Gastroenterology*, vol. 7, no. 1, pp. 249–253, 2014.

[3] P. Heger, T. F. Weber, J. Rehm, A. Pathil, F. Decker, and P. Schemmer, "Cervical esophagotomy for foreign body extraction—case report and comprehensive review of the literature," *Annals of Medicine and Surgery*, vol. 7, pp. 87–91, 2016.

[4] S. O. Ikenberry, T. L. Jue, M. A. Anderson et al., "Management of ingested foreign bodies and food impactions," *Gastrointestinal Endoscopy*, vol. 73, no. 6, pp. 1085–1091, 2011.

[5] A. Burgos, L. Rabago, and P. Triana, "Western view of the management of gastroesophageal foreign bodies," *World Journal of Gastrointestinal Endoscopy*, vol. 8, no. 9, pp. 378–384, 2016.

[6] F. I. Wahid, H. U. Rehman, and I. A. Khan, "Management of foreign bodies of upper digestive tract," *Indian Journal of Otolaryngology and Head and Neck Surgery*, vol. 66, no. 1, pp. 203–206, 2014.

[7] M. Birk, P. Bauerfeind, P. H. Deprez et al., "Removal of foreing bodies on the upper gastrointestinal tract in adults: European society of gastrointestinal endoscopy (ESGE) clinical guideline," *Endoscopy*, vol. 48, pp. 1–8, 2016.

[8] C.-W. Hung, S.-C. Hung, C. J. Lee, W.-H. Lee, and K. H. Wu, "Risk factors for complications after a foreign body is retained in the esophagus," *The Journal of Emergency Medicine*, vol. 43, no. 3, pp. 423–427, 2012.

[9] R. E. Kramer, D. G. Lerner, T. Lin et al., "Management of ingested foreign bodies in children: a clinical report of the NASPGHAN endoscopy committee," *Journal of Pediatric Gastroenterology and Nutrition*, vol. 60, no. 4, pp. 562–574, 2015.

[10] D. Antoniou and G. Christopoulos-Geroulanos, "Management of foreign body ingestion and food bolus impaction in children: a retrospective analysis of 675 cases," *Turkish Journal of Pediatrics*, vol. 53, no. 4, pp. 381–387, 2011.

[11] B. Erbil, M. A. Karaca, M. A. Aslaner et al., "Emergency admissions due to swallowed foreign bodies in adults," *World Journal of Gastroenterology*, vol. 19, no. 38, pp. 6447–6452, 2013.

[12] S. L. W. Sperry, S. D. Crockett, C. B. Miller, N. J. Shaheen, and E. S. Dellon, "Esophageal foreign-body impactions: epidemiology,

time trends, and the impact of the increasing prevalence of eosinophilic esophagitis," *Gastrointestinal Endoscopy*, vol. 74, no. 5, pp. 985–991, 2011.

[13] S. A. Jafari, M. Khalesi, S. Partovi, M. A. Kiani, H. Ahanchian, and H. R. Kianifar, "Ingested foreign bodies removed by lexible endoscopy in pediatric patients: a 10-year retrospective study," *Iranian Journal of Otorhinolaryngology*, vol. 26, no. 76, pp. 175–179, 2014.

[14] S. Dereci, T. Koca, F. Serdaroğlu, and M. Akçam, "Foreign body ingestion in children," *Türk Pediatri Arşivi*, vol. 50, no. 4, pp. 234–240, 2015.

[15] S. Umihanic, F. Brick, and S. Hodzic, "Foreign body impaction in esophagus: experiences at Ear-Nose-Throat Clinic in Tuzla, 2003–2013," *Journal of Ear, Nose and Throat*, vol. 25, no. 4, pp. 214–218, 2015.

[16] T. O. Abbas, N. A. Shahwani, and M. Ali, "Endoscopic management of ingested foreign bodies in children: a retrospective review of cases, and review of the literature," *Open Journal of Pediatrics*, vol. 3, no. 4, pp. 428–435, 2013.

[17] A. Sanei-Moghaddam, A. Sanei-Moghaddam, and S. Kahrobaei, "Lateral soft tissue X-ray for patients with suspected fishbone in oropharynx, a thing in the past," *Iranian Journal of Otorhinolaryngology*, vol. 27, no. 83, pp. 459–462, 2015.

[18] H.-H. Chen, L.-X. Ruan, S.-H. Zhou, and S.-Q. Wang, "The utility of repeated computed tomography to track a foreign body penetrating the esophagus to the level of the thyroid gland," *Oral Radiology*, vol. 30, pp. 196–202, 2014.

[19] C.-C. Yao, I.-T. Wu, L.-S. Lu et al., "Endoscopic management of foreign bodies in the upper gastrointestinal tract of adults," *BioMed Research International*, vol. 2015, Article ID 658602, 6 pages, 2015.

[20] M. Shafique, S. Yaqub, E. S. Lie, V. Dahl, F. Olsbø, and O. Røkke, "New and safe treatment of food impacted in the esophagus: a single center experience of 100 consecutive cases," *Gastroenterology Research and Practice*, vol. 2013, Article ID 142703, 4 pages, 2013.

[21] C.-C. Tseng, T.-Y. Hsiao, and W.-C. Hsu, "Comparison of rigid and flexible endoscopy for removing esophageal foreign bodies in an emergency," *Journal of the Formosan Medical Association*, vol. 115, no. 8, pp. 639–644, 2016.

[22] D. Shreshtha, K. Sikka, C. A. Singh, and A. Thakar, "Foreign body esophagus: when endoscopic removal fails," *Indian Journal of Otolaryngology and Head & Neck Surgery*, vol. 65, no. 4, pp. 380–382, 2013.

37

Postpartum Tuberculosis: A Diagnostic and Therapeutic Challenge

Vijay Kodadhala,[1] Alemeshet Gudeta,[1] Aklilu Zerihun,[1] Odene Lewis,[2] Sohail Ahmed,[3] Jhansi Gajjala,[3] and Alicia Thomas[2]

[1]*Department of Internal Medicine, Howard University Hospital, 2041 Georgia Avenue NW, Washington, DC 20060, USA*
[2]*Division of Pulmonary Medicine, Howard University Hospital, 2041 Georgia Avenue NW, Washington, DC 20060, USA*
[3]*Division of Infectious Diseases, Howard University Hospital, 2041 Georgia Avenue NW, Washington, DC 20060, USA*

Correspondence should be addressed to Vijay Kodadhala; vkodadhala@gmail.com

Academic Editor: Tun-Chieh Chen

Tuberculosis (TB) infection in pregnant women and newborn babies is always challenging. Appropriate treatment is pivotal to curtail morbidity and mortality. TB diagnosis or exposure to active TB can be emotionally distressing to the mother. Circumstances can become more challenging for the physician if the mother's TB status is unclear. Effective management of TB during pregnancy and the postpartum period requires a multidisciplinary approach including pulmonologist, obstetrician, neonatologist, infectious disease specialist, and TB public health department. Current guidelines recommend primary Isoniazid prophylaxis in TB exposed pregnant women who are immune-suppressed and have chronic medical conditions or obstetric risk factors and close and sustained contact with a patient with infectious TB. Treatment during pregnancy is the same as for the general adult population. Infants born to mothers with active TB at delivery should undergo a complete diagnostic evaluation. Primary Isoniazid prophylaxis for at least twelve weeks is recommended for those with negative diagnostic tests and no evidence of disease. Repeated negative diagnostic tests are mandatory before interrupting prophylaxis. Separation of mother and infant is only necessary when the mother has received treatment for less than 2 weeks, is sputum smear-positive, or has drug-resistant TB. This case highlights important aspects for management of TB during the postpartum period which has a higher morbidity. We present a case of a young mother migrating from a developing nation to the USA, who was found to have a positive quantiFERON test associated with multiple cavitary lung lesions and gave birth to a healthy baby.

1. Introduction

Tuberculosis is a widespread, infectious disease caused by various strains of mycobacteria, usually *Mycobacterium tuberculosis*. It is an airborne infection. When patients do not have symptoms, it is known as latent tuberculosis. About ten percent of latent infections eventually progresses to active disease which, if left untreated, kills more than fifty percent of those infected [1]. Worldwide, the burden of TB disease in pregnant women is substantial. In 2011, it was estimated that more than 200,000 cases of active tuberculosis occurred among pregnant women globally; the greatest burdens were in Africa and Southeast Asia [2]. Prenatal care presents a unique opportunity for evaluation and management of latent and active tuberculosis in pregnant women. Individuals with

an increased risk of tuberculosis may seek medical care only during pregnancy such as our patient. Since pregnancy has not been shown to increase the risk of TB, the epidemiology of TB in pregnancy is a reflection of the general incidence of disease [3].

2. Case Presentation

A 31-year-old woman from Columbia with medical history significant for Gestational Diabetes presented to the labor ward without prior prenatal care. She came to the United States eight months prior to presentation. She received cesarean section for fetal distress and gave birth to a healthy baby. Her medical history was negative for cough, shortness

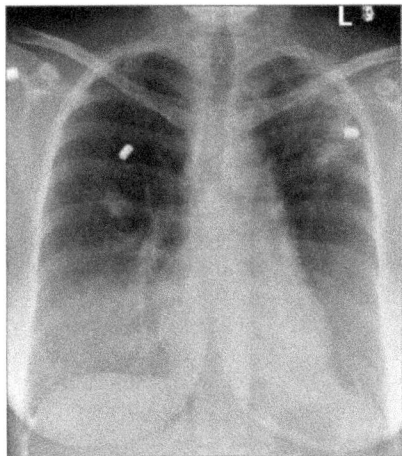

FIGURE 1: Chest X-ray. Increased density over the left upper lung and right middle lobe suspicious for infiltrate/fibrotic change.

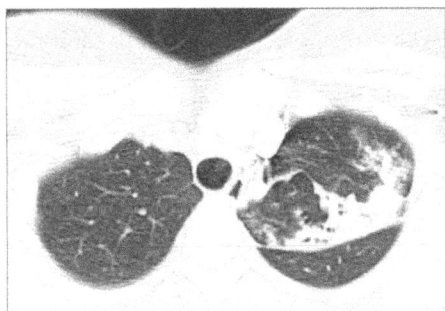

FIGURE 2: CT chest, noncontrast. Multiple cavitary lesions in left upper lobe.

of breath, fever, night sweating or loss of appetite, incarceration or living in institution, and any contact with TB patient or chronically coughing person. She was never diagnosed with active or latent TB. At the time of presentation patient was not actively coughing. Patient did not remember if she received BCG vaccination as a child or not.

Physical examination revealed young healthy looking female patient without any cardiopulmonary distress. Examination was negative for lymphadenopathy; chest was symmetrical, resonant to percussion, clear to auscultation bilaterally. Examination of other systems was within normal limits. BCG vaccination scar was not noted on either of the both upper arms.

The patient's perioperative chest X-ray (Figure 1) showed a small irregular density in the right middle lung and there was a hazy increased density over the left upper lung, which was suspicious for infiltrates versus fibrotic changes. Lucency was also noted within the left upper lobe, which was suspicious for cavitary change and further evaluation with CT was recommended for possible pulmonary tuberculosis. Noncontrast CT (Figure 2) showed patchy and nodular opacity in the apical posterior segment of the left upper lobe and to a lesser extent in the superior segment of the right lower lobe and right lung base as well as a small axillary

node. The differential diagnosis would include mycobacterial infection and pyogenic pneumonia. In light of positive chest X-ray and chest CT scan, TB quantiFERON gold test was requested. All other lab tests including tests for hepatitis B surface antigen, HCV, HIV, work-up for collagen vascular diseases, and sarcoidosis were negative.

QuantiFERON TB gold test was positive. To address further plan of management following the positive quantiF-ERON TB test, a multidisciplinary approach, which included pulmonary diseases specialist, infectious diseases specialist, obstetrician, and pediatrician, was undertaken to address the following areas of concern: (1) isolation of baby from mother, (2) isolation of baby from other babies in nursery, (3) initiating LTBI (latent TB infection) treatment in baby, and (4) initiating four-drug TB regimen in the mother. The panel agreed to respiratory isolation, obtaining three sputum samples for AFB smears, bronchoalveolar lavage (BAL) for mother, starting mother on four-drug anti-TB regimen and the baby on LTBI treatment, while keeping the mother and baby together.

Three induced sputum samples were obtained and were stained for Acid Fast Bacilli (AFB) which did not reveal any Acid Fast Bacilli. Patient initially refused bronchoscopy procedure, but after explaining to her the significance of the procedure, she consented for bronchoscopy. She received bronchoscopy (Figure 3) with biopsy and BAL. Bronchoscopy revealed hyperemic and friable bronchial tree mucosa. BAL was done from both left and right side and biopsy was taken from left upper lobe. Lab data are summarized in Table 1. Biopsy from left upper lobe showed predominantly bronchial mucosa with chronic inflammation and fibrosis. Special stain for Acid Fast Bacilli (Fite Stain) and fungi (GMS stain) were negative. Immunostain for CD-68 highlights few macrophages. BAL from right lower lobe was negative for malignancy and no evidence for infectious organisms and showed lympho/histiocytic infiltrate (primarily histiocytes). Left upper lobe BAL was also negative for malignancy and showed lympho/histiocytic infiltrate.

Sputum and BAL sample analysis with Direct AFB probe and AFB culture was positive for AFB. Public health was notified and mother was continued on full course of TB treatment.

Baby was evaluated by neonatology team, PPD was performed, and it was negative and chest X ray was normal. As per multidisciplinary team plan, baby was started on INH prophylaxis for the possible latent TB infection while awaiting gastric aspirate TB work-up results. Mom and baby are allowed to be together.

2.1. Follow-Up. Patient and the baby were closely followed in pulmonary, infectious diseases, and pediatric clinics. Importance of medication compliance and adverse effects of medication were explained to the patient and she clearly understands the instructions. Two months after commencement of the treatment, patient and baby remained compliant with treatment regimen and did not experience any adverse effects of medications. Baby's growth chart was satisfactory. Patient expressed wish to travel back to her home country.

TABLE 1: Additional lab data.

Connective tissue disease work-up	Bronchial washing	ABG on room air	Summary of TB work-up
ACE level: 41 (9–67) U/L: normal ESR: 30 mm/hr CRP: 1.4 (normal < 0.8) Anti-CCP: normal ANCA: negative ANA: negative	Appearance: clear WBC: 8 RBC: 63 Poly: 7% Mesothelial cells: 6% Culture: normal flora Bronchial washing: AFB PCR was positive Culture was positive for mycobacterium tuberculosis Fungal stain: negative Mycobacterial PCR: positive Culture for bacteria: normal flora	FiO_2 : 0.21 pH: 7.5 $PaCO_2$: 30 PaO_2 : 106 SaO_2 : 99	*Sputum:* AFB stain (3x): negative AFB culture on broth culture: positive for AFB Mycobacterium TB complex identified by direct probe *Broncho alveolar lavage (BAL):* AFB stain: negative Mycobacterium tuberculosis complex identified by direct probe AFB culture on broth: positive for AFB

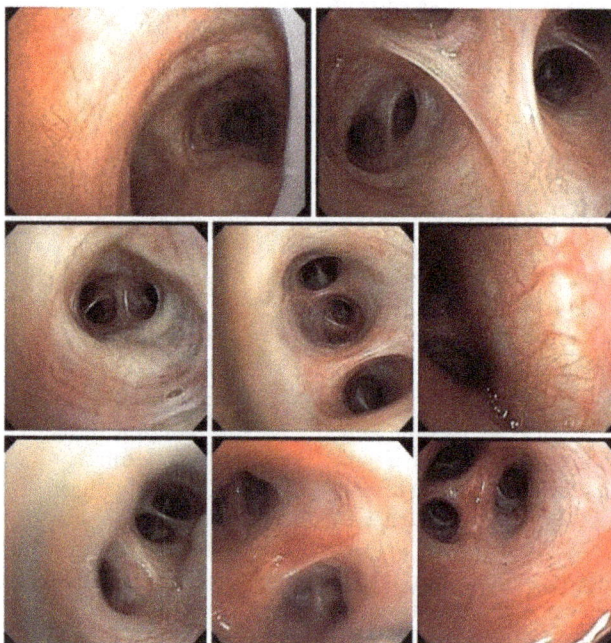

FIGURE 3: Bronchoscopy. Hyperemic and friable bronchial tree mucosa. BAL was done from both left and right side and biopsy was taken from left upper lobe.

We took the opportunity and once again clearly gave her the instructions about the need for regular doctor follow-up of both mother and the baby. Patient has good educational background and she promised to follow our instructions. Sadly, we lost contact with her after she left the USA. We sincerely hope that she followed our instructions and both mother and baby completed treatment and prophylaxis, respectively.

3. Discussion: Tuberculosis in Pregnancy

3.1. Introduction. More than 200,000 cases of TB occur among pregnant women globally. Pregnancy has no influence on pathogenesis, disease progression, and treatment response.

Pathophysiology

(i) Airborne Respiratory Droplets are inhaled and delivered to the terminal airways. Macrophages ingest the mycobacteria, which continue to multiply intracellularly and can potentially spread to other organs through the lymphatics and blood stream.

(ii) LTBI means new reactivity to the tuberculin skin test (or interferon-gamma release assay).

(iii) Progressive TB means primary progressive after initial infection, reactivation of LTBI.

3.2. Pathophysiology of TB. Inhalation of *Mycobacterium tuberculosis* results in one of the four possible outcomes: (1) immediate clearance of the organism, (2) latent infection, (3) the onset of active disease (primary infection), and (4) active disease many years later (reactivation of the disease).

In due course, approximately 10 percent of the infected individuals develop active disease, either primary or reactivation of LTBI. If the host defense mechanism is poor, mycobacteria proliferate within alveolar macrophages and destroy them, resulting in release of cytokines and chemokines. These in return attract other phagocytic cells including monocytes, other alveolar macrophages, and neutrophils resulting in nodular granulomatous structure formation and called the tubercle. Bacteria replication continues leading to lymph nodes involvement called primary TB, involvement of lung parenchyma along with lymph node involvement called Ghon's complex. Unchecked bacterial growth results in hematogenous spread results in disseminated TB (see Pathophysiology in Section 3.1).

3.3. Diagnosis and Treatment of Latent TB in Pregnancy. Routine testing for TB is not indicated but testing is indicated on patients who need prompt treatment such as immunosuppressed patients, because they are at high risk of progression to active TB. Testing for LTBI prior to pregnancy is preferred. If a patient receiving treatment gets pregnant, treatment should be continued. If there are no risks for progression of LTBI, wait three months postpartum to test and treat latent TB.

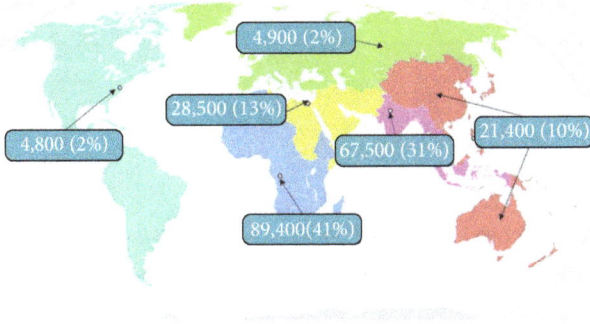

FIGURE 4: Epidemiology of active TB in pregnancy [2].

TABLE 2: American Thoracic Society, CDC, Infectious Disease Society of America recommendations [4].

Medications	Month 1 to month 2	Month 3 to month 9
Isoniazid	√	√
Rifampin	√	√
Ethambutol	√	

TABLE 3: Side effects of anti-TB medications in pregnancy [4].

Medications	Side effects
Isoniazid	Category C: possible increased risk of hepatitis/peripheral neuropathy
Rifampin	Category C: rare cases of fetal abnormalities and hemorrhagic disease
Ethambutol	Category B
Pyrazinamide	Category C: detail teratogenicity data are not available
Fluoroquinolones	Category C: causes arthropathies
Ethionamide	Category C: teratogenic in laboratory animals
Para-aminosalicylic acid	Category C: adverse effects are not certain
Cycloserine	Category C: adverse effects are not certain
Streptomycin	Category D: congenital deafness
Kanamycin/amikacin	Category D: similar side effect with streptomycin

Tools for diagnosis are tuberculin skin testing (TST) and interferon-gamma release assays (IGRAs). Both these tests can be safely performed in pregnancy and pregnancy does have any effect on the results. If the test results are positive further clinical evaluation including clinical features, radiological, microbiological, and immunological investigations should be performed to rule out active TB.

First choice of the treatment of latent TB is Isoniazid (INH) for nine-month duration with daily pyridoxine supplement. However in one of the following circumstances four-month treatment with Rifampin is indicated. (1) INH resistance, (2) intolerance to INH, and (3) poor medication compliance.

3.4. Active Tuberculosis in Pregnancy. Sugarman et al. estimated that 216 500 (95% uncertainty range 192 100–247 000) active tuberculosis cases existed in pregnant women globally in 2011. The greatest burdens were in the WHO African region with 89 400 cases and the WHO South East Asian region with 67 500 cases. Though active tuberculosis in pregnancy burden is concentrated in Africa and South East Asia, Sugarman et al.'s study reveals that active TB in pregnancy is seen worldwide in both developed and developing countries (Figure 4) [2].

3.5. Clinical Manifestation of TB in Pregnancy. Pregnant patients with active TB typically have the same clinical manifestations as nonpregnant patients which include fever, chest pain, fatigue, cough, weight loss, night sweat, and dyspnea. TB symptoms could be masked by physiological symptoms of pregnancy. Malaise and fatigue may be attributed to pregnancy and it is more difficult to recognize weight loss.

3.6. Diagnosis of TB in Pregnancy. The evaluation for active TB in pregnancy should be as in nonpregnancy which includes chest X ray (with appropriate protection of the fetus), sputum for AFB and TB PCR. Evaluation for extrapulmonary disease should be guided by clinical symptoms. Diagnosis of pregnancy should prompt the evaluation for HIV infection.

Transmission of TB from Mother to Newborn Infant. It can occur by vertical transmission (very rare) of TB by transplacental transmission through umbilical veins to the fetal liver and lungs or aspiration and swallowing of infected amniotic fluid in utero- or intrapartum causing primary infection of fetal lungs and gut. Transplacental infection occurs late in pregnancy and aspiration from amniotic fluid occurs in the perinatal period. In the postpartum period a horizontal spread by droplet from mother or undiagnosed family member is most commonly suggested. Transmission of tuberculosis through breast milk does not occur [5].

Effects of Active TB on Pregnant Women and Infants. They include premature birth, low birth weight, intrauterine growth retardation, perinatal death (sixfold risk increase).

3.7. Treatment of Active TB in Pregnancy. Treatment should be initiated if the suspicion of active disease is moderate to high such as persistent upper lobe infiltrate, cough in a high risk individual, and positive AFB smear/PCR as benefits of treatment overweight risks.

The initial treatment regimen should consist of Isoniazid, Rifampicin, and Ethambutol. Although all of these drugs cross the placenta, they do not appear to have teratogenic effects. Streptomycin is the only antituberculosis drug documented to have harmful effects on the human fetus (congenital deafness) and should not be used. Although detailed teratogenicity data are not available, PZA can probably be used safely during pregnancy and is recommended by the World Health Organization (WHO) and the International Union against Tuberculosis and Lung Disease (IUATLD)

TABLE 4: Control of transmission of TB in pregnancy [4].

Mother	Infant	
Active TB on treatment	Active TB on treatment	No separation
Active TB on treatment	Latent TB on treatment	No separation
Active TB on treatment	No active TB or latent TB	Infant should be treated for latent TB for 3 to 4 months until reevaluation
Known or suspected drug resistant TB	No active TB or latent TB	Should be separated until mother is noninfectious
Known or suspected active TB	Has not been evaluated	Should be separated until both have been fully evaluated

(Table 2) [5]. Ethambutol may be discontinued after one month if the results of drug sensitivity showed the organism is susceptible to Isoniazid and Rifampin. Pyrazinamide is not used routinely for pregnant women in the United States because of limited safety data but it is recommended by WHO.

3.8. Side Effects of Anti-TB Medications in Pregnancy. Drug interactions are common and need careful monitoring and appropriate action. It is near impossible to discuss all the adverse effects of anti-TB medications here. We will discuss major adverse effects of first-line anti-TB drugs and second line anti-TB medications (Table 3). *INH* adverse affects result anywhere from mild asymptomatic transaminitis to fatal hepatitis, peripheral neurotoxicity, and lupus like reaction. In pregnancy INH should be prescribed with pyridoxine supplementation. *Rifampin* adverse effects include skin reactions like pruritus, gastrointestinal reactions like nausea, anorexia, abdominal pain, flulike syndrome, hepatotoxicity, severe immunologic reactions like thrombocytopenia, hemolytic anemia, acute renal failure, and thrombotic thrombocytopenic purpura. *Ethambutol* can cause retrobulbar neuritis and peripheral neuritis. *Pyrazinamide* may result in hepatotoxicity, gastrointestinal symptoms, nongouty polyarthralgia, and asymptomatic hyperuricemia among others [4].

3.9. Follow-Up. Treatment can be administered by directly observed therapy (DOT) to improve adherence and to evaluate for drug toxicity. Expert in TB should be consulted for interruptions longer than two weeks or for sporadic adherence. Baseline liver enzymes and monthly liver enzymes should be obtained. Patient should be informed to call if any symptoms or signs of hepatitis occur.

3.10. Toxicity and Monitoring of Anti-TB Medications in Pregnancy. There is increased risk of hepatotoxicity in pregnancy and postpartum. So base line Liver Function Test (LFT) and then monthly LFTs are recommended. Other investigations like HIV, HBV, HCV are also recommended. Avoidance of alcohol use and hepatotoxins exposure is advised. Mild transaminitis should prompt more frequent monitoring. Stop medication in symptomatic patients with ALT greater than three times and asymptomatic patient with ALT greater than five times.

3.11. Breast Feeding in Patient with Active TB. Breastfeeding is not contraindicated if the mother is being treated for active tuberculosis or latent TB with first-line agents. The infant should receive pyridoxine if mother is receiving Isoniazid. Breast feeding is contraindicated if the mother is receiving rifabutin or fluoroquinolone.

3.12. Control of Transmission of TB in Pregnancy. Mother and baby bonding is very important and breast feeding plays significant role in providing immunity to baby in the first few months. So every safe measure should be undertaken to make sure that mother and baby are allowed to be together and if separation is inevitable (Table 4), clinicians have to make the best effort to make it as short as possible. Breast feeding should be continued. It is very important for clinicians to have knowledge about special situations like that of our case where mother was diagnosed with active TB and infant does not have active or latent TB, or as a matter of fact any one of the situations mentioned in Table 4. If mother has active TB and is on treatment and baby has one of the following conditions, either active TB or LTBI or no infection, standard of care therapy should be initiated for the baby and separation is not recommended. Mother should always wear mask until she is no longer infectious. In other situations both mother and baby should be fully evaluated before they are allowed to be together.

4. Conclusion

Diagnosing and treating active or latent TB in pregnancy and during postpartum period is very important as it affects both mother and baby. It can cause significant morbidity and mortality if not correctly diagnosed and treated adequately. Though our patient presented without any risk factors (except a positive travel history) and symptoms of TB, high index of suspicion lead to correct diagnosis and hence appropriate treatment.

Abbreviations

TB: Tuberculosis
BCG: Bacille Calmette-Guerin
CT: Computed tomography
HIV: Human immunodeficiency virus
HCV: Hepatitis C virus
HBV: Hepatitis B virus
LTBI: Latent TB infection
AFB: Acid Fast Bacillus
BAL: Bronchoalveolar Lavage

GMS: Grocott's Methenamine silver
CD: Cluster differentiation
PCR: Polymerase chain reaction
PPD: Purified protein derivative
INH: Isoniazid
ALT: Alanine transaminase
LFT: Liver Function Test
W.H.O: World Health Organization
IUATLD: International Union against Tuberculosis
          and Lung Disease.

Competing Interests

The authors declare that they have no conflict of interests.

Authors' Contributions

Vijay Kodadhala, M.D., Alemeshet Gudeta, M.D., and Aklilu Zerihun, M.D., contributed towards an extensive review of literature as well as paper drafting. Odene Lewis, M.D., and Sohail Ahmed, M.D., also made important contributions to this paper. Jhansi Gajjala, M.D., and Alicia Thomas, M.D., primarily managed the patient and overviewed the paper.

References

[1] WHO, "Tuberculosis," Fact Sheet 104, World Health Organization, 2010.

[2] J. Sugarman, C. Colvin, A. C. Moran, and O. Oxlade, "Tuberculosis in pregnancy: an estimate of the global burden of disease," *The Lancet Global Health*, vol. 2, no. 12, pp. e710–e716, 2014.

[3] G. Schaefer, I. A. Zervoudakis, F. F. Fuchs, and S. David, "Pregnancy and pulmonary tuberculosis," *Obstetrics & Gynecology*, vol. 46, no. 6, pp. 706–715, 1975.

[4] American Thoracic Society, CDC, and Infectious Diseases Society of America, "Treatment of tuberculosis," *Morbidity and Mortality Weekly Report*, vol. 52, no. 11, pp. 1–77, 2003.

[5] H. Mittal, S. Das, and M. M. A. Faridi, "Management of newborn infant born to mother suffering from tuberculosis: current recommendations & gaps in knowledge," *Indian Journal of Medical Research*, vol. 140, pp. 32–39, 2014.

38

A Rare Case of Metastatic Choriocarcinoma of Lung Origin

Parth Rali,[1] Jianwu Xie,[2] Grishma Rali,[3] Mayur Rali,[4] Jan Silverman,[2] and Khalid Malik[1]

[1]*Division of Pulmonary and Critical Care, Allegheny General Hospital, Pittsburgh, PA 15212, USA*
[2]*Division of Pathology, Allegheny General Hospital, Pittsburgh, PA 15212, USA*
[3]*Children's Hospital of Philadelphia, Philadelphia, PA, USA*
[4]*Hofstra Northwell School of Medicine, Department of Family Medicine, Southside Hospital, Bay Shore, NY, USA*

Correspondence should be addressed to Parth Rali; dr_parth_rali@yahoo.com

Academic Editor: Akif Turna

Choriocarcinoma is part of the spectrum of gestational trophoblastic disease that occurs in women of reproductive age. Although the most common metastatic site of choriocarcinoma is the lung, primary pulmonary choriocarcinoma is rare. To diagnose primary pulmonary choriocarcinoma, the patient should have no previous gynecologic malignancy, have elevated human chorionic gonadotropin, and have pathological confirmation of the disease excluding gonadal primary site of the tumor. Due to the paucity of data, there are no guidelines for treatment. Prognosis of this malignancy is extremely poor. We report a rare case of metastatic primary lung choriocarcinoma in a 69-year-old postmenopausal woman who was treated with combination of surgery, chemotherapy, and radiation. The patient had a good outcome and is doing well after 1-year follow-up.

1. Introduction

Choriocarcinoma is a germ cell tumor containing cells of trophoblastic origin. It is usually associated with gestational event like molar pregnancy and secretes human chorionic gonadotropin (b-hCG) [1]. Primary pulmonary choriocarcinoma (PPC) is a rare tumor that generally affects young individuals [2]. It is rarely reported in postmenopausal women [3]. PPC portends a very poor prognosis with a dismal 5-year survival rate of <5% [3]. We report a rare case of metastatic PPC in a 69-year-old postmenopausal woman.

2. Case

69-year-old-woman with history of hypertension, hyperlipidemia, and 50 pack-year smoking presented to our emergency room with 8 days of new onset dizziness, gait instability, and severe occipital headaches. Physical examination was positive for horizontal nystagmus to the right. CT scan of her head demonstrated a right sided inferior cerebellar lesion with minimal hemorrhage which was confirmed on the MRI of the brain (Figure 1). Patient was started on decadron and admitted to neurosurgical intensive care unit.

Patient underwent skull base suboccipital craniectomy with microscopic resection and debulking of the cerebellar mass. Follow-up CT head showed no residual tumor and patient had a complete clinical recovery.

Histologic examination of the brain metastasis was consistent with syncytiotrophoblastic cells. Immunohistochemical stains were positive for cytokeratin 5.2, AE1/AE3, EMA, and CK7 and strongly positive for beta-hCG supportive for choriocarcinoma differentiation (Figure 2). Metastatic workup which included CT chest, abdomen, and pelvis and PET scan showed a right upper lobe (RUL) mass (Figure 3). There was no evidence of any other metastatic disease. The serum b-hCG was elevated to 1668 mIU/ml (normal < 10 mIU/ml).

CT guided core needle biopsy of the RUL lung mass and touch imprint cytology demonstrated poorly differentiated malignant cells, including scattered multinucleated tumor giant cells. Immunohistochemical studies performed on the core biopsy demonstrated positive staining of the malignant cells for PLAP and beta-hCG. The malignant cells were negative for AFP, CD30, OCT 3/4, glypican-3, and CD-117 which supports the diagnosis of a poorly differentiated lung carcinoma with choriocarcinomatous differentiation. The

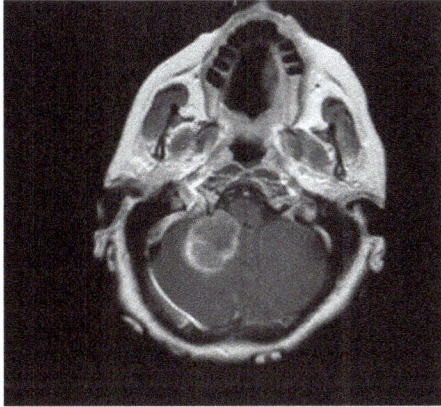

FIGURE 1: T1 weighted MRI of brain showing right cerebellar lesion.

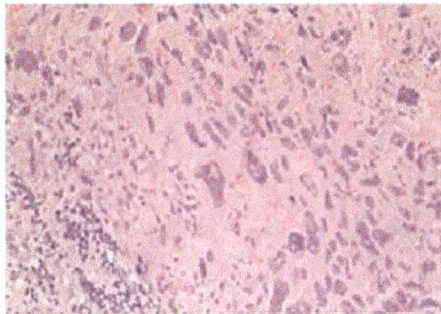

(a)

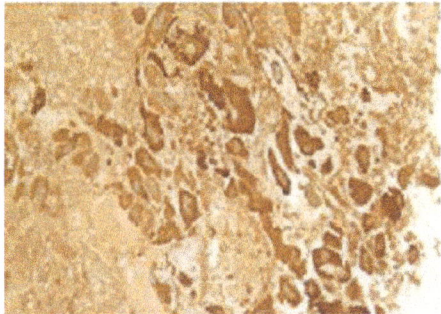

(b)

FIGURE 2: Brain biopsy. (a) Histologic examination of the biopsy reveals a sheet of syncytiotrophoblastic cells characterized by multi-lobulated to multinucleated and spindle shaped cells with a moderate amount of eosinophilic cytoplasm (H&E ×20). (b) Immunohistochemical stain for beta-hCG shows moderate to strong cytoplasmic staining of the syncytiotrophoblastic cells (×20).

negative staining for TTF-1, Napsin-A, CK 5/6, and p63 supports that the poorly differentiated malignancy is neither a conventional adenocarcinoma nor squamous cell carcinoma, respectively (Figure 4).

The patient had a follow-up normal pelvic examination, endometrial biopsy, and pelvic ultrasound. The patient refused to undergo lung resection of her tumor. She was treated with whole brain and lung mass radiation and 6 cycles of chemotherapy with carboplatin and etoposide. With

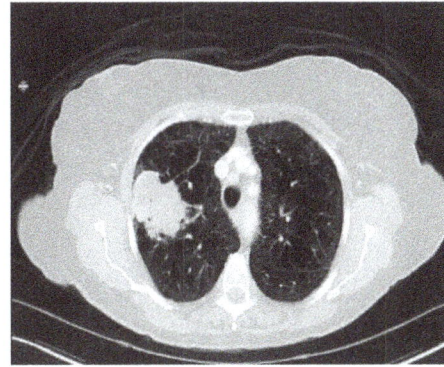

FIGURE 3: CT chest showing right upper lobe mass with emphysema.

chemoradiation, her b-hCG level continued to decrease. She had persistence of the right upper lobe mass without any evidence of metastatic disease on subsequent follow-up imaging. Long-term plans are close clinical follow-up with serial b-hCG and imaging.

3. Discussion

Choriocarcinoma is a malignant proliferation of trophoblastic cells. The histological pattern is characterized by sheets of cytotrophoblasts and syncytiotrophoblast without chorionic villi [4]. Choriocarcinoma is part of the spectrum of gestational trophoblastic disease and it commonly occurs in women of reproductive age [4, 5].

Trophoblastic diseases have affinity for blood vessels and usually metastasize hematogenously [5]. The most common metastatic site is the lung (80%) and the occurrence of respiratory failure requiring intubation is an independent factor for poor outcome. Metastasis to the brain occurs in 10% of patients and virtually all patients with cerebral involvement have a simultaneous pulmonary involvement [4].

Primary lung carcinoma with trophoblastic differentiation is rare. Although cases of PPC have been reported as early as 1950s [6, 7], there are at least 34 cases reported including this case [8], although the exact number of cases is uncertain since similar cases may have been reported with different names.

The diagnostic criteria proposed include [1] no previous gynecologic malignancy, solitary or predominant lung lesion with the exclusion of a gonadal primary site, elevated b-hCG titers that normalize after surgery or chemotherapy, and pathologic confirmation of the disease

The major differential diagnosis is giant cell carcinoma of lung, since both malignancies are composed of a dimorphic population of polygonal mononucleated and pleomorphic, multinucleated giant cells. Some authors considered that the presence of predominant tumor multinucleated giant cells in tumor tissue as a diagnostic feature for a primary lung choriocarcinoma and sheets of polygonal mononucleated tumor cells with scattered giant cells as a feature of giant cell carcinoma of lung [9]. By immunohistochemical stain, the giant cells in primary lung choriocarcinoma show very strong positive staining of b-HCG, as seen in our case [9]. However,

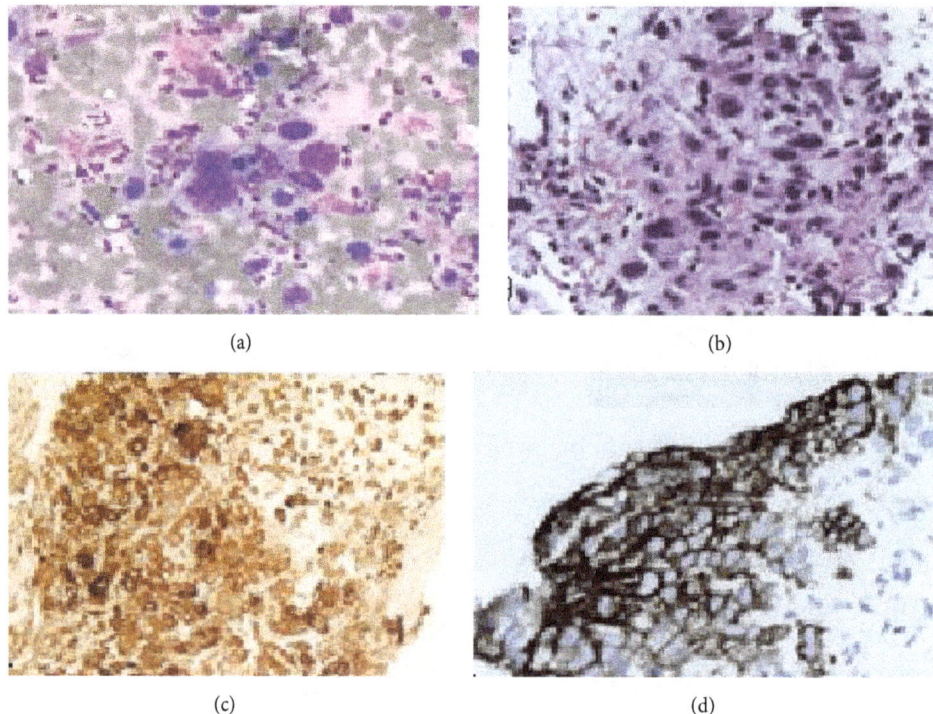

FIGURE 4: RUL mass biopsy. (a) Touch imprint cytology from core needle biopsy demonstrates bizarre, pleomorphic cells arranged in a dissociative fashion. Some of the tumor cells are multilobulated to multinucleated with pleomorphic, hyperchromatic nuclei (Diff-Quik stain ×20). (b) Core needle biopsy reveals bizarre syncytiotrophoblasts characterized by pleomorphic cells, including some that are multilobulated to multinucleated. The cells have a moderate amount of surrounding eosinophilic cytoplasm. Extensive necrosis is noted in the cores (H&E ×20). (c) Immunohistochemical stain for beta-hCG shows intense strong positive cytoplasmic staining (×40). (d) Strong diffuse positive cytoplasmic and membranous staining for PLAP (×40).

the possibility of a mix germ cell tumor cannot be totally excluded based on the lung biopsy, but no other germ cell components were seen in the resected brain metastasis.

The understanding of the cell origin and pathogenesis of primary lung choriocarcinoma is limited, though multiple theories exist [9]. The first popular theory is that it arises from an ectopic primordial germ cell in the lung during the embryonic development. The second theory is that the primary lung choriocarcinoma is a high-grade transformation from a nontrophoblastic lung tumor. The third theory is that the primary lung choriocarcinoma and giant cell carcinoma of lung are the same entity. Although all these theories are reasonable, molecular studies might prove useful to better define the histogenesis of this rare malignancy.

In our case, a negative CT scan of the abdomen and pelvis, cervical cytology, and endometrial biopsy ruled out gynecologic origin of the tumor. The patient's age and clinical presentation also make it unlikely to be from the gynecological tract. Serum b-hCG titer decreased to value of 98 mIU/mL after a one-year follow-up.

Due to paucity of data, there is no guideline for treatment of PPC. Different treatment modalities have been used with varying success. Surgery alone or with chemo and radiation therapy seems to have a better outcome [9, 10].

In our patient, chemotherapy regimen included etoposide and carboplatin. Etoposide served as the primary agent to induce remission in chorionic tumors [4]. Chemotherapy

regimen with etoposide and platinum has been associated with good result. The patients were alive on 1-year follow-up just like our patient [1, 2]; however, the prognosis of PPC remains very poor with a <5% of patients surviving after 5 years [3].

Authors' Contributions

The authors have participated in preparation of this manuscript equally.

References

[1] V. Di Crescenzo, P. Laperuta, F. Napolitano, C. Carlomagno, A. Garzi, and M. Vitale, "An unusual case of primary choriocarcinoma of the lung," *BMC Surgery*, vol. 13, no. 2, article no. S33, 2013.

[2] U. B. M. Kinni, "Primary pulmonary choriocarcinoma: Is it still an enigma," *Indian Journal of Chest Diseases and Allied Sciences*, vol. 47, pp. 216–226, 2007.

[3] J. Serno, F. Zeppernick, J. Jäkel et al., "Primary pulmonary choriocarcinoma: Case report and review of the literature," *Gynecologic and Obstetric Investigation*, vol. 74, no. 2, pp. 171–176, 2012.

[4] R. S. Berkowitz and D. P. Goldstein, "Chorionic tumors," *The New England Journal of Medicine*, vol. 335, no. 23, pp. 1740–1798, 1996.

[5] X. M. Li, X. Y. Liu, and Z. X. Liu, "Choriocarcinoma with multiple lung, skull and skin metastases in a postmenopausal female: A case report," *Oncology Letters*, vol. 10, no. 6, pp. 3837–3839, 2015.

[6] G. Brouet, J. Chretien, J. Marche, and G. Roussel, "Apparently primary pulmonary choriocarcinoma in pregnancy," *Journal français de médecine et chirurgie thoraciques*, vol. 13, no. 2, pp. 211–222, 1959.

[7] M. Schulz, A. Hernandez, and F. Rebora, "Primary choriocarcinoma of the lung; Case report," *Rev Mex Tuberc Enferm Apar Respir*, vol. 17, no. 4, pp. 314–322, 1956.

[8] Y. Ikura, T. Inoue, H. Tsukuda, T. Yamamoto, M. Ueda, and Y. Kobayashi, "Primary choriocarcinoma and human chorionic gonadotrophin-producing giant cell carcinoma of the lung: Are they independent entities?" *Histopathology*, vol. 36, no. 1, pp. 17–25, 2000.

[9] S. Kamata, A. Sakurada, N. Sato, M. Noda, and Y. Okada, "A case of primary pulmonary choriocarcinoma successfully treated by surgery," *General Thoracic and Cardiovascular Surgery*, vol. 65, no. 6, pp. 361–364, 2016.

[10] P. Vaideeswar, J. Mehta, and J. Deshpande, "Primary pulmonary choriocarcinoma - A series of 7 cases," *Indian Journal of Pathology and Microbiology*, vol. 47, no. 4, pp. 494–496, 2004.

39

Primary Pleuropulmonary Synovial Sarcoma

Fatima Zahra Mrabet ⓘ,[1,2] **Hafsa El Ouazzani,**[2,3] **Leila El Akkari,**[1,2] **Sanaa Hammi,**[1,2] **Jamal Eddine Bourkadi,**[1,2] **and Fouad Zouaidia**[2,3]

[1]*Department of Pneumology, Moulay Youssef University Hospital Center, Rabat, Morocco*
[2]*Faculty of Medicine and Pharmacy, Mohammed V University, Rabat, Morocco*
[3]*Department of Pathology, Ibn Sina University Hospital Center, Rabat, Morocco*

Correspondence should be addressed to Fatima Zahra Mrabet; mrabetfatimazahra@gmail.com

Academic Editor: Akif Turna

Primary pleuropulmonary synovial sarcoma is extremely rare. The diagnosis can only be made after having eliminated an extrapleuropulmonary localization in the past and at the time of diagnosis. Our presentation is about a 40-year-old woman having a cough and dyspnea since three weeks ago; imaging had showed a left pleurisy with pleuropulmonary process. Histological study of the biopsy confirmed the diagnosis of pleuropulmonary synovial sarcoma. PET-SCAN had not identified any extrathoracic localization. This tumor is known for its aggressive nature and high risk of metastasis. Its primitive character is retained following a diagnostic procedure of exclusion. Surgical treatment remains the best therapeutic tool when it is technically feasible; otherwise the prognosis is often unfortunate. In this paper, we report a case of primary pleuropulmonary synovial sarcoma. Through this case, we present a rare disease that is often difficult to diagnose.

1. Introduction

Synovial sarcoma is a rare soft tissue sarcoma accounting for 8% of all soft tissue tumors in the body. It is not originating from the synovial tissue, but is arising from pluripotent mesenchymal tissue. In lung, metastatic synovial sarcoma from extremities is the most common in pulmonary parenchyma and pleura [1].

Primary pleuropulmonary synovial sarcoma is a very rare, but highly aggressive, malignant neoplasm. It must be differentiated from other spindle cell tumors that have similar morphological features through the immunohistochemical study [2].

2. Case Report

Mrs. M. K. a 40-year-old woman, with no notable pathological history, just gave birth a month ago; she has had left chest pain, dry cough, and stage III of mMRC dyspnea evolving, since three weeks ago before her admission, in a context of deterioration of the general state. Clinical examination revealed a left fluid effusion syndrome. The posteroanterior chest roentgenogram showed a homogeneous opacity occupying the totality of left thoracic field with the presence of signs of mediastinal discharge in the right side (Figure 1). An evacuation of the pleurisy was performed repeatedly to relieve the patient (about 2 liters every 3 days).

Thoracic ultrasonography confirmed the presence of pleurisy of high abundance and guided the pleural biopsy returned inconclusive. The thoracic CT showed a mediastino pulmonary process localized at the left lobe superior measuring 104 * 102 * 141 mm comes in contact with the artery under Clavier and the left lateral edge of the aorta and surrounded the left branch of the pulmonary artery which stayed permeably associated with pleurisy ipsilateral of high abundance (Figure 2). Bronchial fibroscopy showed a bud in the left upper lobe bronchus with thickening of its spurs, but the histological study was not contributive twice.

Transthoracic biopsy of the pulmonary tumor process was performed (guided by CT) by using the biopsy needle Gelman type (18 G 11 cm). It is concluded from grade II synovial sarcoma of the FNCLCC at the histological study

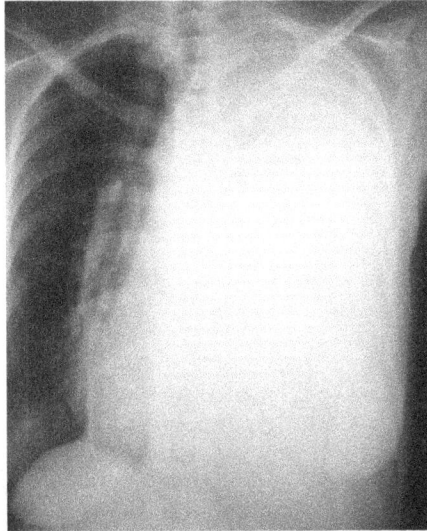

FIGURE 1: Posteroanterior chest roentgenogram showing a homogeneous opacity taking the whole hemi thoracic left field and pushing the mediastinum towards the contralateral side.

of the fragments. The tumor showed spindle-shaped cells forming sheets. The spindle cells are of uniform appearance with oval, dark-staining nuclei and scanty amount of indistinct cytoplasm (Figure 3). On immunohistochemical study, tumor cells were positive for EMA and CD 99. They were negative Cytokeratin AE1/AE3, Desmin, PS 100, and CD34 (Figure 4).

The extension assessment did not show extrathoracic localization, especially a PET SCAN, which did not show extrathoracic hypermetabolism, particularly in the soft tissues, which is, a priori, a fundamental element of the primitive character of the tumor. Unfortunately we could not perform chromosomal studies on this patient; we lack the molecular platform in our instruction because we belong to a low-income country. We retained the diagnosis after eliminating the differential diagnosis.

After the confirmation of the diagnosis, the patient was referred to the oncology center for chemotherapy and died the day after her first cure of treatment.

3. Discussion

Synovial sarcoma is a rare tumor of the young adult. It is located in 90% of the cases in the para-articular regions and in 10% of the cases in various anatomical sites not related to the synovial tissue [3].

Primary pulmonary sarcomas are very rare and comprise only 0.5% of all primary lung malignancies with only a few case reports in the literature. Primary pleuropulmonary and mediastinal synovial sarcomas are more aggressive than soft tissue synovial sarcomas with rare distant metastasis. The diagnosis of primary pleuropulmonary synovial sarcoma (PPSS) requires a combination of clinical, radiological, pathological, and immunohistochemical investigations to exclude alternative primary tumours and metastatic sarcoma [4].

The average age of onset for pleuropulmonary location is 38.5 years. It is not related to cigarette smoking. It affects both sexes with similar incidence on the right and left lungs [4, 5].

Our patient is a nonsmoking woman, and she is 40 years old.

The origin tissue of synovial sarcomas is not well defined; it appears that they develop from a pluripotent mesenchymal cell with synovial differentiation [6]. The term "pleuropulmonary" was first recommended by Essary and colleagues to describe the anatomic subset of primary synovial sarcomas originating from either the lung or the pleura due to inherent difficulties in assigning a precise anatomic origin in most cases. There has been no large series documenting the exact number of repeated pleuropulmonary synovial sarcoma cases worldwide. Ipsilateral pleural effusion was reported, while mediastinal lymphadenopathy was rare [7]. Our patient presented pulmonary and pleural localization at the same time; the presence of an endobronchial bud at bronchial fibroscopy is more in favor of a pulmonary primitive; otherwise double simultaneous localization at the same density at thoracic CT makes it difficult to decide. As described in the literature, the chest CT scan did not show the presence of lymphadenopathy in our presentation, and the pleural location is ipsilateral with respect to pulmonary localization.

The symptomatology as well as the imaging is not characterized by specific sign directing towards a synovial sarcoma. The clinical and radiological data are that of a pleuropulmonary tumor process without histological specificity. So far, four cases of PPSS presenting during pregnancy have been reported [2]. Our patient also had a nonspecific clinical and paraclinical presentation occurring at her first month of postpartum.

Radiologically, compared with soft tissue synovial sarcoma, primary pulmonary and mediastinal synovial sarcoma show less vascularity and a similar "triple sign" (bright, dark, and gray) representing tumor, hemorrhage, and necrosis on magnetic resonance imaging. The presence of significant adenopathy, however, argues against PPSS [8].

The seat is preferentially peripheral but some cases are described at the level of the bronchial tree. The localization of the tumor process in our patient was mediastino-pulmonary with presence of a bud at the level of the lobar bronchus superior to fibroscopy.

Histologically, there are four histologic subtypes: biphasic, monophasic (spindle), monophasic epithelial, and poorly differentiated (round cell) tumors. The most commonly observed subtype is monophasic, and the biphasic subtype is easily diagnosed on the basis of the presence of both epithelial and spindle cells. However, the monophasic subtype can be misdiagnosed as other types of sarcoma [9]. Our patient had a monophasic fusiform subtype at the biopsy.

In the presence of malignant tumor proliferation of spindle-cell sarcomatous aspects, a carcinomatous component should always be sought to eliminate the diagnosis of sarcomatoid carcinoma. Once the pure character of sarcomatous proliferation is established, the possibility of a sarcomatoid carcinoma, which, unlike synovial sarcoma, is always rich in cytonuclear atypia, must be rejected at first sight. In addition, proliferating cells are intensely and

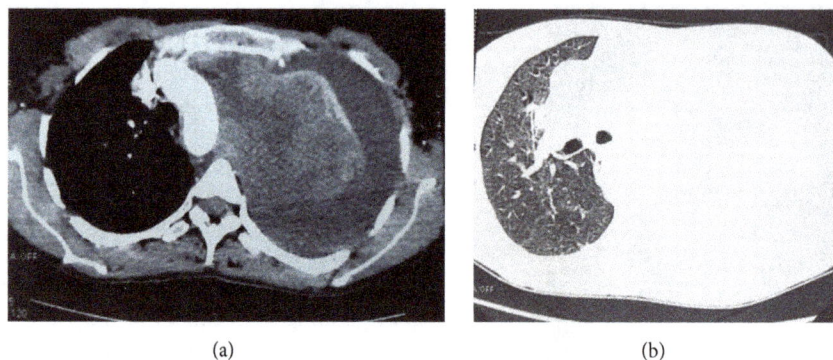

FIGURE 2: CT scan image showing a left mediastinal-pulmonary tumor process [(a) mediastinal window. (b) Parenchymal window].

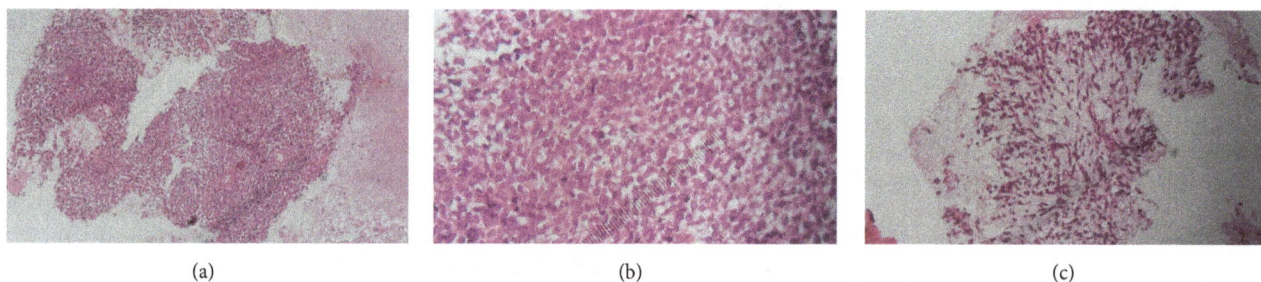

FIGURE 3: Histologically, (a) the tumor showed spindle-shaped cells forming sheets (Hematoxylin Eosin GX10), (b) the spindle cells are of uniform appearance with oval, dark-staining nuclei and scanty amount of indistinct cytoplasm (Hematoxylin Eosin GX20), and (c) we noted a myxoid pattern (Hematoxylin Eosin GX10).

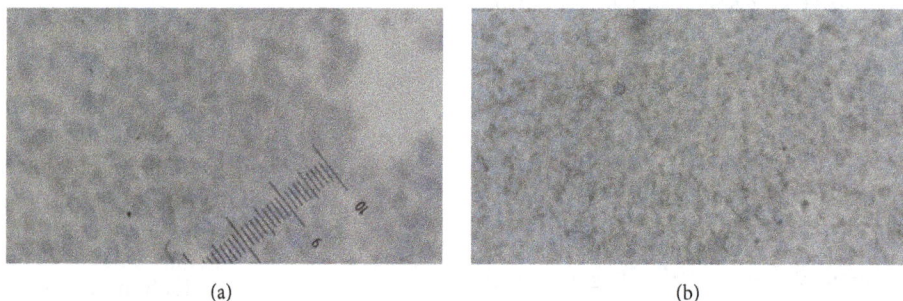

FIGURE 4: On immunohistochemical study, tumor cells were positive for EMA (a) and CD 99 (b).

diffusely positive to epithelial markers. After discarding these 2 more frequent events the diagnosis of sarcoma can be retained [10].

Other differential diagnoses include the fibrous pleural tumor, sarcomatoid subtype of malignant pleural mesothelioma, spindle cell carcinoma, and malignant peripheral nerve sheath tumor [10].

The next question is whether the pleuropulmonary tumor is primitive or secondary. The second eventuality is by far the most frequent. The mother tumor usually sits in the soft tissues. Only the absence of extrapleuropulmonary tumor localization in the past and at the time of diagnosis will attest to the primitive nature of the tumor. In our case, PET SCAN had eliminated an extrathoracic localization of the tumor, so we had retained the diagnosis of primary pleuropulmonary synovial sarcoma.

The recent identification of a chromosomal translocation specific to pleuropulmonary synovial sarcoma has increased the recognition of this particular sarcoma subtype. The chromosomal translocation t(x;18) (p11.2;q11.2) is present in more than 90% of cases of primary PPSS [11]. It produces three types of fusion genes formed in part by SS18 from chromosome 18 and by SSX1, SSX2, or, rarely, SSX4 from the X chromosome [12]. Unusual sites of involvement include the kidney, adrenal gland, retroperitoneum, lung, mediastinum, bone, and nervous system [11]. Despite its high sensitivity, molecular testing is not required if the diagnosis of synovial sarcoma is certain or probable on the basis of clinical, histological, and immunohistochemical evaluations [5].

There is no standardised therapy for PPSS and most patients are treated with surgery alone or surgery with adjuvant radiation therapy. Synovial sarcomas are chemosensitive to ifosfamide and doxorubicin, with an overall response rate of approximately 24 percent. A new drug, pazopanib, seems to provide another option with an improved median progression-free survival and median overall survival in some trials. Radiotherapy has no apparent effect on the control of local disease or overall survival [9, 13].

The prognosis for patients with PPSS is poor, with an overall 5-year survival rate of 50 percent. Factors predicting a worse prognosis for patients with synovial sarcomas include tumour size (>5 cm), male gender, older age (>20 years), extensive tumour necrosis, high grade, large number of mitotic figures (>10 per 10 hpf), neurovascular invasion, and, recently, the *SYT-SSX1* variant [9]. In our observation, approximately 45 days between the appearance of the first clinical signs and the confirmation of the diagnosis, the patient died the day after her first chemotherapy treatment testifying to the aggressiveness of the tumor.

4. Conclusion

Primary pleuropulmonary sarcomas are rare. They first discuss a tumor with double carcinomatous and sarcomatous contingent whose first component is discrete or was not interested in sampling. Once the diagnosis of sarcoma is established, a secondary pulmonary site should be removed, which is more likely. It is therefore only after a diagnostic procedure of exclusion that the primary pulmonary seat of a sarcoma will be retained.

The feature of our observation compared to literature revues is the clinical, radiological, and histological similarity.

Abbreviations

CT: Computed tomography
PPSS: Pleuropulmonary synovial sarcoma
FNCLCC: French Federation Nationale des Centres de Lutte Contre le Cancer
mMRC: Modified Medical Research Council
PET SCAN: Positron-Emission Tomography Scanning.

Disclosure

This case report was written based on clinical observation without any funding.

Authors' Contributions

Fatima Zahra Mrabet drafted this manuscript under Sanaa Hammi's supervision. Hafsa El Ouazzani and Leila El Akkari have made substantial contributions to acquisition of data. Jamal Eddine Bourkadi and Fouad Zouaidia have been involved in drafting the manuscript. All authors read and approved the final manuscript.

References

[1] D. Bhattacharya, S. Datta, A. Das, K. Halder, and S. Chattopadhyay, "Primary pulmonary synovial sarcoma: a case report and review of literature," *International Journal of Applied and Basic Medical Research*, vol. 6, no. 1, pp. 63–65, 2016.

[2] M. K. Panigrahi, G. Pradhan, N. Sahoo, P. Mishra, S. Patra, and P. R. Mohapatra, "Primary pulmonary synovial sarcoma: A reappraisal," *Journal of Cancer Research and Therapeutics*, 2017.

[3] A. Atmane, S. Hammi, A. Regragui et al., "Mode révélateur original et localisation métastatique particulière d'un synovialo-sarcome chez un adulte immunocompétent: à propos d'un cas avec revue de la littérature," *The Pan African Medical Journal*, vol. 28, no. 103, p. 13200, 2017.

[4] R. D. Arun, "A rare primary synovial sarcoma of lung - case report with literature review," *Nursing & Health Sciences*, vol. 3, no. 1, 2017.

[5] L. K. Rajeev, R. Patidar, G. Babu, M. C. Suresh Babu, K. N. Lokesh, and G. V. Patil Okaly, "A rare case of primary synovial sarcoma of lung," *Lung India*, vol. 34, no. 6, pp. 545–547, 2017.

[6] L. Qassimi, W. El Khattabi, H. Lyousfi, A. Aichane, and H. Afif, "Une tumeur rare de la paroi thoracique : le synovialosarcome," *Revue de Pneumologie Clinique*, vol. 71, no. 4, pp. 251-252, 2015.

[7] F. J. Podbielski, T. E. Sambo, A. Salamat, M. J. Blecha, and M. M. Connolly, "Primary Pulmonary Synovial Sarcoma," *PLEURA*, vol. 3, no. 1-2, 2016.

[8] R. C. Ward, A. E. Birnbaum, B. I. Aswad, and T. T. Healey, "Solitary pulmonary nodule: pleuropulmonary synovial sarcoma," *Rhode Island Medical Journal*, vol. 97, no. 5, pp. 40–43, 2014.

[9] C.-C. Chang and P.-Y. Chang, "Primary pulmonary synovial sarcoma," *Journal of Cancer Research and Practice*, vol. 5, no. 1, pp. 24–26, 2018, https://doi.org/10.1016/j.jcrpr.2017.09.002.

[10] W. R. Li, C. Thakur, and S. Gupta, "Primary pulmonary synovial sarcoma: one case report," *Journal of Lung Cancer Diagnosis & Treatment*, vol. 2, p. 114, 2017.

[11] K. Bunch and S. H. Deering, "Primary Pulmonary Synovial Sarcoma in Pregnancy," *Case Reports in Obstetrics and Gynecology*, vol. 2012, 3 pages, 2012.

[12] J. S. Kambo, B. Richardson, D. N. Ionescu, T. Tucker, and G. Kraushaar, "Primary pulmonary synovial sarcoma: A case with unique and impressive computed tomography findings," *Canadian Respiratory Journal*, vol. 22, no. 1, pp. e1–e3, 2015.

[13] A. Ech-Cherrate, N. Zaghba, H. Benjelloun, A. Bakhatar, N. Yassine, and A. Bahlaoui, "Localisation thoracique des synovialosarcomes (à propos de quatre observations)," *Revue des Maladies Respiratoires*, vol. 30, p. A95, 2013.

40

Pulmonary Alveolar Proteinosis in Setting of Inhaled Toxin Exposure and Chronic Substance Abuse

Meirui Li [iD],[1] **Salem Alowami,**[2] **Miranda Schell,**[2] **Clive Davis,**[3] and **Asghar Naqvi** [iD][2]

[1]*Michael G. DeGroote School of Medicine, McMaster University, Hamilton, ON, Canada*
[2]*Department of Pathology and Molecular Medicine, McMaster University, Hamilton, ON, Canada*
[3]*Divisions of Critical Care, Respirology, and General Internal Medicine, Department of Medicine,*
 McMaster University, Hamilton, ON, Canada

Correspondence should be addressed to Asghar Naqvi; anaqvi@stjosham.on.ca

Academic Editor: Shinichiro Ohshimo

Pulmonary alveolar proteinosis (PAP) is a rare lung disorder in which defects in alveolar macrophage maturation or function lead to the accumulation of proteinaceous surfactant in alveolar space, resulting in impaired gas exchange and hypoxemia. PAP is categorized into three types: hereditary, autoimmune, and secondary. We report a case of secondary PAP in a 47-year-old man, whose risk factors include occupational exposure to inhaled toxins, especially aluminum dust, the use of anabolic steroids, and alcohol abuse, which in mice leads to alveolar macrophage dysfunction through a zinc-dependent mechanism that inhibits granulocyte macrophage-colony stimulating factor (GM-CSF) receptor signalling. Although the rarity and vague clinical presentation of PAP can pose diagnostic challenges, clinician awareness of PAP risk factors may facilitate the diagnostic process and lead to more prompt treatment.

1. Introduction

Pulmonary alveolar proteinosis (PAP) is a rare lung disease characterized by the accumulation of proteinaceous material in the alveoli due to decreased clearance of surfactant by alveolar macrophages. First described in 1958, the prevalence of PAP has been estimated to be 6.87 per million [1, 2].

PAP patients can present asymptomatically or with vague complaints of dyspnea and cough [3]. High resolution computed tomography (HRCT) scan of the lungs show either bilateral diffuse ground-glass opacity or the characteristic "crazy-paving" pattern [4]. Bronchoalveolar lavage (BAL) is used in diagnosis in up to 83% of cases in recent years, replacing lung biopsy as the diagnostic tool of choice [5, 6].

There are three types of PAP: hereditary, autoimmune, and secondary. Hereditary PAP mainly affects children, while the latter two occur in adults [3]. Here, we report the case of a patient who developed PAP secondary to environmental exposure in the setting of chronic alcohol and steroid abuse.

2. Case Report

A previously well 47-year-old man presented with progressive dyspnea on exertion and fleeting bouts of sharp precordial chest pain for several months. Echocardiogram showed mild diastolic dysfunction and wall motion abnormalities on Persantine Sestamibi stress test, leading to the diagnosis of heart failure. However, the patient's symptoms worsened in the subsequent months despite being on optimal management for heart failure and he was admitted to the hospital. An in-patient cardiac catheterization showed no significant obstruction in the coronary arteries, prompting investigations for a pulmonary etiology.

The patient was a lifelong nonsmoker who worked as an elevator mechanic with occasional exposure to small quantities of hazardous materials such as aluminum dust, asbestos, paint fumes, hydraulic oil, and cleaning agents. There is no increase in the exposure immediately prior to the onset of dyspnea. He reported a history of chronic alcohol

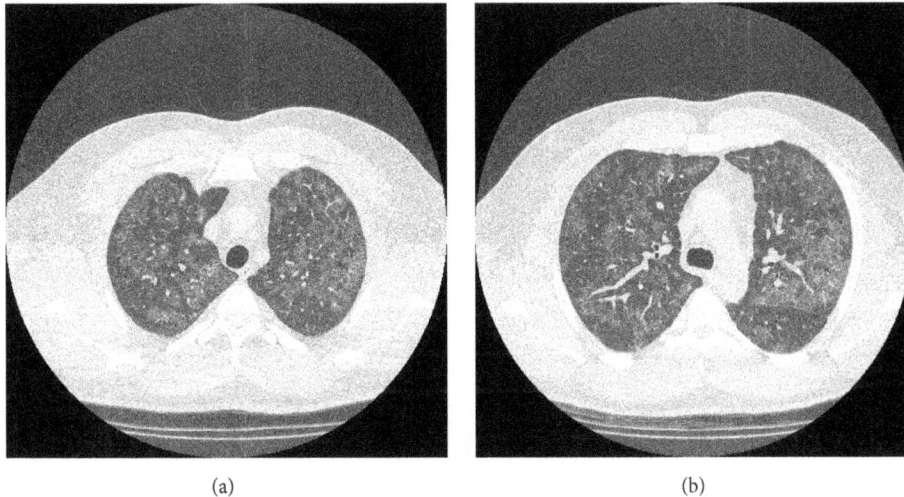

(a)   (b)

FIGURE 1: (a) and (b) Bilateral diffuse ground-glass opacities with thickened interlobular septae were seen in multiple sections of the lungs on HRCT.

consumption of 6–12 beers per day, as well as regular use of anabolic steroids. He had no past history of hematological cancers, chemotherapy, or radiation.

Physical exam revealed a heavily muscled man of 270 lbs with abdominal obesity. There were no audible wheezes or signs suggesting consolidation on auscultation of the lungs. Cardiac exam revealed normal heart sounds, absence of murmurs or rubs, and a nondisplaced apex. Arterial blood gas analysis revealed an alveolar-arterial gradient of 15 mmHg, consistent with gas transfer defect. Except for a mild diffusion defect (DLCO 81% of predicted), spirometry was normal with a FEV1 of 4.52 (110% of predicted) and FVC of 5.5 (103% of predicted), and a FEV1/FVC ratio of 81%. A 6-minute walk test was sufficient to cause dyspnea and a drop in oxygen saturation from 94% to 91%. Diffuse airspace disease was noted on chest X-ray. An HRCT scan demonstrated bilateral diffusely scattered zones of ground-glass opacification with accentuation of the interlobular septae, suggesting alveolar disease. This combination of findings characterizes the so-called "crazy-paving pattern" commonly seen in PAP. There is no convincing evidence of interstitial lung disease, nor any signs of air trapping that would suggest an obstructive etiology (Figure 1).

BAL of the lungs yielded milky and opalescent fluid. Amorphous green, orange, and orange-centred globules and histiocytes containing dense proteinaceous material were seen on Papanicolaou-stained smears of BAL fluid (Figure 2). These globules appeared densely dark blue and basophilic under Diff-Quick stain and were periodic acid-Schiff- (PAS-) positive and diastase-resistant (Figures 3 and 4), consistent with the diagnosis of PAP. Blood sample was tested for antibodies against granulocyte macrophage-colony stimulating factor (GM-CSF) through an outside lab and was reported negative. As standard treatment, the patient was set to undergo whole-lung lavage (WLL). When initial washings did not yield significant amount of secretions, the diagnosis of PAP was questioned and WLL was converted to wedge biopsy of the lung in the operating room. H&E stains of the wedge

biopsy showed intact alveolar structure filled with amorphous granular eosinophilic material and no interstitial pathology, confirming the diagnosis of PAP (Figure 5). Following the result of the biopsy, a second WLL was scheduled for the patient. Pulmonary testing one year later showed that DLCO had improved from 81% to 98% of predicted; FEV1, FVC, and VC were again normal. On exercise testing, the patient was able to achieve a low-normal work capacity of 80% of maximum predicted value, with normal oxygen saturation at rest and on exertion.

3. Discussion

Autoimmune and secondary PAP are the two acquired forms of PAP affecting adults. Autoimmune PAP, which makes up 90% of reported PAP cases [3], is caused by the production of autoantibodies against GM-CSF, a crucial cytokine in the maturation of monocytes into macrophages [7]. Secondary PAP occurs in the setting of macrophage dysfunction caused by infections, hematological disorders, immunosuppression, and exposure to hazardous materials [3]. Hematologic disorders are the most common etiology for secondary PAP, accounting for an estimated 88% of cases [8]. The exact incidence of PAP due to inhalational exposure is unknown. Secondary PAP patients have negative serology for anti-GM-CSF antibodies [3]. The standard therapy for PAP is whole-lung lavage. Although exogenous GM-CSF has been shown to be safe and beneficial for autoimmune PAP, it is not routinely used for secondary PAP [9].

Our patient reported exposure to inhaled toxins such as aluminum dust, organic dust comprised of human sheddings, and fumes of paint and cleaning products. Inhaled dusts and fumes have been described as risk factors for secondary PAP in studies and case reports. Silica dust is the most frequently reported hazardous substance (21% in a single-centre German study), followed by aluminum dust (18%). Exposure to fumes of paint and cleaning products have been reported by 13% and 8% of patients, respectively [6].

(a)

(b)

(c)

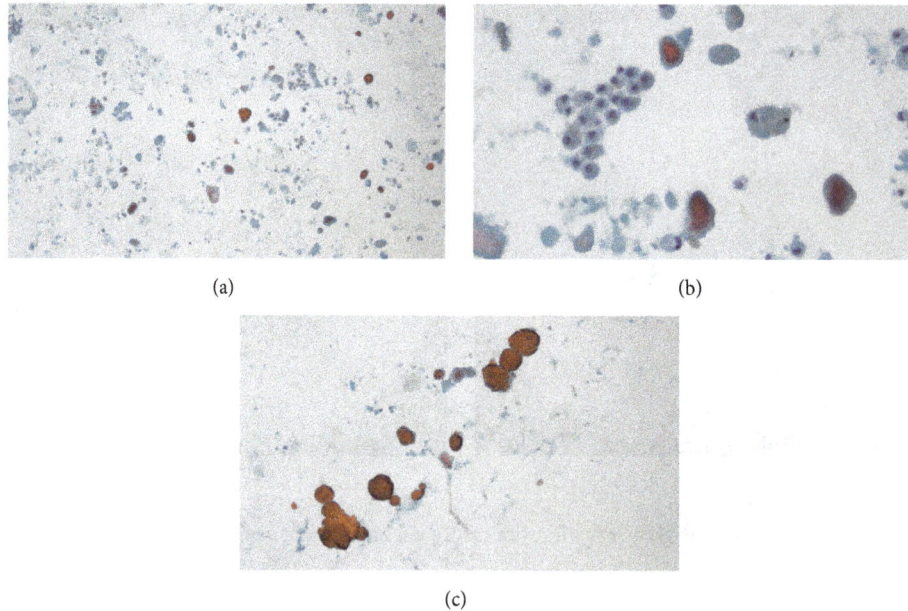

FIGURE 2: (a) Papanicolaou-stained smear of BAL fluid (lower magnification). (b) Papanicolaou-stained smear of BAL fluid (higher magnification) showing amorphous globules and alveolar histiocytes (likely macrophages) with dense intracellular proteinaceous material. (c) Paucicellular, amorphous globules staining orange, green, and green with orange centre under Papanicolaou-stain (higher magnification).

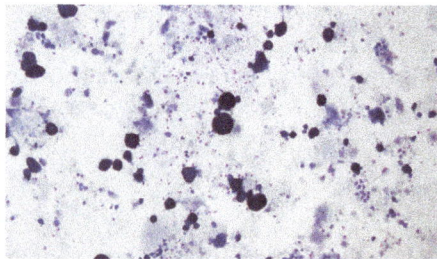

FIGURE 3: Diff-Quick stain of BAL fluid showing densely blue, basophilic globules.

Unlike autoimmune PAP, macrophage dysfunction in secondary PAP occurs through a mechanism that is largely independent of anti-GM-CSF antibodies. This is evident in the case of a Japanese patient who developed secondary PAP two weeks after being exposed to silica and aluminum dust particles following the Great East Japan Earthquake. The patient's serum was observed to have an inhibitory effect on GM-CSF signalling despite the paucity of anti-GM-CSF antibodies [10].

Ongoing controversy exists regarding the association between inhalational exposure and the development of autoimmune PAP. It has been reported that exposure to indium compounds, which are used as transparent conductive coating on flat-screen electronic displays, can lead to the production of autoantibodies against GM-GSF [11]. The percentage of autoimmune PAP patients who also had inhalational exposure varies between 26% and 54% in studies [6, 12, 13]. In one Chinese study, this percentage is not significantly different from the prevalence of inhalational

exposure in non-PAP hospital controls [13]. While it is possible that exposure to inhaled toxins plays a role in the pathogenesis of autoimmune PAP, stronger evidence is needed.

Our patient has a history of alcohol and steroid abuse concomitant to occupational exposure of inhaled hazardous substances. Although there are no previous reports linking alcohol abuse to PAP, alcohol has been demonstrated to inhibit alveolar macrophage function in animal and molecular models. Mice subjected to chronic ethanol ingestion are shown to have suppressed cytokine secretion and macrophage phagocytosis in the alveoli. Ingesting ethanol for six weeks leads to decreased GM-CSF receptor expression on murine alveolar macrophages and impaired binding of transcription factor PU.1 to the receptor [14]. The effect of alcohol on GM-CSF signalling may be zinc-dependent. Zinc is an important cofactor in cellular processes including GM-CSF signalling. Ethanol ingestion in mice leads to decreased expression of zinc transporters on murine alveolar macrophages and increased risk of zinc deficiency through malnutrition [15]. Both GM-CSF therapy and zinc supplementation are able to restore macrophage phagocytic function in ethanol-fed mice, further supporting the link between alcohol and alveolar macrophage dysfunction [15, 16]. Similarly, corticosteroids have not been established as a causative agent of secondary PAP. Corticosteroids are routinely used to treat neonatal respiratory distress syndrome by increasing Type II alveolar cell surfactant production [17]. Macrophage function may also be impaired through the immunosuppressive effect of systemic corticosteroids. A retrospective cohort study done in 2015 found that corticosteroid therapy in autoimmune PAP patients lead to higher disease severity score in a dose dependent manner. Furthermore, the authors concluded that

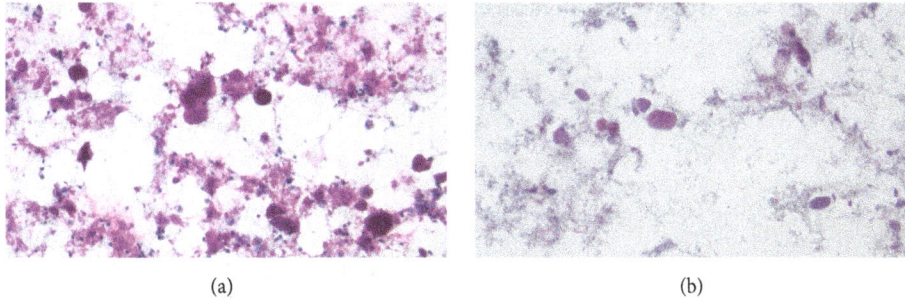

FIGURE 4: (a) PAS stain of BAL fluid. Globules were PAS-positive. (b) The globules were diastase-resistant.

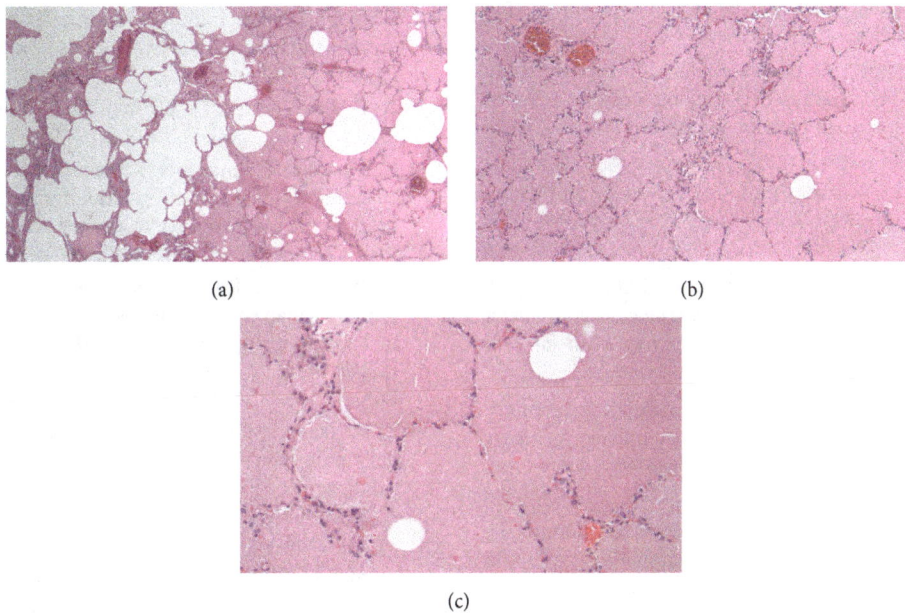

FIGURE 5: H&E stain of lung wedge biopsy sections at 100x (a), 200x (b), and 400x (c) magnifications showing intact alveolar walls, normal interstitium, and amorphous, eosinophilic granular material in the airspace.

the worsening of disease is likely due to corticosteroids exacerbating the pathogenic process of PAP per se and cannot simply be attributed to the increased rates of opportunistic infections secondary to immunosuppression [18]. Therefore, it is possible that steroid abuse also had a synergistic effect on the patient developing PAP.

Although hereditary PAP has been described as a disease affecting children and infants, since 2010 three cases of adult-onset hereditary PAP have been reported in literature. All three patients tested negative for anti-GM-CSF antibodies and had elevated serum GM-CSF levels and mutations in either CSF2RA or CSF2RB gene encoding parts of the GM-CSF receptor. Serum GM-CSF level and genetic testing have not been done on our patient [19–21]. Although it cannot be ruled out, given the extreme rarity of adult-onset hereditary PAP and the presence of risk factors such as inhalational exposure, secondary PAP is a much more likely etiology.

Long-term follow-up is needed to determine whether cessation of exposure prevents future recurrences of PAP.

4. Conclusion

Inhalational exposure to toxic dusts and fumes is a major risk factor for developing secondary PAP. Although a link between alcohol abuse and PAP has not been established, ethanol ingestion has been demonstrated to suppress GM-CSF signalling and macrophage function in mice models. It is possible that alcohol and steroid abuse have played contributory roles in the pathogenesis of PAP in this patient. The rarity and vague clinical presentation of PAP can pose diagnostic challenges. The presence of medical and social risk factors of PAP should raise suspicion for PAP in patients presenting with respiratory symptoms with no clear cause. Increasing clinician awareness for these risk factors can shorten the time to diagnosis and treatment, potentially improving patient outcome.

References

[1] S. H. Rosen, B. Castleman, and A. A. Liebow, "Pulmonary alveolar proteinosis," *The New England Journal of Medicine*, vol. 258, no. 23, pp. 1123–1142, 1958.

[2] R. Avetisyan, B. Carey, W. Zhang et al., "Prevalence of pulmonary alveolar proteinosis (PAP) determined using a large health care claims database," in *Proceedings of the American Thoracic Society International Conference*, San Diego, Calif, USA, May 2014.

[3] R. Borie, C. Danel, M.-P. Debray et al., "Pulmonary alveolar proteinosis," *European Respiratory Review*, vol. 20, no. 120, pp. 98–107, 2011.

[4] H. Ishii, B. C. Trapnell, R. Tazawa et al., "Comparative study of high-resolution CT findings between autoimmune and secondary pulmonary alveolar proteinosis," *CHEST*, vol. 136, no. 5, pp. 1348–1355, 2009.

[5] T. Suzuki and B. C. Trapnell, "Pulmonary alveolar proteinosis syndrome," *Clinics in Chest Medicine*, vol. 37, no. 3, pp. 431–440, 2016.

[6] F. Bonella, P. C. Bauer, M. Griese, S. Ohshimo, J. Guzman, and U. Costabel, "Pulmonary alveolar proteinosis: new insights from a single-center cohort of 70 patients," *Respiratory Medicine*, vol. 105, no. 12, pp. 1908–1916, 2011.

[7] B. C. Trapnell and J. A. Whitsett, "GM-CSF regulates pulmonary surfactant homeostasis and alveolar macrophage-mediated innate host defense," *Annual Review of Physiology*, vol. 64, pp. 775–802, 2002.

[8] H. Ishii, J. F. Seymour, R. Tazawa et al., "Secondary pulmonary alveolar proteinosis complicating myelodysplastic syndrome results in worsening of prognosis: a retrospective cohort study in Japan," *BMC Pulmonary Medicine*, vol. 14, no. 37, pp. 1471–2466, 2014.

[9] R. Tazawa, B. C. Trapnell, Y. Inoue et al., "Inhaled granulocyte/macrophage-colony stimulating factor as therapy for pulmonary alveolar proteinosis," *American Journal of Respiratory and Critical Care Medicine*, vol. 181, no. 12, pp. 1345–1354, 2010.

[10] S. Hisata, H. Moriyama, R. Tazawa, S. Ohkouchi, M. Ichinose, and M. Ebina, "Development of pulmonary alveolar proteinosis following exposure to dust after the great east japan earthquake," *Respiratory Investigation*, vol. 51, no. 4, pp. 212–216, 2013.

[11] K. J. Cummings, W. E. Donat, D. B. Ettensohn, V. L. Roggli, P. Ingram, and K. Kreiss, "Pulmonary alveolar proteinosis in workers at an indium processing facility," *American Journal of Respiratory and Critical Care Medicine*, vol. 181, no. 5, pp. 458–464, 2010.

[12] Y. Inoue, B. C. Trapnell, R. Tazawa et al., "Characteristics of a large cohort of patients with autoimmune pulmonary alveolar proteinosis in Japan," *American Journal of Respiratory and Critical Care Medicine*, vol. 177, no. 7, pp. 752–762, 2008.

[13] Y.-L. Xiao, K.-F. Xu, Y. Li et al., "Occupational inhalational exposure and serum GM-CSF autoantibody in pulmonary alveolar proteinosis," *Occupational and Environmental Medicine*, vol. 72, no. 7, pp. 504–512, 2015.

[14] P. C. Joshi, L. Applewhite, J. D. Ritzenthaler et al., "Chronic ethanol ingestion in rats decreases granulocyte-macrophage colony-stimulating factor receptor expression and downstream signaling in the alveolar macrophage," *The Journal of Immunology*, vol. 175, no. 10, pp. 6837–6845, 2005.

[15] P. C. Joshi, A. Mehta, W. S. Jabber, X. Fan, and D. M. Guidot, "Zinc deficiency mediates alcohol-induced alveolar epithelial and macrophage dysfunction in rats," *American Journal of Respiratory Cell and Molecular Biology*, vol. 41, no. 2, pp. 207–216, 2009.

[16] A. J. Mehta, P. C. Joshi, X. Fan et al., "Zinc supplementation restores PU.1 and Nrf2 Nuclear Binding in alveolar macrophages and improves redox balance and bacterial clearance in the lungs of alcohol-fed rats," *Alcoholism: Clinical and Experimental Research*, vol. 35, no. 8, pp. 1519–1528, 2011.

[17] A. D. Postle and J. O. Warner, "Steroids, surfactant and lung disease," *Thorax*, vol. 51, no. 9, pp. 880-881, 1996.

[18] K. Akasaka, T. Tanaka, N. Kitamura et al., "Outcome of corticosteroid administration in autoimmune pulmonary alveolar proteinosis: a retrospective cohort study," *BMC Pulmonary Medicine*, vol. 15, no. 1, article 88, 2015.

[19] R. Tazawa, K. Ito, T. Ogi et al., "Adult onset hereditary pulmonary alveolar proteinosis caused by CSF2RA deletion," in *Proceedings of the American Thoracic Society International Conference A42 Pathogenesis of Interstitial Lung Disease*, San Diego, Calif, USA, May 2014.

[20] T. Tanaka, N. Motoi, Y. Tsuchihashi et al., "Adult-onset hereditary pulmonary alveolar proteinosis caused by a single-base deletion in CSF2RB," *Journal of Medical Genetics*, vol. 48, no. 3, pp. 205–209, 2011.

[21] M. Ito, K. Nakagome, H. Ohta et al., "Elderly-onset hereditary pulmonary alveolar proteinosis and its cytokine profile," *BMC Pulmonary Medicine*, vol. 17, no. 1, article 40, 2017.

41

Hemoptysis following Talc Pleurodesis in a Pneumothorax Patient

Yusuke Kakiuchi, Fumihiro Yamaguchi, Makoto Hayashi, and Yusuke Shikama

Department of Respiratory Medicine, Showa University Fujigaoka Hospital, 1-30 Fujigaoka, Aoba-ku, Yokohama 227-8501, Japan

Correspondence should be addressed to Fumihiro Yamaguchi; f~y@med.showa-u.ac.jp

Academic Editor: Tun-Chieh Chen

The purpose of this article is to report a case of hemoptysis occurring in combination with secondary spontaneous pneumothorax following chemical pleurodesis by talc. A Japanese male with cancer of renal pelvis was found with the left pneumothorax and multiple lung metastases. A computed-tomography scan revealed severe emphysema throughout the lungs. Talc pleurodesis was employed to arrest air leakage. The patient developed hemoptysis 45 minutes after talc injection into the thorax. This is the first report of hemoptysis following talc pleurodesis. The agent could induce severe inflammation in capillary vessels of the lung following visceral pleura infiltration.

1. Introduction

Spontaneous pneumothorax is a common condition divided into primary and secondary types on the basis of presence or absence of underlying lung diseases such as emphysema and interstitial pneumonia [1, 2]. More specifically, secondary spontaneous pneumothorax occurs especially in elderly patients and causes severe respiratory failure in some cases. Surgical intervention is the procedure of choice in patients with intractable pneumothorax. However, chemical pleurodesis is useful for more elderly patients who generally exhibit poor lung function. The efficacy of chemical pleurodesis in pneumothorax patients is well established in clinical practice [3, 4], and talc is the substance most commonly used worldwide despite the occurrence of severe side effects including acute respiratory distress syndrome (ARDS) [5–7]. This report details the occurrence of hemoptysis in combination with secondary spontaneous pneumothorax following talc pleurodesis, suggesting that talc induced severe inflammation in capillary vessels of the lung.

2. Case Report

A 72-year-old Japanese male with cancer of the renal pelvis and a smoking history of 120 pack-years had continued on two cycles of doublet chemotherapy consisting of cisplatin with gemcitabine for the past year. He was referred to our hospital because of acute dyspnea. A computed-tomography (CT) scan of his chest at diagnosis revealed left pneumothorax, multiple nodules, pleural effusion, and severe emphysema throughout the lungs. Figure 1 shows that some nodules with cavities were located in the edge of the lung. As shown in Table 1, tumor markers CA19-9, SCC, and CYFRA21-1 were elevated with values of 903.4 U/ml, 9.5 ng/ml, and 23.6 ng/ml, respectively. Peripheral blood count was consistent with mild anemia and coagulation parameters were within normal limits. He was therefore diagnosed with lung metastasis. A chest tube was inserted into the seventh intercostal space in the left median axillary line for drainage on day 1; however air leakage continued. Subsequently 70 ml of autologous blood was injected into the left thorax through the chest tube on day 12, but this intervention was unsuccessful. Poor lung function was inferred due to the severe emphysema and surgical intervention was thus deemed inappropriate. In addition left pleural effusion was detected, and it was possible that such effusion could have been increased by lung metastasis. Therefore talc pleurodesis was employed to arrest air leakage and prevent recurrent pleural effusion. 50 ml of saline containing 4 g sterile talc powder was administered into the left thorax on day 17. The patient developed hemoptysis 45 minutes

(a)

(b)

(c)

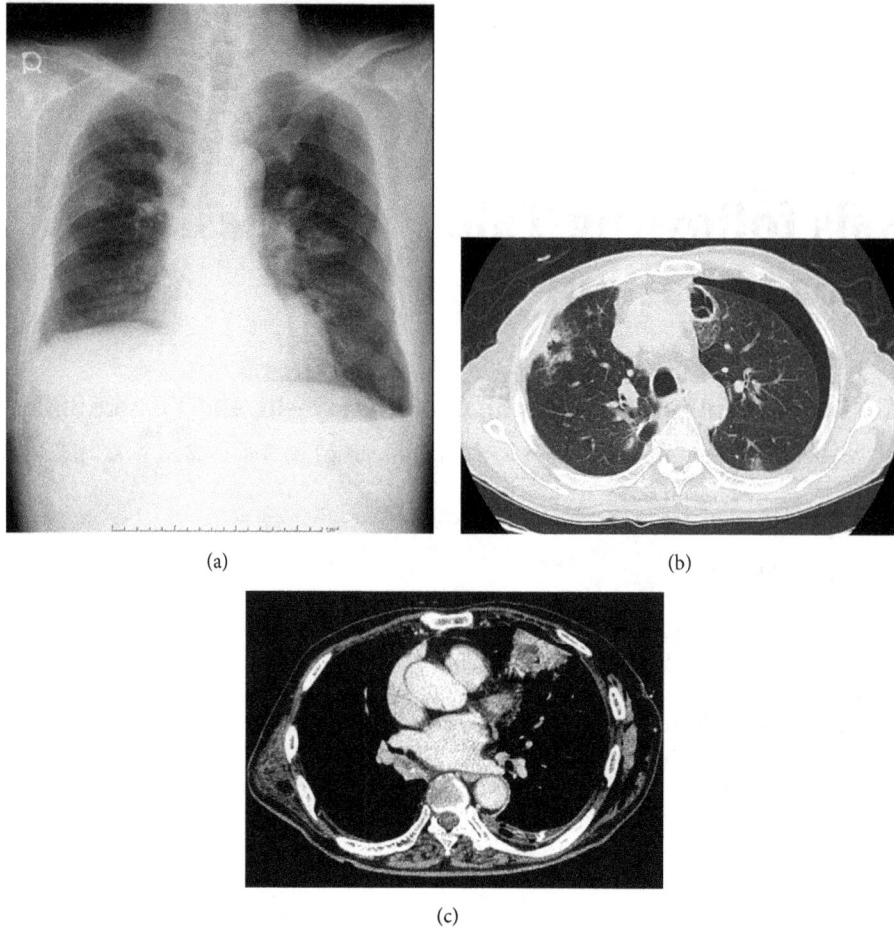

FIGURE 1: (a) A chest X-ray showed a left pneumothorax and multiple metastases in the bilateral lung. (b) A CT scan of the chest revealed that some nodules with cavities were located in the edge of the lung. (c) A contrast enhanced CT scan of the chest revealed a cavity, culprit lesion of hemoptysis, 25 mm in size, in the left upper lobe.

TABLE 1: Laboratory data.

Peripheral blood counts	
WBC	$9600/\mu l$
RBC	$418 \times 10^4/\mu l$
Hb	$12\,g/dl$
Plt	$23.4 \times 10^4/\mu l$
Blood coagulation	
PT	126%
APTT	>120%
Tumor marker	
CA19-9	$903.4\,U/ml$
SCC	$9.5\,ng/ml$
CYFRA21-1	$23.6\,ng/ml$

after talc injection through the chest tube and immediately required a bronchial artery embolization (Figure 2). Talc pleurodesis was eventually successful and the chest tube was then removed.

3. Discussion

Surgical intervention is generally applied for recurrent or complicated pneumothorax. However, chemical pleurodesis is useful in management of inoperable patients. In fact intrapleural adhesion has been described as a treatment for patients with secondary spontaneous pneumothorax according to the clinical guidelines published by the British Thoracic Society [3] and the American College of Chest Physicians [4]. Agents that reportedly induce intrapleural adhesions include tetracycline derivatives, bleomycin, cisplatin, iodopovidone, 50% dextrose in water, autologous blood, and OK-432 [8–12]. In particular, talc is the most commonly used such agent worldwide because of its high efficacy and low cost [13]. Complications of talc pleurodesis were initially reported due to the presence of contaminants such as asbestos [14], but talc in current use is purified and sterilized and its efficacy has been well established [15]. There have been several reports that talc administration into the thorax is more effective in preventing recurrent pneumothorax or reducing malignant pleural effusion than other sclerosing agents [6, 7]. In the present case, both left pneumothorax and pleural effusion

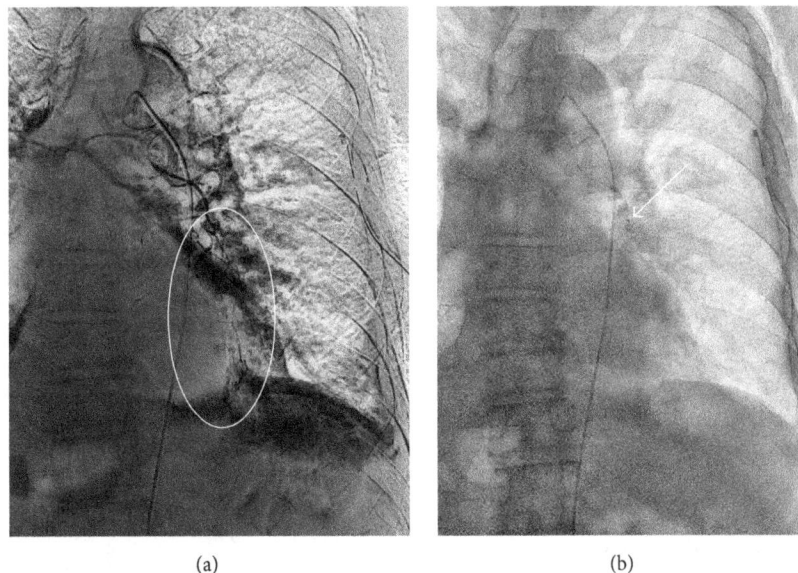

FIGURE 2: (a) A chest X-ray showed bleeding from the left bronchial artery in the left upper lobe (white circle). (b) A chest X-ray indicated the arrest of bleeding after bronchial artery embolization (white arrow).

were detected. Hence talc was selected to arrest air leakage and prevent recurrent pleural effusion following failed pleurodesis with autologous blood. On the other hand it should be noted that intrapleural talc administration can lead to severe side effects. More specifically, many physicians have reported ARDS associated with talc pleurodesis [16–18]. In the present case the patient did not exhibit symptoms of ARDS but developed hemoptysis shortly after establishment of intrapleural adhesion. This is the first report of hemoptysis following talc pleurodesis, whereas hemothorax has previously been reported in a few cases [1]. Such side effects can be related to the size and dose of talc in the preparation. Several previous studies have shown that intrapleural adhesion with low doses of talc (<2-3 g and medium particle size > 6–31.5 μm) did not induce either ARDS or pneumonitis [19, 20]. In a rabbit model, IL-8 and VEGF levels in serum were elevated with decreasing talc particle size; furthermore pleural fluid IL-8 and VEGF levels were higher in the small particle talc group (<5 μm) than in particles of mixed size [21]. Moreover talc deposition in the lung was observed more clearly with small size particles. Talc particles were attached not only to the pleural surface, but also to the alveolar spaces and septa in the lung which was the site of injection with talc. Conversely, talc deposition was detected only in alveolar septa in the opposite lung. In addition, particle migration was demonstrated in spleen, liver, and kidney which were vascularized [21]. These findings suggest that talc circulates throughout the body and can be deposited on capillary vessel walls. As a result, these particles could damage endothelial cells directly, or by producing inflammatory mediators, and thereby develop hemoptysis. In the present case, the patient vomited blood only 45 minutes after talc injection. It is not clear how much time is required for talc particles to infiltrate the pleural surface through mesothelial cells. As shown in Figure 1, cavity-forming cancer nodules were adjacent to

visceral pleura, suggesting the fragile nature of the pleural barrier. An agent could therefore penetrate mesothelial cells on the pleural surface relatively quickly and cause endothelial injury in the cavity. Indeed it has been reported that talc exposure induces prominent damage to mesothelial cells within 15 minutes [22]. In the current study, a bronchial artery embolization was performed for the arrest of bleeding, and it revealed that the culprit vessel was a bronchial artery (Figure 2). There was no formation of a communication between bronchial arteries and pulmonary arteries.

There is no relationship between the success rate of pleurodesis and talc dosage over the range >2–10 g [23]. Low dose talc should therefore be considered, particularly for elderly patients, because dose reduction can potentially suppress adverse effects. In addition small particles of talc could be associated with an increased risk of severe side effects such as ARDS and hemoptysis, and commercial talc is a heterogeneous material whose mean particle size may vary, depending on the location from which it is sourced [24]. The results of this study stress the need for careful attention in patients with secondary spontaneous pneumothorax when using talc for production of intrapleural adhesions.

References

[1] C.-H. How, H.-H. Hsu, and J.-S. Chen, "Chemical pleurodesis for spontaneous pneumothorax," *Journal of the Formosan Medical Association*, vol. 112, no. 12, pp. 749–755, 2013.

[2] P. M. Spieth, A. Güldner, and M. G. De Abreu, "Chronic obstructive pulmonary disease," *Current Opinion in Anaesthesiology*, vol. 25, no. 1, pp. 24–29, 2012.

[3] A. MacDuff, A. Arnold, and J. Harvey, "Management of spontaneous pneumothorax: British Thoracic Society pleural disease guideline 2010," *Thorax*, vol. 65, no. 2, pp. ii18–ii31, 2010.

[4] M. H. Bauman, C. Strange, J. E. Heffner et al., "Management of spontaneous pneumothorax: an American College of Chest Physicians Delphi Consensus Statement," *Chest*, vol. 119, no. 2, pp. 590–602, 2001.

[5] J.-R. Viallat, F. Rey, P. Astoul, and C. Boutin, "Thoracoscopic talc poudrage pleurodesis for malignant effusions: a review of 360 cases," *Chest*, vol. 110, no. 6, pp. 1387–1393, 1996.

[6] Y. C. G. Lee, M. H. Baumann, N. A. Maskell et al., "Pleurodesis Practice for Malignant Pleural Effusions in Five English-Speaking Countries: Survey of Pulmonologists," *Chest*, vol. 124, no. 6, pp. 2229–2238, 2003.

[7] R. W. Light, "Diseases of the pleura: The use of talc for pleurodesis," *Current Opinion in Pulmonary Medicine*, vol. 6, no. 4, pp. 255–258, 2000.

[8] J. Ferrer, J. F. Montes, M. A. Villarino, R. W. Light, and J. García-Valero, "Influence of particle size on extrapleural talc dissemination after talc slurry pleurodesis," *Chest*, vol. 122, no. 3, pp. 1018–1027, 2002.

[9] R. W. Light, N.-S. Wang, C. S. H. Sassoon, S. E. Gruer, and F. S. Vargas, "Comparison of the effectiveness of tetracycline and minocycline as pleural sclerosing agents in rabbits," *Chest*, vol. 106, no. 2, pp. 577–582, 1994.

[10] F. S. Vargas, N.-S. Wang, Hai Minh Lee, S. E. Gruer, C. H. S. Sassoon, and R. W. Light, "Effectiveness of bleomycin in comparison to tetracycline as pleural sclerosing agent in rabbits," *Chest*, vol. 104, no. 5, pp. 1582–1584, 1993.

[11] L. Lang-Lazdunski and A. S. Coonar, "A prospective study of autologous 'blood patch' pleurodesis for persistent air leak after pulmonary resection," *European Journal of Cardio-thoracic Surgery*, vol. 26, no. 5, pp. 897–900, 2004.

[12] M. G. Kim, S. G. Kim, J. H. Lee, Y. G. Eun, and S. G. Yeo, "The therapeutic effect of OK-432 (picibanil) sclerotherapy for benign neck cysts," *Laryngoscope*, vol. 118, no. 12, pp. 2177–2181, 2008.

[13] R. G. C. Inderbitzi, M. Furrer, H. Striffeler, and U. Althaus, "Thoracoscopic pleurectomy for treatment of complicated spontaneous pneumothorax," *Journal of Thoracic and Cardiovascular Surgery*, vol. 105, no. 1, pp. 84–88, 1993.

[14] A. N. Rohl, A. M. Langer, I. J. Selikoff et al., "Consumer talcums and powders: Mineral and chemical characterization," *Journal of Toxicology and Environmental Health*, vol. 2, no. 2, pp. 255–284, 1976.

[15] I. Hunt, B. Barber, R. Southon, and T. Treasure, "Is talc pleurodesis safe for young patients following primary spontaneous pneumothorax?" *Interactive Cardiovascular and Thoracic Surgery*, vol. 6, no. 1, pp. 117–120, 2007.

[16] D. H. Rehse, R. W. Aye, and M. G. Florence, "Respiratory failure following talc pleurodesis," *American Journal of Surgery*, vol. 177, no. 5, pp. 437–440, 1999.

[17] J. R. M. de Campos, F. S. Vargas, E. de Campos Werebe et al., "Thoracoscopy talc poudrage: a 15-year experience," *Chest*, vol. 119, no. 3, pp. 801–806, 2001.

[18] A. Brant and T. Eaton, "Serious complications with talc slurry pleurodesis," *Respirology*, vol. 6, no. 3, pp. 181–185, 2001.

[19] P.-O. Bridevaux, J.-M. Tschopp, G. Cardillo et al., "Short-term safety of thoracoscopic talc pleurodesis for recurrent primary spontaneous pneumothorax: A prospective European multicentre study," *European Respiratory Journal*, vol. 38, no. 4, pp. 770–773, 2011.

[20] J. R. M. Campos, E. C. Werebe, F. S. Vargas, F. B. Jatene, and R. W. Light, "Respiratory failure due to insufflated talc," *Lancet*, vol. 349, no. 9047, pp. 251–252, 1997.

[21] E. H. Genofre, F. S. Vargas, M. M. P. Acencio, L. Antonangelo, L. R. Teixeira, and E. Marchi, "Talc pleurodesis: Evidence of systemic Inflammatory response to small size talc particles," *Respiratory Medicine*, vol. 103, no. 1, pp. 91–97, 2009.

[22] E. H. Genofre, F. S. Vargas, L. Antonangelo et al., "Ultrastructural acute features of active remodeling after chemical pleurodesis induced by silver nitrate or talc," *Lung*, vol. 183, no. 3, pp. 197–207, 2005.

[23] L. Kennedy and S. A. Sahn, "Talc pleurodesis for the treatment of pneumothorax and pleural effusion," *Chest*, vol. 106, no. 4, pp. 1215–1222, 1994.

[24] R. W. Light and F. S. Vargas, "Pleural sclerosis for the treatment of pneumothorax and pleural effusion," *Lung*, vol. 175, no. 4, pp. 213–223, 1997.

42

Use of Extracorporeal Membrane Oxygenation in Postpartum Management of a Patient with Pulmonary Arterial Hypertension

Humna Abid Memon,[1] Zeenat Safdar ⓘ,[2] and Ahmad Goodarzi[3]

[1]Department of Internal Medicine, Houston Methodist Hospital, Houston, TX, USA
[2]Houston Methodist Pulmonary Hypertension Center, Weill Cornell College of Medicine, Houston, TX, USA
[3]Houston Methodist Lung Transplant Center, Houston Methodist Hospital, Houston, TX, USA

Correspondence should be addressed to Zeenat Safdar; zsafdar@houstonmethodist.org

Academic Editor: Reda E. Girgis

Current guidelines do not recommend pregnancy in patients with pulmonary arterial hypertension (PAH). This is due to the associated high mortality, which both dissuades PAH patients from becoming pregnant and encourages termination of pregnancy due to high maternal mortality risk. As a result, there is a lack of data and, consequently, there are only general guidelines available for management of pregnancy in PAH patients. Additionally, novel therapeutic strategies such as extracorporeal membrane oxygenation (ECMO), although used in the management of nonpregnant PAH patients as a bridge to lung transplantation, have not been used to treat cardiopulmonary collapse in pregnant PAH patients. In an attempt to bridge this paucity of data, we report the successful use of ECMO in resuscitation and management of a pregnant PAH patient who experienced cardiopulmonary collapse following a caesarian section.

1. Introduction

Pregnancy in pulmonary arterial hypertension (PAH) patients predictably induces a state of physiologic stress, compounded by increased intravascular volume, that cannot be accommodated by remodeled pulmonary arteries in PAH [1]. Thus, the puerperal state in patients with PAH can precipitate right heart failure (RHF) and hemodynamic collapse. Given this high risk, these patients are counseled against pregnancy [2] However, some women may still choose to become pregnant. Emerging modalities such as extracorporeal membrane oxygenation (ECMO), in the management of pregnant patients with PAH, have not been explored. Herein, we report the novel use of ECMO in the postpartum management of a PAH patient whose pregnancy was complicated by worsening pulmonary arterial hypertension (PAH) and post-caesarian section cardiopulmonary collapse.

2. Case Description

A 20-year-old female, with a known diagnosis of PAH and von Willebrand Disease (vWD), presented to the clinic at 13 weeks of gestation. She was diagnosed with PAH at the age of 5 and had undergone blade followed by balloon atrial septostomy and then subcutaneous (SC) treprostinil was started. On repeat heart catheterization at 14 years of age, tadalafil and bosentan were added to her regimen. At 16 years of age, her care was transitioned to an adult Pulmonary Hypertension (PH) center. An echocardiogram (ECHO) done at that time demonstrated a right ventricular systolic pressure (RVSP) of 88 mm Hg. Bosentan was changed to macitentan due to noncompliance with monthly liver function testing. She was continued on SC infusion of treprostinil at a dose of 38 ng/kg/min, tadalafil 40 mg daily, macitentan 10 mg daily, spironolactone 25 mg daily, digoxin 125 mcg daily, and warfarin.

Despite physicians' recommendations and multiple counseling sessions, the patient became pregnant, citing religious reasons for this decision. On affirmation of her desire to continue her pregnancy, all teratogenic medications such as spironolactone, digoxin, warfarin, and macitentan were stopped while tadalafil and treprostinil were continued. In addition, she was admitted and transitioned from SC

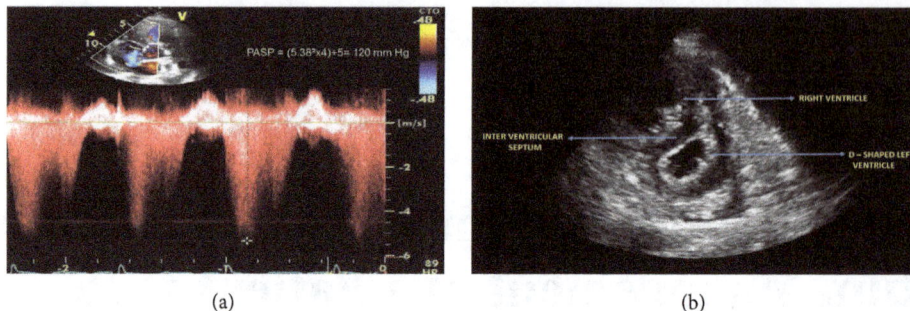

(a)   (b)

FIGURE 1: (a) Tricuspid regurgitation signal on echocardiogram at 25 weeks of gestation showing peak velocity of 5.38 m/s and Pulmonary Artery Systolic Pressure (PASP) of 120 mm Hg. (b) Echocardiogram at 25 weeks of gestation showing enlarged right ventricle and D-shaped left ventricle.

treprostinil to intravenous epoprostenol. She did well on this regimen until 25 weeks of gestation when she presented to the emergency department with complaints of recurrent hemoptysis and acute respiratory distress. She had a respiratory rate of 25/min, blood pressure (BP) of 110/65 mm Hg, and oxygen saturation of 86% in room air. While chest examination was unremarkable, with equal and no additional breath sounds bilaterally, a systolic grade 2/6 murmur was auscultated at the left sternal border and a jugular venous distension of 10 cm was noted on her cardiovascular exam.

The patient was supported with 10 liters (L) of nasal cannula oxygen and an arterial blood gas was obtained, which showed a pH of 7.47, pCO_2 of 27 mm Hg, and pO_2 of 147 mm Hg. Additional laboratory tests, consistent with her history of vWD, revealed thrombocytopenia with a platelet count of $75 \kappa/\mu L$. She was hence admitted to the intensive care unit (ICU) for close monitoring. Following admission, her ECHO showed a RVSP that had increased from 80 mm Hg, noted on her ECHO at 13 weeks of gestation, to 120 mm Hg (Figures 1(a) and 1(b)). In light of these findings and her presentation with acute decompensated PAH, a maternal-fetal specialist team was consulted and she was placed on continuous electronic fetal monitoring. Concurrently, betamethasone and magnesium sulfate were administered for expedition of fetal development and seizure prophylaxis, respectively. In addition, a team of specialists, including neonatal intensivist and cardiovascular surgeon, were assembled.

It was on continuous fetal monitoring at 26 weeks of gestation that fetal bradycardia was discovered, with acceleration and moderate variability between 100 and 110 beats/minute, but no decelerations. Due to concern of further decompensation and imminent danger to the patient and the fetus, an emergent caesarian section was undertaken.

Due to significant thrombocytopenia, the procedure was undertaken under general anesthesia and a healthy male infant was successfully delivered. However, during the closure of the hysterotomy, the patient developed ventricular tachycardia and went into cardiac arrest. Following 15 minutes of successful cardiopulmonary resuscitation (CPR), she was placed on mechanical ventilation. Due to precipitation of RHF, the patient was placed emergently on femoral-femoral venoarterial (VA) ECMO for life support. Using the

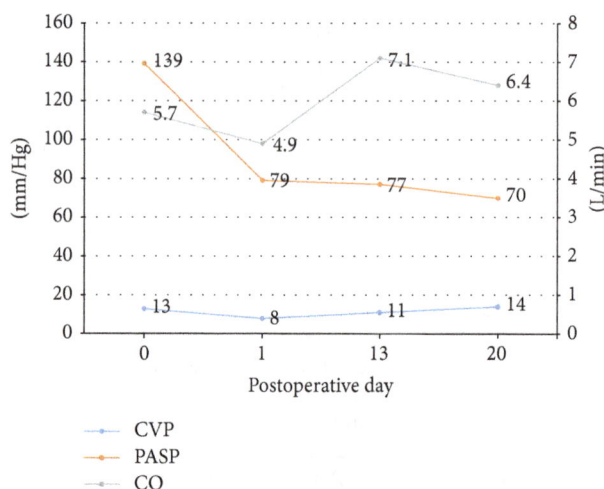

FIGURE 2: Graph representing changes in pulmonary artery systolic pressure, cardiac output, and central venous pressure after initiation of extracorporeal membrane oxygenation. CVP, central venous pressure; PASP, pulmonary artery systolic pressure; CO, cardiac output.

Seldinger technique, a 17-French arterial cannula and a 21-French multistage venous cannula were inserted, and full ECMO support at a flow rate of 3.79 L/min was initiated, in addition to multiple vasopressors, including 5 $\mu g/kg/min$ of dobutamine, 0.04 units/min of vasopressin, and 9 $\mu g/kg/min$ of norepinephrine and milrinone. A Swan Ganz catheter was simultaneously placed at the time of ECMO insertion. Her hemodynamics showed a PAP of 139/85 mm Hg, central venous pressure of 11 mm Hg, pulmonary artery wedge pressure of 10 mm Hg, and cardiac index (CI) of 2.1 L/min/m². The patient had a prolonged stay in the ICU and required continuous inotropes and chronotropes support. Her hospital course was further complicated by recurrent pericardial effusions and consequent cardiac tamponade, for which a pericardial window was undertaken along with hemoptysis that required bronchoscopy and cauterization.

The use of ECMO and reinitiation of PAH specific therapy slowly improved the patient's hemodynamic parameters (Figure 2 and Table 1). PAH specific therapy initially

TABLE 1: Hemodynamic measurements obtained after cardiac arrest and insertion of extracorporeal membrane oxygenation.

Swan Ganz parameters	POD 0	POD 1	POD 13	POD 20
CVP (mm Hg)	13	8	11	14
PASP (mm Hg)	139	110	114	89
PADP (mm Hg)	85	60	59	41
mPAP (mm Hg)	103	79	77	60
CO (l/min)	---	4.9	7.1	6.4
CI (l/m/m2)	----	3.2	4.5	4.1

CVP = central venous pressure, PASP = pulmonary artery systolic pressure, PADP = pulmonary artery diastolic pressure, mPAP = mean pulmonary artery pressure, CO = cardiac output, CI = cardiac index, SVR = systemic venous resistance, and SvO_2 = systemic venous oxygen saturation.

was limited to intravenous epoprostenol, but, upon normalization of LFTs, macitentan was initiated and as PA pressure gradually trended down to 80 mmHg and her blood pressure improved, sildenafil was added. Her requirement for vasopressors declined and she was gradually weaned off. Simultaneously, ECMO flow rates and support through VA ECMO continued to decrease and she was finally removed from ECMO support on postoperative day (POD) 24. With better control of PA pressures along with aggressive diuresis, ventilation improved and her fraction of inspired oxygen (FiO_2) requirements declined. However, due to prolonged intubation and unsuccessful weaning from mechanical ventilation, a tracheostomy was performed on POD 30. A subsequent ECHO demonstrated a RVSP of 69 mm Hg, cardiac output of 4.3 L/min, and CI of 2.5 L/min/m². After switching back to SC treprostinil, she was discharged from the hospital on POD 101, on the following regimen: ambrisentan 10 mg daily, SC treprostinil 30 ng/kg/min, sildenafil 20 mg three times daily, spironolactone 50 mg daily, and digoxin 62.5 mcg daily.

3. Discussion

PAH is defined as resting mPAP ≥ 25 mmHg with pulmonary artery wedge pressure (PCWP) ≤ 15 mm Hg and pulmonary vasculature resistance (PVR) > 3 Woods units [3–5]. Several physiologic changes occur during pregnancy, including an increase in intravascular plasma volume, stroke volume, and cardiac output [1]. Normal pulmonary vasculature responds to these changes to maintain a normal mPAP by decreasing PVR through vasodilation and recruiting previously nonperfused pulmonary vessels [6, 7]. However, in pregnant women with PAH, the pulmonary vasculature lacks the ability to mount this response due to increased endothelin activation along with nitric oxide and prostacyclin deficiency [6]. This places added stress on the already compromised cardiopulmonary system in PAH. The resultant right ventricular failure and cardiovascular collapse are the primary causes of high mortality in gravid patients with PAH [8].

With the use of PAH specific therapy, mortality has decreased in nongravid as well as pregnant females with PAH [7]. Current data suggests that mortality rates in pregnant women with PAH have declined from 50% to 17–33% [7, 9–14]. Despite this decrease, mortality in these patients still remains high, with the highest rates occurring postpartum [15]. Use of ECMO as a bridge to transplantation or recovery in patients with decompensated PAH has been reported in several cases [16–18]. In these patients, not only do targeted drug therapies prove to be inadequate, but their systemic vasodilator effect can potentially compound the worsening right ventricular failure and precipitate impending cardiogenic shock. Although limited, the use of extracorporeal life support in pregnancy and postpartum patients with cardiorespiratory failure has also been on the rise in the last five years [19, 20]. In reviewed cases, the overall maternal and fetal mortality was noted to be around 70% and 80%, respectively [21]. Despite this, there are no designated indications for the use of ECMO in pregnant or postpartum patients with PAH, which has been limited to managing cardiorespiratory collapse arising as a complication of various pathologies, not inclusive of PAH [19–21].

Hence, we report a novel method of managing PAH in the postpartum state. As demonstrated by our case, use of ECMO can help stabilize postpartum patients with PAH during a time when the PA pressures are at their peak and maternal mortality is at its highest. We believe that this can play an integral role in successfully managing the complicated hemodynamics in pregnant or postpartum patients with PAH.

Currently, recommendations for management of PAH in pregnancy and the postpartum state include monitoring by a multidisciplinary team, including PAH expert, high risk obstetrician, cardiothoracic surgeon, and anesthesiologist, along with early initiation of PAH specific therapy and close monitoring of fetus [7, 13]. Notably, while our patient had a favorable outcome, pregnancy in PAH patients carries a high risk to both mother and fetus. This holds true especially if management of pregnancy at an experienced PH center is not possible or accessible. Hence, per current guidelines, at time of diagnosis, PAH patients should be strongly dissuaded from becoming pregnant and be concurrently counseled regarding effective contraceptive methods. ECMO as an ancillary tool has not been explored in the management of the accompanying RHF and cardiopulmonary collapse in these high risk PAH patients. The unique risks associated with ECMO in the partum, peripartum, and postpartum period are not yet known, with concerns of both hypercoagulability and hemorrhage. However, as demonstrated by this case, the use of ECMO in pregnant PAH patients warrants further exploration.

Disclosure

This case report was presented at the annual meeting of American College of Chest Physicians on October 25, 2016.

References

[1] B. P. Madden, "Pulmonary hypertension and pregnancy," *International Journal of Obstetric Anesthesia*, vol. 18, no. 2, pp. 156–164, 2009.

[2] N. Galiè, M. Humbert, J. Vachiery et al., "2015 ESC/ERS Guidelines for the Diagnosis and Treatment of Pulmonary Hypertension: The Joint Task Force for the Diagnosis and Treatment of Pulmonary Hypertension of the European Society of Cardiology (ESC) and the European Respiratory Society (ERS): Endorsed By: Association for European Paediatric and Congenital Cardiology (AEPC), International Society for Heart and Lung Transplantation (ISHLT)," *European Respiratory Journal*, vol. 46, no. 4, pp. 903–975, 2015.

[3] M. M. Hoeper, H. J. Bogaard, and R. Condliffe, "Definitions and diagnosis of pulmonary hypertension," *Journal of the American College of Cardiology*, vol. 62, no. 25, pp. D42–D50, 2013.

[4] V. V. McLaughlin, S. L. Archer, D. B. Badesch et al., "ACCF/AHA 2009 expert consensus document on pulmonary hypertension: a report of the American College of Cardiology Foundation Task Force on Expert Consensus Documents and the American Heart Association: developed in collaboration with the American College of Chest Physicians, American Thoracic Society, Inc., and the Pulmonary Hypertension Association," *Circulation*, vol. 119, no. 16, pp. 2250–2294, 2009.

[5] N. Galiè, M. M. Hoeper, M. Humbert et al., "Guidelines for the diagnosis and treatment of pulmonary hypertension: The Task Force for the Diagnosis and Treatment of Pulmonary Hypertension of the European Society of Cardiology (ESC) and the European Respiratory Society (ERS), endorsed by the International Society of Heart and Lung Transplantation (ISHLT)," *European Heart Journal*, vol. 30, pp. 2493–2537, 2009.

[6] Z. Safdar, "Pulmonary arterial hypertension in pregnant women," *Therapeutic Advances in Respiratory Disease*, vol. 7, no. 1, pp. 51–63, 2013.

[7] A. R. Hemnes, D. G. Kiely, B. A. Cockrill et al., "Statement on pregnancy in pulmonary hypertension from the pulmonary

vascular research institute," *Pulmonary Circulation*, vol. 5, no. 3, pp. 435–465, 2015.

[8] A. Gei and C. Montufar-Rueda, "Pulmonary hypertension and pregnancy: An overview," *Clinical Obstetrics and Gynecology*, vol. 57, no. 4, pp. 806–826, 2014.

[9] B. M. Weiss, L. Zemp, B. Seifert, and O. M. Hess, "Outcome of pulmonary vascular disease in pregnancy: A systematic overview from 1978 through 1996," *Journal of the American College of Cardiology*, vol. 31, no. 7, pp. 1650–1657, 1998.

[10] E. Bédard, K. Dimopoulos, and M. A. Gatzoulis, "Has there been any progress made on pregnancy outcomes among women with pulmonary arterial hypertension?" *European Heart Journal*, vol. 30, no. 3, pp. 256–265, 2009.

[11] D. G. Kiely, R. Condliffe, V. Webster et al., "Improved survival in pregnancy and pulmonary hypertension using a multiprofessional approach," *BJOG: An International Journal of Obstetrics & Gynaecology*, vol. 117, no. 5, pp. 565–574, 2010.

[12] X. Jaïs, K. M. Olsson, J. A. Barbera et al., "Pregnancy outcomes in pulmonary arterial hypertension in the modern management era," *European Respiratory Journal*, vol. 40, no. 4, pp. 881–885, 2012.

[13] A. G. Duarte, S. Thomas, Z. Safdar et al., "Management of pulmonary arterial hypertension during pregnancy: A retrospective, multicenter experience," *CHEST*, vol. 143, no. 5, pp. 1330–1336, 2013.

[14] S. Katsuragi, K. Yamanaka, R. Neki et al., "Maternal outcome in pregnancy complicated with pulmonary arterial hypertension," *Circulation Journal*, vol. 76, no. 9, pp. 2249–2254, 2012.

[15] J. Shaun Smith, J. Mueller, and C. J. Daniels, "Pulmonary arterial hypertension in the setting of pregnancy: A case series and standard treatment approach," *Lung*, vol. 190, no. 2, pp. 155–160, 2012.

[16] E. B. Rosenzweig, D. Brodie, D. C. Abrams, C. L. Agerstrand, and M. Bacchetta, "Extracorporeal membrane oxygenation as a novel bridging strategy for acute right heart failure in group 1 pulmonary arterial hypertension," *ASAIO Journal*, vol. 60, no. 1, pp. 129–133, 2014.

[17] D. C. Abrams, D. Brodie, E. B. Rosenzweig, K. M. Burkart, C. L. Agerstrand, and M. D. Bacchetta, "Upper-body extracorporeal membrane oxygenation as a strategy in decompensated pulmonary arterial hypertension," *Pulmonary Circulation*, vol. 3, no. 2, pp. 432–435, 2013.

[18] M.-T. Tsai, C.-H. Hsu, C.-Y. Luo, Y.-N. Hu, and J.-N. Roan, "Bridge-to-recovery strategy using extracorporeal membrane oxygenation for critical pulmonary hypertension complicated with cardiogenic shock," *Interactive CardioVascular and Thoracic Surgery*, vol. 21, no. 1, pp. 55–61, 2015.

[19] C. Agerstrand, D. Abrams, M. Biscotti et al., "Extracorporeal membrane oxygenation for cardiopulmonary failure during pregnancy and postpartum," *The Annals of Thoracic Surgery*, vol. 102, no. 3, pp. 774–779, 2016.

[20] S. A. Moore, C. A. Dietl, and D. M. Coleman, "Extracorporeal life support during pregnancy," *The Journal of Thoracic and Cardiovascular Surgery*, vol. 151, no. 4, pp. 1154–1160, 2016.

[21] N. S. Sharma, K. M. Wille, S. C. Bellot, and E. Diaz-Guzman, "Modern use of extracorporeal life support in pregnancy and postpartum," *ASAIO Journal*, vol. 61, no. 1, pp. 110–114, 2015.

43

Streptococcus intermedius Causing Necrotizing Pneumonia in an Immune Competent Female: A Case Report and Literature Review

Faris Hannoodi, Israa Ali, Hussam Sabbagh, and Sarwan Kumar

Crittenton Hospital, 1101 W. University Drive, 2 South, Rochester, MI 48307, USA

Correspondence should be addressed to Faris Hannoodi; fh.saint@hotmail.com

Academic Editor: Tun-Chieh Chen

We report a case of a 52-year-old immunocompetent Caucasian female treated for necrotizing *Streptococcus intermedius* pneumonia and review available literature of similar cases. Our patient presented with respiratory failure and required hospitalization and treatment in the intensive care unit. Moreover, she required surgical drainage of right lung empyema as well as decortication and resection. The review of literature revealed three cases of *S. intermedius* pneumonia, one of which was a mortality. Comparison of the published cases showed a highly varied prehospital course and radiological presentations, with a symptomatic phase ranging from 10 days to five months. Radiological findings varied from an isolated pleural effusion to systemic disease with the presence of brain abscesses. Immunocompetence appears to correlate well with the overall prognosis. In addition, smoking appears to be an important risk factor for *S. intermedius* pneumonia. In 2 (50%) of cases, pleural fluid analysis identified *S. intermedius*. In contrast, no organism was found in our patient, necessitating the acquisition of lung tissue sample for the diagnosis. In conclusion, both medical and surgical management are necessary for effective treatment of *S. intermedius* pneumonia. The outcome of treatment is good in immunocompetent individuals.

1. Introduction

Streptococcus intermedius is part of the *Streptococcus anginosus* subgroup (formerly *Streptococcus milleri*) [1–4]. It is a Gram-positive, catalase negative coccus that is nonmotile and is a facultative anaerobe [5]. They are normally found as part of the oral cavity and the gastrointestinal tract [4, 6, 7]. Although bacteria of the *S. anginosus* group are known to cause abscesses and systemic infections, *S. intermedius* pneumonia is rare and there are very few reported cases. We report an interesting case of necrotizing pneumonia in an immunocompetent patient caused by *S. intermedius* and we also review published cases in the reported literature.

2. Case Summary

A 52-year-old immunocompetent Caucasian female with a past medical history of asthma, that is only treated with albuterol rescue inhaler, and who is also an ex-smoker was transferred from the urgent care clinic to the emergency department (ED). She presented with shortness of breath with minimal activity and low oxygen saturation. Her prior symptoms were coughing and sputum production (greenish, thick, and nonbloody) for 6 weeks. She had been treated for community acquired pneumonia as an outpatient by her primary care physician and in an urgent care clinic. She was initially treated with oral erythromycin for a week. Two weeks following that, she received a week's course of ciprofloxacin. Her symptoms, however, failed to improve.

Her vitals at presentation were temperature: 99.8°F, HR: 130 BPM, BP: 113/59 mmHg, RR: 36, and SpO2: 84% on room air. She was in severe respiratory distress and unable to complete a sentence without pausing or coughing. Lung exam findings included diminished breath sounds on the right lung base and rhonchi and crackles throughout both lungs on auscultation. ABGs showed pH 7.32, pCO_2 33, and pO_2 69 on 36% FiO_2. The blood test results can be seen in Table 1, most significant of which is the leukocytosis. The extent of the pneumonic process is demonstrated in the images presented in Figure 1.

(a)

(b)

(c)

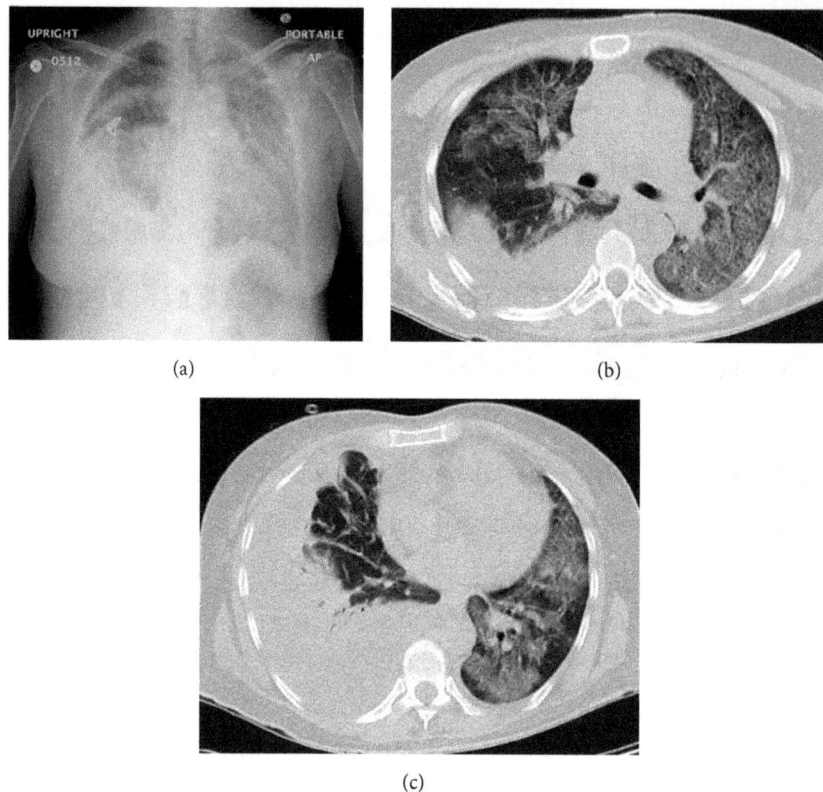

Figure 1: Chest X-ray (a) shows bilateral multilobar lung infiltrate with the appearance of loculated right pleural effusion. CT scan of the chest shows patchy airway disease throughout the upper lung lobes (b) as well as lower lung lobes (c).

Table 1: Blood test results.

Glu	108	mg/dL
Na	142	mEq/L
K	3.0	mEq/L
Cl	108	mEq/L
HCO_3^-	14.5	mEq/L
AG	19.5	
BUN	27.0	mg/dL
Cr	1.1	mg/dL
GFR	52	
Lactate	1.9	mmol/L
WBC	29.2	$10^3/\mu L$
Neu	95	%
Lym	3.5	%
Mon	1.3	%
Eos	0.2	%
Hgb	11.4	g/dL
Plt	428	$10^3/\mu L$

AG: anion gap and GFR: glomerular filtration rate.

The patient was transferred to the intensive care unit and started empirically on aztreonam, vancomycin, and azithromycin with high flow oxygen. The patient's blood cultures, fungal cultures, legionella antigen and pleural fluid Gram staining, acid fast staining, and culture were all negative. Decortication, resection of the right upper lung lobe, and drainage of the empyema were performed on the third day of hospitalization and a chest tube was inserted.

Histology of the lung tissue sample showed acute and chronic pneumonitis with large areas of organization, focal abscess formation, and palisaded necrotizing granulomata. Special staining did not show any organisms. Culture of the tissue sample did grow *Streptococcus intermedius*, however. The organism was penicillin sensitive, but the patient has penicillin allergy. She was therefore given IV ceftriaxone, since beta-lactams have higher efficacy against streptococci than vancomycin. The patient was treated for a total of 14 days in hospital with IV antibiotics, of which, 7 days were in the intensive care unit.

3. Discussion

A search through PubMed and Google Scholar yielded only three reported cases of pneumonia caused by *S. intermedius*. All of the published cases are of male patients. 2 (67%) of the published cases are for patients in their 50s. Our case appears to be the only female patient. The immunocompetence of two of the reported cases is not mentioned. One case states the patient denies having risk factors for HIV [10]. Alcoholic liver cirrhosis is noted to be one of the conditions in one of the patients [9], which is a predisposing factor to infection as it

TABLE 2: Published cases of *Streptococcus intermedius* data.

Case	Our case	1 [8]	2 [9]	3 [10]
Age	52	79	55	52
Gender	F	M	M	M
Radiological diagnosis	Bilateral pneumonia, loculated right pleural effusion	Left upper lobe pneumonia and left pleural empyema	Right upper lobe pneumonia, bilateral brain abscesses	Loculated left pleural effusion
Duration of respiratory symptoms	6 weeks	—	10 days	5 months
Past medical history	Asthma	Surgical drainage of right empyema 4 months prior	Alcoholic liver cirrhosis	Hypertension, hyperlipidemia, and poor dental hygiene
Smoker status	Ex-smoker	Ex-smoker	—	Active smoker
Systolic blood pressure (mmHg)	113	104	—	125
Heart rate	110	118	—	93
Respiratory rate	36	—	—	—
Oxygen saturations	84% on room air	93% on 3 L	—	—
Temperature	99.8°F (37.7°C)	101.1°F (38.4°C)	101.3°F (38.5°C)	98.0°F (36.7°C)
Initial WBC	29.2	39.6	—	Normal (no number given)
Initial empiric antibiotics	Aztreonam, vancomycin + azithromycin	Meropenem	Ceftriaxone + ampicillin	Levofloxacin + clindamycin
Targeted antibiotics	Ceftriaxone	Meropenem	—	Levofloxacin
Total duration of antibiotics	14 days	14 days	—	24
Surgical intervention	Decortication, resection of right upper lung lobe and chest tube insertion	Left pleurectomy and chest tube insertion	Video-assisted thoracoscopic biopsy	Thoracocentesis and chest tube insertion
Outcome	Survived	Survived	Died	Survived

leads to immune system dysfunction and relative immunoincompetence [11] (*refer to Table 2*).

The duration of symptoms for *S. intermedius* prior to hospitalization is highly variable, ranging from 10 days to 5 months. In one of the cases, the patient had empyema drained 4 months prior to presentation, though the responsible organism is not mentioned [8]. The radiological findings were also varied, ranging from presence of isolated pleural effusion to pneumonia with abscesses. This is consistent with the organism's property of causing local as well as systemic abscesses [6, 7].

As we can see in Table 2, there is one risk factor that most of the cases appear to share: a history of smoking. In general, smoking is a risk factor for pulmonary infections as it impairs ciliary function and increases mucous increases [12]. The patients appear to be hemodynamically stable on presentation, but they also have respiratory compromise and meet the criteria for a positive systemic inflammatory response. Fever is not always present even in severe respiratory disease as demonstrated in our case, neither is an elevated WBC as seen in one of the reported cases [10].

Treatment duration with antibiotics in our case and in one of the reported cases was 14 days, though in another it was 24 days [10]. *S. intermedius* appears to be sensitive to beta-lactam antibiotics, though some cases of resistance have been reported [13]. In penicillin allergic patients, vancomycin is suggested as an alternative [14]. All the patients had a form of procedural intervention performed. This is expected as 3 (75%) of the patients had empyema with some form of loculation that necessitated drainage. Only one (25%) of the patients in the reported cases died from the pneumonia. This may be attributable to the concomitant presence of brain abscesses and liver cirrhosis [9].

As presented in Table 3, all of the cases that had a pleural fluid sample from the patient show it to be an exudate as LDH is >1000, meeting Light's criteria as well as the two-test and three-test rules [15, 16]. In both cases 1 and 3, organisms were identified in pleural fluid culture. In case 1, *S. intermedius* was identified following PCR and a homology search on the culture of the pleural fluid. In contrast, no organisms were identified in either pleural fluid microscopy or culture from the sample taken from our patient. The diagnosis was

TABLE 3: Published cases of *Streptococcus intermedius* pleural fluid and tissue analysis.

Case	Our case	1 [8]	2 [9]	3 [10]
Total protein (g/dL)	4.0	4.3	—	4.2
LDH	1372	2873	—	6280
Glucose (mg/dL)	93	1.0	—	10
Gram staining	No organisms	No organisms	—	—
Pleural fluid culture	No growth	*S. anginosus* group	—	*S. intermedius*
Tissue histology	Necrotizing pneumonia, culture: *S. intermedius*	—	Necrotizing pneumonia, culture: *S. intermedius*	—

Case 2 did not have a pleural fluid sample; *S. anginosus*: *Streptococcus anginosus*.

instead made by lung tissue sample culture. This shows that even when no organism is identified in the pleural fluid, *S. intermedius* can still be the etiologic agent. In both case 2 and in our case, histology of the lung tissue revealed necrotizing pneumonia, signifying the severity of disease caused by this organism (*refer to Table 3*).

4. Conclusion

To sum up, *Streptococcus intermedius* pneumonia has a wide-ranging prehospital incubation period, presentation, and radiological findings. Nonetheless, it is clear from both our case and the reported cases that *S. intermedius* causes severe disease that requires medical as well as surgical management to be treated effectively. Moreover, if pleural fluid microscopy and culture are negative, efforts should be made to obtain a lung tissue sample for microscopy and culture to identify the bacterium. Despite the severity of the disease, *S. intermedius* pneumonia shows good sensitivity to broad-spectrum antibiotics such as beta-lactams. As a result, patients have a good prognosis provided that they are immunocompetent.

Competing Interests

The authors declare no competing interests.

Authors' Contributions

Faris Hannoodi was the main author, drafted most of the manuscript, and reviewed published literature, Israa Ali helped in drafting manuscript, Hussam Sabbagh helped in drafting manuscript, and Sarwan Kumar helped in drafting manuscript and revised its material. All authors read and approved the final manuscript.

References

[1] K. L. Ruoff, "Streptococcus anginosus ('Streptococcus milleri'): the unrecognized pathogen," *Clinical Microbiology Reviews*, vol. 1, no. 1, pp. 102–108, 1988.

[2] R. A. Whiley and D. Beighton, "Emended descriptions and recognition of *Streptococcus constellatus*, *Streptococcus intermedius*, and *Streptococcus anginosus* as distinct species,"

International Journal of Systematic and Evolutionary Microbiology, vol. 41, no. 1, pp. 1–5, 1991.

[3] R. A. Whiley, D. Beighton, T. G. Winstanley, H. Y. Fraser, and J. M. Hardie, "Streptococcus intermedius, *Streptococcus constellatus*, and *Streptococcus anginosus* (the Streptococcus milleri group): association with different body sites and clinical infections," *Journal of Clinical Microbiology*, vol. 30, no. 1, pp. 243–244, 1992.

[4] J. E. Clarridge III, S. Attorri, D. M. Musher, J. Hebert, and S. Dunbar, "Streptococcus intermedius, *Streptococcus constellatus*, and *Streptococcus anginosus* ('Streptococcus milleri group') are of different clinical importance and are not equally associated with abscess," *Clinical Infectious Diseases*, vol. 32, no. 10, pp. 1511–1515, 2001.

[5] R. A. Whiley, H. Fraser, J. M. Hardie, and D. Beighton, "Phenotypic differentiation of *Streptococcus intermedius*, *Streptococcus constellatus*, and *Streptococcus anginosus* strains within the 'Streptococcus milleri group'," *Journal of Clinical Microbiology*, vol. 28, no. 7, pp. 1497–1501, 1990.

[6] B. Mejàre, "Characteristics of Streptococcus milleri and Streptococcus mitior from infected dental root canals," *Odontologisk Revy*, vol. 26, no. 4, pp. 291–308, 1975.

[7] M. T. Parker and L. C. Ball, "Streptococci and aerococci associated with systemic infection in man," *Journal of Medical Microbiology*, vol. 9, no. 3, pp. 275–302, 1976.

[8] S. Noguchi, K. Yatera, T. Kawanami et al., "Pneumonia and empyema caused by *Streptococcus intermedius* that shows the diagnostic importance of evaluating the microbiota in the lower respiratory tract," *Internal Medicine*, vol. 53, no. 1, pp. 47–50, 2014.

[9] R. Khatib, J. Ramanathan, and J. Baran Jr., "Streptococcus intermedius: a cause of lobar pneumonia with meningitis and brain abscesses," *Clinical Infectious Diseases*, vol. 30, no. 2, pp. 396–397, 2000.

[10] S. B. Iskandar, M. A. Al Hasan, T. M. Roy, and R. P. Byrd Jr., "Streptococcus intermedius: an unusual cause of a primary empyema," *Tennessee Medicine: Journal of the Tennessee Medical Association*, vol. 99, no. 2, pp. 37–39, 2006.

[11] M. Dirchwolf, A. Podhorzer, M. Marino et al., "Immune dysfunction in cirrhosis: distinct cytokines phenotypes according to cirrhosis severity," *Cytokine*, vol. 77, pp. 14–25, 2016.

[12] T. W. Marcy and W. W. Merrill, "Cigarette smoking and respiratory tract infection," *Clinics in Chest Medicine*, vol. 8, no. 3, pp. 381–391, 1987.

[13] M. Tracy, A. Wanahita, Y. Shuhatovich, E. A. Goldsmith, J. E. Clarridge III, and D. M. Musher, "Antibiotic susceptibilities of

genetically characterized *Streptococcus milleri* group strains," *Antimicrobial Agents and Chemotherapy*, vol. 45, no. 5, pp. 1511–1514, 2001.

[14] C. Bantar, L. F. Canigia, S. Relloso, A. Lanza, H. Bianchini, and J. Smayevsky, "Species belonging to the 'Streptococcus milleri' group: antimicrobial susceptibility and comparative prevalence in significant clinical specimens," *Journal of Clinical Microbiology*, vol. 34, no. 8, pp. 2020–2022, 1996.

[15] R. W. Light, M. I. Macgregor, P. C. Luchsinger, and W. C. Ball Jr., "Pleural effusions: the diagnostic separation of transudates and exudates," *Annals of Internal Medicine*, vol. 77, no. 4, pp. 507–513, 1972.

[16] J. E. Heffner, L. K. Brown, and C. A. Barbieri, "Diagnostic value of tests that discriminate between exudative and transudative pleural effusions," *Chest*, vol. 111, no. 4, pp. 970–980, 1997.

44

Subcutaneous and Pulmonary Dirofilariasis with Evidence of Splenic Involvement

Adarsha Selvachandran and Raymond J. Foley

Division of Pulmonary/Critical Care, UConn Health, 263 Farmington Avenue, Farmington, CT 06030-1321, USA

Correspondence should be addressed to Raymond J. Foley; rfoley@uchc.edu

Academic Editor: Tatsuo Kawashima

Cases of human dirofilariasis have been reported in several countries around the world, including a large number in the Atlantic and Gulf Coast regions of the United States. Most commonly, these cases have subcutaneous or pulmonary involvement; however, there have been few reports of dirofilariasis involving structures such as large vessels, mesentery, the spermatic cord, and liver. We present a case of an unusual presentation of human dirofilariasis presenting as a shoulder abscess and what is presumed to be pulmonary and splenic involvement in a 55-year-old female.

1. Introduction

Dirofilaria immitis, colloquially known as the dog heartworm, is a nematode that utilizes dogs as its natural host. Humans serve as a dead-end host for *D. immitis*. In dogs, *D. immitis* exists as a mature worm in the right ventricle and pulmonary arteries. Cases of human dirofilariasis have been reported in several countries [1]. These case reports have described dirofilariasis involvement in multiple anatomic structures [2]. The mature female adult produces microfilariae that can be found in the dog's blood. When mosquitos feed on the dog, the microfilariae are ingested with the blood meal. The microfilariae then mature into larvae within the mosquito and ultimately migrate to the mosquito's proboscis. When the mosquito takes its next blood meal, it acts as a vector. The larvae leave the proboscis and enter the bite wound. When the vector mosquito takes a blood meal from a human, transmission of *D. immitis* to a dead-end human host would occur, provided the larva finds its way into the bite wound (see Figure 1) [3].

2. Case Presentation

A 55-year-old female initially sought medical attention for abdominal pain following a hernia repair. On presentation, her physical exam and routine bloodwork (including a complete blood count and chemistry profile) were entirely normal. She subsequently underwent additional diagnostic testing. The abdominal computerized tomography (CT) scan demonstrated multiple splenic hypodensities along with a left lower lobe nodule (see Figure 2). For this reason, the patient subsequently underwent a dedicated chest CT scan for further evaluation. The chest CT scan revealed multiple nodules involving the right and left lung (see Figure 3). Based upon these imaging findings, our initial differential diagnosis included hemangiomas, lymphoma, fungal infection, sarcoidosis, splenic infarctions, and metastatic nodules. The patient's past medical history was positive for a surgical excision of a right shoulder mass 2 years earlier. The pathology report revealed evidence of *D. immitis* within the shoulder mass. Additionally, she was a lifetime nonsmoker who resided in Connecticut and had no exposure to dogs at home. Her family history was noncontributory.

After the acute episode of her abdominal pain resolved, the patient underwent additional evaluation. Her laboratory data showed that the liver function tests were within normal limits. Serum protein electrophoresis was within normal limits. Serologic testing including *Aspergillus* antigen, *Cryptococcus* antigen, and *Histoplasma* antigen was negative.

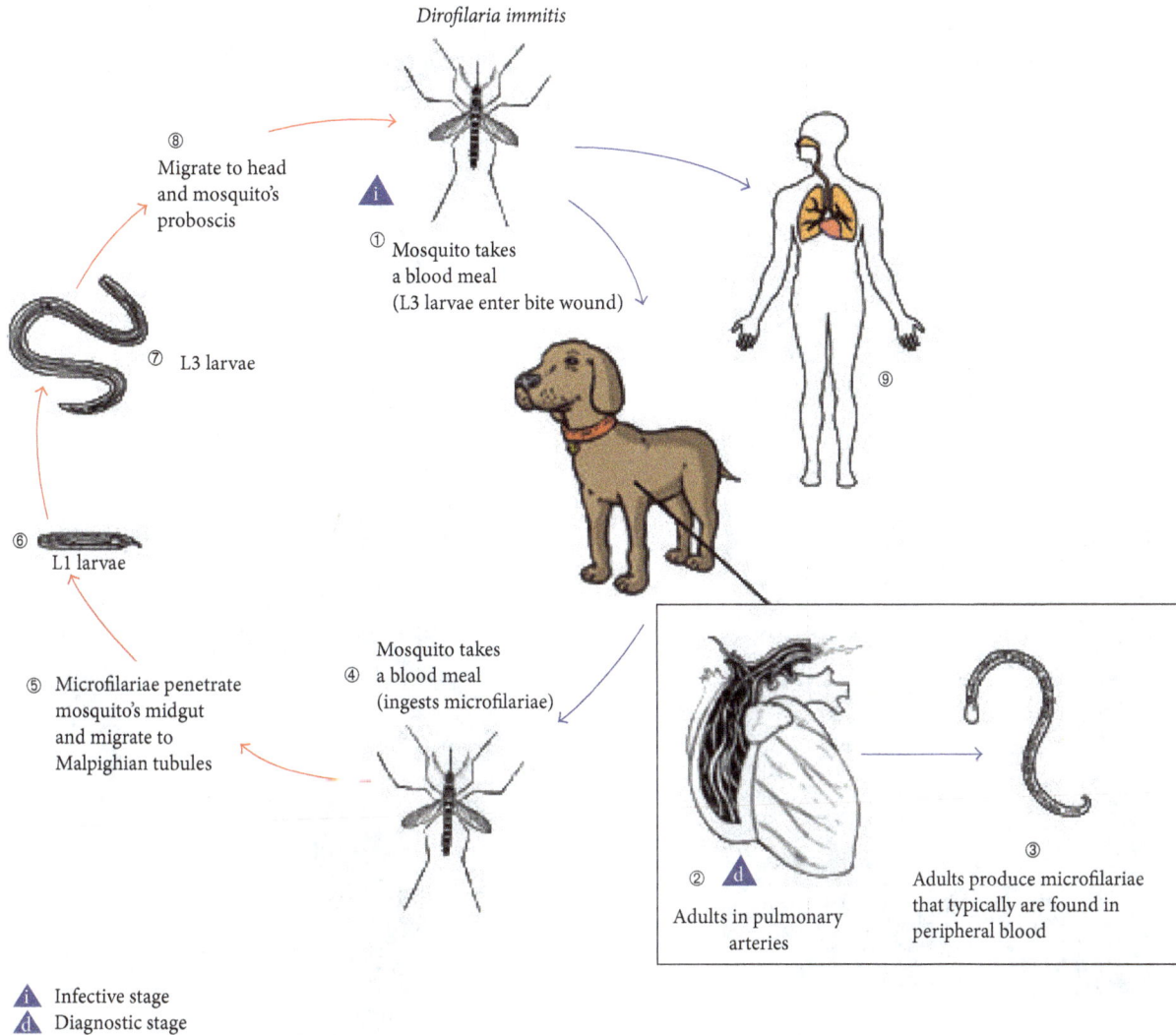

Dirofilaria immitis

⑧ Migrate to head and mosquito's proboscis

ⓘ

① Mosquito takes a blood meal (L3 larvae enter bite wound)

⑦ L3 larvae

⑥ L1 larvae

⑤ Microfilariae penetrate mosquito's midgut and migrate to Malpighian tubules

④ Mosquito takes a blood meal (ingests microfilariae)

② Adults in pulmonary arteries

ⓓ

③ Adults produce microfilariae that typically are found in peripheral blood

⑨

ⓘ Infective stage
ⓓ Diagnostic stage

FIGURE 1: Biology-life cycle of *D. immitis* [1].

Bone marrow aspiration and biopsy showed normal cellular bone marrow with maturing trilineage hematopoiesis. There was no evidence of any granulomatous or lymphoproliferative processes.

A transthoracic echocardiogram showed normal left and right ventricular size and function. There were also findings of minimal tricuspid valve regurgitation and mitral valve thickening. A repeated transthoracic echocardiogram with bubble study did not reveal a patent foramen ovale (PFO) or atrial septal defect. Although not conclusively proven by a splenic biopsy, the cardiologist consultant's impression was that there was no cardiac cause for the presence of *D. immitis* in the splenic system. Follow-up chest, abdomen, and pelvis CT scan 6 months later showed stable to slightly decreased size and appearance of the splenic hypodensities and no evidence of new active disease in the abdomen or pelvis. Chest CT showed stable right and left nodules.

Following this extensive evaluation, the patient was deemed to be clinically and radiologically stable. A repeated chest CT scan was ordered 1 year later in order to ensure stability. The CT scan confirmed the stability of the pulmonary nodules with no changes to heart size and no evidence of mediastinal or hilar lymphadenopathy.

3. Discussion

The interesting aspect of this patient's presentation is the presence of the splenic hypodensities and multiple pulmonary nodules. Published reviews have shown that 75–95% of pulmonary dirofilariasis presents as a single granuloma, which was not the case in this patient [4]. As previously described, *D. immitis* normally enters the blood stream as larvae and migrates to the right ventricle where it develops into a sexually immature worm. When it dies, it is washed into the pulmonary artery and embolizes [5]. Typically the embolization of the deceased worm into the pulmonary arterial tree results in lesions at the lung periphery [6]. In this case, however, the splenic hypodensities indicate that the

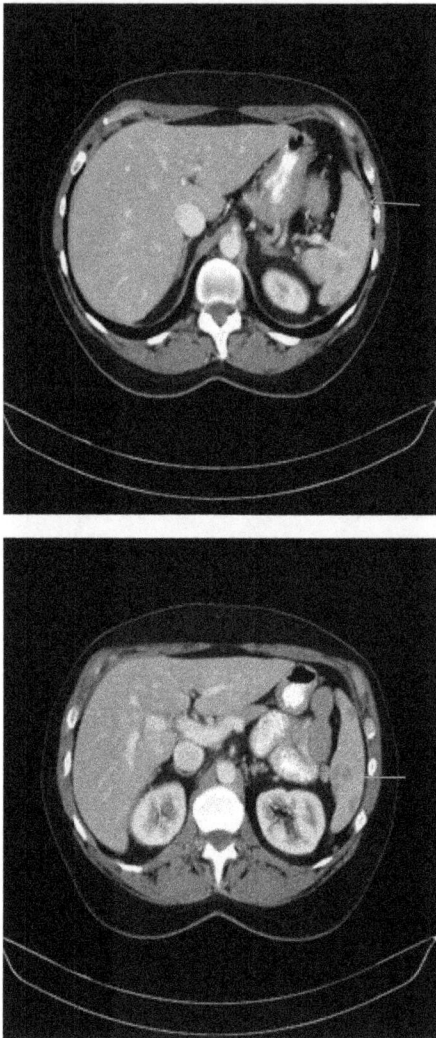

FIGURE 2: Abdominal imaging, revealing multiple splenic hypodensities.

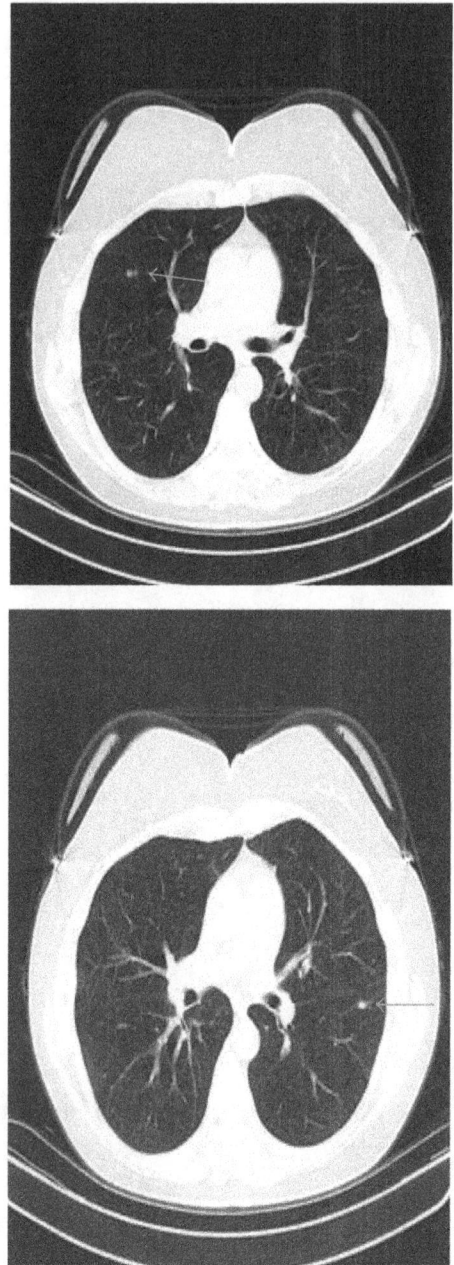

FIGURE 3: Chest CT scan, revealing bilateral nodules.

embolization of the immature adult worm somehow entered the systemic circulation rather than remaining isolated to the pulmonary circulation. The cause of this unusual finding has yet to be reported in the medical literature.

The first explanation under consideration is a cardiac defect, which is why an echocardiogram was pursued. The thought process was that if the patient had PFO or a septal defect, there would be a venue through which an adult worm in the right ventricle could be embolized and enter both the pulmonary circulation and the systemic circulation to end up in the spleen. As reported, the patient had no evidence of such defect on color Doppler or on bubble study, making this explanation less likely. A second explanation could be that there was dissemination of the worm during surgical excision of the patient's right shoulder mass.

Although in this case neither the splenic nor pulmonary lesions were biopsied, the stability of the lesions in conjunction with the patient's history of subcutaneous dirofilariasis makes dirofilariasis the most likely explanation. These lesions have been described in the literature to be well circumscribed

and yellowish-grey in color, with normal lung parenchyma surrounding the lesion when biopsied. Microscopic pathology has been reported to show a central zone of necrosis, with a granulomatous zone with epithelial cells, plasma cells, lymphocytes, and a few scattered giant cells and an outer layer of fibrous tissue. Additionally, fragmented, necrotic portions of the embolized worm have been reported (see Figure 4) [7].

The most common symptom reported has been cough, with a lesser incidence of chest pain, fever, and hemoptysis. [7] In cases of human pulmonary dirofilariasis, medical treatment against the parasite is not indicated as the fragment of the worm has already been encapsulated by the immune system.

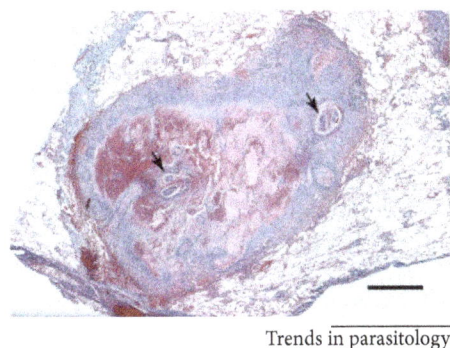

Trends in parasitology

FIGURE 4: Courtesy of trends in parasitology: a coin lesion excised from a human lung showing a well-demarcated granuloma. Cross sections of the worm are highlighted by the black arrows [8].

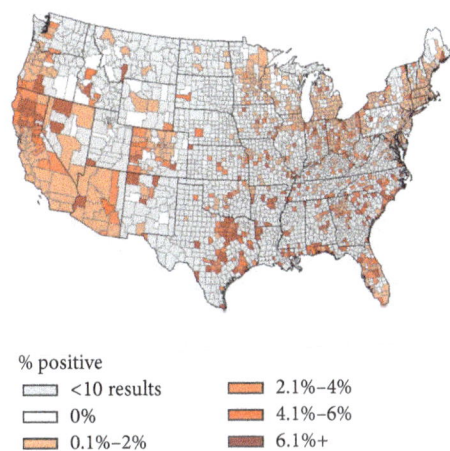

% positive
- <10 results
- 0%
- 0.1%–2%
- 2.1%–4%
- 4.1%–6%
- 6.1%+

FIGURE 5: Courtesy of veterinary parasitology: US distribution of dogs testing positive for *D. immitis* antigen [8].

A literature search for cases of human splenic dirofilariasis yielded no results to date. Although not conclusively proven, the splenic hypodensities can be assumed to be related to the presence of *Dirofilaria* in the splenic system. In the literature, other sites (including liver, lung, subcutaneous tissue, large vessels, peritoneal cavity, and spermatic cord) [2] have been reported.

Ethical Approval

Adarsha Selvachandran and Dr. Foley vouch for scientific integrity of the study and explicitly confirm that the paper meets the highest ethical standards for authorship.

Competing Interests

The authors have stated that they have no competing interests.

Authors' Contributions

Dr. Foley is the sole contributor to this paper.

References

[1] A. Biswas, P. Reilly, A. Perez, and M. H. Yassin, "Human pulmonary dirofilariasis presenting as a solitary pulmonary nodule: a case report and a brief review of literature," *Respiratory Medicine Case Reports*, vol. 10, pp. 40–42, 2013.

[2] M. K. Kim, C. H. Kim, B. W. Yeom, S. H. Park, S. Y. Choi, and J. S. Choi, "The first human case of hepatic dirofilariasis," *Journal of Korean Medical Science*, vol. 17, no. 5, pp. 686–690, 2002.

[3] "Biology-Life Cycle of D. immitis," Centers for Disease Control and Prevention, 2012, http://www.cdc.gov/parasites/dirofilariasis/biology_d_immitis.html.

[4] A. C. Y. Lee, S. P. Montgomery, J. H. Theis, B. L. Blagburn, and M. L. Eberhard, "Public health issues concerning the widespread distribution of canine heartworm disease," *Trends in Parasitology*, vol. 26, no. 4, pp. 168–173, 2010.

[5] J. R. M. de Campos, C. S. V. Barbas, L. T. B. Filomeno et al., "Human pulmonary dirofilariasis: analysis of 24 cases from Sao Paulo, Brazil," *Chest*, vol. 112, no. 3, pp. 729–733, 1997.

[6] T. Miyoshi, H. Tsubouchi, A. Iwasaki, T. Shiraishi, K. Nabeshima, and T. Shirakusa, "Human pulmonary dirofilariasis: a case report and review of the recent Japanese literature," *Respirology*, vol. 11, no. 3, pp. 343–347, 2006.

[7] P. J. Asimacopoulos, A. Katras, and B. Christie, "Pulmonary dirofilariasis: the largest single-hospital experience," *Chest*, vol. 102, no. 3, pp. 851–855, 1992.

[8] D. Bowman, S. E. Little, L. Lorentzen, J. Shields, M. P. Sullivan, and E. P. Carlin, "Prevalence and geographic distribution of *Dirofilaria immitis, Borrelia burgdorferi, Ehrlichia canis*, and *Anaplasma phagocytophilum* in dogs in the United States: results of a national clinic-based serologic survey," *Veterinary Parasitology*, vol. 160, no. 1-2, pp. 138–148, 2009.

From a diagnostic perspective, video-assisted thoracoscopic biopsy is the most direct technique for diagnosing human pulmonary dirofilariasis as less invasive serologic testing is not currently available [4]. In the past, thoracotomy with wedge resection was employed in cases where malignancy was considered and needed to be ruled out.

Risk factors for dirofilariasis in humans are dependent on the size of the dog population, the prevalence of canine dirofilariasis in the population (see Figure 5), and the density of vector mosquitos in the area. Most reported cases of human dirofilariasis are in areas where there is a high prevalence of canine dirofilariasis. As such, clinicians in these areas should be aware of the presence of dirofilariasis and entertain this entity on their differential diagnosis of pulmonary nodules. Awareness of dirofilariasis is important as it may decrease the amount of invasive testing and procedures the patient may undergo and thereby decrease healthcare-related costs.

As the patient was asymptomatic at follow-up, surgical intervention for these stable pulmonary and splenic lesions was deemed to be unnecessary (unlike the subcutaneous lesion in her right shoulder which required surgical resection for both diagnostic purposes and resolution of her pain).

45

Primary Pulmonary Meningioma Simulating a Pulmonary Metastasis

Chun-Mao Juan,[1] Mei-Ling Chen,[2] Shang-Yun Ho,[1] and Yuan-Chun Huang[1]

[1]*Department of Medical Imaging, Changhua Christian Hospital, No. 135 Nanxiao St., Changhua 500, Taiwan*
[2]*Department of Pathology, Changhua Christian Hospital, No. 135 Nanxiao St., Changhua 500, Taiwan*

Correspondence should be addressed to Yuan-Chun Huang; 168we888@gmail.com

Academic Editor: Daniel T. Merrick

Primary pulmonary meningiomas represent a rare tumor entity. Few cases have been reported in the English medical literature, and they have almost all been solitary and benign in nature, with the exception of several extremely rare cases. We report herein a case of PPM that raised suspicion of a pulmonary metastatic tumor initially, as it was depicted as a single, round, small, ground-glass opacity pulmonary nodule on a chest computed tomography scan, in a 55-year-old man with a history of buccal cancer. Increased awareness of the clinical and radiologic characteristics of this rare category can assist a multidisciplinary team to perform adequate management.

1. Introduction

Primary pulmonary meningiomas (PPMs) are rare tumors and only sporadic cases have been reported. Most PPMs are solitary pulmonary nodules, incidentally detected on chest plain film or chest computed tomography (CT). We report a case of PPM herein, which raised suspicion of a pulmonary metastatic tumor initially.

2. Case Report

A 55-year-old man was referred to our Chest Department due to abnormal pulmonary nodules located in the left upper and lower lung lobes, which were detected on a chest CT scan. He had a past history of left buccal cancer without distant metastasis more than ten years ago, for which he received surgery and local radiotherapy. He underwent regular follow-up by contrast-enhanced CT scanning of the head and neck without local recurrence. With the exception of buccal cancer, the patient denied any history of other neurologic or pulmonary disorders. He underwent a health examination, and a chest CT scan revealed a 4.5 mm ground-glass opacity nodule in the left upper lobe and a 16 mm part-solid ground-glass nodule in the left lower lobe of the lung (Figure 1). Three

months later, the pulmonary lesions did not show regression in a follow-up chest CT. Due to a history of buccal cancer, the patient underwent thoracoscopic wedge resection of the pulmonary nodules owing to concern regarding pulmonary metastasis, with an uneventful recovery.

In histopathological study, the nodular lesion in the left lower lobe of the lung proved to be granulomatous inflammation. Microscopically, the tumor in the left upper lobe of the lung was composed of nests of round to spindle-shaped cells, which presented in a focal whorl pattern (Figure 2). The tumor cells showed clear cytoplasm and round and oval nuclei, with a delicate chromatin distribution and some intranuclear inclusions. They did not demonstrate mitotic figures nor atypia. Immunohistochemical staining demonstrated consistent expressions of epithelial membrane antigen (EMA), progesterone receptors (PR), and CD56 in the tumor cells. Conversely, the results of tests for S-100 protein, human melanin black 45 (HMB45), synaptophysin, and melan-A were negative. Finally, a histological diagnosis of pulmonary meningioma without characteristics of malignancy was made according to the above-described morphological and immunohistochemical features. Central nervous system surveys revealed negative findings. No tumor recurrence was observed in the 6-month follow-up CT study.

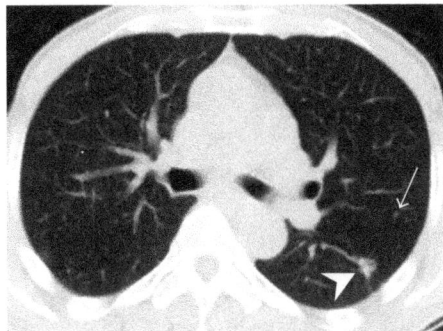

FIGURE 1: Axial chest computed tomography scan at subcarinal level demonstrates a 4.5 mm ground-glass opacity nodule in left upper lobe of lung (arrow) and a 16 mm part-solid ground-glass nodule in left lower lobe of lung (arrowhead). They are proved to be a pulmonary meningioma in left upper lobe of lung and granulomatous inflammation in left lower lobe of lung in histologic diagnosis, respectively.

3. Discussion

PPM, defined by the typical histological features of meningioma in the absence of CNS lesions, is a rare neoplasm. Only 45 cases were described in the English medical literature to 2015 [1]. Most of these were solitary and benign in nature, and fewer than five cases have been reported to be malignant, with only one case of autopsy-proven liver metastasis [2–4]. Only one case was reported to consist of multiple primary pulmonary meningiomas. According to a review in 2008, this neoplasm appears to have a mild preponderance in older women [5]. The female/male ratio is 14 : 11, and the tumor size of the PPM ranges from 0.4 cm to 6.5 cm.

Most PPMs present as an asymptomatic solitary lung nodule and are detected incidentally on chest plain film or chest CT. Few cases have been reported to be symptomatic and present with hemoptysis [6]. On chest CT, a PPM usually presents as a single noncalcified pulmonary tumor with a circumscribed margin. Except in the case of endobronchial PPM, the bronchi or pleurae are not involved [7]. After contrast medium administration, the enhancement pattern is variable. Strong and homogeneous enhancement has been reported [1]. As in our case and in previously reported cases, when patients have a history of malignant tumor, PPM or isolated metastasis may not be distinguishable only on radiologic images. In a scenario of a pulmonary small nodular lesion which was detected in chest CT in a patient with history of malignancy like our patient, a metastatic tumor should be listed in the differential diagnosis. It was not distinguishable only on radiologic study if the lesion is small, because many tumors may present as a small round nodule initially. A tissue proof of the small pulmonary nodule with pathohistological study is needed if a definite diagnosis is required in this scenario [8].

Histologically, PPMs appear as well-circumscribed tumors without any bronchial or pleural involvement. Microscopically, these tumors usually present with spindle-shaped or ovoid cells arranged in lobules or a whorl pattern [9].

Absence of mitoses is most common in benign cases; conversely, mitoses are prominent in malignant cases. Psammoma bodies have often been reported. Immunohistochemistry demonstrates positivity for vimentin and EMA [10]. The incidence of extracranial meningioma metastasis is about 0.1%. The lungs (60%) are the most commonly involved locations of metastases of meningioma, followed by the abdomen (34%), cervical lymph nodes (18%), skeletal system (11%), pleura (9%), brain and spine (7%), and mediastinum (5%) [11]. Metastatic pulmonary meningioma is usually detected after diagnosis of central nervous system meningioma and may arise many years after excision of the primary meningioma. The interval from diagnosis of central nervous system meningioma to diagnosis of pulmonary metastases ranges between 2 months and 26 years [12]. Malignant histology results, a papillary morphology of tumor cells, the presence of venous sinus invasion, and local tumor recurrence are risk factors for distant metastasis. A histological diagnosis of pulmonary meningioma could represent a primary or secondary pulmonary meningioma, because PPM and metastatic meningioma share a similar histological appearance which presents as spindle-shaped or ovoid cells arranged in lobules or a whorl pattern [9, 13]. It is not possible to distinguish between primary and metastatic meningioma only by histologic study. Radiological study of the central nervous system is required to exclude an intracranial or spinal meningioma. Otherwise, magnetic resonance imaging is preferred to CT owing to its greater sensitivity [14].

Two hypotheses regarding the pathogenesis of PPMs have been proposed: they may arise from pluripotential subpleural mesenchyma or from minute pulmonary meningothelial-like nodules (MPMNs) [5]. Recently, some authors have performed studies that support the hypothesis that PPMs and MPMNs are related, because they may be derived from the same precursor cells [15]. MPMNs are small interstitial lesions (100 μm to 3 mm) that maintain the original architecture of lung parenchyma, whereas PPMs present as nodular lesions that substitute for the parenchyma. MPMNs may have a relationship with chronic lung disease, whereas they may not be congenital cases due to absence in pediatric lung specimens [16]. Immunohistochemistry of MPMNs demonstrates positivity for CD56, progesterone receptor, epithelial membrane antigen, and vimentin, which is similar to PPMs. In fact, it may be difficult to distinguish MPMNs from PPMs, with the exception of clues by their size. Some authors have hypothesized that PPMs might be a giant form of MPMNs [17]; however, it is not known whether there is a great difference between the incidence of MPMNs (0.3 to 9.5% at autopsy or surgical resection) and that of PPMs.

The treatment for pulmonary meningioma is most commonly surgical resection. Wedge resection is ideal for peripheral lesions. On the contrary, lobectomy is suitable for lesions located in the central lung [5]. Recent widely accepted techniques such as CT-guided dye injection or coil placement could assist with localization of pulmonary nodules before wedge resection of small pulmonary nodules, guiding video-assisted thoracic surgery and minimizing sacrifice of pulmonary tissue to achieve an adequate diagnostic yield for

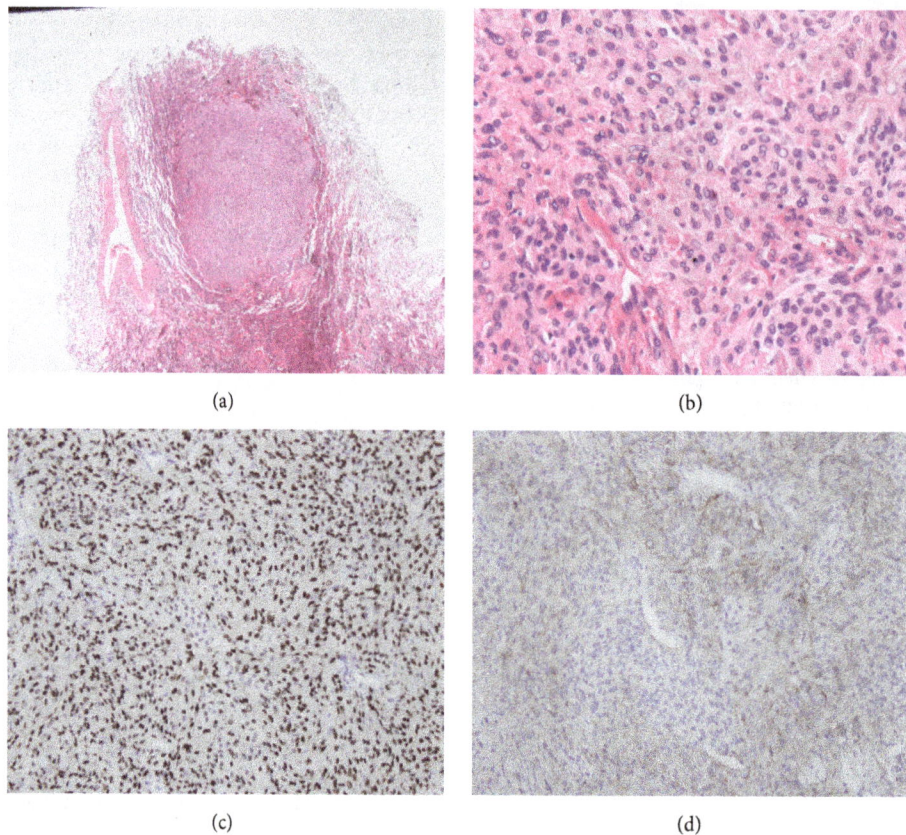

FIGURE 2: Histological features of the case (surgical lung biopsy specimen). (a) Microscopic examination revealed a well-defined nodule that compressed surrounding lung parenchyma. Hematoxylin-eosin (HE) 40x. (b) At high power view, the tumor includes nests of round to spindle shape cells that present focal whorls pattern. The tumor cells showed clear cytoplasm and round and oval nuclei with delicate chromatin distribution and some intranuclear inclusions. Mitotic figures are not present. Hematoxylin-eosin (HE) 200x. (c) In immunohistochemistry study, the tumor cells showed positive staining for PR (100x) and (d) CD56 (100x).

histopathologic assessment. Surgical resection provides not only a conclusive pathologic diagnosis but an excellent long-term prognosis. No tumor recurrence has been reported in benign cases. Therefore, some authors consider that these tumors may be suitable for surgical resection due to their benign biological nature [18].

In conclusion, a greater knowledge of the clinical and radiological features of this rare entity is important to achieve more accurate and improved management. PPM should be listed in the differential diagnoses of single or multiple pulmonary nodules, even though it may present as a ground-glass opacity nodule on a CT scan.

Competing Interests

The authors declare that they have no competing interests.

References

[1] Y. Y. Kim, Y. K. Hong, J.-H. Kie, and S. J. Ryu, "Primary pulmonary meningioma: an unusual cause of a nodule with strong and homogeneous enhancement," *Clinical Imaging*, vol. 40, no. 1, pp. 170–173, 2016.

[2] J. J. C. van der Meij, K. A. Boomars, J. M. M. van den Bosch, W. J. van Boven, P. C. de Bruin, and C. A. Seldenrijk, "Primary pulmonary malignant meningioma," *Annals of Thoracic Surgery*, vol. 80, no. 4, pp. 1523–1525, 2005.

[3] R. A. Prayson and C. F. Farver, "Primary pulmonary malignant meningioma," *The American Journal of Surgical Pathology*, vol. 23, no. 6, pp. 722–726, 1999.

[4] C. Weber, S. Pautex, G. B. Zulian, M. Pusztaszeri, and J. A. Lobrinus, "Primary pulmonary malignant meningioma with lymph node and liver metastasis in a centenary woman, an autopsy case," *Virchows Archiv*, vol. 462, no. 4, pp. 481–485, 2013.

[5] M. Incarbone, G. L. Ceresoli, L. Di Tommaso et al., "Primary pulmonary meningioma: report of a case and review of the literature," *Lung Cancer*, vol. 62, no. 3, pp. 401–407, 2008.

[6] N. Izumi, N. Nishiyama, T. Iwata et al., "Primary pulmonary meningioma presenting with hemoptysis on exertion," *Annals of Thoracic Surgery*, vol. 88, no. 2, pp. 647–648, 2009.

[7] A. Fidan, B. Caglayan, B. Arman, and N. Karadayi, "Endobronchial primary pulmonary meningioma," *Saudi Medical Journal*, vol. 29, no. 10, pp. 1512–1513, 2008.

[8] J. Picquet, I. Valo, Y. Jousset, and B. Enon, "Primary pulmonary meningioma first suspected of being a lung metastasis," *Annals of Thoracic Surgery*, vol. 79, no. 4, pp. 1407–1409, 2005.

[9] A. Cesario, D. Galetta, S. Margaritora, and P. Granone, "Unsuspected primary pulmonary meningioma," *European Journal of Cardio-Thoracic Surgery*, vol. 21, no. 3, pp. 553–555, 2002.

[10] Y.-J. Cheng, J.-T. Wu, H.-Y. Chen et al., "Coexistence of intracranial meningioma, pulmonary meningiomas, and lung cancer," *The Annals of Thoracic Surgery*, vol. 91, no. 4, pp. 1283–1285, 2011.

[11] E. Yekeler, M. Dursun, D. Yilmazbayhan, and A. Tunaci, "Multiple pulmonary metastases from intracranial meningioma: MR imaging findings (case report)," *Diagnostic and Interventional Radiology*, vol. 11, no. 1, pp. 28–30, 2005.

[12] M. Wang, R. Zhan, C. Zhang, and Y. Zhou, "Multiple pulmonary metastases in recurrent intracranial meningioma: case report and literature review," *Journal of International Medical Research*, vol. 44, no. 3, pp. 742–752, 2016.

[13] M. Chiarelli, M. De Simone, M. Gerosa, A. Guttadauro, and U. Cioffi, "An incidental pulmonary meningioma revealing an intracranial meningioma: primary or secondary lesion?" *Annals of Thoracic Surgery*, vol. 99, no. 4, pp. e83–e84, 2015.

[14] I. R. Whittle, C. Smith, P. Navoo, and D. Collie, "Meningiomas," *The Lancet*, vol. 363, no. 9420, pp. 1535–1543, 2004.

[15] A. Weissferdt, X. Tang, S. Suster, I. I. Wistuba, and C. A. Moran, "Pleuropulmonary meningothelial proliferations: evidence for a common histogenesis," *American Journal of Surgical Pathology*, vol. 39, no. 12, pp. 1673–1678, 2015.

[16] S. Mukhopadhyay, O. A. El-Zammar, and A.-L. A. Katzenstein, "Pulmonary meningothelial-like nodules: new insights into a common but poorly understood entity," *The American Journal of Surgical Pathology*, vol. 33, no. 4, pp. 487–495, 2009.

[17] K. Masago, W. Hosada, E. Sasaki et al., "Is primary pulmonary meningioma a giant form of a meningothelial-like nodule? A case report and review of the literature," *Case Reports in Oncology*, vol. 5, no. 2, pp. 471–478, 2012.

[18] Y. Satoh and Y. Ishikawa, "Primary pulmonary meningioma: ten-year follow-up findings for a multiple case, implying a benign biological nature," *Journal of Thoracic and Cardiovascular Surgery*, vol. 139, no. 3, pp. e39–e40, 2010.

46

Pulmonary Artery Pseudoaneurysm: A Rare Cause of Fatal Massive Hemoptysis

Himaja Koneru,[1] Sreeja Biswas Roy,[2] Monirul Islam,[1]
Hesham Abdelrazek,[2] Debabrata Bandyopadhyay,[1] Nikhil Madan,[2]
Pradnya D. Patil,[3] and Tanmay S. Panchabhai [iD][2]

[1]*Department of Thoracic Medicine, Geisinger Medical Center, Danville, PA, USA*
[2]*Norton Thoracic Institute, St. Joseph's Hospital and Medical Center, Phoenix, AZ, USA*
[3]*Taussig Cancer Institute, Department of Hematology and Oncology, Cleveland Clinic, Cleveland, OH, USA*

Correspondence should be addressed to Tanmay S. Panchabhai; tanmay.panchabhai@dignityhealth.org

Academic Editor: Javier de Miguel-Díez

Pulmonary artery pseudoaneurysm (PAPA), an uncommon complication of pyogenic bacterial and fungal infections and related septic emboli, is associated with high mortality. The pulmonary artery (PA) lacks an adventitial wall; therefore, repeated endovascular seeding of the PA with septic emboli creates saccular dilations that are more likely to rupture than systemic arterial aneurysms. The most common clinical presentation of PAPA is massive hemoptysis and resultant worsening hypoxemia. Computed tomography angiography is the preferred diagnostic modality for PAPA; typical imaging patterns include focal outpouchings of contrast adjacent to a branch of the PA following the same contrast density as the PA in all phases of the study. In mycotic PAPAs, multiple synchronous lesions are often seen in segmental and subsegmental PAs due to ongoing embolic phenomena. The recommended approach for a mycotic PAPA is prolonged antimicrobial therapy; for massive hemoptysis, endovascular treatment (e.g., coil embolization, stenting, or embolization of the feeding vessel) is preferred. PAPA resection and lobectomy are a last resort, generally reserved for patients with uncontrolled hemoptysis or pleural hemorrhage. We present a case of a 28-year-old woman with necrotizing pneumonia from intravenous drug use who ultimately died from massive hemoptysis and shock after a ruptured PAPA.

1. Introduction

Pulmonary artery pseudoaneurysms (PAPAs) are associated with high mortality; therefore, early detection is of paramount importance. Massive hemoptysis from a ruptured PAPA is fatal in over 50% of patients, and a high index of suspicion is required for the diagnosis. These aneurysms frequently occur in patients with necrotizing infections of the lung or heart and those who are at high risk of septic embolism. We present the case of a 28-year-old woman who was admitted to our institution with prolonged respiratory failure. She was an intravenous drug user, and she had necrotizing pneumonia that led to development of multiple PAPAs, which in turn led to massive hemoptysis, shock, and death.

2. Case Report

A 28-year-old woman with a recent history of intravenous drug use presented with insomnia, generalized pain, and anxiety. Her physical examination was significant for tachycardia (heart rate: 130 beats per minute), hypoxia with oxygen saturation of 82% on room air, bilateral diffuse crackles over both lung fields, and confusion. Her initial laboratory evaluation revealed acute kidney damage (creatinine: 5.8 mg/dL). A chest radiograph demonstrated bilateral patchy alveolar opacities, indicating an acute alveolar process such as pulmonary edema or pneumonia. Ensuing hypoxic respiratory failure required endotracheal intubation. Given the patient's history of intravenous drug use, an emergent transesophageal echocardiogram was performed. This showed a large, bulky vegetation on the tricuspid valve that appeared to involve

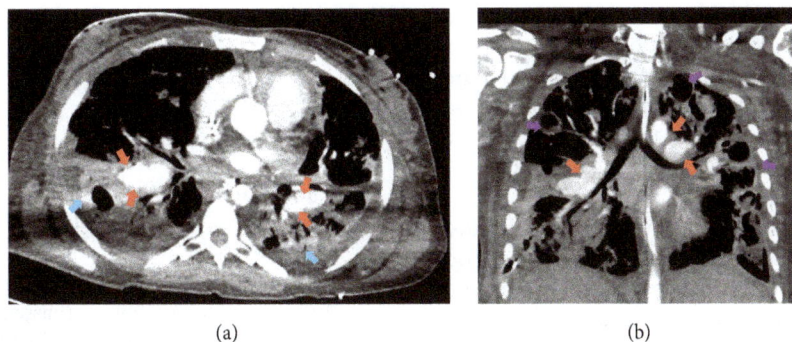

(a)   (b)

FIGURE 1: Computed tomogram angiography of the chest in (a) axial plane and (b) coronal plane depicting multiple saccular, contrast-enhanced structures close to the branches of the pulmonary arteries. These were found to be mycotic pulmonary artery pseudoaneurysms (red arrows). Bilateral, bibasilar dense consolidations from necrotizing *Staphylococcus aureus* pneumonia (blue arrows) and cavities secondary to necrotizing *S. aureus* pneumonia (purple arrows) are also seen.

more than one leaflet, as well as possible pulmonic valve endocarditis with a small mobile echogenicity attached to the pulmonic valve, consistent with infective endocarditis.

Broad antimicrobial therapy was initiated with vancomycin and piperacillin-tazobactam. Blood cultures grew *Staphylococcus aureus*, as did the tracheal aspirate. Computed tomography (CT) of the chest, abdomen, and pelvis revealed numerous pulmonary septic emboli with hepatosplenomegaly. On day 4, antimicrobial coverage was changed to a daptomycin-based regimen on the sensitivities, but the patient's fever and tachycardia persisted.

Repeat CT of the chest, abdomen, and pelvis revealed interval worsening pulmonary opacities, new cavitary lesions, new bilateral lower-lobe-predominant consolidations, and a complicated right pleural effusion. Right thoracoscopy was performed and an intercostal drain was placed for the right empyema. Flexible fiber-optic bronchoscopy revealed copious purulent material in both lungs. Anticipating prolonged weaning from mechanical ventilation, a tracheostomy was performed on day 10. Repeat blood cultures on days 7, 9, and 20 showed no signs of bacterial infection, and the patient's overall clinical condition improved. She was weaned off mechanical ventilation on day 20.

On days 25 through 27, the patient began experiencing intermittent, self-limited episodes of hemoptysis via her tracheostomy tube. Fiber-optic bronchoscopy revealed small blood clots, but overall her clinical condition was improving. On day 34, the patient developed massive hemoptysis, and copious amounts of blood were suctioned from her mouth, nostrils, and tracheostomy tube. She rapidly developed progressive hypoxemia that was unresponsive to 100% supplemental oxygen; mechanical ventilation was therefore initiated. Hypoxic cardiorespiratory arrest ensued and after several rounds of cardiopulmonary resuscitation, return of spontaneous circulation was achieved.

Another fiber-optic bronchoscopy demonstrated massive blood clots throughout the patient's airways bilaterally, but no active source of bleeding was identified. She developed refractory shock that required multiple vasoactive agents, as well as blood products delivered via massive transfusion protocol. An emergent CT angiogram of the chest revealed bilateral PAPAs and a dilated right heart, likely related to pulmonary

hypertension (Figure 1). After multidisciplinary review of her case with interventional radiology experts and thoracic surgeons, embolization was deemed inappropriate due to the size of the PAPAs. Bilateral lower lobe resection was considered, but it was thought to be futile given her unstable hemodynamics and underlying poor lung reserve from the ongoing *S. aureus* pneumonia. Moreover, such a procedure involved a high risk of massive hemorrhage of the large PAPAs. The patient's grim prognosis was discussed with her family, and she was transitioned to comfort care. She died on day 35.

3. Discussion

Although they are rare, the mortality of PAPAs is as high as 50% in diagnosed cases [1, 2]. PAPAs may be congenital or acquired, and the most common cause of acquired PAPA is infection [3]. Tuberculosis and syphilis were the former main infectious causes of PAPA; however, in the current era of efficacious antibiotic therapy, the incidence of PAPA due to tuberculosis or syphilis has greatly decreased [3]. Organisms implicated in causing modern-day PAPA include pyogenic bacteria (e.g., *S. aureus*, *S. pyogenes*, *Klebsiella*, and *Actinomyces*), *Mycobacterium tuberculosis* (rare), and various fungi (*Mucor*, *Aspergillus*, and *Candida*) [4]. Successive endovascular seeding of the PA lumen from multiple emboli or microemboli has been proposed as the pathogenesis of PAPAs in the infectious setting [5]. Such repeated seeding gradually destroys the vessel wall from the inside (i.e., the luminal side) outward, causing PAPA formation. Other rare causes of PAPAs include chest wall trauma and iatrogenic trauma from PA catheters. Several case reports have described PAPAs resulting from lung cancer (including primary squamous cell cancer, primary sarcoma, and metastatic sarcoma) [4, 6–8].

Patients with PAPA commonly present with hemoptysis and hypoxemia and sometimes experience chest pain. Chest radiography can show focal consolidation, solitary pulmonary nodules, or multiple pulmonary nodules near the central or peripheral pulmonary vasculature [9]. Definitive diagnosis is made via CT angiography—a modality that not only establishes diagnosis, but also helps plan therapy with endovascular treatment modalities. On CT angiography,

PAPAs appear as focal outpouchings of contrast adjacent to a PA branch following the same contrast density as the PA in all phases of the study [10]. Pulmonary angiography demonstrates delayed emptying of contrast material from the sac [10]. In the case of a mycotic PAPA, multiple synchronous lesions are usually seen in segmental and subsegmental PAs due to ongoing embolic phenomena.

Because the PA lacks an adventitial wall, PAPAs are more likely to rupture than true arterial aneurysms. Therefore, hemoptysis due to a ruptured PAPA is often fatal and must be promptly recognized and treated. Antimicrobial therapy remains an important component of managing mycotic PAPAs. Empiric intravenous antimicrobial therapy targeting broad gram-negative and gram-positive coverage should be instituted as soon as PAPA is suspected. In addition, antifungal, antimycobacterial, and antitreponemal coverage must be considered in immunocompromised patients. Although no overall consensus exists regarding the optimal duration and type of antimicrobial therapy in patients with PAPA, prolonged therapy similar to infective endocarditis is considered appropriate.

Urgent endovascular treatment is the preferred approach in managing hemoptysis resulting from PAPAs, and such treatment should not be delayed. Direct coil embolization, endovascular stents, or embolization of the aneurysm's feeding vessel are the reported effective occlusion modalities [11–14]. In the case of a small pseudoaneurysm, occluding the feeding vessel might be adequate; however, coil embolization is preferred for larger aneurysms [11–14]. It is important to note that successful embolization of the PAPA not only requires successful coil placement, but also an intact coagulation cascade and reduced arterial pressure to promote thrombosis. This is a challenge, especially in mycotic PAPAs, as patients usually present with sepsis and associated coagulopathy. Balloon embolization can be considered as an alternative in these cases [15]. In wide-necked PAPAs, endovascular stenting has been described as successful treatment [16, 17]. Potential graft infection due to ongoing septic embolic phenomena must be considered as a possible complication of graft stent placements and this treatment should be avoided in patients with active bacteremia, due to the high chances of graft seeding. Another less preferred approach in the management of PAPAs that are not amenable to endovascular treatment is direct percutaneous thrombin injection [18].

Operative repair for PAPAs involves open thoracotomy and aneurysm resection, with lobectomy for the involved lobes. Surgical treatment, however, is associated with increased mortality and morbidity compared with endovascular treatment, especially because patients with mycotic PAPAs are acutely ill and often have poor pulmonary reserve [19, 20]. Surgical approaches should be reserved for patients with pleural hemorrhage, uncontrolled hemoptysis, or aggressive infections that may not respond to medical therapy alone (e.g., mucormycosis). Surgery is also preferred in patients who have a high chance of endovascular graft or coil infection, such as patients with active bacteremia or resistant organisms [19, 20]. In conclusion, PAPAs are rare complications of infective endocarditis. A high degree of suspicion is needed for diagnosing PAPAs on imaging. Timely recognition can improve outcomes, as it allows for earlier intervention.

References

[1] E. Jean-Baptiste, "Clinical assessment and management of massive hemoptysis," *Critical Care Medicine*, vol. 28, no. 5, pp. 1642–1647, 2000.

[2] E. D. Santelli, D. S. Katz, A. M. Goldschmidt, and H. A. Thomas, "Embolization of multiple rasmussen aneurysms as a treatment of hemoptysis," *Radiology*, vol. 193, no. 2, pp. 396–398, 1994.

[3] Y. Chen, M. D. Gilman, K. L. Humphrey et al., "Pulmonary artery pseudoaneurysms: Clinical features and CT findings," *American Journal of Roentgenology*, vol. 208, no. 1, pp. 84–91, 2017.

[4] C. S. Restrepo and A. P. Carswell, "Aneurysms and Pseudoaneurysms of the Pulmonary Vasculature," *Seminars in Ultrasound, CT and MRI*, vol. 33, no. 6, pp. 552–566, 2012.

[5] T. Bartter, R. S. Irwin, and G. Nash, "Aneurysms of the pulmonary arteries," *CHEST*, vol. 94, no. 5, pp. 1065–1075, 1988.

[6] J. D. J. Camargo, S. M. Camargo, T. N. Machuca, and R. M. Bello, "Large Pulmonary Artery Pseudoaneurysm Due to Lung Carcinoma: Pulmonary Artery Pseudoaneurysm," *Journal of Thoracic Imaging*, vol. 25, no. 1, pp. W4–W5, 2010.

[7] A. Koch, G. Mechtersheimer, U. Tochtermann, and M. Karck, "Ruptured pseudoaneurysm of the pulmonary artery - Rare manifestation of a primary pulmonary artery sarcoma," *Interactive CardioVascular and Thoracic Surgery*, vol. 10, no. 1, pp. 120-121, 2010.

[8] E. T. Nguyen, C. I. S. Silva, J. M. Seely, S. Chong, K. S. Lee, and N. L. Müller, "Pulmonary artery aneurysms and pseudoaneurysms in adults: findings at CT and radiography.," *AJR. American journal of roentgenology*, vol. 188, no. 2, pp. W126–134, 2007.

[9] A. R. Abreu, M. A. Campos, and B. P. Krieger, "Pulmonary artery rupture induced by a pulmonary artery catheter: a case report and review of the literature," *Journal of Intensive Care Medicine*, vol. 19, no. 5, pp. 291–296, 2004.

[10] G. Sundar, M. Ahmed, S. Keshava, D. Boddu, and N. K. Chaudhary, "Mycotic Pulmonary Artery Pseudoaneurysm in a Child Treated by Endovascular Coil Embolization," *Vascular Disease Management*, vol. 12, no. 12, pp. E242–E246, 2015.

[11] Y. Matsumura, S. Shiono, K. Saito, and T. Sato, "Pulmonary artery pseudoaneurysm after lung resection successfully treated by coil embolization," *Interactive CardioVascular and Thoracic Surgery*, vol. 11, no. 3, pp. 364-365, 2010.

[12] S. Shin, T.-B. Shin, H. Choi et al., "Peripheral pulmonary arterial pseudoaneurysms: Therapeutic implications of endovascular treatment and angiographic classifications," *Radiology*, vol. 256, no. 2, pp. 656–664, 2010.

[13] T.-B. Shin, S.-K. Yoon, K.-N. Lee et al., "The Role of Pulmonary CT Angiography and Selective Pulmonary Angiography in Endovascular Management of Pulmonary Artery Pseudoaneurysms Associated with Infectious Lung Diseases," *Journal of Vascular and Interventional Radiology*, vol. 18, no. 7, pp. 882–887, 2007.

[14] K. Yamakado, H. Takaki, M. Takao et al., "Massive hemoptysis from pulmonary artery pseudoaneurysm caused by lung radiofrequency ablation: Successful treatment by coil embolization," *CardioVascular and Interventional Radiology*, vol. 33, no. 2, pp. 410–412, 2010.

[15] W. A. Renie, R. J. Rodeheffer, S. Mitchell, W. C. Balke, and R. I. White Jr., "Balloon embolization of a mycotic pulmonary artery aneurysm," *The American Review of Respiratory Disease*, vol. 126, no. 6, pp. 1107–1110, 1982.

[16] M.-C. Chou, H.-L. Liang, H.-B. Pan, and C.-F. Yang, "Percutaneous stent-graft repair of a mycotic pulmonary artery pseudoaneurysm," *CardioVascular and Interventional Radiology*, vol. 29, no. 5, pp. 890–892, 2006.

[17] A. Park and W. Cwikiel, "Endovascular treatment of a pulmonary artery pseudoaneurysm with a stent graft: Report of two cases," *Acta Radiologica*, vol. 48, no. 1, pp. 45–47, 2007.

[18] C. L. Hovis and P. T. Zeni Jr., "Percutaneous thrombin injection of a pulmonary artery pseudoaneurysm refractory to coil embolization," *Journal of Vascular and Interventional Radiology*, vol. 17, no. 12, pp. 1943–1946, 2006.

[19] M. J. Coffey, J. Fantone 3rd., M. C. Stirling, and J. P. Lynch 3rd., "Pseudoaneurysm of pulmonary artery in mucormycosis. Radiographic characteristics and management.," *American Journal of Respiratory and Critical Care Medicine (Salma)*, vol. 145, no. 6, pp. 1487–1490, 1992.

[20] C. Savage, J. B. Zwischenberger, K. C. Ventura, and G. R. Wittich, "Hemoptysis secondary to pulmonary pseudoaneurysm 30 years after a gunshot wound," *The Annals of Thoracic Surgery*, vol. 71, no. 3, pp. 1021–1023, 2001.

47

Multifocal Pulmonary Granular Cell Tumor Presenting with Postobstructive Pneumonia

Samid M. Farooqui,[1] **Muhammad S. Khan,**[1,2] **Laura Adhikari,**[3] **and Viral Doshi**[1,2]

[1]*Department of Internal Medicine, University of Oklahoma Health Sciences Center, Oklahoma City, OK, USA*
[2]*Section of Pulmonary, Critical Care and Sleep Medicine, University of Oklahoma Health Sciences Center, Oklahoma City, OK, USA*
[3]*Department of Pathology, University of Oklahoma Health Sciences Center, Oklahoma City, OK, USA*

Correspondence should be addressed to Samid M. Farooqui; samid-farooqui@ouhsc.edu

Academic Editor: Daniel T. Merrick

Granular cell tumor (GCT) is a neoplasm of Schwann cell origin. Its presence in the aerodigestive tract is uncommon and becomes a diagnostic challenge on initial presentation. Our case is of a 59-year-old woman who presented to the emergency department with a history of productive cough and dyspnea associated with fever and chest pain. An initial chest X-ray (CXR) showed a right middle lobe consolidation with follow-up Computed Tomography (CT) scan showing a mass in the right bronchus. Bronchoscopy revealed a polypoid, sessile granular mass in the right bronchus intermedius with multiple white lesions in trachea, left main bronchus, and right upper bronchi. Histology revealed a benign GCT. Bronchoalveolar lavage from the right middle lobe grew *Streptococcus pneumoniae*. Patient was treated with intravenous levofloxacin during hospital stay and discharged on a 7-day course of oral antibiotics to be followed as outpatient but was lost to follow-up. GCT can present as a polypoid tumor causing recurrent postobstructive pneumonia. Surgical resection is the most successful treatment option. The tumor is more common in third and fourth decade of life and our patient is the oldest patient, according to our knowledge, to have a GCT.

1. Introduction

Granular cell tumor (GCT) is a rare lesion of Schwann cell origin which frequently occurs in the upper aerodigestive tract but can potentially affect all parts of the body, including the skin. The head and neck area is affected 45%–65% of the time with more than two-thirds of the lesions occurring intraorally—tongue, mucosa and hard palate being the most common sites [1]. Involvement of the bronchi and lower respiratory tract is much less common, with the lesions typically being solitary, submucosal origin nodules [2]. We present here the case of a rare large polypoid GCT causing postobstructive pneumonia.

2. Case

Our patient is a 59-year-old African American female with a past medical history of asthma who presented to the emergency department with shortness of breath, fever, and persistent right-sided chest pain with a cough productive of purulent sputum for the last 1 week. Physical examination was unremarkable except for crackles in the right lung base. Blood workup was significant for leukocytosis of 28,760/mm^3 (4.00–11.00 K/mm^3), with normal hemoglobin level, platelet count, and chemistry panel. Chest X-ray (CXR) performed was significant for a right middle lobe consolidation. A subsequent CT chest showed a right middle lobe consolidation, with an endobronchial lesion within the right bronchus intermedius, concerning for postobstructive pneumonia (Figures 1 and 2). She was started on levofloxacin for treatment and admitted for further workup.

A bronchoscopy was performed which showed multiple flat white colored lesions in the trachea, left main-stem bronchi, right upper lobe bronchi (Figure 3), and a large polypoid, sessile, and white colored tumor located just distal to the secondary carina causing near-complete obstruction (>80%) of the right proximal bronchus intermedius (Figures 4 and 5). Several endobronchial biopsies were obtained from

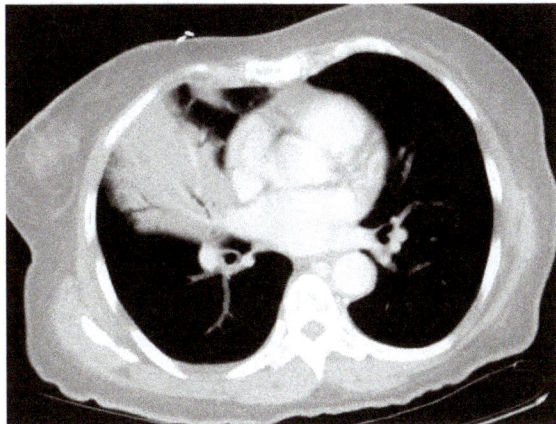

FIGURE 1

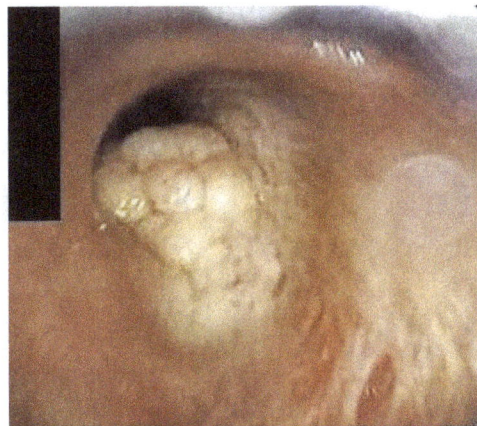

FIGURE 2

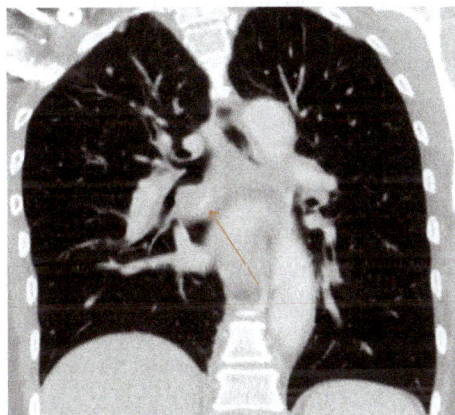

FIGURE 3

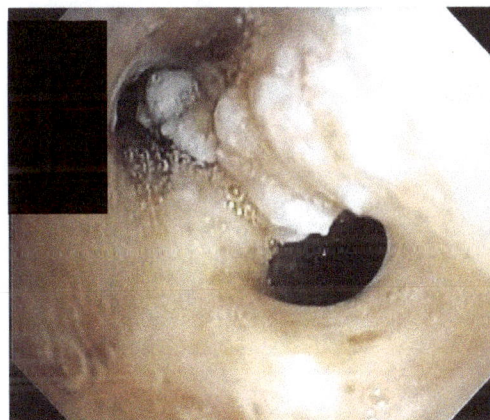

FIGURE 4

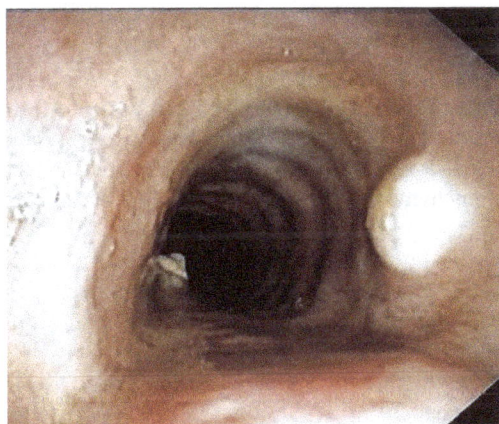

FIGURE 5

the large polypoid tumor located in bronchus intermedius and from the lesion in left main bronchus. Histopathological examination was consistent with granular cell tumor with tumor markers S-100 (Figure 6), Sox-10 (Figure 7), and CD-68 positive. Immunohistochemical analysis for pancytokeratin, cytokeratin 8/18, and synaptophysin was negative.

Notably, sputum culture and right middle lobe bronchoalveolar lavage culture grew *Streptococcus pneumoniae*. The patient improved over the course of 4 days and was discharged home with a course of oral antibiotics for a total of 7 days, and follow-up was arranged in pulmonary clinic. However, patient was lost to follow-up.

3. Discussion

Granular cell tumors (GCTs), first described by Abrikosov in 1926 [3], are now believed to be of neurogenic (Schwann cell) origin [4]. Pulmonary GCTs comprise approximately 6–10% of all GCTs with majority being found in the lower respiratory tract as polypoid, endobronchial masses [2]. The tumor commonly occurs in middle-aged patients, with mean age reported to be in the fourth decade of life (36-37 years) and an equal prevalence in males and females [5]. Our patient is the oldest individual reported in literature, per our knowledge. Common symptoms at presentation include hemoptysis (17%), chronic cough (13%), chest pain (6%), and unexplained dyspnea (3%). Patients can also present with an asymptomatic lung nodule (8%) on imaging or as an incidental finding on bronchoscopy (8%) [6]. Our patient

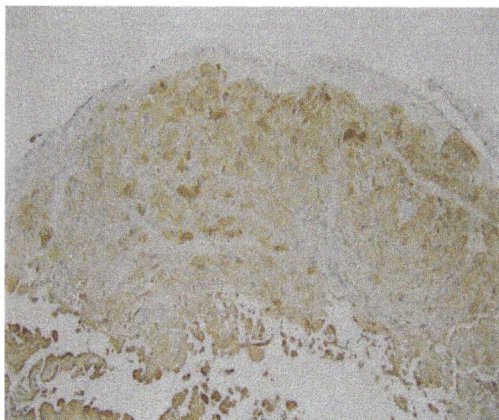

FIGURE 6

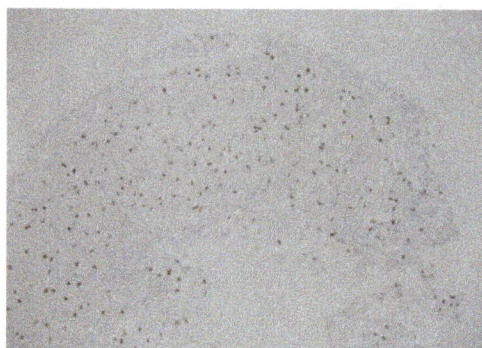

FIGURE 7

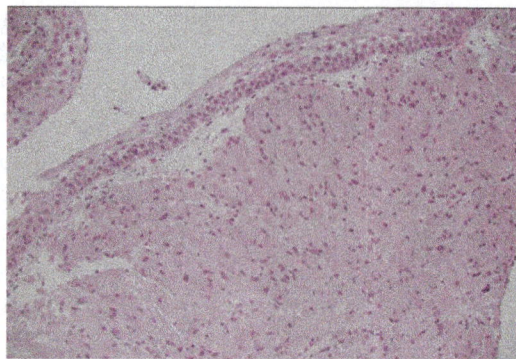

FIGURE 8

presented with multiple respiratory tract GCTs, including a large polypoid granular cell tumor causing postobstructive pneumonia with cultures positive for *Streptococcus pneumoniae*.

Pulmonary GCTs, like their extrapulmonary counterparts, can rarely be multifocal and have been reported to be associated with genetic mutations in PTPN11 as part of LEOPARD syndrome [2, 7]. In one case series, multifocal GCTs were reported to arise from all lobes of the lung and from the main-stem bronchi [2]. In up to 25% of cases there can be multiple GCTs, but the presence of multifocal GCT in lung does not necessarily indicate malignancy [2]. The presence of metastatic malignant GCT from extrapulmonary sites has been described in the settings of multifocal pulmonary GCT [8, 9] and metastasis should be ruled out. In our patient, despite the presence of multifocal GCT in the lungs, CT scan of chest abdomen and pelvis did not reveal any extrapulmonary focus of the disease decreasing suspicion for metastasis.

The infiltrative nature of pulmonary GCTs is a well-established feature for this benign tumor [2]. Peribronchial tissue extension has been reported in up to 40% of tumors as these tumors like to grow along muscle fibers, fibrous septa, and nerve sheath bundles [2]. Pseudoepitheliomatous hyperplasia, an overgrowth or thickening of the overlying squamous epithelium (Figure 8), is a diagnostic feature seen for these tumors. Microscopically, the tumor is composed

of abundant eosinophilic granular cytoplasm, with fairly uniform arrangement of small nuclei. GCT is mostly benign, with malignant course occurring in 2% of cases [10]. Differentiation between benign and malignant GCTs is often difficult. Six histologic features have been described which can predict malignant potential of GCTs. These features include spindling of the tumor cells, the presence of vesicular nuclei with large nucleoli, increased mitotic rate (>2 mitoses/10 high-power fields at 200x magnification), a high nuclear-to-cytoplasm (N : C) ratio, pleomorphism, and necrosis. Histologically, malignant GCT is diagnosed when three or more of the six criteria are fulfilled [11]. Our case did not fulfill the criteria for malignant GCT.

Treatment of patients with endobronchial GCT has not been clearly defined. Current therapeutic options include surgical resection, endoscopic removal, YAG laser, and fulguration [2]. Overall, surgical excision has the highest cure rate. Of the 20 surgically treated patients followed for a mean of 3.3 years, only one patient was reported to have had symptomatic recurrence. The extent of surgical resection is unclear; however most authors agree that when postobstructive parenchymal damage has occurred, segmental or lobar resection is indicated [6]. Sleeve resection is considered when local resection of a mass is anatomically feasible [2]. The tumors can be observed in some cases. Spontaneous resolution has been documented in only one case. If distal lung parenchyma is preserved, then bronchoscopic extirpation and laser therapy can be considered [2].

GCT can be associated with other neoplasms in approximately 13% of cases [12]. The most common neoplasm associated with pulmonary GCT is lung carcinoma. Esophageal cancer and renal cell carcinomas have also been observed in patients with pulmonary GCT [2]. Nonneoplastic diseases reported in patients with pulmonary GCT include sarcoidosis and HIV infection [1, 13].

In conclusion, pulmonary GCT is a rare entity, which can present as a large polypoid tumor causing recurrent postobstructive pneumonia and can be found throughout the bronchial tree and in peripheral lung fields in the form of multifocal GCTs, as in our case. Even though risk of malignancy is very rare, if multiple lung lesions are present, metastatic GCT should be ruled out by appropriate imaging. The patients should be followed at regular interval to assess for recurrence.

Disclosure

Dr. Doshi is the attending physician on record. This case was presented as a poster presentation at the American Thoracic Society International Conference held in Washington, DC, USA, in May 2017.

References

[1] J. C. Garancis, R. A. Komorowski, and J. F. Kuzma, "Granular cell myoblastoma," *Cancer*, vol. 25, no. 3, pp. 542–550, 1970.

[2] M. Deavers, D. Guinee, M. N. Koss, and W. D. Travis, "Granular cell tumors of the lung: Clinicopathologic study of 20 cases," *The American Journal of Surgical Pathology*, vol. 19, no. 6, pp. 627–635, 1995.

[3] A. Abrikosov, "Ueber Myome ausgehend von quergestreifter willkiirlicher Muskulatur," *Virchows Archiv*, 1926.

[4] A. M. Al-Ghamdi, J. D. A. Flint, N. L. Muller, and K. C. Stewart, "Hilar pulmonary granular cell tumor: A case report and review of the literature," *Annals of Diagnostic Pathology*, vol. 4, no. 4, pp. 245–251, 2000.

[5] E. Szczepulska-Wójcik, R. Langfort, W. Kupis et al., "Granular cell tumor - A rare, benign neoplasm of respiratory tract. Analysis of cases diagnosed in institute of tuberculosis and lung diseases," *Pneumonologia i Alergologia Polska*, vol. 72, no. 5-6, pp. 187–191, 2004.

[6] O. G. Hernandez, E. F. Haponik, and W. R. Summer, "Granular cell tumour of the bronchus: Bronchoscopic and clinical features," *Thorax*, vol. 41, no. 12, pp. 927–931, 1986.

[7] K. A. Schrader, T. N. Nelson, A. De Luca, D. G. Huntsman, and B. C. Mcgillivray, "Multiple granular cell tumors are an associated feature of LEOPARD syndrome caused by mutation in PTPN11," *Clinical Genetics*, vol. 75, no. 2, pp. 185–189, 2009.

[8] M. Klima and J. Peters, "Malignant granular cell tumor," *Archives of Pathology & Laboratory Medicine*, vol. 111, no. 11, pp. 1070–1073, 1987.

[9] J. W. Steffelaar, M. Nap, and V. U. J. G. M. Haelst, "Malignant granular cell tumor. Report of a case with special reference to carcinoembryonic antigen," *The American Journal of Surgical Pathology*, vol. 6, no. 7, pp. 665–672, 1982.

[10] S. Aksoy, H. Abali, S. Kilickap, H. Harputluoglu, and M. Erman, "Metastatic granular cell tumor: A case report and review of the literature," *Acta Oncologica*, vol. 45, no. 1, pp. 91–94, 2006.

[11] M. Jiang, T. Anderson, C. Nwogu, and D. Tan, "Pulmonary malignant granular cell tumor," *World Journal of Surgical Oncology*, vol. 1, article 22, 2003.

[12] G. R. McSwain, R. Colpitts, A. Kreutner, P. H. O'Brien, and S. Spicer, "Granular cell myoblastoma," *Surgery, Gynecology and Obstetrics*, vol. 150, no. 5, pp. 703–710, 1980.

[13] J. Liebman and C. M. Linthicum, "Granular cell myoblastoma (schwannoma) of the carina in a patient with sarcoidosis," *Southern Medical Journal*, vol. 69, no. 12, pp. 1613-1614, 1976.

48

Smoking Relapse Causing an Acute Exacerbation of Desquamative Interstitial Pneumonia with Pleural Effusions and Mediastinal Adenopathies

Tyler Pickell [ID],[1] Jamie Donnelly,[2] and Francois Abi Fadel[1,3]

[1]*Marian University College of Osteopathic Medicine, Indianapolis, IN, USA*
[2]*Ameripath, Indianapolis, IN, USA*
[3]*Respiratory Institute, Cleveland Clinic, Cleveland, OH, USA*

Correspondence should be addressed to Tyler Pickell; tpickell988@marian.edu

Academic Editor: Reda E. Girgis

Desquamative interstitial pneumonia (DIP) is a rare interstitial pneumonia often caused by smoking. DIP is typically regarded as a chronic disease, but acute DIP exacerbations can occur, and some have resulted in death. Factors that can provoke a DIP exacerbation are not well described in the literature. We present a case of a 58-year-old male with DIP, who after being treated successfully with smoking cessation and steroids for 7 months, required hospitalization for acute hypoxemic respiratory failure. This acute episode was very likely an exacerbation of his DIP after a smoking relapse period of 6 weeks prior to this acute presentation. This report also highlights unique CT findings in a DIP case of pleural effusions and mediastinal adenopathies seen chronically and relapsing acutely. To the best of our knowledge, CT findings of pleural effusions and mediastinal adenopathies concurrently have not been described in a case of DIP in chronic or acute conditions.

1. Introduction

Desquamative interstitial pneumonia (DIP) is one of the rarest interstitial pneumonias originally described by Liebow in 1965 [1, 2]. Liewbow et al.'s paper first described DIP cases with acute exacerbations that resulted in death. Currently, literature is lacking on potential causes leading to DIP exacerbations, and very few cases of DIP exacerbations have been described [3–7].

We are reporting a case of a 58-year-old male with proven DIP on prior surgical lung biopsy, who presented with acute fulminant respiratory failure. Unique features of this case are first that the respiratory failure resulted most likely from a DIP exacerbation, which was very likely due to smoking relapse. In addition, our patient had significant pleural effusions and mediastinal adenopathies that were not explained by any other etiologies and we believe were due to an acute decline of DIP.

2. Case Report

Our patient is a 58-year-old Caucasian male referred initially to the pulmonary clinic for an abnormal high resolution computed tomography (HRCT) of the chest (Figure 1) showing ground glass opacities (GGOs), thickening of the interlobular septa primarily in the bases with minimal honeycombing, mediastinal adenopathies, and small bilateral pleural effusions. He had complaints of progressive shortness of breath and an unproductive cough. Medical history was relevant for 31-pack-year smoking history, asbestos exposure, uncontrolled Diabetes Mellitus type II, and obesity. His oxygen saturation was 93% on room air. Lung auscultation revealed bibasilar crackles with poor air entry but no clubbing or cyanosis. Pulmonary function test demonstrated an obstructive lung disease with mildly decreased forced vital capacity (FVC) at 76% and forced expiratory volume in one second (FEV1) at 70%, borderline FEV1/FVC ratio at 72%, and excellent effort. Lung volumes also revealed a

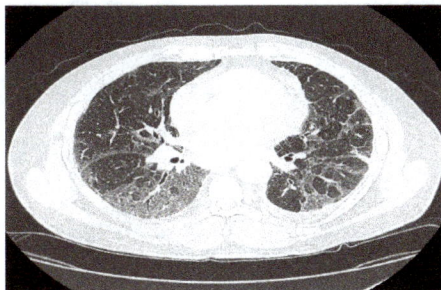

FIGURE 1: CT-high resolution chest without contrast. Taken 15 months before acute exacerbation. Ground glass opacities with thickening of the interlobular septa, predominantly in the lung bases.

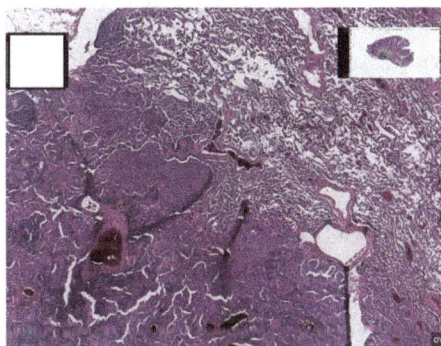

FIGURE 3: 10x lung view showing dense accumulation of intra-alveolar macrophages. Classic histological DIP findings.

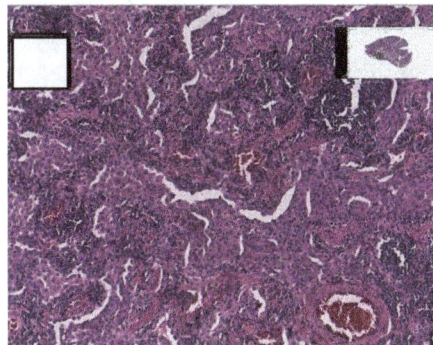

FIGURE 2: Low power overview showing DIP and RB-ILD with adjacent normal but slightly inflamed lung.

restrictive lung disease with moderately decreased total lung capacity (TLC) at 64%. Finally, the diffusion capacity of carbon monoxide (DLco) was severely reduced at 44%.

The initial outpatient workup included a complete blood count (CBC), comprehensive metabolic panel (CMP), erythrocyte sedimentation rate (ESR), N-terminal probrain natriuretic peptide (NT-proBNP), urinalysis, lactate dehydrogenase (LDH), C-reactive protein (CRP), erythrocyte sedimentation rate (ESR), creatine kinase (CK), angiotensin converting enzyme (ACE) level, antineutrophil cytoplasmic antibodies (ANCA), rheumatoid factor (RF), anti-cyclic citrullinated peptide immunoglobulin G (Anti-CCP), histoplasmosis antibodies, human leukocyte antigen B27 (HLA-B27), aspergillus galactomannan antigen, interferon-gamma release assay for tuberculosis, anti-SCL-70 antibody, beta D-glucan, and antinuclear antibodies (ANA). All were negative except a borderline nonspecific elevation in ACE, LDH, and CK levels and positive ANCA antibodies.

To address the interstitial lung disease pattern, a video-assisted thoracoscopic surgery (VATS) lung biopsy was performed. Right lower and right upper lobe wedge excisions revealed classic desquamative interstitial pneumonia, along with foci of respiratory bronchiolitis interstitial pneumonia, mild interstitial fibrosis, and emphysematous changes (Figures 2 and 3).

The patient's history of lifelong smoking along with asbestos exposure [8] likely contributed to these histological changes and DIP diagnosis.

To treat DIP, he was started on a tapered dose of glucocorticoids (starting at 40 mg of prednisone) along with nicotine replacement therapy for smoking cessation. Over a 7-month treatment course, the prednisone dose was lowered to 10mg with improvement in his dyspnea and cough. With assistance from the nicotine replacement, the patient successfully quit smoking for 6 months. Repeat CT images showed improvement in GGOs and resolution of prior small pleural effusions.

After 7 months of DIP treatment and with minimal respiratory symptoms, he restarted smoking one pack of cigarettes a day. Six weeks after restarting smoking, respiratory issues quickly developed, and he required hospitalization for acute hypoxemic respiratory failure. Upon admission the patient was tachypneic with labored breathing, worsening bibasilar crackles, decreased air entry, and an unproductive cough. Given his presentation and dropping oxygen saturation to 84% on room air, he was given 100% FiO2 (fraction of inspired oxygen) by nonrebreather mask.

After discussing treatment options for respiratory failure, the patient refused intubation and mechanical ventilation with complete understanding that his condition could be life-threatening. His breathing was therefore supported with alternating 100% FiO2 by nonrebreather mask and noninvasive ventilator support to maintain oxygen saturation above 90%.

A chest X-ray (Figure 4) and a chest CT angiogram (Figure 5) were ordered. No pulmonary emboli were found. However, imaging did show significant worsening bilateral GGOs, bibasilar consolidations, mediastinal adenopathies, and a new moderate right pleural effusion. The patient was started on broad spectrum antibiotics with vancomycin, piperacillin/tazobactam, and azithromycin. Laboratory workup was unremarkable for infection however. White blood cell count was slightly elevated at 12,600 without a left shift. Procalcitonin level was borderline at 0.14 ng/mL, C-reactive protein was elevated initially but then normalized, and the patient was afebrile at 98.4 Fahrenheit. NT-proBNP was normal which excluded congestive heart failure as a cause for the pleural effusion and GGOs. Repeated arterial blood gas measurements displayed no abnormalities in pH or carbon dioxide levels despite his labored breathing.

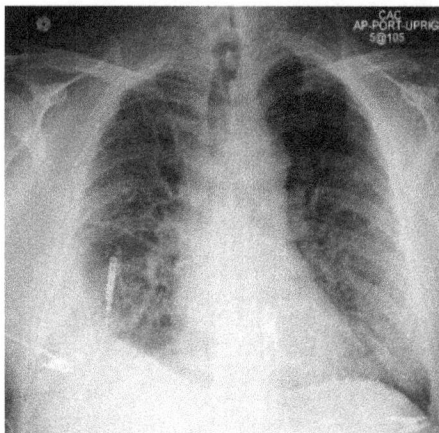

FIGURE 4: Anteroposterior chest X-ray taken at the hospital admission during acute exacerbation of DIP. Right pleural effusion and bilateral lung interstitial opacities.

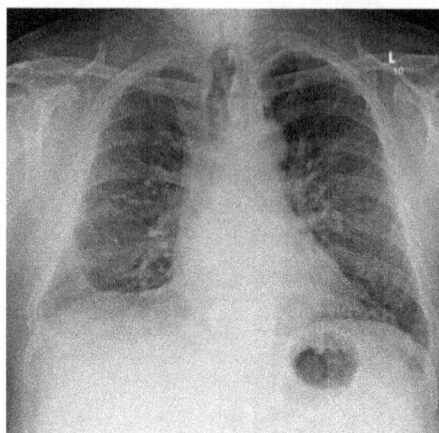

FIGURE 6: Anteroposterior chest X-ray 10 days after acute exacerbation and treatment with glucocorticoids. Right pleural effusion resolved with improvement in interstitial opacities.

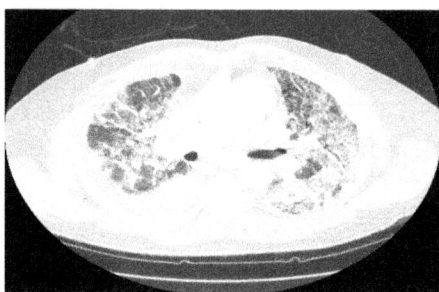

FIGURE 5: Chest CT angiogram taken during the acute exacerbation. Right pleural fluid filling 1/4 of chest, bilateral interstitial, and airspace disease. Ground glass opacities, pathological adenopathies in the mediastinum, cardiomegaly, and no pulmonary embolus.

He was given 40 mg methylprednisolone every 8 hours. Within hours, his shortness of breath and oxygen saturation drastically improved. All respiratory symptoms dissipated, and he was stable to be treated as an outpatient after 48 hours of starting treatment. His discharge plan included oxygen support by nasal cannula and oral prednisone. He agreed to a smoking cessation plan with nicotine patches.

Ten days after discharge, an office-visit chest X-ray (Figure 6) showed complete resolution of the pleural effusion and bilateral interstitial and airspace diseases markedly improved. His oxygen saturation climbed to 96% on room air indicating supplemental oxygen was no longer needed.

3. Discussion

DIP and respiratory bronchiolitis interstitial lung disease (RB-ILD) are the two interstitial pneumonias associated with smoking [1]. While 90% of DIP is primarily due to smoking, 10% is a result of other causes [1, 11–13]. Other causes include drugs (i.e., sirolimus and nitrofurantoin) [12], infections (i.e., cytomegalovirus, hepatitis C, and aspergillus) [12], connective tissue diseases, environmental exposures (i.e., asbestos, beryllium, and copper) [1, 11, 12], and in children with a surfactant protein mutation [12, 14]. Some documented causes of DIP exacerbations include lung biopsy with VATS and lung transplantation [5, 15, 16].

Common symptoms of DIP are dyspnea on exertion and a dry cough [1, 11]. Physical exam findings in DIP typically consist of bibasilar crackles and sometimes cyanosis or digital clubbing [11]. The typical age of onset is 40-60 [1, 11].

Despite similarities in presentation with other interstitial pneumonias, especially RB-ILD, histological as well as clinical correlation can be utilized to differentiate DIP [11, 13, 17]. The gold standard for DIP and RB-ILD diagnosis is surgical lung biopsy though both may exist together [1]. Histological features unique to DIP are as follows: accumulation of brown-yellow pigmented "smokers pigment" macrophages diffusely within alveolar spaces including distal airways, with

Additional negative tests included respiratory polymerase chain reaction viral panel, fungal serology, blood cultures, sputum acid-fast bacilli testing, urine streptococcus, and legionella. Sputum fungal and bacterial cultures grew *Candida dubliniensis* and *Pseudomonas fluorescens*. Although, these organisms are not generally considered pathogens in humans unless severely immunocompromised and have been found in normal oral flora [9, 10].

To further investigate a cause for the acute decompensation, the patient was offered a bronchoscopy and thoracentesis for mediastinal sampling and pleural effusion, respectively. After an extensive discussion, he refused all invasive diagnostic procedures.

Four days passed after being given broad spectrum antibiotics and no improvement was observed. Repeat imaging showed a persistence of bilateral interstitial opacities and pleural effusion. His oxygen saturation level still required 100% FiO2 supplementation to maintain above 90%. Because initial workup for the acute respiratory failure was inconclusive, less common etiologies were considered including DIP exacerbation.

On the fourth hospitalization day, treatment for possible DIP exacerbation was initiated and antibiotics were stopped.

associated interstitial inflammation and/or fibrosis, however without or with very few honeycomb changes [11, 12, 18, 19]. CT findings in DIP include patchy GGOs that are usually symmetric and in the mid and lower zones [11–13, 18]. PFTs demonstrate a restrictive lung defect with a decreased DLco [1, 12].

Though this patient was a heavy lifelong smoker, 6 months of smoking cessation followed by 6 weeks of smoking relapse was enough to significantly flare his DIP into a life-threatening event. To our knowledge, this is the first case to describe smoking relapse as a likely cause for DIP exacerbation. Research shows 54-67% of smokers who attempt to quit in the first-year relapse [20]. Given relapse is so prevalent among smokers attempting to quit, relapse smoking as a possible cause for DIP exacerbation is significant.

Additionally, there are only one prior case reporting mediastinal adenopathies [21] and no cases reporting pleural effusions with DIP as observed in our patient.

The two main treatments for DIP are smoking cessation and glucocorticoids. The DIP mortality rate is 30% at 10 years [17]. Appropriate treatment for an acute DIP episode may lead to complete recovery to baseline as illustrated in our case. Avoidance of possible causes for DIP exacerbations, such as relapse smoking, may lead to improved mortality outcomes in this patient population.

4. Conclusion

Desquamative Interstitial Pneumonia (DIP) can present with fulminant near fatal exacerbations. We believe that smoking relapse has contributed to the acute exacerbation of our patient's DIP. This underlines the importance of smoking cessation and preventing smoking relapse in all DIP patients as one of the few treatments that could alter the course and prevent exacerbations. Glucocorticoids remain the other treatment for chronic and fulminant cases of DIP. Although not previously described, our case demonstrates that pleural effusions and mediastinal adenopathies may exist in both acute and chronic DIP presentations.

Disclosure

This research did not receive any specific grant from funding agencies in the public, commercial, or not-for-profit sectors. This case report has not been published previously, is not under consideration for publication elsewhere, and has been approved for submission by all authors and the institutional affiliate.

References

[1] S. H. Bak and H. Y. Lee, "Overlaps and uncertainties of smoking-related idiopathic interstitial pneumonias," *International Journal of Chronic Obstructive Pulmonary Disease*, vol. Volume 12, pp. 3221–3229, 2017.

[2] A. A. Liebow, A. Steer, and J. G. Billingsley, "Desquamative interstitial pneumonia," *American Journal of Medicine*, vol. 39, no. 3, pp. 369–404, 1965.

[3] G. Flusser, G. Gurman, H. Zirkin, I. Prinslo, and D. Heimer, "Desquamative interstitial pneumonitis causing acute respiratory failure, responsive only to immunosuppressants," *Respiration*, vol. 58, no. 5-6, pp. 324–326, 1991.

[4] A. Churg, J. L. Wright, and H. D. Tazelaar, "Acute exacerbations of fibrotic interstitial lung disease," *Histopathology*, vol. 58, no. 4, pp. 525–530, 2011.

[5] J. M. Sánchez Varilla, M. Vázquez Martín, H. García Dante, J. Peñas del Castillo, and T. Domínguez Plata, "Exacerbación aguda de un caso de neumonitis intersticial descamativa tras biopsia pulmonar por videotoracoscopia," *Anales de Medicina Interna*, vol. 22, no. 12, pp. 604-605, 2005.

[6] T. H. Gould, M. D. Buist, D. Meredith, and PD. Thomas, "Fulminant desquamative interstitial pneumonitis," *Anaesthesia and Intensive Care Journal*, vol. 26, pp. 677–679, 1998.

[7] D. W. Park, T. H. Kim, J. W. Shon et al., "Near fatal desquamative interstitial pneumonia with bilateral recurrent tension pneumothorax," *Sarcoidosis Vasculitis and Diffuse Lung Disease*, vol. 32, no. 2, Article ID 26278697, pp. 167–171, 2015.

[8] B. Corrin and A. B. Price, "Electron microscopic studies in desquamative interstitial pneumonia associated with asbestos," *Thorax*, vol. 27, no. 3, pp. 324–331, 1972.

[9] E. Svobodová, P. Staib, J. Losse, F. Hennicke, D. Barz, and M. Józsi, "Differential interaction of the two related fungal species Candida albicans and Candida dubliniensis with human neutrophils," *The Journal of Immunology*, vol. 189, no. 5, pp. 2502–2511, 2012.

[10] B. S. Scales, R. P. Dickson, J. J. Lipuma, and G. B. Huffnagle, "Microbiology, genomics, and clinical significance of the Pseudomonas fluorescens species complex, an unappreciated colonizer of humans," *Clinical Microbiology Reviews*, vol. 27, no. 4, pp. 927–948, 2014.

[11] B. Godbert, M.-P. Wissler, and J.-M. Vignaud, "Desquamative interstitial pneumonia: An analytic review with an emphasis on aetiology," *European Respiratory Review*, vol. 22, no. 128, pp. 117–123, 2013.

[12] H. D. Tazelaar, J. L. Wright, and A. Churg, "Desquamative interstitial pneumonia," *Histopathology*, vol. 58, no. 4, pp. 509–516, 2011.

[13] G. A. Margaritopoulos, S. Harari, A. Caminati, and K. M. Antoniou, "Smoking-related idiopathic interstitial pneumonia: A review," *Respirology*, vol. 21, no. 1, pp. 57–64, 2016.

[14] S. Bressieux-Degueldre, S. Rotman, G. Hafen, J.-D. Aubert, and I. Rochat, "Idiopathic desquamative interstitial pneumonia in a child: A case report," *BMC Research Notes*, vol. 7, no. 1, article no. 383, 2014.

[15] M. B. King, J. Jessurun, and M. I. Hertz, "Recurrence of desquamative interstitial pneumonia after lung transplantation," *American Journal of Respiratory and Critical Care Medicine*, vol. 156, no. 6, pp. 2003–2005, 1997.

[16] Y. Yogo, Y. Oyamada, M. Ishii et al., "A case of acute exacerbation of desquamative interstitial pneumonia after video-assisted thoracoscopic surgery (VATS)," *Nihon Kokyuki Gakkai Zasshi*, vol. 41, no. 6, pp. 386–391, 2003.

[17] C. B. Carrington, E. A. Gaensler, R. E. Coutu, M. X. Fitzgerald, and R. G. Gupta, "Natural History and Treated Course of Usual and Desquamative Interstitial Pneumonia," *The New England Journal of Medicine*, vol. 298, no. 15, pp. 801–809, 1978.

[18] C. Dias, P. Mota, I. Neves, S. Guimarães, C. Souto Moura, and A. Morais, "Transbronchial cryobiopsy in the diagnosis of desquamative interstitial pneumonia," *Revista Portuguesa de Pneumologia (English Edition)*, vol. 22, no. 5, pp. 288–290, 2016.

[19] J. H. Ryu, J. L. Myers, S. A. Capizzi, W. W. Douglas, R. Vassallo, and P. A. Decker, "Desquamative interstitial pneumonia and respiratory bronchiolitis- associated interstitial lung disease," *CHEST*, vol. 127, no. 1, pp. 178–184, 2005.

[20] D. S. Hasin and B. F. Grant, "The National Epidemiologic Survey on Alcohol and Related Conditions (NESARC) Waves 1 and 2: Review and summary of findings," *Social Psychiatry and Psychiatric Epidemiology*, vol. 50, no. 11, pp. 1609–1640, 2015.

[21] N. Sato, Y. Kawabata, N. Takayanagi et al., "A case of desquamative interstitial pneumonia with bilateral hilar and mediastinal lymphadenopathy," *Nihon Kokyūki Gakkai zasshi = the journal of the Japanese Respiratory Society*, vol. 42, no. 5, pp. 446–453, 2004.

49

Daptomycin-Induced Acute Eosinophilic Pneumonia: Late Onset and Quick Recovery

Mohamad Rachid, Khansa Ahmad, Meghan Saunders-Kurban, Aelia Fatima, Aditya Shah, and Anas Nahhas

Internal Medicine, Advocate Christ Medical Center, Oak Lawn, IL, USA

Correspondence should be addressed to Mohamad Rachid; mohammedrachid98@gmail.com

Academic Editor: Shih-Yi Lee

Background. Daptomycin is a cyclic lipopeptide antibiotic that provides great coverage for gram positive cocci. From the early years of daptomycin use, concerns were raised regarding the pulmonary side effects of daptomycin and potential development of acute eosinophilic pneumonia (AEP) secondary to daptomycin therapy. *Discussion.* AEP could be idiopathic or induced by drugs or toxins. It is a distinct entity from atopic diseases and autoimmune, parasitic, or fungal infections that can also cause pulmonary eosinophilia. Multiple medications are associated with acute eosinophilic pneumonia. Multiple cases of daptomycin-induced AEP have been reported in the literature. Diagnosis of AEP is based on clinical history, laboratory tests, and radiographic studies. Obtaining bronchoalveolar lavage or lung biopsy is needed to confirm the diagnosis. Timing of the drug use and clinical presentation is crucial in the diagnosis of drug-induced AEP. Discontinuation of the offending drug and systemic corticosteroids are the mainstay treatment with great outcomes and recovery. *Conclusion.* We present a case of AEP caused by daptomycin, with complete recovery after discontinuation of daptomycin and administration of steroids. The patient had AEP after almost 6 weeks of daptomycin therapy which has never been reported in literature and our patient achieved complete recovery with appropriate management.

1. Introduction

Daptomycin is a cyclic lipopeptide antibiotic approved by the FDA in 2003. Daptomycin provides great coverage for gram positive cocci. Shortly after its approval, concerns were raised regarding the pulmonary side effects of daptomycin and potential development of acute eosinophilic pneumonia (AEP) secondary to daptomycin therapy. About 35 cases were reported in the literature. We present a case of AEP caused by daptomycin, with complete recovery after discontinuation of daptomycin and administration of steroids. The patient had AEP after almost 6 weeks of daptomycin therapy which has not been reported in the literature. The patient achieved complete recovery in less than 48 hours of appropriate management.

2. Case Report

A 64-year-old male, with past medical history of peripheral arterial disease, had a left groin graft placement that was complicated with Methicillin Resistant *Staphylococcus Aureus* (MRSA) infection. Intravenous vancomycin was initiated which was complicated by the red man syndrome. Vancomycin was discontinued and the patient was switched to intravenous daptomycin 6 mg/kg/day for six weeks.

After almost six weeks of daptomycin therapy, the patient presented with progressive shortness of breath of two-day duration with associated fever and productive cough. Initial vital signs upon presentation were temperature 38.6°C (101.5°F), heart rate 100 beats per minute, respiratory rate 22 breaths per minute, oxygen saturation 93% on room air, and blood pressure 92/66 mmHg. Chest exam revealed coarse rhonchi bilaterally.

The initial white blood cells count was 18.0 K/UL, elevated eosinophil count 1 K/UL, and elevated erythrocyte sedimentation rate (ESR) 60 mm/hr. Initial chest-X-ray showed acute bilateral interstitial infiltrates.

The patient was admitted for presumed hospital acquired pneumonia (HCAP) and started on intravenous piperacillin-tazobactam and levofloxacin. However, his clinical condition

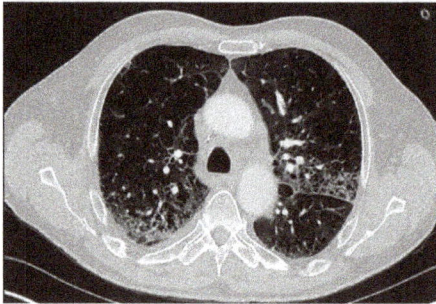

FIGURE 1: Chest Computed Tomography (CT) angiogram obtained to rule out pulmonary embolism (PE) showed diffuse bilateral pulmonary infiltrates, mediastinal lymphadenopathy, and small bilateral pleural effusions.

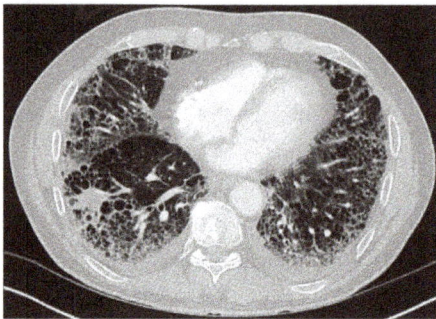

FIGURE 2: Chest Computed Tomography (CT) angiogram obtained to rule out pulmonary embolism (PE) showed diffuse bilateral pulmonary infiltrates, mediastinal lymphadenopathy, and small bilateral pleural effusions.

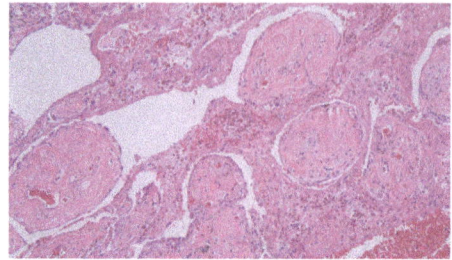

FIGURE 3: Picture of the lung tissue obtained showing chronic inflammatory changes, dense fibrinous airspace exudates, areas of organization, and prominent eosinophils, consistent with eosinophilic pneumonia.

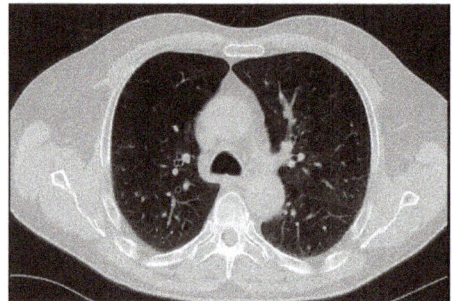

FIGURE 4: Repeat Chest CT, after one week of the initial CT, showing almost complete resolution of previous infiltrates, disappearance of mediastinal lymphadenopathy, and resolution of bilateral pleural effusions.

did not improve. He had progressive cough and increasing oxygen requirements. Chest Computed Tomography (CT) angiogram obtained to rule out pulmonary embolism (PE) showed diffuse bilateral pulmonary infiltrates, mediastinal lymphadenopathy, and small bilateral pleural effusions (Figures 1 and 2). The study was negative for PE. Suspicion for daptomycin-induced eosinophilic pneumonia was raised. Daptomycin was discontinued and intravenous methylprednisolone 80 mg every 8 hours was started.

Bronchoscopy to obtain bronchoalveolar lavage could not be done due to high oxygen requirements the patient needed and the patient was not intubated at that point to do it safely. Thus, the patient was sent for open lung biopsy via video assisted thoracoscopic surgery (VATS). The lung biopsy revealed chronic inflammatory changes, dense fibrinous airspace exudates, areas of organization, and prominent eosinophils, consistent with eosinophilic pneumonia (Figure 3).

The patient improved within 48 hours after discontinuation of daptomycin and initiation of intravenous methylprednisolone. The patient was oxygenating well on room air on day 2 of steroids therapy. IV methylprednisolone was tapered gradually to oral prednisone 40 mg daily then prednisone was stopped in five days. Repeat Chest CT, after one week of the initial CT, showed almost complete resolution of previous infiltrates, disappearance of mediastinal lymphadenopathy, and resolution of bilateral pleural effusions (Figure 4). The left groin wound was well healed upon discharge.

3. Discussion

AEP is a subtype of acute pneumonia which is idiopathic or induced by drugs or toxins. It is distinct from atopic diseases and autoimmune, parasitic, or fungal infections that can also cause pulmonary eosinophilia. Multiple medications are associated with acute eosinophilic pneumonia including nonsteroidal anti-inflammatory drugs, minocycline [1], antidepressants, and antipsychotics [2].

Daptomycin is a cyclic lipopeptide antibiotic which was approved by the FDA in 2003. Daptomycin inhibits DNA, RNA, and protein synthesis by causing depolarization of the membrane potential when it binds the bacterial membrane [3]. It has excellent spectrum for gram positive bacteria [4]. Daptomycin is usually used against Methicillin Resistant *Staphylococcus Aureus* (MRSA) as a second line agent after vancomycin in treating skin, soft tissue infections, and bacteremia [5].

Early after the approval of daptomycin by the FDA, multiple cases of daptomycin-induced eosinophilic pneumonia have been reported. Hayes Jr. et al. reported the first case of daptomycin-induced eosinophilic pneumonia in 2007 [6]. Kim and colleagues reviewed the reported cases in the FDA

Adverse Event Reporting System (AERS) submitted from 2004 to 2010. They put forth criteria to classify these cases as definite, probable, possible, or unlikely [7]. Based on their criteria, our patient had a definitive diagnosis of daptomycin-induced eosinophilic pneumonia.

Diagnosis of daptomycin-induced AEP is based on clinical history, laboratory results, and radiographic findings. Usually these patients present with dyspnea and cough with or without fever. The clinical presentation may vary from mild respiratory complaints to minimal requirement of oxygen, up to acute respiratory distress syndrome (ARDS). Laboratory workup may reveal peripheral eosinophilia, leukocytosis, or elevated markers of inflammation such as erythrocyte sedimentation rate (ESR) and C-reactive protein (CRP). Chest X-ray reveals bilateral pulmonary infiltrates. Chest CT may reveal bilateral consolidation, infiltrates, pulmonary nodules [3], ground glass opacity [8], and bilateral pleural effusions [2]. In our case, bilateral peripheral infiltrates were abundant which is consistent with eosinophilic pneumonia. Definitive diagnosis necessitates bronchoalveolar lavage (BAL) to obtain cell count. BAL with more than 25% of eosinophilic is diagnostic of eosinophilic pneumonia. Sometimes, a lung biopsy is needed to confirm the diagnosis. It is crucial to exclude other causes of eosinophilic lung disease such as parasitic infections, fungal infections, or vasculitis, before making the final diagnosis of any drug-induced AEP, including daptomycin. The Department of Pulmonary and Intensive Care at University Hospital in Dijon, France is maintaining a helpful website to report medications and drugs associated with lung injuries. The website is: http://www.pneumotox.com [9].

The criteria to diagnose AEP consist of 4 components: presence of febrile illness of less than 5-day duration, diffuse bilateral pulmonary infiltrates, hypoxemia defined as partial pressure of oxygen of less than 60 mmHg or oxygen saturation less than 90% on room air, and bronchoalveolar lavage with greater than 25% eosinophils or eosinophilic pneumonia on lung biopsy [10]. Solomon and Schwarz created criteria to diagnose drug-induced AEP, consisting of (1) presence of AEP confirmed by criteria mentioned earlier, (2) presence of causative drug with appropriate temporal relationship, (3) other causes of AEP excluded like fungal or parasitic infections, (4) clinical improvement after cessation of the drug, and (5) the recurrence of AEP with rechallenge to the drug [11]. Rechallenging with the drug is not recommended.

In Idiopathic AEP, most of the time, the peripheral eosinophil count is not elevated in the early phases but may become elevated later on during the course of the disease [12]. Our patient did have peripheral eosinophilia. We reviewed 28 reported cases of daptomycin-induced AEP and we found that 23 out of 28 cases did have peripheral eosinophilia. Peripheral eosinophilia is not necessary to diagnose AEP and it is not part of the current diagnostic criteria [10] but peripheral eosinophilia may suggest eosinophilic pneumonia. Yusuf et al. [13] suggested using the peripheral eosinophils count as a marker to monitor for daptomycin-induced AEP. They suggested obtaining baseline eosinophils count before starting daptomycin therapy then following up the count during treatment course to monitor for peripheral eosinophilia.

The pathophysiology of daptomycin-induced AEP is unclear. Daptomycin binds the lung surfactant irreversibly and may act like an antigen taken up by alveolar macrophages which then leads to inflammatory cascade and tissue damage. Alveolar macrophages present the antigen to T-helper 2 lymphocytes, which release multiple inflammatory factors like IL-5 and Eotaxin. IL-5 is known to induce production of eosinophils in bone marrow and recruit them to inflammatory sites. Eotaxin is a chemokine and acts as a chemoattractant which causes migration and recruitment of eosinophils [14, 15]. In case this theory is truly the cause of AEP in patients on daptomycin therapy, the question is why are only some patients affected by AEP on daptomycin therapy? Why is it uncommon to see this side effect from daptomycin therapy? These questions have yet to be answered with further research.

The histologic findings of drug-induced eosinophilic pneumonia have been described in multiple case reports. Most of the reported cases diagnosed daptomycin-induced AEP based on BAL findings. In cases where lung biopsies were obtained, the majority revealed organizing pneumonia with eosinophilic infiltrates and chronic inflammatory changes [3, 14, 16]. In our case, we confirmed the diagnosis by lung biopsy. Hayes Jr. et al. [6] reported alveolar and interstitial eosinophils with minimal edema in the biopsy results. Our patient's lung biopsy revealed chronic inflammatory changes, diffuse fibrinous airspace exudates, and prominent admixed eosinophils.

The mainstay treatment of daptomycin-induced AEP, and any other drug-induced AEP, is to give corticosteroids and to stop the offending drug. This practice is based on previous case reports of daptomycin-induced AEP and other medication induced lung injuries. Steroids are recommended to patients with acute lung injuries caused by amiodarone, cocaine, and bleomycin [17]. Our patient had a dramatic recovery within 36 hours after stopping daptomycin and starting steroid therapy. In most reported cases, daptomycin was stopped and patients received steroid therapy. In a few cases, daptomycin was stopped and steroids were not given. All of these patients had a complete recovery without relapse [3, 8, 13, 14, 18]. AEP is an acute inflammatory process and giving steroids is a reasonable treatment option. With reported cases of complete recovery by discontinuing daptomycin alone, is giving steroids warranted or not? There are no guidelines that address this question and further research is needed. However, it is reasonable to give steroids in patients with severe hypoxemia and respiratory failure. A systematic review was recently published on 35 reported cases in the literature [19].

4. Conclusion

Daptomycin is not widely used, yet physicians should be aware of daptomycin-induced AEP in any patient actively on daptomycin and presenting with respiratory complaints. Daptomycin-induced AEP is not related to therapy timing. It may occur as early as day three of treatment and as late as week six of the treatment course. AEP is a serious side effect of daptomycin but easily treatable if diagnosed early during the course of the disease. High clinical suspicion and thorough workup are needed for diagnosis of AEP. The current mainstay therapy is stopping daptomycin with or without steroid therapy. Further research is needed to assess the role of steroids in the treatment of AEP, including the optimal dose and duration of therapy.

This case is unique because the patient had daptomycin-induced AEP after almost six weeks of daptomycin therapy, which has not been previously reported in the literature. As long as the patient is undergoing daptomycin therapy, the risk of AEP still exists, even after a considerable amount of time has passed.

References

[1] S. W. Hung, "Minocycline-induced acute eosinophilic pneumonia: A case report and review of the literature," *Respiratory Medicine Case Reports*, vol. 15, pp. 110–114, 2015.

[2] J. J. Patel, A. Antony, M. Herrera, and R. J. Lipchik, "Daptomycin-induced acute eosinophilic pneumonia," *Wisconsin Medical Society*, vol. 113, pp. 199–201, 2014.

[3] E. Cobb, R. C. Kimbrough, K. M. Nugent, and M. P. Phy, "Organizing pneumonia and pulmonary eosinophilic infiltration associated with daptomycin," *Annals of Pharmacotherapy*, vol. 41, no. 4, pp. 696–701, 2007.

[4] C. F. Carpenter and H. F. Chambers, "Daptomycin: another novel agent for treating infections due to drug-resistant gram-positive pathogens," *Clinical Infectious Diseases*, vol. 38, no. 7, pp. 994–1000, 2004.

[5] Cubicin1 (daptomycin) [package insert]. Lexington, MA, USA: Cubist Pharmaceuticals; Revised January 2013.

[6] D. Hayes Jr., M. I. Anstead, and R. J. Kuhn, "Eosinophilic pneumonia induced by daptomycin," *Infection*, vol. 54, no. 4, pp. e211–e213, 2007.

[7] P. W. Kim, A. F. Sorbello, R. T. Wassel, T. M. Pham, J. M. Tonning, and S. Nambiar, "Eosinophilic pneumonia in patients treated with daptomycin: Review of the literature and US FDA adverse event reporting system reports," *Drug Safety*, vol. 35, no. 6, pp. 447–457, 2012.

[8] A. S. Kalogeropoulos, S. Tsiodras, D. Loverdos, P. Fanourgiakis, and A. Skoutelis, "Eosinophilic pneumonia associated with daptomycin: A case report and a review of the literature," *Journal of Medical Case Reports*, vol. 5, article 13, 2011.

[9] P. Camus and P. Foucher, *The drug-induced respiratory disease website [Internet]*, 2012, Dijon, France; 2012. Published June 10, 2012. Updated July 11, 2014. Web site. http://www.pneumotox.com/.

[10] F. Philit, B. Etienne-Mastroïanni, A. Parrot, C. Guérin, D. Robert, and J.-F. Cordier, "Idiopathic acute eosinophilic pneumonia: A study of 22 patients," *American Journal of Respiratory and Critical Care Medicine*, vol. 166, no. 9, pp. 1235–1239, 2002.

[11] J. Solomon and M. Schwarz, "Drug-, toxin-, and radiation therapy-induced eosinophilic pneumonia," *Seminars in Respiratory and Critical Care Medicine*, vol. 27, no. 2, pp. 192–197, 2006.

[12] B. W. Jhun, S. J. Kim, K. Kim, and J. E. Lee, "Clinical implications of initial peripheral eosinophilia in acute eosinophilic pneumonia," *Respirology*, vol. 19, no. 7, pp. 1059–1065, 2014.

[13] E. Yusuf, N. Perrottet, C. Orasch, O. Borens, and A. Trampuz, "Daptomycin-associated eosinophilic pneumonia in two patients with prosthetic joint infection," *Surgical Infections*, vol. 15, no. 6, pp. 834–837, 2014.

[14] B. A. Miller, A. Gray, T. W. Leblanc, D. J. Sexton, A. R. Martin, and T. G. Slama, "Acute eosinophilic pneumonia secondary to daptomycin: A report of three cases," *Clinical Infectious Diseases*, vol. 50, no. 11, pp. e63–e68, 2010.

[15] J. N. Allen, "Drug-induced eosinophilic lung disease," *Clinics in Chest Medicine*, vol. 25, no. 1, pp. 77–88, 2004.

[16] A. Shinde, A. Seifi, S. DelRe, W. H. Moustafa Hussein, and J. Ohebsion, "Daptomycin-induced pulmonary infiltrates with eosinophilia," *Infection*, vol. 58, no. 2, pp. 173-174, 2009.

[17] M. A. Jantz and S. A. Sahn, "Corticosteroids in acute respiratory failure," *American Journal of Respiratory and Critical Care Medicine*, vol. 160, no. 4, article 1079-100, 1999.

[18] M. Hatipoglu, A. Memis, V. Turhan, M. Mutluoglu, and K. Canoglu, "Possible daptomycin-induced acute eosinophilic pneumonia in a patient with diabetic foot infection," *International Journal of Antimicrobial Agents*, vol. 47, no. 5, pp. 414-415, 2016.

[19] P. Uppal, K. L. LaPlante, M. M. Gaitanis, M. D. Jankowich, and K. E. Ward, "Daptomycin-induced eosinophilic pneumonia - a systematic review," *Antimicrobial Resistance and Infection Control*, vol. 5, no. 1, article 55, 2016.

50

Primary Pulmonary Amebiasis Complicated with Multicystic Empyema

Ali Zakaria, Bayan Al-Share, and Khaled Al Asad

Istishari Hospital, Department of Internal Medicine, Division of Pulmonology, Amman 11183, Jordan

Correspondence should be addressed to Ali Zakaria; alizakaria86@hotmail.com

Academic Editor: Reda E. Girgis

Amebiasis is a parasitic infection caused by the protozoan *Entamoeba histolytica*. While most infections are asymptomatic, the disease could manifest clinically as amebic dysentery and/or extraintestinal invasion in the form of amebic liver abscess or other more rare manifestations such as pulmonary, cardiac, or brain involvement. Herein we are reporting a case of a 24-year-old male with history of Down syndrome who presented with severe right side pneumonia complicated with multicystic empyema resistant to regular medical therapy. Further investigation revealed a positive pleural fluid for *E. histolytica* cysts and trophozoites. The patient was diagnosed with primary pleuropulmonary amebiasis and he responded promptly to surgical drainage and metronidazole therapy. In patients from endemic areas all physicians should keep a high index of suspicion of amebiasis as a cause of pulmonary disease.

1. Introduction

Amebiasis occurs worldwide; it is estimated that approximately 40 to 50 million people develop colitis or extraintestinal disease annually with 40,000 deaths [1]. The prevalence is disproportionately increased in developing countries because of poor socioeconomic conditions and sanitation levels. In most cases the infections are asymptomatic yet; it can manifest clinically as intestinal disease or rarely as extraintestinal invasion in the form of liver abscess, pleuropulmonary, cardiac, or brain disease. The lungs are the second most common site of extraintestinal infection, with pleural invasion accounting for 2-3% of patients with invasive disease.

2. Case Presentation

The patient is a 24-year-old male with a history of Down syndrome who was brought to our hospital from Yemen by his brother after 10 days of fever (39.5°C), productive cough, shortness of breath, and right side chest pain. He developed the symptoms after few days of being found eating a sandwich that he hid in an organic fertilized soil of his house backyard. He was brought to our hospital in Jordan after he failed a course of moxifloxacin for assumed diagnosis of community acquired pneumonia.

On presentation he was still complaining of same symptoms, and he denied any jaundice, abdominal pain, nausea, vomiting, or diarrhea. On physical examination he was alert, oriented, sweaty, and in mild respiratory distress. His vital signs were as follows: temperature 38.3°C; pulse 110 bpm; respiratory rate 26 bpm; blood pressure 90/45 mmHg; and O_2% of 82% on room air. He had cracked lips, protruded tongue, erythematous, and dry mucous membranes of the oropharynx. Chest exam revealed significant decreased air entry and tactile vocal fremitus with crackles and minimal wheezes on the right side and normal heart sounds with no murmurs or rubs or gallops. His abdomen was soft and nontender with no evidence of organomegaly.

He was immediately resuscitated with IVF bolus and oxygen supplementation; his chest X-ray revealed right sided obliteration of costophrenic angle and displaced right lung (Figure 1). CT scan showed right sided pleural effusion with pocket mainly in lateral aspect and in the oblique fissure, multiple gas bubbles with air fluid levels, and partial atelectasis of right middle and lower lobes that are medially displaced (Figure 2). Abdomen ultrasound and CT scan showed no evidence of obvious gross liver pathology.

He was diagnosed with right sided pneumonia complicated with multicystic empyema, and he underwent thoracotomy with drainage, decortication, and chest tube placement.

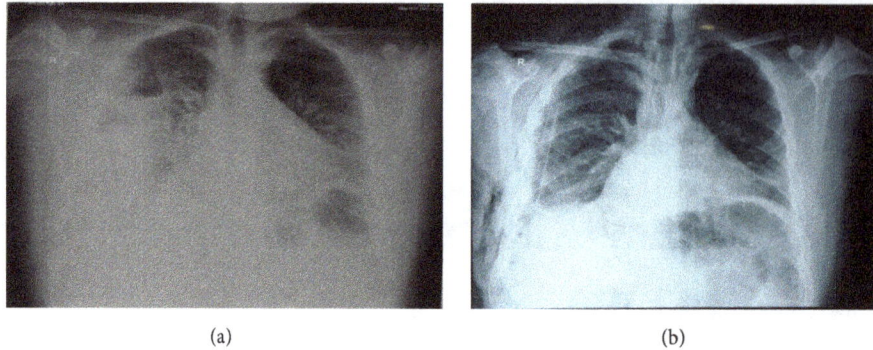

(a)   (b)

FIGURE 1: (a) Preoperative chest X-ray shows right sided obliteration of costophrenic angle and displaced right lung. (b) Postoperative resolution of the empyema (note chest tube).

Light microscopic examination of both pleural fluid and bronchoalveolar lavage sample revealed *Entamoeba* cysts and trophozoites. Microbiology revealed negative acid-fast stain or fungal infection. Aerobic and anaerobic blood culture showed no growth.

Colonoscopy was done and biopsy revealed mixed inflammatory infiltrate suggestive of infection with no demonstrable amoeba. And stool analysis ×3 was also negative for *Entamoeba* cyst or trophozoites. Serological test was not done due to unavailability.

The patient was treated with metronidazole 750 mg three times daily; luminal agent was not given due to unavailability in Jordan. His clinical condition significantly improved after 48 hours of antibiotic treatment. On one-month follow-up visit he was free of symptoms, and he returned back to Yemen.

3. Discussion

Amebiasis is defined by the World Health Organization (WHO) and Pan American Health Organization (PAHO) as a parasitic infection with the protozoan *Entamoeba histolytica* regardless of symptomatology. It is considered the third most common parasitic infection worldwide with around 500 million infections per year and a leading cause of parasite-related mortality with over 100,000 deaths annually. This protozoal infection has an especially high prevalence in subtropical and tropical countries where poor socioeconomic and sanitary conditions predominate, while in resource-rich nations infections may be seen in travelers to and emigrants from endemic areas [2–5].

The majority of *Entamoeba* infections are asymptomatic. Factors that influence whether infection leads to asymptomatic or invasive disease include the *E. histolytica* strain and host factors such as genetic susceptibility, age, and immune status, where young age, pregnancy, corticosteroid treatment, malignancy, malnutrition, and alcoholism are considered risk factors for severe disease [4].

Clinical manifestation of amebiasis generally occurs in the form of intestinal involvement as acute or subacute colitis, with symptoms range from mild diarrhea to severe dysentery producing abdominal pain, diarrhea, and bloody stools, to fulminant amebic colitis. It can also present as extraintestinal

disease in the form of amebic liver abscess and even more rare as pulmonary, cardiac, and brain involvement.

Pleuropulmonary complications (i.e., pleural effusion, lung abscess, and, rarely, pleural empyema) are the second most frequent extraintestinal complication; they occur in 7–20% of patients with amebic liver abscesses and in 2-3% of those with invasive disease [6]. The presentation of pleuropulmonary amebiasis is variable and depends on the type of pulmonary involvement whether it is primary simulating bronchopneumonia or tuberculosis or secondary to rupture giving the characteristic suppurative syndrome. The most common symptoms include pain, cough, hemoptysis, and dyspnea. The pain may be pleuritic or localized to the right upper quadrant. Cough can be nonproductive but more often is associated with expectoration of material ranging from small amounts of sputum to large amounts of amebic pus. If a hepatobronchial fistula develops, the patient may expectorate necrotic material that can include liver abscess contents; such material may have a reddish brown or "anchovy sauce" appearance [1].

The theoretical mechanisms of thoracic amebiasis are as follows. First, the infection usually spreads to the lung by direct rupture of an amoebic liver abscess through the diaphragm. Second, the infection may disseminate to the thorax directly from the primary intestinal lesion through hematogenous or lymphatic spread. And finally, inhalation of dust containing cysts of *E. histolytica* is also a hypothetical route (which is the most probable route in our case) [6, 7].

Pleuropulmonary amebiasis is easily confused with other illnesses which makes the differential diagnosis rather a complex one, involving and not limited to (1) pulmonary TB, (2) bacterial lung abscess, (3) carcinoma of the lung, and (4) in endemic areas malaria and schistosomiasis considered common causes of parasitic deaths that can present with unremitting fevers and hepatic or lung disease [8, 9].

The diagnosis of pleuropulmonary amebiasis may be supported by the clinical manifestation and radiographic imaging such as homogenous opacity or cavitating lesion most commonly involving the right lower and middle lobes, elevated right hemidiaphragm, basilar pulmonary infiltrates with areas of focal atelectasis, and pleural effusions. In the setting of suggestive findings on imaging studies, confirmatory

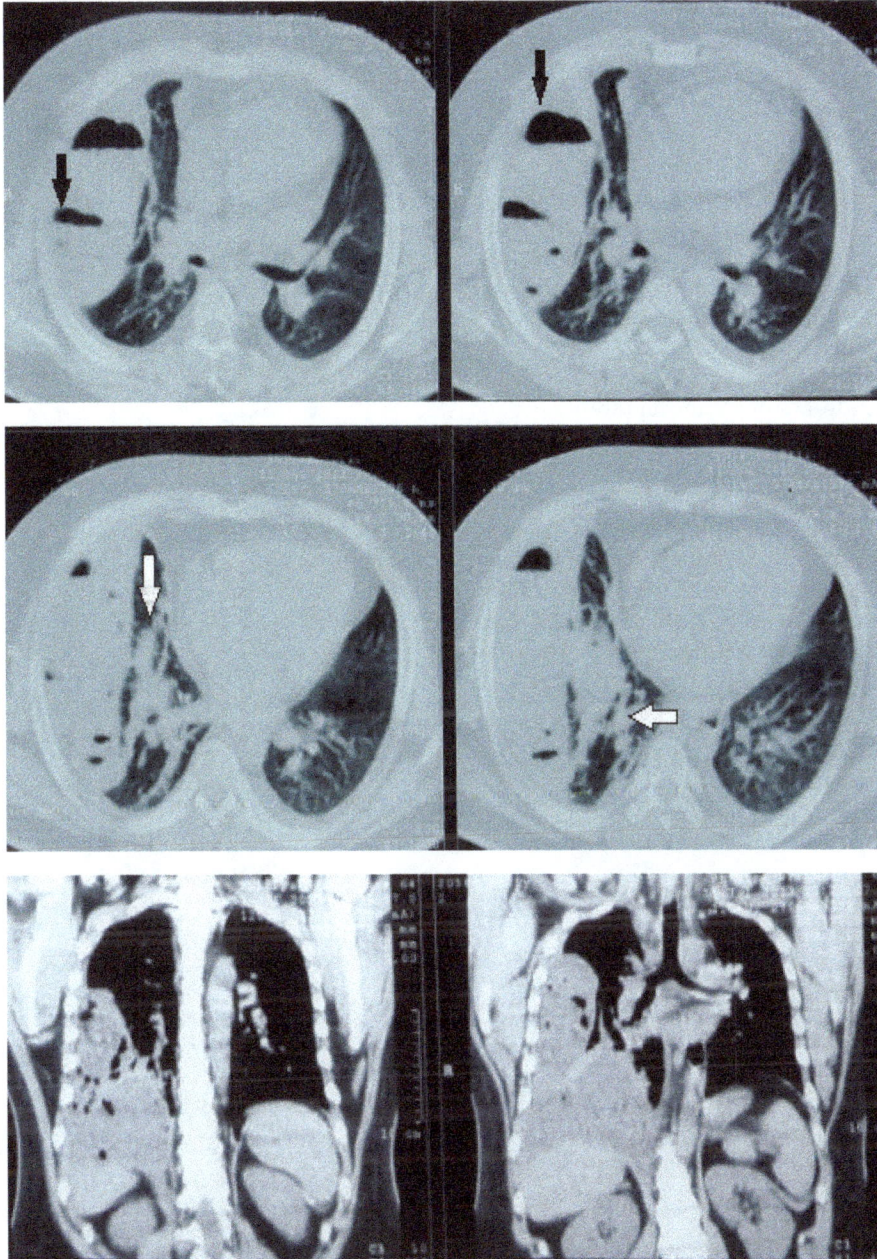

FIGURE 2: Chest CT scan right sided pleural effusion with pocket mainly in lateral aspect and in the oblique fissure, multiple gas bubbles with air fluid levels (black arrow), and partial atelectasis of right middle and lower lobes that are medially displaced (white arrow).

serologic or antigenic testing should be pursued and perhaps supplemented with stool microscopy or antigenic testing of stool [10, 11].

Light microscopic examination can often identify characteristic trophozoites and cysts through direct, concentrated, and/or permanently stained smears. Keeping in mind that the organisms may appear intermittently, specimens from patients with disseminated disease may not contain cysts and trophozoites despite repeated examinations [5]. Immunological tests such as indirect hemagglutination assay (IHA) and enzyme-linked immunosorbent assay (ELISA) for *E.*

histolytica antibodies are characterized by high sensitivity. The primary disadvantage of serologic tests is that they cannot distinguish between past and current infection unless IgM is detected; IgM antibodies to *E. histolytica* are short-lived and rarely detected. In contrast, IgG antibodies are long-lived but highly prevalent in endemic settings. New serologic tests based on recombinant *E. histolytica* antigens have been developed; such assays may be especially useful in endemic areas [5, 12].

In general, amebic pleural effusions should be aspirated. Drained pleural effusions resolve rapidly with drainage and antimicrobial therapy, which consists of metronidazole (750 mg orally three times daily for 7 to 10 days) or alternatively tinidazole (2 g once daily for five days) [13]. Most patients respond to a single course of treatment with resolution of symptoms before the end of therapy. In rare cases, a second course is needed because of failure to achieve complete resolution after the initial regimen. Treatment with a luminal agent such as paromomycin (25–30 mg/kg/day orally in three divided doses for seven days), diiodohydroxyquin (650 mg orally three times daily for 20 days), or diloxanide furoate (500 mg orally three times daily for 10 days) to eliminate intraluminal cysts is also warranted.

The mortality rate of amebic pleural empyema is as high as 16%, which can increase to 42% due to the rupture of a hepatic abscess into the pleural space. Empyema requires chest tube thoracostomy and decortication to prevent recurrence and chronic infection [8, 10, 14].

In conclusion, pleuropulmonary amebiasis is the second most frequent extraintestinal complication that can be easily treated with drainage and antimicrobial therapy. Inhalation of dust containing cysts of *E. histolytica* is a possible route of primary infection. In patients from endemic areas all physicians should keep a high index of suspicion of amebiasis as a cause of pulmonary disease.

Competing Interests

The authors declare that they have no competing interests.

References

[1] D. Kennedy and O. P. Sharma, "Hemoptysis in a 49-year-old man: an unusual presentation of a sporadic disease," *Chest*, vol. 98, no. 5, pp. 1275–1278, 1990.

[2] "WHO/PAHO/UNESCO report. A consultation with experts on amoebiasis. Mexico City, Mexico 28-29 January, 1997," *Epidemiological Bulletin*, vol. 18, no. 1, pp. 13–14, 1997.

[3] C. Ximénez, P. Morán, L. Rojas, A. Valadez, and A. Gómez, "Reassessment of the epidemiology of amebiasis: state of the art," *Infection, Genetics and Evolution*, vol. 9, no. 6, pp. 1023–1032, 2009.

[4] S. L. Stanley Jr., "Amoebiasis," *The Lancet*, vol. 361, no. 9362, pp. 1025–1034, 2003.

[5] R. Fotedar, D. Stark, N. Beebe, D. Marriott, J. Ellis, and J. Harkness, "Laboratory diagnostic techniques for *Entamoeba* species," *Clinical Microbiology Reviews*, vol. 20, no. 3, pp. 511–532, 2007.

[6] S. M. Shamsuzzaman and Y. Hashiguchi, "Thoracic amebiasis," *Clinics in Chest Medicine*, vol. 23, no. 2, pp. 479–492, 2002.

[7] X.-Y. Meng and J.-X. Wu, "Perforated amebic liver abscess: clinical analysis of 110 cases," *Southern Medical Journal*, vol. 87, no. 10, pp. 985–990, 1994.

[8] S. M. Shamsuzzaman and Y. Hashiguchi, "Thoracic amebiasis," *Clinics in Chest Medicine*, vol. 23, no. 2, pp. 479–492, 2002.

[9] J. M. Salles, L. A. Moraes, and M. C. Salles, "Hepatic amebiasis," *Brazilian Journal of Infectious Diseases*, vol. 7, no. 2, pp. 96–110, 2003.

[10] K. D. Lyche and W. A. Jensen, "Pleuropulmonary amebiasis," *Seminars in Respiratory Infections*, vol. 12, no. 2, pp. 106–112, 1997.

[11] B. S. Pritt and C. Graham Clark, "Amebiasis," *Mayo Clinic Proceedings*, vol. 83, no. 10, pp. 1154–1160, 2008.

[12] S. L. Stanley Jr., T. F. Jackson, L. Foster, and S. Singh, "Longitudinal study of the antibody response to recombinant *Entamoeba histolytica* antigens in patients with amebic liver abscess," *American Journal of Tropical Medicine and Hygiene*, vol. 58, no. 4, pp. 414–416, 1998.

[13] H. B. Fung and T.-L. Doan, "Tinidazole: a nitroimidazole antiprotozoal agent," *Clinical Therapeutics*, vol. 27, no. 12, pp. 1859–1884, 2005.

[14] K. R. Kubitschek, J. Peters, D. Nickeson, and D. M. Musher, "Amebiasis presenting as pleuropulmonary disease," *Western Journal of Medicine*, vol. 142, no. 2, pp. 203–207, 1985.

51

Plastic Bronchitis in an AIDS Patient with Pulmonary Kaposi Sarcoma

Sheila A. Habib ⓘ,[1,2] Robert C. Vasko,[3] Jack Badawy,[4] and Gregory M. Anstead ⓘ[5,6]

[1]*Department of Medicine, Division of Pulmonary Diseases and Critical Care Medicine,*
 University of Texas Health at San Antonio (UTH-SA), San Antonio, TX 78229, USA
[2]*Medical Service, Division of Pulmonary Diseases and Critical Care Medicine,*
 South Texas Veterans Health Care System (STVHCS), San Antonio, TX 78229, USA
[3]*Department of Pediatrics, Children's Hospital Los Angeles, Los Angeles, CA 90027, USA*
[4]*Department of Medicine, Division of General and Hospital Medicine, UTH-SA, San Antonio, TX 78229, USA*
[5]*Department of Medicine, Division of Infectious Diseases, UTH-SA, San Antonio, TX 78229, USA*
[6]*Medical Service, Division of Infectious Diseases, STVHCS, San Antonio, TX 78229, USA*

Correspondence should be addressed to Sheila A. Habib; habibs@uthscsa.edu

Academic Editor: Fabio Midulla

Plastic bronchitis is the expectoration of bronchial casts in the mold of the tracheobronchial tree. It is a rare occurrence of unknown etiology that has been primarily described in children with congenital heart disease. In this case report, we present the first reported case of plastic bronchitis in a patient with pulmonary Kaposi sarcoma and underlying HIV infection.

1. Introduction

Plastic bronchitis (PB) is the formation of casts in the mold of the tracheobronchial tree, leading to airway obstruction. It has been described in association with a variety of coexisting disorders, but most commonly in children with cyanotic congenital heart disease following the Fontan procedure. To our knowledge, we describe the first case of PB in the setting of human immunodeficiency virus (HIV) infection and pulmonary Kaposi sarcoma (KS).

2. Case Presentation

A 25-year-old Hispanic male with HIV infection (CD4 count <40 cells/μL, viral load 307 copies/mL on antiretroviral therapy) and pulmonary KS on chemotherapy presented with progressive dyspnea and cough productive of rubbery red and white material (Figure 1). Physical examination revealed hypoxia, coarse crackles to the bilateral lower lung fields, and multiple violaceous cutaneous plaques. Chest computed tomography showed diffuse peribronchovascular consolidative opacities with surrounding ground glass opacities, interlobular septal thickening, and infiltrative soft

tissue densities throughout the mediastinum (Figure 2). Blood and sputum cultures, autoimmune serologic tests, and serologic tests for *Coccidioides* and *Cryptococcus* were negative. Bronchoscopy revealed "tissue-like" material within the tracheobronchial tree, forming casts (Figures 3 and 4). On histopathological analysis, the casts were composed of fibrin with sparse leukocytic infiltrate, consistent with a diagnosis of PB (Figure 5).

Attempts made to clear the fibrinous material from the lung with nebulized dornase alfa, high-frequency oscillation treatments (MetaNeb System (Hill-Rom, Chicago, IL)), and a percussion vest were unsuccessful. Nebulized ipratropium and albuterol and supplemental oxygen by nasal cannula afforded occasional symptomatic relief. Multiple bronchoscopic procedures were performed to remove the fibrinous material from the lung, but it quickly reaccumulated. The expectorated material did not dissolve with tissue plasminogen activator (TPA) *ex vivo*, and thus a trial of nebulized TPA was not conducted. A prednisone taper provided only transient improvement.

In some cases, PB has been due to lymphatic leakage into the bronchi either from surgical trauma or pulmonary

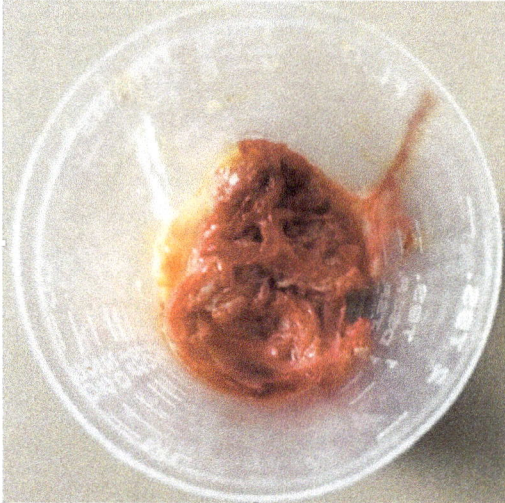

FIGURE 1: The rubbery red and white material expectorated by the patient.

lymphatic abnormalities, with resolution of the condition after ligation of the thoracic duct [1]. In this patient, KS of the intrapulmonary lymphatics was likely causing a chyle leakage. Thus, a lymphangiogram was attempted to determine sites of lymphatic leakage that might be amenable to surgical intervention; however, tracer injected into the lymph vessels in the groin area failed to migrate, likely due to lymphatic involvement with KS. Lymphoscintigraphy was also performed, using the hands as injection sites, but no abnormal uptake of tracer within the lungs was demonstrated. Although thoracic duct embolization was offered to the patient, he declined the procedure.

Over approximately three months, the patient was repeatedly readmitted for respiratory distress and ultimately required endotracheal intubation and mechanical ventilation. Repeated bronchoscopy was performed in an effort to clear the casts, but it was unsuccessful. While on the ventilator, he empirically received multiple therapies for the reduction of lymphatic flow (including total parenteral nutrition (TPN), midodrine, and octreotide) and the treatment of KS (with sirolimus) to curb cast production. Unfortunately, the patient developed refractory respiratory failure and was transitioned to comfort measures. An autopsy revealed extensive pulmonary KS with hepatization of the lung and near obliteration of the normal alveolar architecture with copious mucin and cellular debris within the airways (Figures 6, 7, and 8).

3. Discussion

Plastic bronchitis is a rare condition of unclear pathogenesis characterized by the expectoration of casts in the mold of the tracheobronchial tree. It was first described by Galen in the second century AD as *venae arteriosae expectorantii*, which translates literally to "expectorated arteries and veins" [1, 2]. Since that time, PB has been described in association with bronchial inflammation (due to asthma [3–5],

allergic bronchopulmonary aspergillosis (ABPA) [6], cystic fibrosis [7], influenza [8], and pneumonia); cardiac anomalies (especially following the palliative Fontan procedure [9]); and disorders of lymphatic drainage (lymphangiectasia and lymphangiomatosis [10–13]). Patients with PB typically present with nonspecific symptoms of cough, wheezing, dyspnea, and hypoxemia [1, 14]. In a minority of patients, *ventilgeraeusch* ("sound of a fan") or *bruit de drapeau* ("sound of a flag snapping") may be present and indicate subtotal airway obstruction [1]. Diagnosis is made by visualization of casts, either in expectorated material or via bronchoscopy. Casts typically appear as a white branching mold of the tracheobronchial tree. In our case, we suspect the white-red coloration to be secondary to the vascular nature of KS and the propensity for bleeding. Multiple classification schemes have been proposed for PB [2, 15]. Seear et al. reviewed nine cases with bronchial cast formation and characterized two distinct groups. Type 1 (or inflammatory) casts are composed of fibrin and have a dense eosinophilic infiltrate. They are typically observed in the setting of underlying bronchial disease (such as asthma, cystic fibrosis, and ABPA). Type 2 (or acellular) casts consist mainly of mucin with little cellular infiltrate. These are most commonly observed following the Fontan procedure but may also be seen in noninflammatory causes of PB [15, 16]. Therapeutic approaches to PB are largely anecdotal and focus on (1) facilitating the removal or expectoration of casts and (2) treatment of the underlying etiology. Cast removal may be achieved mechanically (by bronchoscopy [17, 18] and chest physiotherapy) and/or by pharmacologic therapies. PB with type 1/inflammatory casts may respond to anti-inflammatory therapies such as oral and inhaled corticosteroids, bronchodilators, mucolytics [19, 20], and macrolide antibiotics [21]. On the other hand, those with type 2/acellular casts may benefit from optimization of hemodynamics, aerosolized fibrinolytics [14, 16, 19, 22], or thoracic duct ligation [1]. In both cases, aggressive treatment of the underlying etiology provides the most durable relief.

The development of PB has not been previously described in patients with KS, an angioproliferative disorder of the vascular and lymphatic endothelium. KS is well known to cause lymphatic obstruction and lymphedema of the extremities but lymphatic stasis in the lungs has not been well described [23, 24]. Other disorders of the pulmonary lymphatic system (such as lymphangiectasia and lymphangiomatosis) have been associated with the development of PB [11, 12]. Treatment of these disorders focuses on decreasing chyle production by dietary modifications (i.e., a low fat diet excluding long-chain triglycerides, TPN [25]), pharmacologic therapies (including octreotide [26], midodrine [27]), and/or surgical intervention (i.e., thoracic duct ligation) [1]. In this case, the patient empirically received TPN and trials of pharmacologic therapies; however, he continued to produce bronchial casts with frequent airway obstruction. Thoracic duct ligation was considered but was ultimately deferred due to critical illness. Despite empiric aggressive treatment, our patient had persistent bronchial obstruction due to ongoing cast formation and developed refractory respiratory failure. Postmortem analysis revealed extensive pulmonary

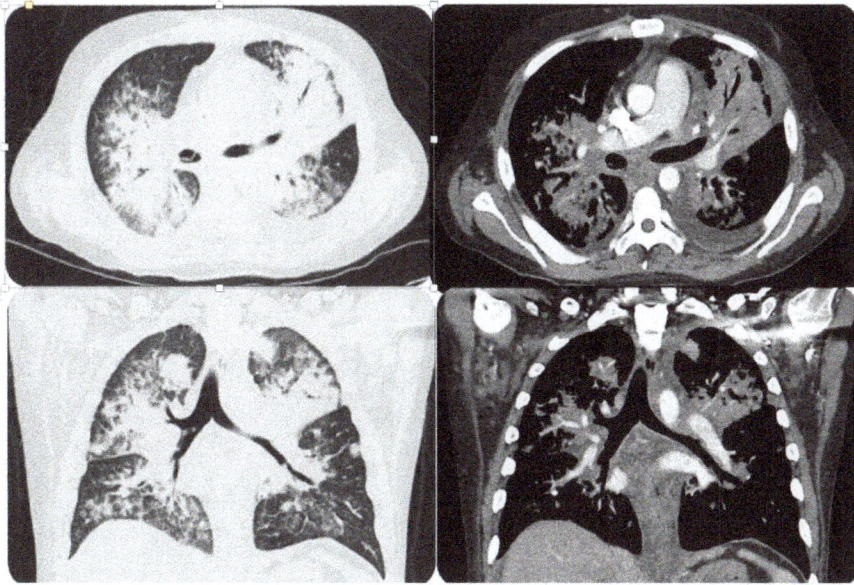

FIGURE 2: Computed tomography of the chest showed diffuse peribronchovascular consolidative opacities with surrounding ground glass opacities, interlobular septal thickening, and infiltrative soft tissue densities throughout the mediastinum. There is also a linear filling defect in the bronchus intermedius.

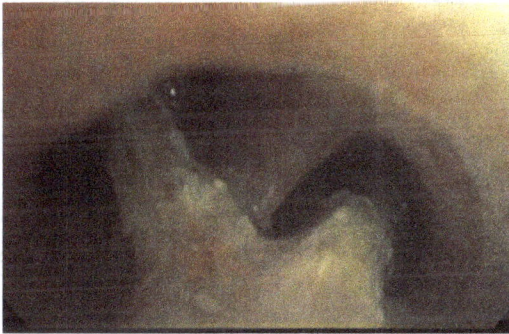

FIGURE 3: Bronchoscopic image at the level of the main carina with "tissue-like" material evident.

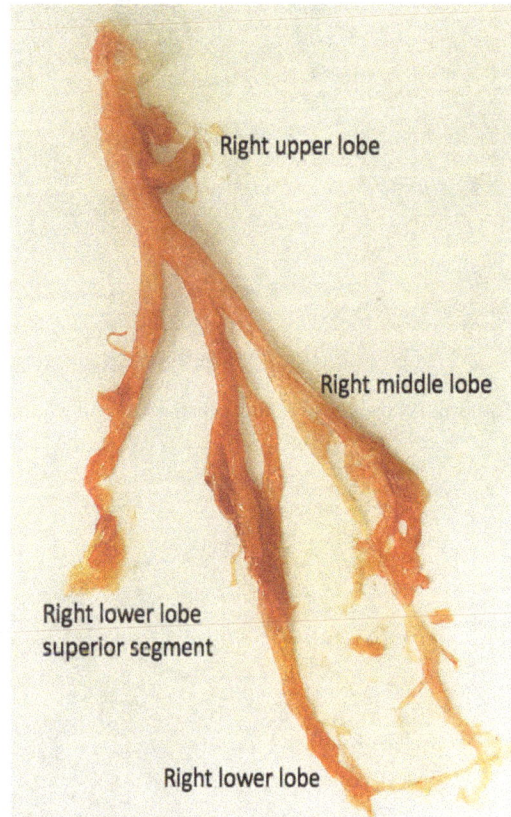

FIGURE 4: Bronchial cast obtained by flexible bronchoscopy fitting the mold of the right bronchial tree.

KS and loss of alveolar architecture that ultimately resulted in refractory respiratory failure.

Plastic bronchitis, although rare, is a life-threatening condition that has been seen in multiple underlying pulmonary conditions. This case report highlights an unusual cause of PB and the need for further investigation into its pathogenesis and therapeutic measures.

Disclosure

This case was presented in the 'Lung Pathology' case report session under the title "The Casts that Take Your Breath Away" at the CHEST 2015 meeting in Montréal, Canada, on Tuesday October 27, 2015.

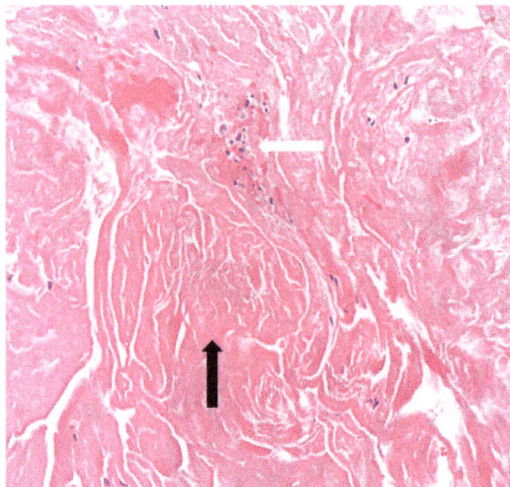

FIGURE 5: Histopathology of the bronchial cast shows fibrin (black arrow) with few leukocytes (white arrow).

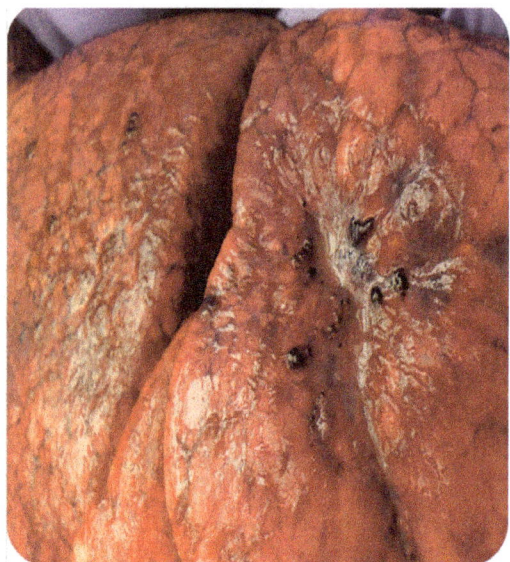

FIGURE 6: Postmortem finding: hepatization of the lung.

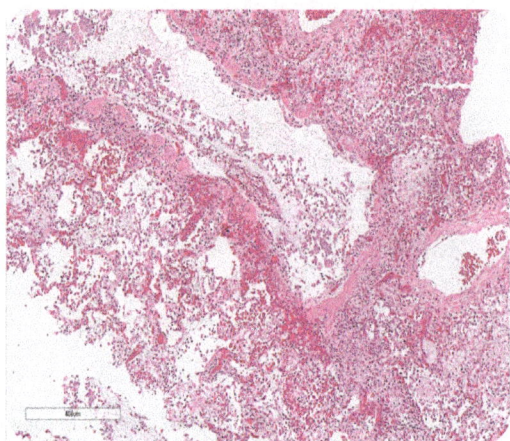

FIGURE 7: Postmortem finding: longitudinal cross section of a terminal bronchiole filled with mucin and cellular debris.

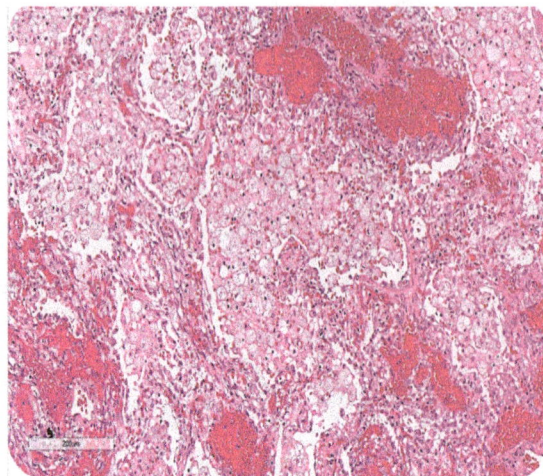

FIGURE 8: Postmortem finding: mucin-filled alveoli surrounded by angiomatous features of Kaposi sarcoma.

Acknowledgments

Special thanks go to Shohei Ikoma, MD, and Francis Sharkey, MD, for assistance with pathology interpretation and pictures.

References

[1] M. H. Eberlein, M. B. Drummond, and E. F. Haponik, "Plastic bronchitis: A management challenge," *The American Journal of the Medical Sciences*, vol. 335, no. 2, pp. 163–169, 2008.

[2] P. Madsen, S. A. Shah, and B. K. Rubin, "Plastic bronchitis: New insights and a classification scheme," *Paediatric Respiratory Reviews*, vol. 6, no. 4, pp. 292–300, 2005.

[3] S. S. Pawar, R. H. Chun, A. R. Rao, and J. E. Kerschner, "Management of plastic bronchitis in a child with mild intermittent asthma," *Annals of Otology, Rhinology & Laryngology*, vol. 120, no. 11, pp. 697–699, 2011.

[4] M. Tonan, M. Sawada, K. Tsuchiya et al., "Successful treatment of severe asthma-associated plastic bronchitis with extracorporeal membrane oxygenation," *Journal of Anesthesia & Clinical Research*, vol. 26, no. 2, pp. 265–268, 2012.

[5] E. J. Kim, J. E. Park, D. H. Kim, and J. Lee, "Plastic Bronchitis in an Adult with Asthma," *Tuberculosis and Respiratory Diseases*, vol. 73, no. 2, pp. 122–126, 2012.

[6] N. G. Sanerkin, R. M. Seal, and J. G. Leopold, "Plastic bronchitis, mucoid impaction of the bronchi and allergic bronchopulmonary aspergillosis, and their relationship to bronchial asthma.," *Annals of Allergy, Asthma & Immunology*, vol. 24, no. 11, pp. 586–594, 1966.

[7] D. Mateos-Corral, E. Cutz, M. Solomon, and F. Ratjen, "Plastic bronchitis as an unusual cause of mucus plugging in cystic fibrosis," *Pediatric Pulmonology*, vol. 44, no. 9, pp. 939–940, 2009.

[8] J. Zhang and X. Kang, "Plastic bronchitis associated with influenza virus infection in children: A report on 14 cases," *International Journal of Pediatric Otorhinolaryngology*, vol. 79, no. 4, pp. 481–486, 2015.

[9] M. Larue, J. G. Gossett, R. D. Stewart, C. L. Backer, C. Mavroudis, and M. L. Jacobs, "Plastic Bronchitis in Patients

With Fontan Physiology: Review of the Literature and Preliminary Experience With Fontan Conversion and Cardiac Transplantation," *World Journal for Pediatric and Congenital Heart Surgery*, vol. 3, no. 3, pp. 364–372, 2012.

[10] A. Stoddart, H. E. Dincer, C. Iber, R. Tomic, and M. Bhargava, "Chyloptysis causing plastic bronchitis," *Respiratory Medicine Case Reports*, vol. 13, pp. 4–6, 2014.

[11] J. Wiggins, E. Sheffield, P. K. Jeffery, D. M. Geddes, and B. Corrin, "Bronchial casts associated with hilar lymphatic and pulmonary lymphoid abnormalities," *Thorax*, vol. 44, no. 3, pp. 226-227, 1989.

[12] L. G. Nair and C. P. Kurtz, "Lymphangiomatosis presenting with bronchial cast formation," *Thorax*, vol. 51, no. 7, pp. 765-766, 1996.

[13] J. Languepin, P. Scheinmann, B. Mahut et al., "Bronchial casts in children with cardiopathies: The role of pulmonary lymphatic abnormalities," *Pediatric Pulmonology*, vol. 28, no. 5, pp. 329–336, 1999.

[14] C. M. Avitabile, D. J. Goldberg, K. Dodds, Y. Dori, C. Ravishankar, and J. Rychik, "A multifaceted approach to the management of plastic bronchitis after cavopulmonary palliation," *The Annals of Thoracic Surgery*, vol. 98, no. 2, pp. 634–640, 2014.

[15] M. Seear, H. Hui, F. Magee, D. Bohn, and E. Cutz, "Bronchial casts in children: A proposed classification based on nine cases and a review of the literature," *American Journal of Respiratory and Critical Care Medicine*, vol. 155, no. 1, pp. 364–370, 1997.

[16] B. K. Rubin, "Plastic Bronchitis," *Clinics in Chest Medicine*, vol. 37, no. 3, pp. 405–408, 2016.

[17] N. Sriratanaviriyakul, F. Lam, B. M. Morrissey, N. Stollenwerk, M. Schivo, and K. Y. Yoneda, "Safety and Clinical Utility of Flexible Bronchoscopic Cryoextraction in Patients with Non-neoplasm Tracheobronchial Obstruction," *Journal of Bronchology & Interventional Pulmonology*, vol. 22, no. 4, pp. 288–293, 2015.

[18] S. Ishman, D. T. Book, S. F. Conley, and J. E. Kerschner, "Plastic bronchitis: An unusual bronchoscopic challenge associated with congenital heart disease repair," *International Journal of Pediatric Otorhinolaryngology*, vol. 67, no. 5, pp. 543–548, 2003.

[19] E. Gibb, R. Blount, N. Lewis et al., "Management of plastic bronchitis with topical tissue-type plasminogen activator," *Pediatrics*, vol. 130, no. 2, pp. e446–e450, 2012.

[20] G. Lis, E. Cichocka-Jarosz, U. Jedynak-Wasowicz, and E. Glowacka, "Add-on treatment with nebulized hypertonic saline in a child with plastic bronchitis after the Glenn procedure," *Jornal Brasileiro de Pneumologia*, vol. 40, no. 1, pp. 82–85, 2014.

[21] K. D. Schultz and C. M. Oermann, "Treatment of cast bronchitis with low-dose oral azithromycin," *Pediatric Pulmonology*, vol. 35, no. 2, pp. 139–143, 2003.

[22] L. Heath, S. Ling, J. Racz et al., "Prospective, longitudinal study of plastic bronchitis cast pathology and responsiveness to tissue plasminogen activator," *Pediatric Cardiology*, vol. 32, no. 8, pp. 1182–1189, 2011.

[23] T. D. Gasparetto, E. Marchiori, S. Lourenço et al., "Pulmonary involvement in Kaposi sarcoma: Correlation between imaging and pathology," *Orphanet Journal of Rare Diseases*, vol. 4, no. 1, article no. 18, 2009.

[24] P. K. Ramdial, R. Chetty, B. Singh, R. Singh, and J. Aboobaker, "Lymphedematous HIV-associated Kaposi's sarcoma," *Journal of Cutaneous Pathology*, vol. 33, no. 7, pp. 474–481, 2006.

[25] K. Sriram, R. A. Meguid, and M. M. Meguid, "Nutritional support in adults with chyle leaks," *Nutrition Journal*, vol. 32, no. 2, pp. 281–286, 2016.

[26] R. D. Helin, S. T. V. Angeles, and R. Bhat, "Octreotide therapy for chylothorax in infants and children: A brief review," *Pediatric Critical Care Medicine*, vol. 7, no. 6, pp. 576–579, 2006.

[27] D. Z. Liou, H. Warren, D. P. Maher et al., "A novel therapeutic for refractory chylothorax," *CHEST*, vol. 144, no. 3, pp. 1055–1057, 2013.

52

Symptomatic Patent Foramen Ovale with Hemidiaphragm Paralysis

Hussain Ibrahim, Adnan Khan, Shawn P. Nishi, Ken Fujise, and Syed Gilani

University of Texas Medical Branch, 301 University Boulevard, 5.106 John Sealy Annex, Galveston, TX 77555-0553, USA

Correspondence should be addressed to Hussain Ibrahim; huibrahi@utmb.edu

Academic Editor: Samer Al-Saad

Dyspnea accounts for more than one-fourth of the hospital admissions from Emergency Department. Chronic conditions such as Chronic Obstructive Pulmonary Disease, Congestive Heart Failure, and Asthma are being common etiologies. Less common etiologies include conditions such as valvular heart disease, pulmonary embolism, and right-to-left shunt (RLS) from patent foramen ovale (PFO). PFO is present in estimated 20–30% of the population, mostly a benign condition. RLS via PFO usually occurs when right atrium pressure exceeds left atrium pressure. RLS can also occur in absence of higher right atrium pressure. We report one such case that highlights the importance of high clinical suspicion, thorough evaluation, and percutaneous closure of the PFO leading to significant improvement in the symptoms.

1. Introduction

In evaluation of a patient with a chief complaint of dyspnea, a potential pitfall would be to neglect rarer etiologies in favor of more common causes. Dyspnea accounts for 28.6% of the admissions to the hospital from Emergency Department (ED), common etiologies being chronic conditions such as Asthma, Heart Failure, and Chronic Obstructive Pulmonary Disease (COPD) [1]. In light of the number of patients visiting the ED with dyspnea-related complaints, it would be easy to overlook the less common cause of dyspnea. This can impact patient outcomes. Less common causes of dyspnea including valvular heart disease, pulmonary embolism, and intracardiac shunt are curable if the proper diagnosis is made in a timely fashion. We present one such case of treatable dyspnea due to patent foramen ovale (PFO) related right-to-left shunt (RLS) in setting of right hemidiaphragm paralysis. Our review of literature revealed only eleven cases with RLS via PFO in presence of right hemidiaphragm (Table 1) [2–10].

2. Case Presentation

59-year-old female with past medical history of long standing primary hypertension, chronic kidney disease Stage III, and Diabetes Mellitus type II started experiencing gradual worsening shortness of breath (SOB) after self-limiting bout of viral pneumonia three months priorly. Her CXR showed right hemidiaphragm elevation that was confirmed with a sniff test (Figure 1).

Detailed pulmonary evaluation for continued SOB also showed moderate COPD and elevated Alveolar-arterial (A-a) gradient on pulmonary function test. Ventilation-Perfusion scan did not show any evidence of pulmonary embolism. Sleep study with apnea-hypopnea index (AHI) of 110 per hour confirmed severe obstructive sleep apnea (OSA) and sleep efficiency of 63.4%.

She was started on continuous positive airway pressure (CPAP) for OSA and on 4 liters/minute (L/min) oxygen via nasal cannula (NC) for continued hypoxia. As part of workup for headaches and hemidiaphragm paralysis, MRI of the brain showed intracranial aneurysm that required craniotomy and clipping. Postoperatively, patient was difficult to extubate due to continued hypoxemia. Therefore, transthoracic echocardiogram (TTE) was performed that showed right-to-left intracardiac shunt on saline bubble study. Transesophageal echocardiogram confirmed a PFO with continuous RLS, normal right ventricle, and right atrium size (Figure 2). Over the next few months, patient

TABLE 1: Literature review: reported cases of PFO and hemidiaphragm.

Patient #	Author, year	Age and gender	SOB duration	Hemidiaphragm diagnosis	Probable cause of paralysis	Side of hemidiaphragm	RAP (M/A/V) mmHg	PA Pressure (M/A/V) mmHg	PFO closure improving hypoxia	PaO2 correction on arterial blood gases on PFO closure
(1)	Murray et al., 1991 [2]	72, male	3 months	CXR, fluoroscopy	Idiopathic/Viral	Right	Normal	—	Yes	60 to 71 mmHg
(2)	Cordero et al., 1994 [3]	57, male	1 month	Chest X-ray, sniff test, EMG	Neurapraxia	Right	—	—	Not closed	37 to 78 mmHg
(3)	Ghamande et al., 2001 [4]	79, female	6 weeks	CT, sniff test	Postsurgical	Right	7/9/7	30/15/21	Yes	55 mmHg before closure
(4)	López Gastón et al., 2005 [5]	75, male	7 days	CXR, chest CT, fluoroscopy	L central line placement	Right	2	19.4	Yes	50 to 63 mmHg
(5)	Maholic and Lasorda, 2006 [6]	84, female	1 month	Chest X-ray, sniff test	Guillain Barre	Right	5, mean	22/5	Yes	48 to 67 mmHg
(6)	Perkins et al., 2008 [7]	73, female	2 weeks	Chest X-ray, Sniff Test	Idiopathic	Right	5, mean	14 mean	Yes	65 mmHg before closure
(7)	Fabris et al., 2015 [8]	66, female	Few weeks	Chest X-ray	Idiopathic	Right	3	12 mean	Yes	—
(8)	Sakagianni et al., 2012 [9]	72, female	3 weeks	Chest X-ray	After surgery	Right	14	36/19/24	Yes	Patient on vent at time of closure
(9)	Darchis et al., 2007 [10]	79, female	3 weeks	Chest X-ray	Liver mets and enlarged liver	Right	4	—	Yes	60 to 78 mmHg
(10)	Darchis et al., 2007 [10]	61, female	Acute	Chest X-ray	Postsurgical (phrenic nerve injury)	Right	5	—	Yes	61 to 84 mmHg
(11)	Darchis et al., 2007 [10]	84, female	3 weeks	Chest X-ray	Idiopathic	Right	—	—	Yes	49 to 74 mmHg

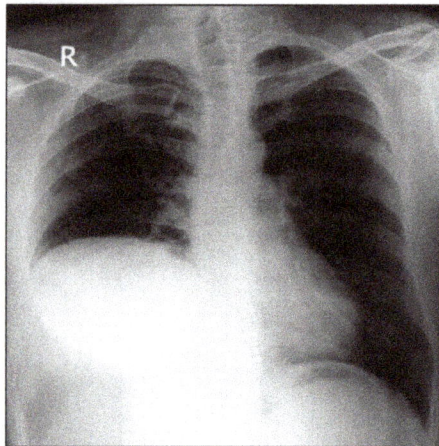

FIGURE 1: Chest X-ray with right hemidiaphragm paralysis.

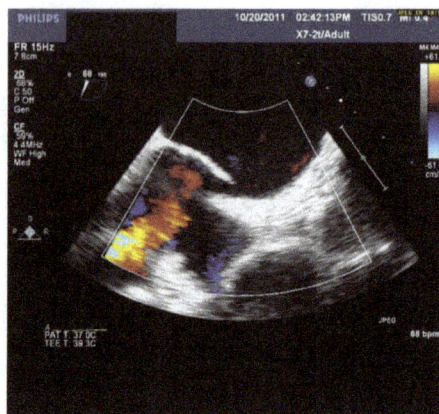

FIGURE 2: Transesophageal echocardiogram with Doppler demonstrating right-to-left interatrial shunting through the patent foramen ovale.

required multiple hospitalizations for repeat episodes of SOB presenting to the hospital with oxygen saturations in low 80% despite using continuous 4 L/min oxygen via NC therefore requiring high flow oxygen and continuous positive airway pressure (CPAP) to stabilize her. Acute exacerbation episodes were treated with CPAP and diuresis, and these measures would improve the dyspnea but did not alleviate. Due to persistent hypoxia and lifestyle limiting dyspnea despite oxygen supplementation patient was referred for PFO closure. As part of evaluation for hypoxia and PFO, patient underwent right and left heart catheterization (RHC and LHC) that showed normal coronaries, normal pulmonary pressure and resistance, normal LV filling pressure, and femoral artery O2 saturation of 87% on room air. After heart team discussion including pulmonologist, percutaneous PFO closure was recommended. Patient underwent successful percutaneous PFO closure using 30 mm Amplatzer Cribriform Septal Occluder (ST Jude Medical). She had immediate improvement in her SOB after PFO closure. She was taken off continuous oxygen after 6-minute walk test prior to discharge. Furosemide requirement reduced from 40 mg oral twice daily to 40 mg

oral once daily after PFO closure. Her status is at five years after PFO closure with no hospitalization related to SOB. She is currently NYHA Class II, walks > 300 yards, and performs all the activities of daily life without any limitations.

3. Discussion

In patients with refractory SOB and hypoxia that fails to resolve with oxygen therapy, a physiologic or anatomic RLS should be considered as part of the differential diagnosis. Workup should include echocardiogram with a bubble study and right heart catheterization. Statistically, the most common cause of an interatrial communication is a patent foramen ovale (PFO), present in estimated 20–30% of the adult population [11, 12]. PFO is mostly asymptomatic and functions as a flap-like valve that transiently opens when right atrial pressure gets higher than the left atrial pressure during maneuvers like having bowel movement, coughing, or sneezing. However, a PFO can facilitate a new onset RLS in cases in which the pressure gradient across the atria is reversed (right atrial pressure > left atrial pressure). Conditions such as OSA, COPD, and other causes of pulmonary hypertension (PH) can lead to reversal of atrial pressure. The findings of normal right sided pressures with an accompanying RLS across a PFO appear to be a paradox. In our patient, RHC revealed normal right and left fillings pressures and normal pulmonary artery pressure and resistance, suggesting optimized COPD and OSA treatment, excluding reversal of atrial pressures as mechanism for RLS.

Hypoxemia secondary to RLS with normal pulmonary artery pressure has been extensively documented after right pneumonectomy whereas only few case reports have documented hypoxemia secondary to a RLS through a PFO in the presence of an elevated right hemidiaphragm, which our patient had due to viral pneumonia [11, 12]. We agree with the proposed mechanism by Zanchetta et al. for the paradoxical shunt based on an anatomical and embryological review of the flow dynamics from the inferior vena cava (IVC) into right atrium. Normally, blood enters the right atrium in upward and backward direction from IVC towards the foramen ovale (FO) to avoid collision with blood entering in downward and forward direction from the superior vena cava. In setting of right hemidiaphragm paralysis, blood flow from IVC is further directed towards the FO resulting in RLS through the PFO even in absence of reversed atrial pressures [10, 13]. Therefore, patient may not present with typical platypnea-orthodeoxia symptoms. Presence of exuberant Eustachian valve can also exacerbate the RLS via redirecting the flow towards the PFO in absence of reversed atrial pressures [14].

4. Conclusion

Right-to-left shunting through a PFO can occur due to multiple etiologies that either increase the right atrial pressure, reduce the left atrial pressure, or facilitate the IVC flow to be directed to the PFO. In some patients, PFO related RLS can lead to significant hypoxia and SOB. As in our case, high clinical suspicion and thorough evaluation helped reach the diagnosis of significant RLS via PFO in setting of right hemidiaphragm paralysis. Percutaneous PFO closure led to significant improvement in patient symptoms.

References

[1] A. Elixhauser and P. Owens, "Reasons for being admitted to the hospital through the emergency department," *Agency for Healthcare Research and Quality Statistical Brief #2*, 2003, http://www.hcup-us.ahrq.gov/reports/statbriefs/sb2.pdf.

[2] K. D. Murray, L. K. Kalanges, J. E. Weiland et al., "Platypnea-orthodeoxia: an unusual indication for surgical closure of a patent foramen ovale," *Journal of Cardiac Surgery*, vol. 6, no. 1, pp. 62–67, 1991.

[3] P. J. Cordero, P. Morales, J. Vallterra et al., "Transient right-to-left shunting through a patent foramen ovale secondary to unilateral diaphragmatic paralysis," *Thorax*, vol. 49, no. 9, pp. 933-934, 1994.

[4] S. Ghamande, R. Ramsey, J. F. Rhodes, and J. K. Stoller, "Right hemidiaphragmatic elevation with a right-to-left interatrial shunt through a patent foramen ovale: a case report and literature review," *CHEST*, vol. 120, no. 6, pp. 2094–2096, 2001.

[5] O. D. López Gastón, O. Calnevaro, C. Gallego et al., "Platypnea-orthodeoxia syndrome, atrial septal aneurysm and right hemidiaphragmatic elevation with a right-to left shunt through a patent foramen ovale," *Medicina*, vol. 65, no. 3, pp. 252–254, 2005 (Spanish).

[6] R. Maholic and D. Lasorda, "Successful percutaneous closure of a patent foramen ovale causing hypoxia in the setting of an elevated hemidiaphragm due to guillian-barre syndrome," *The Journal of Invasive Cardiology*, vol. 18, no. 9, pp. 434-435, 2006.

[7] L. A. Perkins, S. M. Costa, C. D. Boethel, and M. E. Lawrence, "Hypoxemia secondary to right-to-left interatrial shunt through a patent foramen ovale in a patient with an elevated right hemidiaphragm," *Respiratory Care*, vol. 53, no. 4, pp. 462–465, 2009.

[8] T. Fabris, P. Buja, U. Cucchini et al., "Right-to-left interatrial shunt secondary to right hemidiaphragmatic paralysis: An unusual scenario for urgent percutaneous closure of patent foramen ovale," *Heart, Lung and Circulation*, vol. 24, no. 4, pp. e56–e59, 2015.

[9] K. Sakagianni, D. Evrenoglou, D. Mytas, and M. Vavuranakis, "Platypnea-orthodeoxia syndrome related to right hemidiaphragmatic elevation and a stretched patent foramen ovale," *BMJ Case Rep*, vol. 2012, Article ID 007735, 2012.

[10] J. S. Darchis, P. V. Ennezat, C. Charbonnel et al., "Hemidiaphragmatic paralysis: An underestimated etiology of right-to-left shunt through patent foramen ovale?" *European Heart Journal - Cardiovascular Imaging*, vol. 8, no. 4, pp. 259–264, 2007.

[11] P. T. Hagen, D. G. Scholz, and W. D. Edwards, "Incidence and size of patent foramen ovale during the first 10 decades of life: an autopsy study of 965 normal hearts," *Mayo Clinic Proceedings*, vol. 59, no. 1, pp. 17–20, 1984.

[12] D. C. Fisher, E. A. Fisher, J. H. Budd, S. E. Rosen, and M. E. Goldman, "The incidence of patent foramen ovale in 1,000 consecutive patients: a contrast transesophageal echocardiography study," *CHEST*, vol. 107, no. 6, pp. 1504–1509, 1995.

[13] M. Zanchetta, G. Rigatelli, and S. Y. Ho, "A mystery featuring right-to-left shunting despite normal intracardiac pressure," *CHEST*, vol. 128, no. 2, pp. 998–1002, 2005.

[14] M. El Tahlawi, B. Jop, B. Bonello et al., "Should we close hypoxaemic patent foramen ovale and interatrial shunts on a systematic basis?" *Archives of Cardiovascular Diseases*, vol. 102, no. 11, pp. 755–759, 2009.

53

Pulmonary Sequestration with Renal Aplasia and Elevated SUV Level in PET/CT

Serdar Şen,[1] Nilgün Kanlıoğlu Kuman,[1] Ekrem Şentürk,[1] Engin Pabuşcu,[2] and Ertan Yaman[3]

[1] Thoracic Surgery Department, Faculty of Medicine, Adnan Menderes University, Aydın 09000, Turkey
[2] Thoracic Surgery Department, Osmaniye State Hospital, Toprakkale, Turkey
[3] Thoracic Surgery Department, Çorum State Hospital Corum, Turkey

Correspondence should be addressed to Nilgün Kanlıoğlu Kuman, nilkanlioglu@gmail.com

Academic Editors: J. Bordon, W. Gao, and N. Yoshimura

Extralobar sequestration with other bronchopulmonary malformations is commonly seen; however, the association of extralobar sequestration with renal aplasia is very rare. A 75-year-old female patient was admitted with back pain. Ultrasonography revealed aplasia of the left kidney and tomography showed 6×4.5 cm sized tumor in the left hemithorax at the posterobasal area. The lesion has focally increased glycolytic activity (SUVmax: 3.2) at the left upper pole on positron emission tomography scan (PET/CT). Sequestrectomy was performed after the confirmation by frozen section that the lesion was benign and of extrapulmonary sequestration. No complication occurred during postoperative and 50-month follow-up period.

1. Introduction

Pulmonary sequestration (PS) is a rare anomaly in the spectrum of congenital bronchopulmonary malformations that occur by any given impairment of embryonic development.

Two forms of pulmonary sequestration are described depending on whether or not the abnormal lung tissue possesses its own pleural covering, such as intralobar and extralobar sequestration. The ratio of intralobar to extralobar sequestration is about 3 : 1 [1].

Extralobar pulmonary sequestration (ELS) has its own sac that is anatomically separated from the rest of the lung and usually obtains its blood supply from systemic vessels [2]. The arterial supply to 80% ELS comes directly from the thoracic or abdominal aorta, with approximately 15% receiving blood via another systemic artery and 5% via the pulmonary artery [3].

2. Case Report

A seventy-five-year-old female patient was admitted to our hospital with back and abdominal pain. Routine laboratory tests were in normal limits and yielded no differential diagnosis. There was a tenderness in right upper abdomen in physical examination. Abdominal ultrasonography revealed aplasia of left kidney and an increased density was observed in the left lower zone on chest radiography. The patient had not suffered from kidney related disease formerly. Chest tomography (CT) showed 6×4.5 cm sized tumor with regular shape that had millimetric calcification in the left hemithorax in the lower lobe in posterobasal area (Figure 1).

Homogeneous and hypodense tumor has focal increase of glycolytic activity (SUVmax; 3.2) at the left upper pole of the lesion on PET/CT (Figure 2).

A cystic, 8 cm sized intrathoracic extrapulmonary lesion with benign characteristics was observed in operation. Sequestrectomy was performed following confirmation that the lesion was benign and was of extrapulmonary sequestration with frozen section examination. Arterial supply was from the centrum tendineum of the left diaphragm. (Figure 3).

Cystic sequestrectomy material was filled with mucous and haemorrhagic fluid. Microscopic examination revealed ectatic bronchial structures in which there were overall inflammation and microcalcification (Figure 4).

There was no evidence of malignant transformation. No complication occurred during early postoperative and 50-month follow-up period.

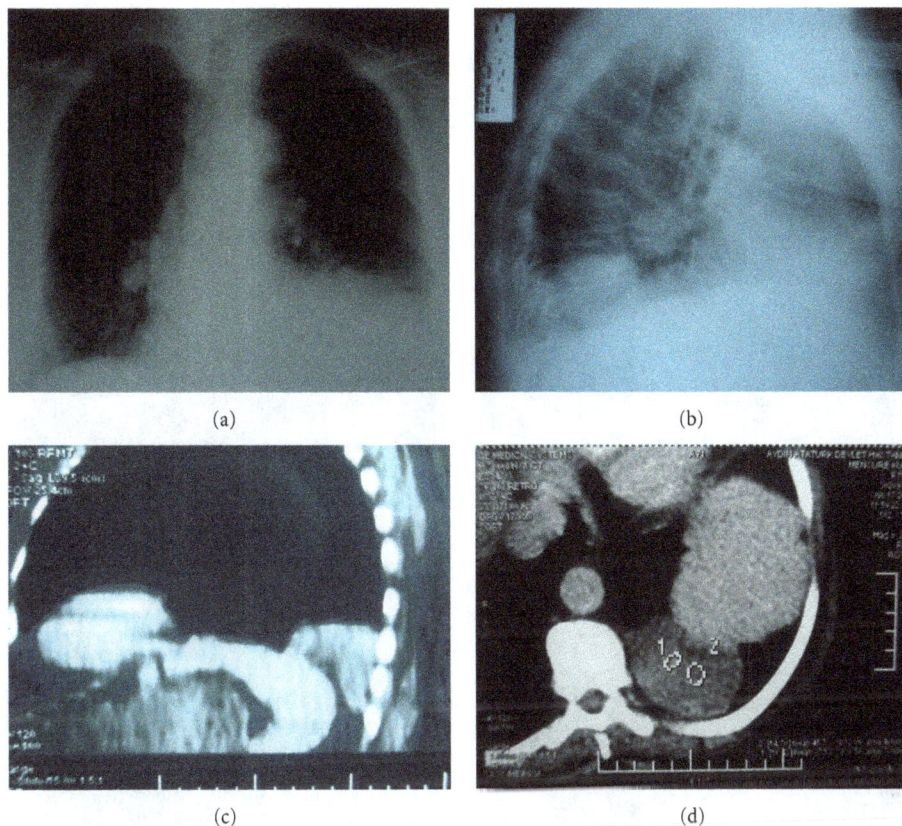

FIGURE 1: (a and b) Lesion can be seen in left hemithorax at inferior zone above diaphragm in chest radiographies (c and d) Thorax CT showing thatthe lesion has microcalcifications and close relationship with diaphragm and posterior costophrenic sinus.

3. Discussion

More than 60% of patients with ELS have coexisting congenital anomalies and congenital diaphragmatic hernia that consists of the most common anomaly of these (16%). About 25% of ELS were found in association with other congenital lung abnormality such as hypoplasia, congenital cystic adenomatoid malformation (CCAM), congenital lobar emphysema, or bronchogenic cyst [3]. In the present study we found unilateral renal aplasia, which is an extremely rare experience. Aplasia of left kidney revealed via abdominal ultrasonography and decreased glycolytic activity viewed on PET CT. As to our knowledge, there is no kidney aplasia associated with ELS in related publications.

Clinical manifestations of ELS are quite variable. Recurrent infections and respiratory distress or an asymptomatic mass can be clinically manifested [4]. Also back pain can be observed if torsion of ELS was occurred [5]. In our case there was no evidence of torsion; however, back pain might depend on diaphragmatic irritation or preexisting abdominal illness.

In some adults, ELS may occur in an unusual mediastinal location, which might be suspected to be malignancy [1]. PET/CT examination showed moderate SUV elevation in a part of the lesion which depended on chronic inflammation in our case and which was initially considered as a malignant degeneration.

ELS was diagnosed preoperatively in 9% of the cases [1]. Pulmonary angiography, magnetic resonance imaging, computed tomography scanning, bronchography, and ultrasonography have all been used in selected cases to confirm preoperative diagnosis [1]. Scar tissue due to recurrent infections may obscure the artery in sequestration. These adhesions can be very dense, and scar tissue may mimic the artery [6].

Typical radiologic appearance is a homogeneous soft-tissue mass in the lower hemithorax [7]. The other localizations of the ELS were mediastinum and interior of diaphragm, although localizations below the diaphragm are seldom [7]. Numerous reports have described severe complications due to pulmonary sequestration, such as fungal infection, tuberculosis, fatal hemoptysis, massive hemothorax, cardiovascular problems, and even malignant degeneration of ELS [8]. Main treatment of pulmonary sequestration is resection, especially in symptomatic cases [1]. The resection can be made due to thoracotomy or video-assisted thoracic surgery (VATS) [5]. The intraoperative blood loss is relatively high in VATS series because of the dense and wide adhesions and inflammation especially in the cases with pulmonary abscess. Serious hemorrhage and even death have been reported when this condition is not recognized at surgery [6].

Some groups have also reported that the use of coil embolisation in infants is a less invasive manner to eliminate

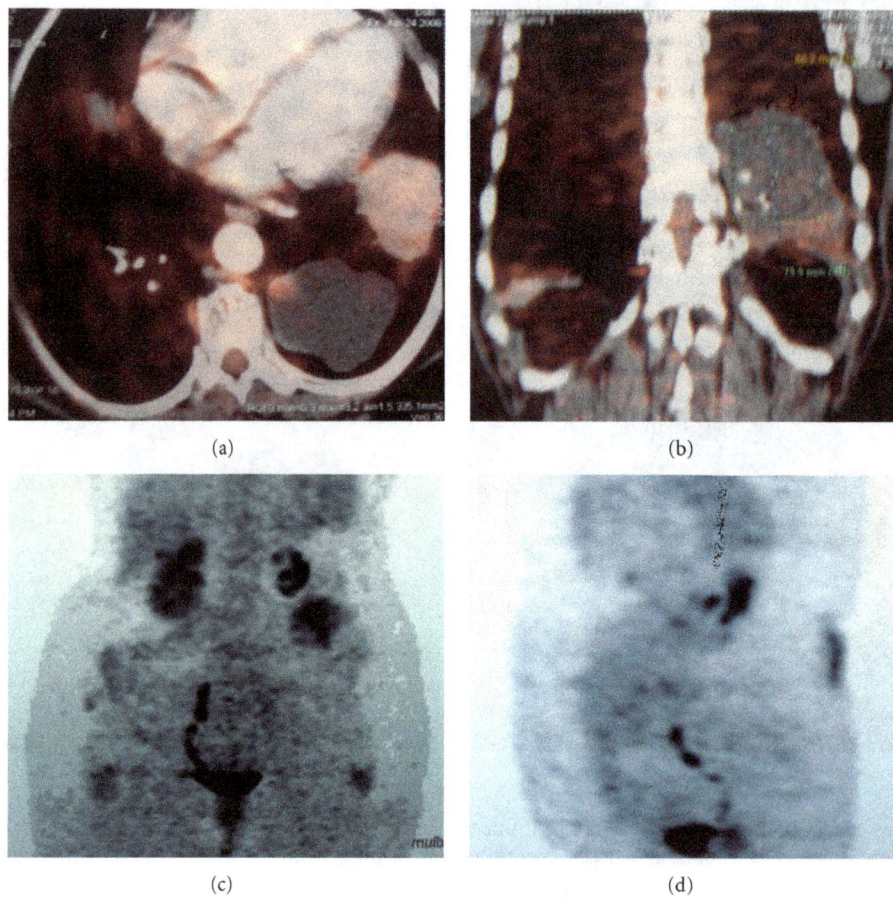

(a)   (b)

(c)   (d)

FIGURE 2: (a and b) Focally increased glycolytic activity in the lesion detected on PET CT. (c and d) Decreased glycolytic activity of the left kidney was seen on PET CT.

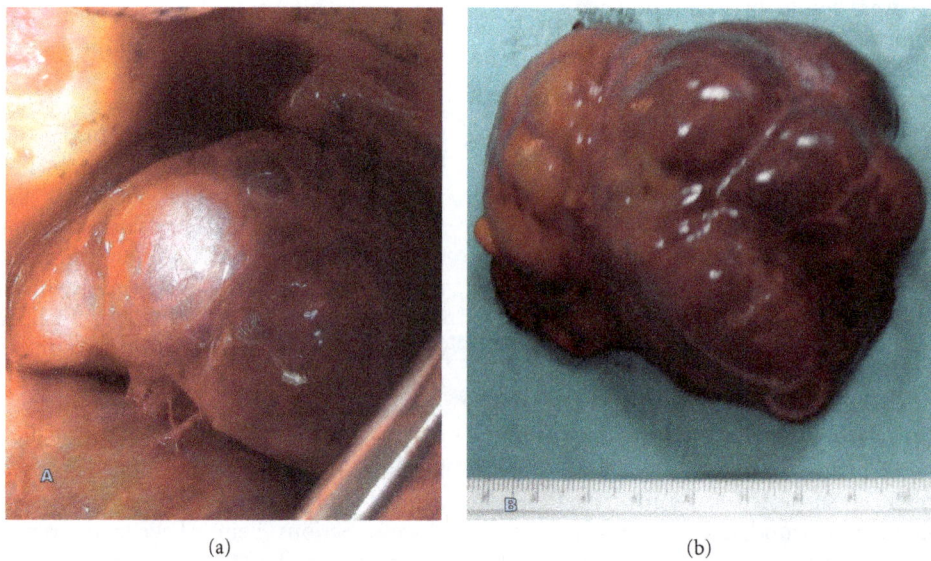

(a)   (b)

FIGURE 3: (a) Blood supply of the lesion comes from the left diaphragm. (b) Smooth, lobulated, sequestrated lung tissue is seen on macroscopic image.

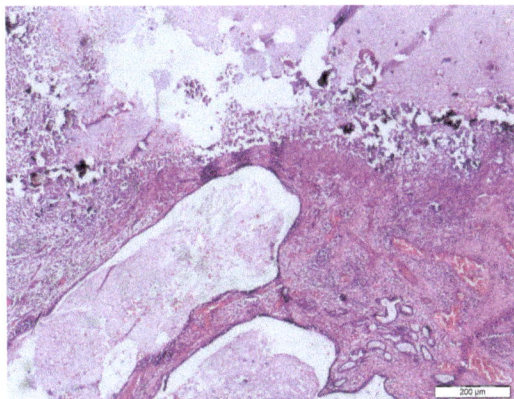

FIGURE 4: Microscopic examination revealed ectatic bronchial structures, inflammation, and microcalcification (HE, ×100).

the feeding artery [6]. Overlook of a large systemic blood vessel may result in lethal hemorrhage due to retraction of the vessel below the diaphragm [5].

We prefer the resection of pulmonary malformations in order to establish a definitive diagnosis and also to prevent potentially serious complications and late infections.

References

[1] J. M. Sippel, P. S. Ravichandran, R. Antonovic, and W. E. Holden, "Extralobar pulmonary sequestration presenting as a mediastinal malignancy," *Annals of Thoracic Surgery*, vol. 63, no. 4, pp. 1169–1171, 1997.

[2] R. W. Lupinski, T. Agasthian, C. H. Lim, and Y. L. Chua, "Extralobar pulmonary sequestration simulates posterior neurogenic tumor," *Annals of Thoracic Surgery*, vol. 77, no. 6, pp. 2203–2204, 2004.

[3] H. J. Corbett and G. M. Humphrey, "Pulmonary sequestration," *Paediatric Respiratory Reviews*, vol. 5, pp. 59–68, 2004.

[4] E. Y. Huang, H. L. Monforte, and D. B. Shaul, "Extralobar pulmonary sequestration presenting with torsion," *Pediatric Surgery International*, vol. 20, no. 3, pp. 218–220, 2004.

[5] J. A. Taylor, T. Laor, and B. W. Warner, "Extralobar pulmonary sequestration," *Surgery*, vol. 143, no. 6, pp. 833–834, 2008.

[6] P. B. Kestenholz, D. Schneiter, S. Hillinger, D. Lardinois, and W. Weder, "Thoracoscopic treatment of pulmonary sequestration," *European Journal of Cardio-Thoracic Surgery*, vol. 29, no. 5, pp. 815–818, 2006.

[7] M. L. Rosado-de-Christenson, A. A. Frazier, J. T. Stocker, and P. A. Templeton, "From the archives of the AFIP. Extralobar sequestration: radiologic-pathologic correlation," *Radiographics*, vol. 13, no. 2, pp. 425–441, 1993.

[8] D. Van Raemdoncka, K. De Boeckb, H. Devliegerb et al., "Pulmonary sequestration: a comparison between pediatric and adult patients," *European Journal Cardio-Thoracic Surgery*, vol. 19, pp. 388–395, 2001.

54

Interstitial Lung Disease of the UIP Variant as the Only Presenting Symptom of Rheumatoid Arthritis

Abhinav Agrawal, Braghadheeswar Thyagarajan, Sidney Ceniza, and Syed Hasan Yusuf

Department of Internal Medicine, Monmouth Medical Center, Long Branch, NJ 07740, USA

Correspondence should be addressed to Braghadheeswar Thyagarajan; bthyag@barnabashealth.org

Academic Editor: Fabio Midulla

Rheumatoid arthritis is a chronic inflammatory disease primarily manifesting with symptoms of joint pain. It also involves multiple organ systems in the body, including the lungs. Interstitial lung disease (ILD) is the most common form of pulmonary involvement in rheumatoid arthritis (RA). Without the typical symptoms such as chronic joint pain, establishing the diagnosis of RA could be quite challenging and a high index of suspicion is thereby required to diagnose ILD in patients with RA, thereby delaying treatment and increasing morbidity and mortality. We report a case of a 67-year-old Hispanic male with no previous history of rheumatoid arthritis or symptoms of typical joint pain who comes to the hospital only with the chief complaints of progressive worsening of shortness of breath for a duration of 6 months and was eventually diagnosed with ILD of the usual interstitial pneumonia variant with serologies positive for rheumatoid arthritis.

1. Introduction

Rheumatoid arthritis affects about 1% of the population [1]. Respiratory symptoms in rheumatoid arthritis can be due to a variety of conditions that affect the parenchyma, pleura, airways, or vasculature. The majority of respiratory manifestations occur within the first 5 years of disease [2]. Respiratory symptoms may precede onset of articular symptoms in 10–20% of cases [3]. Interstitial lung disease (ILD) is the primary pulmonary involvement in RA with prevalence ranging from 4% to 68% mostly in the age group of 50 to 60 years [4].

2. Case Presentation

Our patient is a 67-year-old Hispanic male who presented to our hospital for the chief complaint of progressive worsening of shortness of breath of 3 weeks duration and was admitted for acute respiratory distress due to interstitial lung disease of unknown etiology. His medical history includes coronary artery disease, status postpercutaneous coronary intervention in 2010, hypertension, hyperlipidemia, and diabetes mellitus type 2. He has a significant smoking history of 20 to 30 pack-years and a significant history of alcohol drinking consuming 12 cans of beer per day for 30 years. He has quit smoking and drinking for 10 to 15 years. He works as a janitor and has no significant occupational exposure to asbestos or silicone.

Six months prior to the day of admission, the patient had complaints of dry cough for which he visited his primary care physician and was prescribed over-the-counter cough suppressants with no relief. The patient had a chest X-ray done at this time which showed mild hazy changes in bilateral lung fields (Figure 1 dry cough and eventually developed progressive shortness of breath with no dyspnea at rest. The patient continued to ignore his symptoms until few weeks prior to the day of admission he had significant shortness of breath to the point to which he could not walk to the bathroom in his house. Concerned of this he came to the hospital for further evaluation.

In the ED, the patient was brought in by his daughter and he had significant shortness of breath during ambulation which caused him to rest after every few steps. His initial SpO2 on room air was 77% and he was put on 3-litre O2 on nasal canula and his SpO2 improved to 93%. His blood

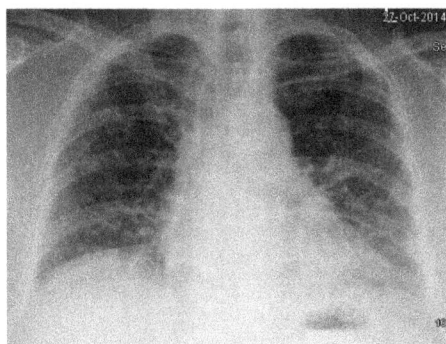

FIGURE 1: Chest X-ray taken 6 months prior to the day of admission showing mild hazy changes in bilateral lung fields.

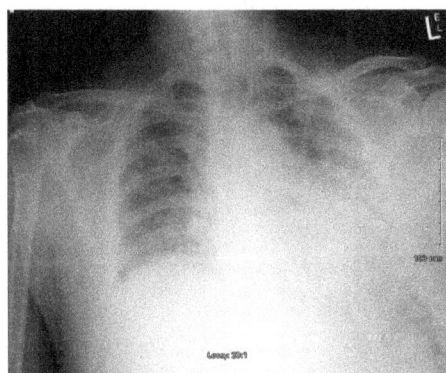

FIGURE 2: Chest X-ray showing worsening reticular and hazy markings throughout bilateral lung fields compared to the previous chest X-ray.

pressure was 134/76 mm of hg, heart rate was 78/min, and respiratory rate was 22/min. On physical examination the patient was awake, alert and oriented, his neck was supple with no jugular venous distension, his heart sounds were audible with no murmurs or gallops, and auscultation of his chest revealed bilateral breath sounds with significant velcro rales on all the lung fields bilaterally. Abdomen was soft and nontender and the patient had no focal neurological deficits. Examination of his extremities revealed no pedal edema but grade 3 clubbing of his finger nails. The patient denied fever, chills, hemoptysis, orthopnea or paroxysmal nocturnal dyspnea, recent travel, or sick contacts.

Chest X-ray in the emergency department showed reticular and hazy markings throughout the both lungs, being worse compared to the previous chest X-ray (Figure 2). A CT scan of the chest showed extensive honeycombing and bronchiectasis of both lungs which were markedly worse when compared to a CT scan done 4 years ago (Figure 3). X-rays of both hands and wrists showed early inflammatory arthropathy but the patient denied joint pain (Figure 4). 2D echocardiogram showed ejection fraction of 59% with mild mitral regurgitation and no pulmonary hypertension, which was not consistent with CHF.

Concerning his chest X-ray and CT scan findings, ILD was now the working diagnosis. The differential at this time was idiopathic versus rheumatoid arthritis. Laboratory data showed elevated erythrocyte sedimentation rate 98 (N 0–20), elevated C-reactive protein 17.4 ($N \leq 7.0$), elevated rheumatoid factor 275 ($N \leq 10$), and elevated cyclic citrullinated peptide >250 ($N < 20$). To exclude causes of falsely elevated rheumatoid factor, hepatitis C Ab was done which was negative. ANA and DsDNA were both negative.

The complete blood count, electrolytes, and renal and liver functions were within normal limits. Lung biopsy was avoided due to the complications of an invasive procedure.

A diagnosis of interstitial lung disease of the usual interstitial pneumonia (UIP) variant due to rheumatoid arthritis was made. The patient was given intravenous solumedrol 40 mg TID which was tapered and changed to oral prednisone 60 mg daily upon discharge. During his hospital stay he was on nasal O2 3 litres and had episodes of desaturation on ambulation; hence he was discharged with home oxygen. He was advised to continue the rest of his medications for his comorbidities and to follow up with his primary care physician and pulmonologist as outpatient. Eventually the patient was referred to a tertiary care center for lung transplant. The patient is currently on the waiting list for his lung transplant.

3. Discussion

Rheumatoid arthritis (RA) is a chronic and systemic inflammatory response, primarily affecting the joints [1]. Interstitial lung disease (ILD) is a well-established and debilitating extra-articular manifestation of RA with a median survival of 2.6 years versus 9.9 years of RA without ILD [5]. This is as a resultant of progressive pulmonary deterioration with lung fibrosis and RA's inherent complications. RA-ILD affects up to 20–30% of RA patients with a 2 : 1 predilection for males as compared to females [6].

RA-ILD, lacking its own agreed classification, is generally subdivided on the basis of its radiographic and histopathological identification, which correlates well with the 7 subtype seen in idiopathic interstitial pneumonia appearances. The usual interstitial pneumonia (UIP) histopathological pattern is more commonly seen in RA as compared to other connective tissue disorders (CTD) where nonspecific interstitial pneumonia (NSIP) is the more prevalent pattern [7]. The patient mentioned above has the UIP type of ILD. The UIP pattern of RA appears to predict poor outcome and apparent clinical deterioration (disease progression), in contrast to idiopathic UIP (a.k.a. idiopathic pulmonary fibrosis) where its lack of response to medical treatment is generally recognized. However data comparing the two groups is limited, revealing somewhat improved 5-year survival rate in RA-UIP as compared to IPF [8]. The other RA-ILD subtype, NSIP pattern, which usually is seen more in women and nonsmokers, seems to be more favorable in terms of survival and response to treatment based on limited studies [9].

Despite the lack of clarity in the pathogenesis of RA-ILD, several predisposing risk factors have been implicated in the possible development of ILD including male gender, smoking, older age, high RA disease activity, long duration

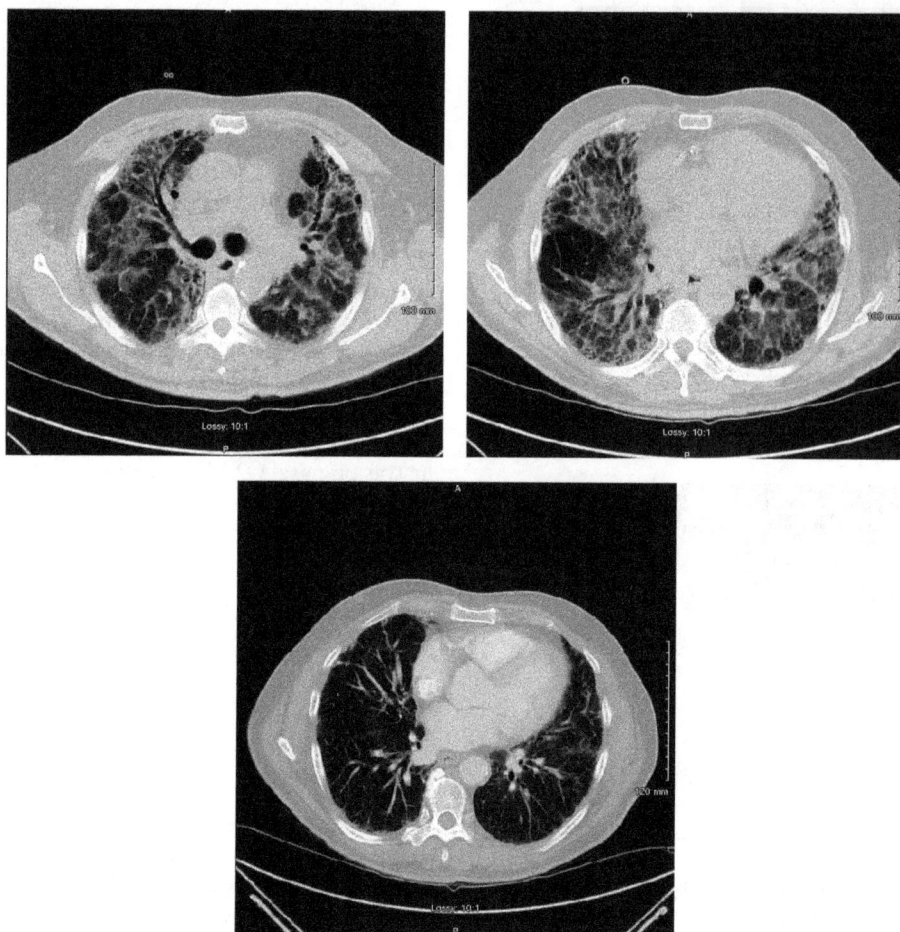

FIGURE 3: CT scan of the chest showing extensive honeycombing consistent with UIP.

of disease, genetic carriers of HLA-DRB1*1502, HLA-B40, anti-trypsin, anti-CCP, and RF; however other studies reveal conflicting data on these associations [10–14]. It has been observed that there is a convincing association tobacco usage with the development of RA-ILD [15]. It was interesting to note that our patient was a long-standing smoker. Anti-CCP is highly specific for RA (about 98%) and multiple studies are showing it can appear prior to the development of arthritis [16]. An interesting cohort of patients is being increasingly recognized for the development of RA-ILD and positive anti-CCP serology w/o synovitis, which initially presented with dyspnea only like our patient. One theory for such subjects is that they belong to a pre-RA state, which could then accelerate to develop RA if genetically and environmentally susceptible. Thus, the clinical implication of positive CCP and RF serology in a patient with lung fibrosis but without RA, which we have described in our case report, remains even more so challenging.

To date, no cost-effective screening has been validated but a detailed history (including environmental exposure, pets) and physical exam remain the most valuable tool in the assessment of patients inflicted with this condition. PFTs are considered highly sensitive in particular, a reduced DLCO (diffusing capacity of the lung for carbon monoxide),

seen even if other pulmonary function indices do no reveal restrictive abnormalities for instance in pseudo-normal PFTs created by combination of pulmonary fibrosis and coexisting emphysema [17]. Thus the specificity of DLCO is also reduced as emphysema can also affect the DLCO. The diagnosis and histopathological subtype of RA-ILD are best established with lung biopsy but due to its invasive risks, an acceptable and equally effective mode for diagnosing is utilizing HRCT where CT features, for instance, bilateral subpleural reticulation with or without honeycombing (UIP) and predominant ground glass appearance (NSIP), would be consistent with interstitial lung disease [18, 19] and a respectable 70% concordance with its histological diagnosis [20]. The CT chest of our patient had honeycombing (Figure 3) which was consistent with UIP pattern of ILD and an invasive procedure such as biopsy and its complications was avoided.

Treatment with anti-inflammatory and/or immunosuppressive agents is recommended regardless of the pattern of fibrosis [21]. Corticosteroids are the mainstay of therapy, particularly for cases of ILD where they may lead to regression on imaging and potential clinical improvement [22]. Similarly, our patient was treated with corticosteroids. Cyclophosphamide and azathioprine have been used with varying success [23]. Methotrexate, a first-line agent in the treatment

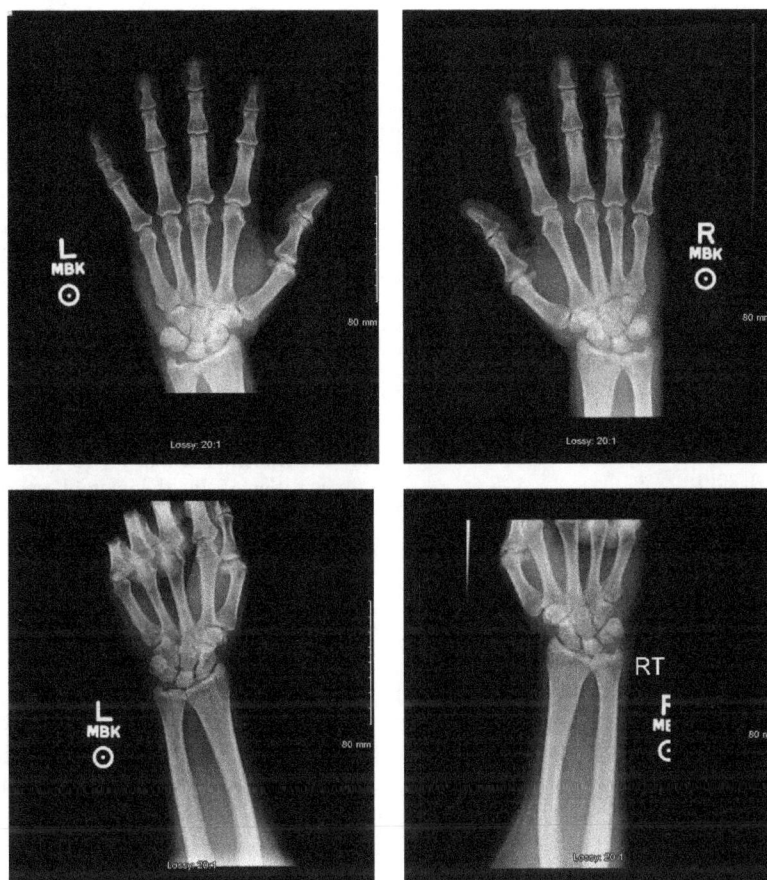

FIGURE 4: X-ray of the bilateral hands showing early inflammatory arthropathy.

of rheumatoid arthritis joint disease, is known to be associated with drug-induced pneumonitis, but fortunately this is rare. However, there is no evidence that this agent leads to progression of ILD [24]. There is considerable controversy as to whether antitumour necrosis factor (TNF) agents improve or worsen ILD. Studies evaluating this issue tend to be confounded by older age and prior use of methotrexate among participants. Similar controversy also exists for rituximab, with some studies reporting improvement [25] and other studies reporting development of ILD [26].

Adjuvant therapy for RA-ILD includes smoking cessation, management of gastroesophageal reflux disease, referral to pulmonary rehabilitation, supplemental oxygen, and vaccination against influenza and pneumococcal disease. All of this was implemented in the care of our patient. In the absence of active rheumatoid arthritis, patients with rheumatoid arthritis lung disease who fail to respond to therapy should be considered for lung transplant. In patients with a UIP pattern, work-up for transplant should be considered early. A retrospective review of Canadian patients with advanced lung disease found no difference in outcomes between patients with RA-ILD and those with IPF at 1 year following lung transplant, suggesting that transplant is a reasonable option for these patients [27]. Similarly our patient had absence of active RA and given the UIP pattern of ILD he was referred for lung transplant program.

4. Conclusion

The diagnosis of RA becomes quite challenging without the usual symptoms of joint pain. It is critical for a physician to assess the patient for systemic and articular signs and symptoms of connective tissue disease when evaluating a patient with pulmonary disease of unknown etiology as patients may initially present with pulmonary symptoms. Early diagnosis can lead to early initiation of treatment and early referral to lung transplant centers in qualifying patients, thereby decreasing morbidity and mortality.

Acknowledgments

This work was supported by Department of Pulmonary Critical Care and Department of Radiology at Monmouth Medical Center.

References

[1] S. E. Gabriel, "The epidemiology of rheumatoid arthritis," *Rheumatic Disease Clinics of North America*, vol. 27, no. 2, pp. 269–281, 2001.

[2] B. Marigliano, A. Soriano, D. Margiotta, M. Vadacca, and A. Afeltra, "Lung involvement in connective tissue diseases: a comprehensive review and a focus on rheumatoid arthritis," *Autoimmunity Reviews*, vol. 12, no. 11, pp. 1076–1084, 2013.

[3] D. N. O'Dwyer, M. E. Armstrong, G. Cooke, J. D. Dodd, D. J. Veale, and S. C. Donnelly, "Rheumatoid arthritis (RA) associated interstitial lung disease (ILD)," *European Journal of Internal Medicine*, vol. 24, no. 7, pp. 597–603, 2013.

[4] L. Carmona, I. González-Álvaro, A. Balsa, M. A. Belmonte, X. Tena, and R. Sanmartí, "Rheumatoid arthritis in Spain: occurrence of extra-articular manifestations and estimates of disease severity," *Annals of the Rheumatic Diseases*, vol. 62, no. 9, pp. 897–900, 2003.

[5] T. Bongartz, C. Nannini, Y. F. Medina-Velasquez et al., "Incidence and mortality of interstitial lung disease in rheumatoid arthritis—a population-based study," *Arthritis & Rheumatism*, vol. 62, no. 6, pp. 1583–1591, 2010.

[6] U. A. Gauhar, A. L. Gaffo, and G. S. Alarcón, "Pulmonary manifestations of rheumatoid arthritis," *Seminars in Respiratory and Critical Care Medicine*, vol. 28, no. 4, pp. 430–440, 2007.

[7] B. W. Kinder, H. R. Collard, L. Koth et al., "Idiopathic nonspecific interstitial pneumonia: lung manifestation of undifferentiated connective tissue disease?" *American Journal of Respiratory and Critical Care Medicine*, vol. 176, no. 7, pp. 691–697, 2007.

[8] A. Rajasekaran, D. Shovlin, V. Saravanan, P. Lord, and C. Kelly, "Interstitial lung disease in patients with rheumatoid arthritis: comparison with cryptogenic fibrosing alveolitis over 5 years," *Journal of Rheumatology*, vol. 33, no. 7, pp. 1250–1253, 2006.

[9] H.-K. Lee, D. S. Kim, B. Yoo et al., "Histopathologic pattern and clinical features of rheumatoid arthritis-associated interstitial lung disease," *Chest*, vol. 127, no. 6, pp. 2019–2027, 2005.

[10] A. Bilgici, H. Ulusoy, O. Kuru, Ç. Çelenk, M. Ünsal, and M. Danaci, "Pulmonary involvement in rheumatoid arthritis," *Rheumatology International*, vol. 25, no. 6, pp. 429–435, 2005.

[11] E. Gabbay, R. Tarala, R. Will et al., "Interstitial lung disease in recent onset rheumatoid arthritis," *The American Journal of Respiratory and Critical Care Medicine*, vol. 156, no. 2, pp. 528–535, 1997.

[12] P. J. Charles, M. C. Sweatman, J. R. Markwick, and R. N. Maini, "HLA-B40: a marker for susceptibility to lung disease in rheumatoid arthritis," *Disease Markers*, vol. 9, no. 2, pp. 97–101, 1991.

[13] H. M. Habib, A. A. Eisa, W. R. Arafat, and M. A. Marie, "Pulmonary involvement in early rheumatoid arthritis patients," *Clinical Rheumatology*, vol. 30, no. 2, pp. 217–221, 2011.

[14] K. Migita, T. Nakamura, T. Koga, and K. Eguchi, "HLA-DRB1 alleles and rheumatoid arthritis-related pulmonary fibrosis," *Journal of Rheumatology*, vol. 37, no. 1, pp. 205–207, 2010.

[15] K. G. Saag, S. Kolluri, R. K. Koehnke et al., "Rheumatoid arthritis lung disease: determinants of radiographic and physiologic abnormalities," *Arthritis and Rheumatism*, vol. 39, no. 10, pp. 1711–1719, 1996.

[16] J. Avouac, L. Gossec, and M. Dougados, "Diagnostic and predictive value of anti-cyclic citrullinated protein antibodies in rheumatoid arthritis: a systematic literature review," *Annals of the Rheumatic Diseases*, vol. 65, no. 7, pp. 845–851, 2006.

[17] V. Cottin, H. Nunes, P.-Y. Brillet et al., "Combined pulmonary fibrosis and emphysema: a distinct underrecognised entity," *European Respiratory Journal*, vol. 26, no. 4, pp. 586–593, 2005.

[18] E. J. Kim, B. M. Elicker, F. Maldonado et al., "Usual interstitial pneumonia in rheumatoid arthritis-associated interstitial lung disease," *European Respiratory Journal*, vol. 35, no. 6, pp. 1322–1328, 2010.

[19] J. Biederer, A. Schnabel, C. Muhle, W. L. Gross, M. Heller, and M. Reuter, "Correlation between HRCT findings, pulmonary function tests and bronchoalveolar lavage cytology in interstitial lung disease associated with rheumatoid arthritis," *European Radiology*, vol. 14, no. 2, pp. 272–280, 2004.

[20] S. N. Mink and B. Maycher, "Comparative manifestations and diagnostic accuracy of high-resolution computed tomography in usual interstitial pneumonia and nonspecific interstitial pneumonia," *Current Opinion in Pulmonary Medicine*, vol. 18, no. 5, pp. 530–534, 2012.

[21] M. Shaw, B. F. Collins, L. A. Ho, and G. Raghu, "Rheumatoid arthritis-associated lung disease," *European Respiratory Review*, vol. 24, no. 135, pp. 1–16, Mar 2015.

[22] R. W. Hallowell and M. R. Horton, "Interstitial lung disease in patients with rheumatoid arthritis: spontaneous and drug induced," *Drugs*, vol. 74, no. 4, pp. 443–450, 2014.

[23] D. P. Ascherman, "Interstitial lung disease in rheumatoid arthritis," *Current Rheumatology Reports*, vol. 12, no. 5, pp. 363–369, 2010.

[24] J. Rojas-Serrano, E. González-Velásquez, M. Mejía, A. Sánchez-Rodríguez, and G. Carrillo, "Interstitial lung disease related to rheumatoid arthritis: evolution after treatment," *Reumatologia Clinica*, vol. 8, no. 2, pp. 68–71, 2012.

[25] G. J. Keir, T. M. Maher, D. Ming et al., "Rituximab in severe, treatment-refractory interstitial lung disease," *Respirology*, vol. 19, no. 3, pp. 353–359, 2014.

[26] R. Perez-Alvarez, M. Perez-de-Lis, C. Diaz-Lagares et al., "Interstitial lung disease induced or exacerbated by TNF-targeted therapies: analysis of 122 cases," *Seminars in Arthritis and Rheumatism*, vol. 41, no. 2, pp. 256–264, 2011.

[27] A. Yazdani, L. G. Singer, V. Strand, A. C. Gelber, L. Williams, and S. Mittoo, "Survival and quality of life in rheumatoid arthritis-associated interstitial lung disease after lung transplantation," *Journal of Heart and Lung Transplantation*, vol. 33, no. 5, pp. 514–520, 2014.

55

Mycobacterium interjectum Lung Infection

M. C. Mirant-Borde,[1] **S. Alvarez,**[2] **and M. M. Johnson**[1]

[1] *Division of Pulmonary Medicine, Mayo Clinic Florida, 4500 San Pablo Road, Jacksonville, FL 32224, USA*
[2] *Division of Pulmonary Medicine and Infectious Disease, Mayo Clinic Florida, USA*

Correspondence should be addressed to M. M. Johnson; johnson.margaret2@mayo.edu

Academic Editors: D. Franzen and C. Y. Tu

A 62-year-old male presented with productive cough, weight loss, and night sweats. CXR revealed a right upper lobe cavitary lesion. Evaluation was negative for *Mycobacterium tuberculosis*, and sputum revealed *Mycobacterium avium intracellulare* (MAI). Since his clinical course was atypical for MAI, further investigations were pursued which identified *Mycobacterium interjectum* in lung specimens, a very rarely described etiology of pulmonary disease. Appropriate therapy with rifampin, intravenous amikacin, trimethoprim/sulfamethoxazole (TMP/SMX), and ethambutol resulted in clinical and radiographic improvement. This is the third case described over a period of 20 years of destructive lung disease in an immunocompetent adult due to *M. interjectum*.

1. Introduction

Various species of *Mycobacterium* lead to human lung disease. *M. tuberculosis* has historically been the most common mycobacterial pulmonary pathogen, but numerous nontuberculous mycobacteria (NTM) are increasingly identified as a cause of pulmonary infections.

2. Case Description

A 64-year-old male presented to his local physician with drenching night sweats, sixteen-pound unintentional weight loss, and cough productive of dark green sputum for two months. Pertinent negatives included the absence of fever, hemoptysis or dyspnea. Initial chest X-ray (CXR) (Figure 1) demonstrated a right upper lobe cavitary lesion. A 10-day course of ciprofloxacin was provided for a provisional diagnosis of pneumonia without improvement of symptoms. CXR demonstrated progressive cavitation leading to a computed tomography (CT) of the chest (Figure 2) which revealed an 8.6 × 5.9 cm cavity with thick, irregular borders in the right upper lobe with tree-in-bud opacities scattered through the remaining right lung. A sputum sample was negative for *M. tuberculosis* by RNA amplification analysis, and Quantiferon-Gold test was negative. Sputum samples ultimately grew

Mycobacterium avium intracellulare (MAI) prompting treatment with azithromycin, ethambutol, and rifampin which was started almost five months after the onset of symptoms. He presented to our clinic for a second opinion. Further history was notable for current tobacco abuse of 40 pack-year duration and no obvious risk factors for HIV infection. He reported that one of his coworkers was recently placed on isolation for presumed tuberculosis, but this diagnosis was subsequently excluded. He denied any other exposure to tuberculosis or recent travel. Upon presentation, the patient looked well, without respiratory distress, and was afebrile. Physical examination was unremarkable.

Pertinent laboratory testing revealed normal complete blood count, renal and hepatic panel, negative HIV serology, and normal CD4 helper cells and immunoglobulin levels. CD8 lymphocytes were slightly decreased to 169/μL (normal values were between 180 and 1170/μL).

A bronchoscopy with bronchoalveolar lavage (BAL) was performed because his clinical course was atypical for MAI infection, and he had not responded to therapy. *Scopulariopsis* spp. and acid fast bacilli were present on direct examination of smears, but RNA amplification was negative for *M. tuberculosis*. No MAI was isolated.

Based on the initial BAL results, voriconazole, was added and azithromycin was replaced by clarithromycin. Repeated

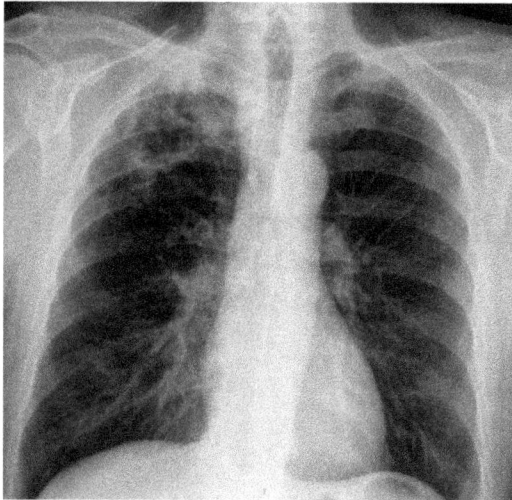

FIGURE 1: Chest X-ray at presentation.

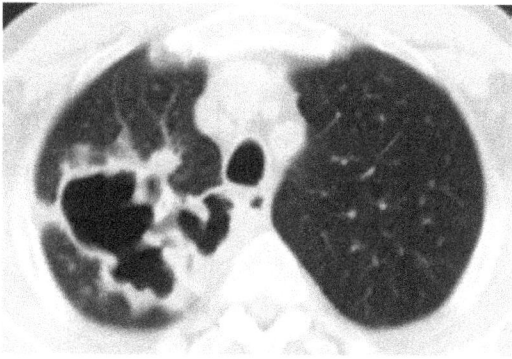

FIGURE 2: Computed tomography of the chest at presentation.

chest CT scans showed disease progression with new involvement of the left lung.

Ultimately, *Mycobacterium interjectum* was identified in the BAL cultures through DNA sequencing 2 months after presentation to our clinic, and levofloxacin was added to his antibiotic regimen. Susceptibility testing showed sensitivity to rifampin (MIC < 0.5 mcg/mL), rifabutin (MIC < 0.12 mcg/mL), ethambutol (MIC = 4 mcg/mL), clarithromycin (MIC < 4 mcg/mL), streptomycin, and clofazimine and resistance to ciprofloxacin. Rifampin and ethambutol demonstrated synergy. Further susceptibility testing differed in that the isolate was resistant to ethambutol and sensitive to Trimethoprim/sulfamethoxazole (TMP/SMX) and amikacin. Thus, treatment was changed to rifampin, intravenous amikacin, TMP/SMX, and voriconazole. Ethambutol was discontinued but subsequently restarted by his local physician in view of the discrepant results in susceptibility testing between the 2 laboratories. Voriconazole was later discontinued due to its interaction with rifampin and the impression that *Scopulariopsis* most likely represented a saprophyte or contaminant. Amikacin was discontinued after 2 months in face of radiologic and clinical improvement.

Following antimicrobial therapy, night sweats and weight loss resolved, and cough and sputum production markedly decreased. Chest CT scan performed after six months of current therapy showed stability of the right apical cavity and substantial improvements in the remaining parenchymal disease. Sputum was negative for acid fast bacilli and fungus at 6 months. The patient has continued to improve clinically and is planned to continue therapy with rifampin, ethambutol, clarithromycin, and TMP/SMX for one year after the first negative sputum culture for mycobacteria. He has tolerated drug therapy well with no recognized complications of treatment. The patient declined consideration of surgical resection of the persistent cavity.

3. Discussion

M. interjectum is a rare and newly described cause of human infection. It was first described in 1993, causing cervical lymphadenitis in an 18-month-old German boy [1]. It was subsequently reported in 9 pediatric cases of necrotizing lymphadenitis [2–6]. It has also been isolated in the sputum of patients with chronic obstructive lung disease or HIV infection, in the urine of an asymptomatic elderly female, and in the stool of an AIDS patient with diarrhea [7, 8]. Fukuoka et al. described a case of an immunosuppressed Japanese woman with polyangiitis who developed multiple cutaneous abscesses infected with *M. interjectum* requiring repeated surgical resection [9]. In one case of a female alcoholic patient with meningoencephalitis, the cerebrospinal fluid culture presented coisolation of *M. malmoense* and *M. interjectum*. Most of the pediatric cases failed antibiotic therapy and required total resection for definite cure. In most cases of isolation of *M. interjectum* in adult patients, the organism was considered clinically insignificant and did not require treatment.

Only 2 cases of cavitary lung disease in immunocompetent adults have been reliably described. The first was reported in 1994, in nonsmoker Moroccan woman aged 52 years at the onset of symptoms with progressive destructive lung disease. There was repeated isolation of *M. interjectum* over a period of 10 years, which was refractory to several antibiotic regimens [10]. Another case of cavitary lung disease mimicking tuberculosis was described by Lacasa et al. in 2005, in Spain. The patient responded to an initial 6-month empiric treatment with rifampicin, isoniazid, and pyrazinamide. He relapsed after 18 months showing resistance to all of the previously used antibiotics and, again, responded to a regimen of combined clarithromycin, levofloxacin, and streptomycin [11]. Another male patient from El Salvador with stable pulmonary opacities had *M. interjectum* isolated from sputum, but we lack information about his clinical background [12].

M. interjectum is phylogenetically found between the fast and slow growing nontuberculous mycobacteria (NTM), leading to its nomenclature, and is similar in its phenotypical and biochemical characteristics to *M. scrofulaceum* (except for hydrolysis of urea which is positive in most cases of *M. scrofulaceum*) and *M. gordonae* [12, 13]. It produces inconsistent reactions for pyrazinamidase, urease, and heat stable catalase [12]. Misclassifications have involved both of these organisms, and accurate diagnosis requires sequencing of the 16S rDNA that codes the ribosomal RNA or high-performance liquid chromatography (HPLC) of the mycolic acids of the cell wall, a more time-consuming and cumbersome technique [2]. Although commonly there is agreement between these tests, discrepant results have been reported [12, 14], and it appears that variants within the *M. interjectum* species may express different HPLC patterns [12]. However, closely related mycobacteria may not be differentiated by 16S rDNA locus polymorphisms, and an algorithm presented by Harmsen et al. is available for this purpose [15]. A newly developed technique that analyzes variations of the heat shock protein (hsp65) gene by PCR restriction fragment polymorphisms has recently described the patterns of rarely isolated mycobacteria, including a new species of *M. interjectum* [16]. Lack of standardization and incomplete pattern libraries may prove to be problematic. In many cases, combination of techniques may be necessary for correct identification of the mycobacterial species [16].

Routes of transmission and susceptibility to pulmonary infection from *M. interjectum* are incompletely understood. It is hypothesized that unrecognized immune abnormalities or structural lung disease may predispose to disease. It is known that tumor necrosis factor (TNF) and interferon (INF) are key regulators of mycobacterial defense [17]. Animal data supports a role for deficiencies in INF γ monocyte release in *M. interjectum* infection [13].

Susceptibility testing has demonstrated multidrug resistance, including resistance to one or more of the following: isoniazid, para-aminosalicylic acid (PAS), pyrazinamide, streptomycin, fluoroquinolones, clarithromycin, and rifampin. Primary isoniazid resistance appears to be commonly encountered. The reported variability in drug sensitivity mandates susceptibility testing when this agent is identified as a human pathogen.

To the best of our knowledge, our case is the third reliably described of destructive lung disease in an immunocompetent adult due to *M. interjectum* since the original report 20 years earlier. We believe the coisolation of *Scopulariopsis* represented saprophytic growth or contaminant. The patient's clinical course improved, and subsequent sputum cultures were negative for fungi, despite only receiving a brief course of voriconazole, further supporting this hypothesis.

An ever increasing spectrum of pathogenic NTM is recognized to cause human lung infection. The clinical manifestations vary from indolent to very aggressive. Clinicians must be aware of the difficulties in accurately identifying distinct NTM species as misidentification may lead to inappropriate therapy. Although the advent of 16s rDNA sequencing, a more rapid and reliable technique for NTM identification, will likely decrease misclassification, failure to improve on therapy should prompt reexamination.

This case describes cavitary lung disease due to *M. interjectum*, a rare NTM species causing lung disease. It is possible that many cases of *M. interjectum* producing destructive lung disease have been misdiagnosed in the past

and that the prevalence of disease is higher than previously suspected. Outgrowth by other NTM could have also contributed to underdiagnosis, a problem that is overcome by DNA sequencing [2]. Due to phenotypic similarities with other NTM but different drug susceptibility patterns, accurate identification of this organism is necessary. More importantly, this case illustrates the need for repeat investigations in the absence of clinical improvement on presumed appropriate therapy.

References

[1] B. Springer, P. Kirschner, G. Rost-Meyer, K. H. Schröder, R. M. Kroppenstedt, and E. C. Böttger, "Mycobacterium interjectum, a new species isolated from a patient with chronic lymphadenitis," *Journal of Clinical Microbiology*, vol. 31, no. 12, pp. 3083–3089, 1993, Erratum in *Journal of Clinical Microbiology*, vol. 32, no. 5, p. 1417, 1994.

[2] D. Tuerlinckx, M. Fauville-Dufaux, E. Bodart, P. Bogaerts, B. Dupont, and Y. Glupczynski, "Submandibular lymphadenitis caused by Mycobacterium interjectum: contribution of new diagnostic tools," *European Journal of Pediatrics*, vol. 169, no. 4, pp. 505–508, 2009.

[3] T. de Baere, M. Moerman, L. Rigouts et al., "Mycobacterium interjectum as causative agent of cervical lymphadenitis," *Journal of Clinical Microbiology*, vol. 39, no. 2, pp. 725–727, 2001.

[4] M. A. Remacha, A. Esteban, M. I. Parra, and M. S. Jiménez, "Case report—cervical lymphadenitis due to mycobacterium interjectum," *Pediatric Pulmonology*, vol. 42, no. 4, pp. 398–399, 2007.

[5] M. Rose, R. Kitz, A. Mischke, R. Enzensberger, V. Schneider, and S. Zielen, "Lymphadenitis cervicalis due to Mycobacterium interjectum in immunocompetent children," *Acta Paediatrica*, vol. 93, no. 3, pp. 424–426, 2004.

[6] S. Rustscheff, L. Maroti, M. Holberg-Petersen, M. Steinbakk, and S. E. Hoffner, "Mycobacterium interjectum: a new pathogen in humans?" *Scandinavian Journal of Infectious Diseases*, vol. 32, no. 5, pp. 569–571, 2000.

[7] B. A. Green and B. Afessa, "Isolation of Mycobacterium interjectum in an AIDS patient with diarrhea," *AIDS*, vol. 14, no. 9, pp. 1282–1284, 2000.

[8] E. Tortoli, P. Kirschner, A. Bartoloni et al., "Isolation of an unusual mycobacterium from an AIDS patient," *Journal of Clinical Microbiology*, vol. 34, no. 9, pp. 2316–2319, 1996.

[9] M. Fukuoka, Y. Matsumura, S. Kore-Eda, Y. Iinuma, and Y. Miyachi, "Cutaneous infection due to Mycobacterium interjectum in an immunosuppressed patient with microscopic polyangiitis," *The British Journal of Dermatology*, vol. 159, no. 6, pp. 1382–1384, 2008.

[10] S. Emler, T. Rochat, P. Rohner et al., "Chronic destructive lung disease associated with a novel mycobacterium," *American Journal of Respiratory and Critical Care Medicine*, vol. 150, no. 1, pp. 261–265, 1994.

[11] J. M. Lacasa, E. Cuchi, and R. Font, "Mycobacterium interjectum as a cause of lung disease mimicking tuberculosis," *International Journal of Tuberculosis and Lung Disease*, vol. 13, no. 8, p. 1048, 2009.

[12] R. Lumb, A. Goodwin, R. Ratcliff, R. Stapledon, A. Holland, and I. Bastian, "Phenotypic and molecular characterization of three clinical isolates of Mycobacterium interjectum," *Journal of Clinical Microbiology*, vol. 35, no. 11, pp. 2782–2785, 1997.

[13] S. Ehlers and E. Richter, "Differential requirement for inter-feron-γ to restrict the growth of or eliminate some recently identified species of nontuberculous mycobacteria in vivo," *Clinical and Experimental Immunology*, vol. 124, no. 2, pp. 229–238, 2001.

[14] E. Tortoli, A. Bartoloni, C. Burrini et al., "Characterization of an isolate of the newly described species Mycobacterium interjectum," *Zentralblatt für Bakteriologie*, vol. 283, no. 3, pp. 286–294, 1996.

[15] D. Harmsen, S. Dostal, A. Roth et al., "RIDOM: comprehensive and public sequence database for identification of Mycobac-terium species," *BMC Infectious Diseases*, vol. 3, article 26, 2003.

[16] B. Häfner, H. Haag, H.-K. Geiss, and O. Nolte, "Different molecular methods for the identification of rarely isolated non-tuberculous mycobacteria and description of new hsp65 restriction fragment length polymorphism patterns," *Molecular and Cellular Probes*, vol. 18, no. 1, pp. 59–65, 2004.

[17] S. M. Holland, "Immunotherapy of mycobacterial infections," *Seminars in Respiratory Infections*, vol. 16, no. 1, pp. 47–59, 2001.

56

Lymphoepithelioma-Like Carcinoma of the Lung: An Unusual Case and Literature Review

Yuan-Chun Huang,[1,2] Ching Hsueh,[1] Shang-Yun Ho,[1] and Chiung-Ying Liao[1]

[1] Department of Medical Imaging, Changhua Christian Hospital, No. 135 Nanxiao Street, Changhua 500, Taiwan
[2] Department of Radiology, Changhua Christian Hospital, Erlin Branch, No. 558, Section 1, Dacheng Road, Erlin Township, Changhua 526, Taiwan

Correspondence should be addressed to Chiung-Ying Liao; cyliaomed@gmail.com

Academic Editors: S. Al-Saad, G. Hillerdal, and N. Reinmuth

We described a case of lymphoepithelioma-like carcinoma (LELC) of the lung of a 65-year-old man with initial symptoms of intermittent chest pain and mild shortness of breath for 2 weeks. A right-lung mass was noted on chest computed tomography (CT) scan and was proved histopathologically as LELC of lung after video-assisted thorascopic lobectomy. He was successfully treated with lobectomy with postoperative adjuvant chemotherapy and is alive without signs of recurrence for 36 months after the diagnosis. It is important for clinicians, pathologists, and radiologists to understand the clinical, pathological, and radiological presentations of this neoplasm to avoid improper clinical decision making and misdiagnosis.

1. Introduction

LELC of the lung was first reported in 1987 [1]. Primary LELC of the lung is a rare entity that has recently been included as a subtype of variants of large cell carcinoma in the World Health Organization's histologic classification of lung tumors [2]. Being a rare entity and mostly seen in Asians, few cases have been described previously [3]. The behavior of LELC of the lung is reported to be highly variable [4]. LELC has been reported in pharyngeal and foregut derivatives including the oral cavity, salivary glands, thymus, lungs, and stomach [5]. The association with Epstein-Barr virus (EBV) is variable [6]. Primary LELC of the lung is rare. The literature of LELC of the lung involves just more than 150 cases until 2006 [3]. In majority, those patients are Orientals, with nearly two-thirds arising from Taiwan, Southern China, and Hong Kong [3].

We present an unusual case with a pulmonary mass on CT scan of the thorax which was subsequently proved as a LELC of the lung and a brief review of the relevant literature.

2. Case Report

The patient is a 65-year-old Taiwanese man, a businessman with initial symptoms of intermittent chest pain with mild shortness of breath for two weeks. Chest X-ray showed a mass lesion in the right lower lung field. Chest CT scan showed a 30 × 29 mm heterogeneously enhanced mass lesion with well-defined margin and lobulated contour in the right middle lobe of lung, abutting the mediastinum (Figure 1). Bronchoscopy showed no endobronchial lesion. He received video-assisted thorascopic lobectomy of right middle lobe of lung and mediastinal lymph nodes dissection.

The pathology, immunohistochemical staining, and in situ hybridization results confirmed LELC of lung. Microscopically, the tumor cells are surrounded by abundant lymphoplasmacytic cells in the stroma. The tumor cells show indistinct cell borders with prominent nucleoli and are closely admixed with infiltrating inflammatory cells. Using in situ hybridization with exhibition of abundant EBV-encoded small nuclear RNA (EBER) in the majority of tumor cells is done, which has become a standard test to display tumor-specific association of EBV. Immunohistochemical staining was positive for cytokeratin (CK), a marker which was almost always positive in LELC of lung [7]. Immunohistochemical staining for P63 was positive. P63 protein as homologue of the p53 protein, being a powerful marker for squamous

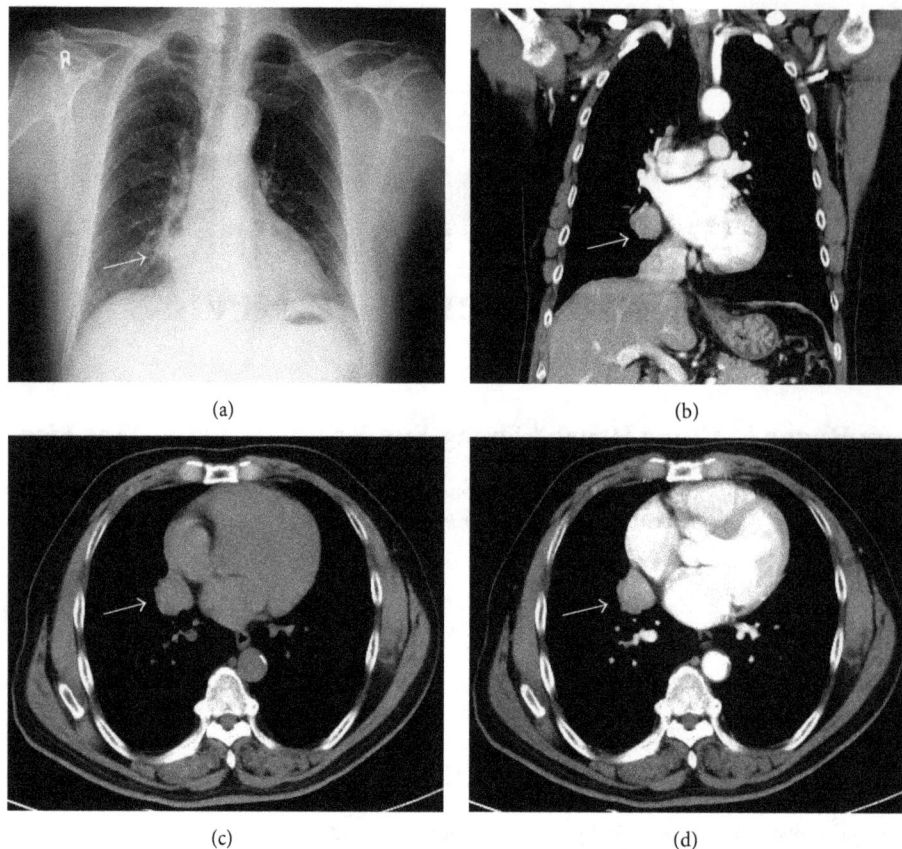

FIGURE 1: (a) Chest X-ray showed a mass lesion in the right paramediastinal region (arrow); (c) Noncontrast-enhanced CT scan: an isodensity lobulated mass lesion in the right middle lobe of lung; ((b) and (d)) Chest CT scan showed a 30 × 29 mm heterogenously enhanced mass lesion with well-defined lobulated margin in the right middle lobe of lung, abutting the mediastinum.

differentiation, was expressed, which excluded a glandular or neuroendocrine differentiation (Figure 2).

Head and neck CT scan and nasopharyngeal fiberscopy were performed and no obvious tumor was found. The patient's postoperative course was uncomplicated, and he was discharged 7 days after operation. Due to advanced stage with parietal pleura invasion and presence of subcarinal lymph node metastasis, postoperative adjuvant chemotherapy was performed on schedule.

3. Discussion

In the literature, most imaging characters of advanced primary pulmonary LELC have been reported in several small clinicopathologic studies en passant [8–10]. Ooi et al. brought out a comparison of CT features between advanced-stage patients (stages III and IV) with LELC of lung and non-small cell lung carcinoma [11]. Those authors stated that LELC of lung was inclinable to demonstrate the following features: central location, large size, smooth margin, vascular encasement, and peribronchovascular nodal spread. Ooi and colleagues stated that if large pulmonary lesions were closely associated with the mediastinum, especially during the occurrence of vascular encasement and peribronchovascular

nodal spread, the diagnosis of primary LELC of lung is more likely than non-LELC neoplasms. Notwithstanding, these features observed by Ooi et al. may be present in patients with bronchogenic carcinoma. Moreover, Chan et al. and Han et al. studied late-stage lesions, and therefore their findings could not be applied completely to earlier-stage patients [9, 10].

The results of Chan et al. [9], Han et al. [10], and Hoxworth et al. [12] suggested that primary LELC of lung most often manifests itself as a peripheral poorly marginated nodule, smaller than 3.5 cm in size, and usually is not associated with lymphadenopathy. However, Ooi et al. declare that primary LELC of lung usually presents as a large pulmonary mass in the central third of the lung with circumscribed borders and associated with lymphadenopathy. The CT scan findings of our case in this report were compatible with the latter descriptions.

Hoxworth et al. [12] first described the MRI features of LELC of the lung. MRI findings of primary pulmonary LELC include intense enhancement with iso- to hypointensity on T1-weighted sequences and iso- to hyperintensity on T2-weighted sequences. Unfortunately, these MRI signal features are nonspecific. As a consequence, the role of MRI in evaluating LELC will be limited as preoperative planning and staging tool with detection of adjacent structures invasion.

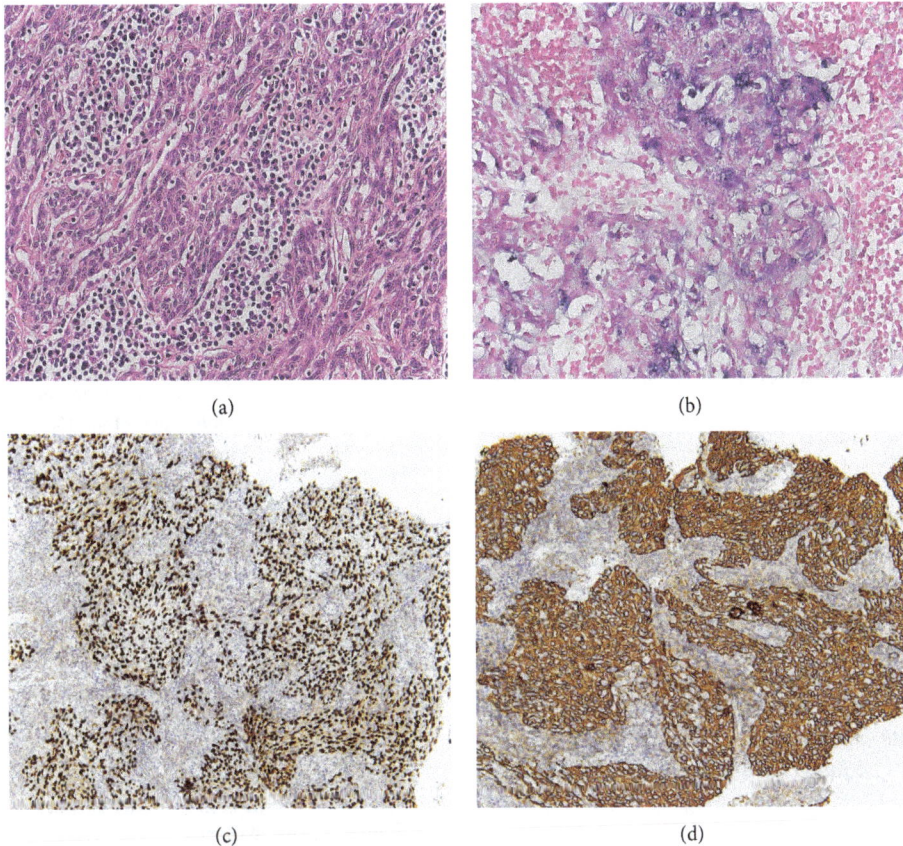

FIGURE 2: (a) Hematoxylin- and Eosin-stained cell block section shows non-small cell carcinoma consisting of syncytial tumor cells with focal necrosis and lymphocytic infiltrate in the background (original magnification, ×400); (b) The immunohistochemical study: EBER(+) (original magnification, ×400); (c) The immunohistochemical study: P63(+) (original magnification, ×200); (d) The immunohistochemical: CK(+) (original magnification, ×200).

In Oriental populations, there is a close relationship between EBV infection and pulmonary LELC. EBV infection may have an essential role in the tumorigenesis of pulmonary LELC [13]. The presence of EBV in LELC has been demonstrated by polymerase chain reaction for EBV DNA, in situ hybridization for EBV DNA and RNA, and immunohistochemistry for EBV-associated proteins [14, 15]. However, it is suggested that there is no association between EBV and LELC in the Western population [16]. Furthermore, a detail expression profile of EBV viral proteins in pulmonary LELC has not been reported.

LELC is pathologically a distinct entity which was classified as a type of non-small cell lung cancer [9]. In histology, it is indistinguishable between primary LELC of the lung and the prototypical LELC occurring in the nasopharynx [9]. Consequently, a nasopharyngeal origin needs to be excluded in all cases. A thorough evaluation of other primary sites such as the nasopharynx should be carried out. The incidence of metastasis to local lymph nodes is 25%; although hematogenous metastasis occurs seldom, the skeletal system is the preferred site [17, 18].

Metastatic nasopharyngeal carcinoma and non-Hodgkin's lymphoma are two main differential diagnoses for LELC [8]. The latter commonly receives nonsurgical management. Incorrect diagnosis will lead to inaccurate staging and inappropriate management. Identification of primary pulmonary LELC will allow precise staging and proper patient management. In the subject of differentiation between lymphoma and LELC, immunohistochemical staining plays a significant role [9]. Neck magnetic resonance imaging or computed tomography scan cooperatively with endoscopic biopsy of the nasopharynx is essential to exclude primary nasopharyngeal carcinoma.

Surgery is the major curative method for stage I non-small cell carcinoma of the lung; patients with late stage non-small cell carcinoma of the lung such as stage II or higher are treated by combination therapy including postoperative radiotherapy, chemotherapy, or both.

LELC in the nasopharynx is radiosensitive, and increasingly it is being perceived as chemosensitive [19]. Ho et al. observed 7 patients with LELC of the lung for response to chemotherapy and found that 5 (71%) had a partial response and 2 (29%) had progressive disease [20]. Evidence about the role of radiotherapy and chemotherapy for LELC of the lung needs further study owing to the relatively small number of cases. However, chemotherapy and radiotherapy have been employed with some success [10, 21].

From limited data available, the behavior of LELC of lung is highly variable nevertheless aggressive malignancy is reported in the minority of cases [5, 22].

Han et al. asserted that the overall survival rate is more favorable in LELC of the lung compared with non-LELC type of non-small cell lung carcinoma; furthermore, it was found that tumor recurrence and necrosis were poor prognostic factors for survival [10]. However, other factors inherent to the nature of the carcinoma may play a part in its relatively good prognosis. The presence of abundant CD8-positive cytotoxic T lymphocytes adjacent to LELC cells and the underexpression of p53 and c-erb B-2 oncoproteins in tumor cells have been postulated to account for the better prognosis in LELC of the lung [21].

4. Conclusion

Conclusively, the CT and MRI image findings of primary pulmonary LELC are similar to those of bronchogenic carcinomas in the majority of cases. LELC of lung may be mistaken histopathologically for metastatic nasopharyngeal carcinoma or lymphoma, resulting in improper patient management. LELC should be considered in the differential diagnosis of primary lung tumors, particularly when an extensive lymphocytic infiltrate is observed. Clinicians, pathologists, and radiologists may encounter primary pulmonary LELC on imaging or at biopsy procedure; consequently familiarity with this distinctive entity is required.

References

[1] L. R. Begin, J. Eskandari, J. Joncas, and L. Panasci, "Epstein-Barr virus related lymphoepithelioma-like carcinoma of lung," *Journal of Surgical Oncology*, vol. 36, no. 4, pp. 280–283, 1987.

[2] W. A. Franklin, "Diagnosis of lung cancer: pathology of invasive and preinvasive neoplasia," *Chest*, vol. 117, no. 4, pp. 80–89, 2000.

[3] J. C. Ho, M. P. Wong, and W. K. Lam, "Lymphoepithelioma-like carcinoma of the lung," *Respirology*, vol. 11, no. 5, pp. 539–545, 2006.

[4] F. F. Chen, J. J. Yan, W. W. Lai et al., "Epstein-Barr virus-associated nonsmall cell lung carcinoma: undifferentiated "lymphoepithelioma-like" carcinoma as a distinct entity with better prognosis," *Cancer*, vol. 82, pp. 2334–2342, 1998.

[5] D. Shibata and L. M. Weiss, "Epstein-Barr virus-associated gastric adenocarcinoma," *The American Journal of Pathology*, vol. 140, no. 4, pp. 769–794, 1992.

[6] K. Oda, J. Tamaru, T. Takenouchi et al., "Association of Epstein-Barr virus with gastric carcinoma with lymphoid stroma," *The American Journal of Pathology*, vol. 143, no. 4, pp. 1063–1071, 1993.

[7] D. S. Zander, H. Popper, J. Jagirdar, A. Haque, and R. Barrios, "Large cell carcinoma," in *Molecular Pathology of Lung Diseases*, Springer, New York, NY, USA, 2008.

[8] A. E. Butler, T. V. Colby, L. Weiss, and C. Lombard, "Lymphoepithelioma-like carcinoma of the lung," *The American Journal of Surgical Pathology*, vol. 13, no. 8, pp. 632–639, 1989.

[9] J. K. Chan, P. K. Hui, W. Y. Tsang et al., "Primary lymphoepithelioma-like carcinoma of the lung: a clinicopathologic study of 11 cases," *Cancer*, vol. 76, pp. 413–422, 1995.

[10] A. J. Han, M. Xiong, Y. Y. Gu, S. X. Lin, and M. Xiong, "Lymphoepithelioma-like carcinoma of the lung with a better prognosis: a clinicopathologic study of 32 cases," *The American Journal of Clinical Pathology*, vol. 115, no. 6, pp. 841–850, 2001.

[11] G. C. Ooi, J. C. Ho, P. L. Khong, M. P. Wong, W. K. Lam, and K. W. T. Tsang, "Computed tomography characteristics of advanced primary pulmonary lymphoepithelioma-like carcinoma," *European Radiology*, vol. 13, no. 3, pp. 522–526, 2003.

[12] J. M. Hoxworth, D. K. Hanks, P. A. Araoz et al., "Lymphoepithelioma-like carcinoma of the lung: radiologic features of an uncommon primary pulmonary neoplasm," *The American Journal of Roentgenology*, vol. 186, no. 5, pp. 1294–1299, 2006.

[13] A. J. Han, M. Xiong, and Y. S. Zong, "Association of Epstein-Barr virus with lymphoepithelioma-like carcinoma of the lung in southern China," *The American Journal of Clinical Pathology*, vol. 114, no. 2, pp. 220–226, 2000.

[14] K. Kasai, Y. Sato, T. Kameya et al., "Incidence of latent infection of Epstein-Barr virus in lung cancers—an analysis of EBER1 expression in lung cancers by in situ hybridization," *Journal of Pathology*, vol. 174, no. 4, pp. 257–265, 1994.

[15] M. Higashiyama, O. Doi, K. Kodama et al., "Lymphoepithelioma-like carcinoma of the lung: analysis of two cases for Epstein-Barr virus infection," *Human Pathology*, vol. 26, no. 11, pp. 1278–1282, 1995.

[16] C. Y. Castro, M. L. Ostrowski, R. Barrios et al., "Relationship between Epstein-Barr virus and lymphoepithelioma-like carcinoma of the lung: a clinicopathologic study of 6 cases and review of the literature," *Human Pathology*, vol. 32, no. 8, pp. 863–872, 2001.

[17] W. Wockel, G. Hofler, H. H. Popper, and A. Morresi-Hauf, "Lymphoepithelioma-like lung carcinomas," *Der Pathologe*, vol. 18, no. 2, pp. 147–152, 1997.

[18] A. T. Chan, P. M. Teo, K. C. Lam et al., "Multimodality treatment of primary lymphoepithelioma-like carcinoma of the lung," *Cancer*, vol. 83, pp. 925–929, 1998.

[19] T. C. Chan, M. L. Teo, W. T. Leung et al., "Role of chemotherapy in the management of nasopharyngeal carcinoma," *Cancer*, vol. 82, pp. 1003–1012, 1998.

[20] J. C. Ho, W. K. Lam, G. C. Ooi, B. Lam, and K. W. Tsang, "Chemoradiotherapy for advanced lymphoepithelioma-like carcinoma of the lung," *Respiratory Medicine*, vol. 94, no. 10, pp. 943–947, 2000.

[21] Y. L. Chang, C. T. Wu, J. Y. Shih, and Y. C. Lee, "New aspects in clinicopathologic and oncogene studies of 23 pulmonary lymphoepithelioma-like carcinomas," *The American Journal of Surgical Pathology*, vol. 26, no. 6, pp. 715–723, 2002.

[22] J. C. Ho, W. K. Lam, G. C. Ooi et al., "Lymphoepithelioma-like carcinoma of the lung in a patient with silicosis," *European Respiratory Journal*, vol. 22, no. 2, pp. 383–386, 2003.

Permissions

List of Contributors

E.Wierda
Departments of Cardiology, Onze Lieve Vrouwe Gasthuis, 1090 HM Amsterdam, The Netherlands

H. J. Reesink
Department of Respiratory Medicine, St. Antonius Ziekenhuis, 3430 EM Nieuwegein, The Netherlands
Department of Pulmonology, Academic Medical Center of the University of Amsterdam, 1105 AZ Amsterdam, The Netherlands
Department of Respiratory Medicine, Onze Lieve Vrouwe Gasthuis, 1090 HM Amsterdam, The Netherlands

H. Bruining
Department of Psychiatry, Rudolf Magnus Institute of Neuroscience, 3584 CG Utrecht, The Netherlands

O.M. van Delden
Department of Radiology, Academic Medical Center of the University of Amsterdam, 1105 AZ Amsterdam, The Netherlands

J. J. Kloek
Department of Cardiothoracic Surgery, Academic Medical Center of the University of Amsterdam, Amsterdam, The Netherlands

P. Bresser
Department of Pulmonology, Academic Medical Center of the University of Amsterdam, 1105 AZ Amsterdam, The Netherlands
Department of Respiratory Medicine, Onze Lieve Vrouwe Gasthuis, 1090 HM Amsterdam, The Netherlands
Department of Cardiothoracic Surgery, Academic Medical Center of the University of Amsterdam, Amsterdam, The Netherlands

René Agustín Flores-Franco and Dahyr Alberto Olivas-Medina
Departamento de Medicina Interna, Christus Muguerza Hospital Del Parque, Calle Dr. Pedro Leal Rodriguez 1802, Colonia Centro, 31000 Chihuahua, CHIH, Mexico

Cesar Francisco Pacheco-Tena
Facultad de Medicina, Universidad Aut´onoma de Chihuahua, Circuito Universitario Campus II, 31240 Chihuahua, CHIH, Mexico

Jorge Duque-Rodríguez
Servicios de Salud de Chihuahua, Sistema Estatal de Salud, Calle Tercera No. 604, Piso 3 Colonia Centro, 31000 Chihuahua, CHIH, Mexico

Jarred Burkart and Gregory A. Otterson
Department of Internal Medicine,The Ohio State University College of Medicine, Columbus, OH 43210, USA

Konstantin Shilo and Weiqiang Zhao
Department of Pathology, The Ohio State University College of Medicine, Columbus, OH 43210, USA

Efe Ozkan and Amna Ajam
Department of Radiology, The Ohio State University College of Medicine, Columbus, OH 43210, USA

Petre V. H. Botianu and Alexandru M. Botianu
Surgical Clinic 4, M5 Department, University of Medicine and Pharmacy of Tirgu Mures, Gheorghe Marinescu 1, 540139 Tirgu Mures, Romania

Anda Mihaela Cerghizan
Medical Clinic 3, M3 Department, University of Medicine and Pharmacy of Tirgu Mures, Revolutiei 35, 540043 Tirgu Mures, Romania

Inderjit Singh, FrancesMae West, Abraham Sanders and Dana Zappetti
Department of Medicine, Division of Pulmonary and Critical Care,Weill Cornell Medical College, New York, NY 10065, USA

Barry Hartman
Department of Medicine, Division of Infectious Diseases,Weill Cornell Medical College, New York, NY 10065, USA

Kubra Erol Kalkan
Department of Internal Medicine, Sisli Etfal Education and Research Hospital, 34377 Istanbul, Turkey

Ahmet Bilici and Fatih Selcukbiricik
Department of Medical Oncology, Sisli Etfal Education and Research Hospital, 34377 Istanbul, Turkey

Nurcan Unver
Department of Pathology, Yedikule Education and Research Hospital, 34020 Istanbul, Turkey

Mahmut Yuksel
Department of Nuclear Medicine, Medical Park Bahcelievler Hospital, 34160 Istanbul, Turkey

Vijay Hadda, Karan Madan, Anant Mohan, Umasankar Kalai and Randeep Guleria
Department of Pulmonary Medicine and Sleep Disorders, All India Institute of Medical Sciences, New Delhi 110029, India

Shweta Sharma, R. K. Mahajan and Nandini Duggal
Department of Microbiology, Dr. Ram Manohar Lohia Hospital and PGIMER, New Delhi 110001, India

V. P. Myneedu
SAG Grade, Department of Microbiology, LRS, Institute of Tuberculosis and Respiratory Disease, Delhi 110030, India

B. B. Sharma
Department of Radiology, Dr. Ram Manohar Lohia Hospital and PGIMER, New Delhi, India

Gladis Isabel Yampara Guarachi, Valeria Barbosa Moreira, Angela Santos Ferreira, Selma M. De A. Sias, Cristovão C. Rodrigues and Graça Helena M. do C. Tcixeira
Department of Pulmonology, Faculty of Medicine, Fluminense Federal University, Pedro Antonio University Hospital, Rua Marques de Paraná, 303 Center, 24033-900 NiterÓi, RJ, Brazil

Shadi Rezai, Ramses Posso, Tiffany Mapp, Crystal Santiago and Manisha Jain
Department of Obstetrics and Gynecology, Lincoln Medical and Mental Health Center, Bronx, NY 10451, USA

Stephen LoBue, Daniel Adams and Yewande Oladipo
St. George's University, School of Medicine, Grenada

William D. Marino
Coney Island Hospital, Pulmonary Medicine, Brooklyn, NY 11235, USA

Cassandra E. Henderson
Department of Obstetrics and Gynecology, Lincoln Medical and Mental Health Center, Bronx, NY 10451, USA
Cornell Medical College, NY 10065, USA

Lauren Tada
Corpus Christi Medical Center, 7002William Drive, Corpus Christi, TX 78412, USA

Humayun Anjum
Pulmonary and Critical Care, Bay Area Medical Center, 7002William Drive, Corpus Christi, TX 78412, USA

W. Kenneth Linville
Pathology Department, Bay Area Medical Center, 7002William Drive, Corpus Christi, TX 78412, USA

Salim Surani
Texas A and M University, 1177 West Wheeler Avenue, Aransas Pass, TX 78336, USA
University of North Texas, 1177 West Wheeler Avenue, Suite 1, Aransas Pass, TX 78336, USA

Gyanendra Kumar Acharya and AjibolaMonsur Adedayo
Department of Internal Medicine,Wyckoff Heights Medical Center, Brooklyn, NY 11237, USA

Hejmadi Prabhu
Division of Cardiology, Department of Internal Medicine,Wyckoff Heights Medical Center, Brooklyn, NY 11237, USA

Derek R. Brinster
Department of Cardiothoracic Surgery, Lenox Hill Hospital,North Shore-Long Island Jewish Health System, New York, NY 10075, USA

Parvez Mir
Division of Pulmonary and Critical Care Medicine, Department of Internal Medicine,Wyckoff Heights Medical Center, Brooklyn, NY 11237, USA

Selvi AGker
Department of Chest Disease, Van Training and Research Hospital, Van, Turkey

Müntecep AGker
Department of Cardiology, Van Training and Research Hospital, Van, Turkey

Özgür Gürsu
Department of Cardiovascular Surgery, Van Training and Research Hospital, Van, Turkey

RJdvan Mercan
Division of Rheumatology, Department of Internal Medicine, Gazi University, Ankara, Turkey

Özgür Bülent Timuçin
Department of Ophthalmology, 'Istanbul Hospital, Van, Turkey

Anirban Das, Sabyasachi Choudhury, Sumitra Basuthakur, Sibes Kumar Das and Angshuman Mukhopadhyay
Department of Pulmonary Medicine, Medical College, Kolkata, West Bengal, India

Salim Surani
Pulmonary, Critical Care and Sleep Medicine, Texas A and M University, Corpus Christi, 1177WestWheeler Avenue, Suite 1, Aransas Pass, TX 78336, USA

Jennifer Tan
Corpus Christi Medical Center, 7101 South Padre Island Drive, Corpus Christi, TX 78412, USA

Alexandra Ahumada
Universidad Autonoma de Baja California, Avenue Álvaro ObregÓn Sn, Nueva, 21100 Mexicali, BC, Mexico
Dorrington Medical Associates, 2219 Dorrington Street, Houston, TX 77030, USA

Saherish S. Surani
Pulmonary Associates, 1177West Wheeler Avenue, Aransas Pass, TX 78336, USA

Sivakumar Sudhakaran
Texas A and M University Health Science Center, 8447 State Highway 47, Bryan, TX 77807, USA

Joseph Varon
The University of Texas Health Science Center, 7000 Fannin Street, Houston, TX 77030, USA
University General Hospital, 7501 Fannin Street, Houston, TX 77054, USA

Anirban Das, Sudipta Pandit, Sibes k. Das, Sumitra Basuthakur and Somnath Das
Department of Pulmonary Medicine, Medical College, 88 College Street, Kolkata, West Bengal 700 073, India

Miguel Angel Ariza-Prota, Ana Pando-Sandoval, Marta García-Clemente, Ramón Fernández and Pere Casan
Hospital Universitario Central de Asturias (HUCA), Instituto Nacional de Silicosis (INS), Area del PulmÓn, Facultad de Medicina, Universidad de Oviedo, 33011 Oviedo, Spain

Yang Xia
Chronic Airways Diseases Laboratory, Department of Respiration, Nanfang Hospital, Southern Medical University, Guangzhou 510515, China
Division of Pulmonary and Critical Care Medicine, Department of Medicine, Johns Hopkins University School of Medicine, Baltimore, MD, USA

Zhenyu Liang, Laiyu Liu and Shaoxi Cai
Chronic Airways Diseases Laboratory, Department of Respiration, Nanfang Hospital, Southern Medical University, Guangzhou 510515, China

Zhenzhen Fu and Omkar Paudel
Division of Pulmonary and Critical Care Medicine, Department of Medicine, Johns Hopkins University School of Medicine, Baltimore, MD, USA

Balaji Saibaba and Prateek Behera
Department of Orthopaedics, SMS Medical College, Jaipur, Rajasthan 302004, India

Umesh Kumar Meena and Ramesh Chand Meena
Department of Orthopaedics, SMS Medical College and Hospital, Jaipur 302004, India

Dipti Baral, Daniel Zaccarini and Birendra Sah
SUNY Upstate Medical University, East Adams Street, Syracuse, NY 13210, USA

Bindu Adhikari and RajMan Dongol
College of Medical Sciences, Bharatpur 44207, Nepal

Amiya Kumar Dwari and Abhijit Mandal
Department of Pulmonary Medicine, Bankura SammilaniMedical College, Bankura, West Bengal 722101, India

Sibes Kumar Das
Department of Pulmonary Medicine, Medical College, 88 College Street, Kolkata,West Bengal 700073, India

Sudhansu Sarkar
Department of Surgery, Bankura Sammilani Medical College, Bankura 722101, India

Kiyoshi Moriyama, Akira Motoyasu, Tomoki Kohyama, Mariko Kotani, Riichiro Kanai, Tadao Ando and Tomoko Yorozu
Department of Anesthesiology, Kyorin University School of Medicine, 6-20-2 Shinkawa, Mitaka, Tokyo 181-8611, Japan

Toru Satoh
Second Department of Internal Medicine, Kyorin University School of Medicine, 6-20-2 Shinkawa, Mitaka, Tokyo 181-8611, Japan

Maxime Maignan and Guillaume F. Bouvet
Institut de Recherches Cliniques de Montréal, Université de Montréal, Montréal, QC, Canada H2W1R7

Colin Verdant
Département de M´edecine, Université de Montréal, Montréal, QC, Canada H3T 1J4

Département de Médecine, Hôpital Sacré Coeur,Université de Montréal, Montréal, QC, Canada H4J 1C5

Michael Van Spall
Centre de Recherche du Centre hospitalier de l'Université de Montréal, Montréal, QC, Canada H2W1T8

Yves Berthiaume
Institut de Recherches Cliniques de Montréal, Université de Montréal, Montréal, QC, Canada H2W1R7
Département de Médecine, Université de Montréal, Montréal, QC, Canada H3T 1J4
Service de Pneumologie, Centre Hospitalier de l'Université de Montréal, Montréal, QC, Canada H2W1T8

A. Potalivo, L. Finessi, F. Facondini, A. Lupo, C. Andreoni, G. Giuliani and C. Cavicchi
Department of Emergency, Anaesthesia and Intensive Care Section, Infermi Hospital, Viale Luigi Settembrini 2, 47923 Rimini, Italy

ErdoLan Çetinkaya, Mehmet Akif Özgül, Fule Gül and Ertan Cam,
Department of Chest Diseases, Yedikule Chest Disease and Chest Surgery Education and Research Hospital, Istanbul, Turkey

Hilal Boyacı
Amasya Merzifon Kara Mustafa Pasa State Hospital, Amasya, Turkey

Emine Kamiloglu
Dr. Burhan Nalbantoğlu State Hospital, Lefkose, Northern Cyprus, Turkey

Mustafa Çörtük
Karabük University Education and Research Hospital, Karabuk, Turkey

Yannick Taverne
Department of Cardiothoracic Surgery, Erasmus Medical Center, 's-Gravendijkwal 230, 3015 CE Rotterdam, Netherlands
Department of Anatomy (ERCATHAN), Erasmus Medical Center, 's-Gravendijkwal 230, 3015 CE Rotterdam, Netherlands

Gert-Jan Kleinrensink
Department of Anatomy (ERCATHAN), Erasmus Medical Center, 's-Gravendijkwal 230, 3015 CE Rotterdam, Netherlands

Peter de Rooij
Department of General Surgery, MaasstadHospital, Olympiaweg 350, 3078 RT Rotterdam, Netherlands

Ercan Kurtipek
Department of Chest Diseases, Konya Training and Research Hospital, 42090 Konya, Turkey

Meryem Elkay Eren Karanis
Department of Pathology, Konya Training and Research Hospital, 42090 Konya, Turkey

Nuri Düzgün and Hıdır Esme
Department of Thoracic Surgery, Konya Training and Research Hospital, 42090 Konya, Turkey

Mustafa Çaycı
Department of Nuclear Medicine, Konya Training and Research Hospital, 42090 Konya, Turkey

Zehra YaGar and Fahrettin Talay
Department of Chest Diseases, Abant Izzet Baysal University School of Medicine, Gölköy, 14280 Bolu, Turkey

Murat Acat
Department of Chest Diseases, Karabuk University School of Medicine, 78000 Karabuk, Turkey

Hilal Onaran, Mehmet Akif Özgül and ErdoLan Çetinkaya
Pulmonary Division, Yedikule Chest Diseases and Surgery Teaching and Research Hospital, 34010 Istanbul, Turkey

Neslihan Fener
Yedikule Chest Diseases and Surgery Teaching and Research Hospital, 34010 Istanbul, Turkey

Nader Abdel-Rahman, Shimon Izhakain, Oren Fruchter and Mordechai R. Kramer
The Pulmonary Institute, Rabin Medical Center, Beilinson Hospital, 49100 Petah Tikva, Israel
The Sackler Faculty of Medicine, Tel Aviv University, 69978 Tel Aviv, Israel

Walter G. Wasser
Mayanei HaYeshua Medical Center, 51544 Bnei Brak, Israel
Rambam Health Care Campus, 3109601 Haifa, Israel

Ahmed Abu-Zaid
College of Medicine, Alfaisal University, Riyadh 11533, Saudi Arabia

Shamayel Mohammed
Department of Pathology and Laboratory Medicine, King Faisal Specialist Hospital and Research Center (KFSH and RC), Riyadh 11211, Saudi Arabia

Ali Cheraghvandi and Logman Cheraghvandi
Chronic Respiratory Diseases Research Center, National Research Institute of Tuberculosis and Lung Diseases (NRITLD), Shahid Beheshti University of Medical Sciences, Tehran 19558 41452, Iran

Majid Marjani
Clinical Tuberculosis and Epidemiology Research Center, National Research Institute of Tuberculosis and Lung Disease (NRITLD), Masih Daneshvari Hospital, Shahid Beheshti University of Medical Sciences, Tehran 19558 41452, Iran

Saeid Fallah Tafti
Nursing and Respiratory Health Management Research Center, National Research Institute of Tuberculosis and Lung Diseases (NRITLD), Shahid Beheshti University of Medical Sciences, Tehran 19558 41452, Iran

Davoud Mansouri
Lung Transplantation Research Center, National Research Institute of Tuberculosis and Lung Diseases (NRITLD), Shahid Beheshti University of Medical Sciences, Tehran 19558 41452, Iran

Calvin Chao and Karl Uy
Division of Thoracic Surgery, UMass Memorial Medical Center, University of Massachusetts Medical School,Worcester, MA, USA

Vijay Vanguri
Department of Pathology, UMass Memorial Medical Center, University of Massachusetts Medical School,Worcester, MA, USA

Mitchell D. Ross and Sreeja Biswas Roy
Department of Internal Medicine, St. Joseph's Hospital and Medical Center, Phoenix, AZ, USA

Pradnya D. Patil
Department of Hematology and Oncology, Taussig Cancer Institute, Cleveland Clinic, Cleveland, OH, USA

Nitika Thawani
Department of Radiation Oncology, University of Arizona Cancer Center, St. Joseph'sHospital andMedical Center, Phoenix, AZ, USA

Ralph Drosten
Department of Radiology, St. Joseph's Hospital and Medical Center, Phoenix, AZ, USA

Vishnu Vasanthan and Jayan Nagendran
Department of Surgery, University of Alberta, Edmonton, AB, Canada
Mazankowski Alberta Heart Institute, Edmonton, AB, Canada

Kieran Halloran and Lakshmi Puttagunta
Department of Medicine, University of Alberta, Edmonton, AB, Canada
University of Alberta Hospital, Edmonton, AB, Canada

Nikolaos Tasis, Ioannis Tsouknidas and Argyrios Ioannidis
Department of Anatomy and Surgical Anatomy, Medical School, National and Kapodistrian University of Athens, Athens, Greece

Konstantinos Nassiopoulos
Hopital Daler, Fribourg, Switzerland

Dimitrios Filippou
Department of Anatomy and Surgical Anatomy, Medical School, National and Kapodistrian University of Athens, Athens, Greece
Department of Surgical Oncology, Laparoscopic Surgery and Laser Surgery, N Athinaio Hospital, Athens, Greece

Ismael Garcia
Facultad de Medicina Tampico, Universidad Autónoma de Tamaulipas, Tampico, TAMPS, Mexico

Joseph Varon
Dorrington Medical Associates, Houston, TX, USA
Foundation Surgical Hospital, Houston, TX, USA
The University of Texas Health Science Center at Houston, Houston, TX 77030, USA

Salim Surani
Texas A and M University, Corpus Christi, TX 78413, USA

Vijay Kodadhala, Alemeshet Gudeta and Aklilu Zerihun
Department of Internal Medicine, Howard University Hospital, 2041 Georgia Avenue NW, Washington, DC 20060, USA

Odene Lewis and Alicia Thomas
Division of Pulmonary Medicine, Howard University Hospital, 2041 Georgia Avenue NW, Washington, DC 20060, USA

Sohail Ahmed and Jhansi Gajjala
Division of Infectious Diseases, Howard University Hospital, 2041 Georgia Avenue NW, Washington, DC 20060, USA

Parth Rali and Khalid Malik
Division of Pulmonary and Critical Care, Allegheny General Hospital, Pittsburgh, PA 15212, USA

Jianwu Xie and Jan Silverman
Division of Pathology, Allegheny General Hospital, Pittsburgh, PA 15212, USA

Grishma Rali
Children's Hospital of Philadelphia, Philadelphia, PA, USA

Mayur Rali
Hofstra Northwell School of Medicine, Department of Family Medicine, Southside Hospital, Bay Shore, NY, USA

Fatima Zahra Mrabet, Leila El Akkari, Sanaa Hammi and Jamal Eddine Bourkadi
Department of Pneumology, Moulay Youssef University Hospital Center, Rabat, Morocco
Faculty of Medicine and Pharmacy, Mohammed V University, Rabat, Morocco

Hafsa El Ouazzani and Fouad Zouaidia
Faculty of Medicine and Pharmacy, Mohammed V University, Rabat, Morocco
Department of Pathology, Ibn Sina University Hospital Center, Rabat, Morocco

Meirui Li
Michael G. DeGroote School of Medicine, McMaster University, Hamilton, ON, Canada

Salem Alowami, Asghar Naqvi and Miranda Schell
Department of Pathology and Molecular Medicine, McMaster University, Hamilton, ON, Canada

Clive Davis
Divisions of Critical Care, Respirology, and General Internal Medicine, Department of Medicine, McMaster University, Hamilton, ON, Canada

Yusuke Kakiuchi, Fumihiro Yamaguchi, Makoto Hayashi and Yusuke Shikama
Department of Respiratory Medicine, Showa University Fujigaoka Hospital, 1-30 Fujigaoka, Aoba-ku, Yokohama 227-8501, Japan

Humna Abid Memon
Department of Internal Medicine, Houston Methodist Hospital, Houston, TX, USA

Zeenat Safdar
Houston Methodist Pulmonary Hypertension Center,Weill Cornell College of Medicine, Houston, TX, USA

Ahmad Goodarzi
Houston Methodist Lung Transplant Center, Houston Methodist Hospital, Houston, TX, USA

Faris Hannoodi, Israa Ali, Hussam Sabbagh and Sarwan Kumar
Crittenton Hospital, 1101W. University Drive, 2 South, Rochester, MI 48307, USA

Adarsha Selvachandran and Raymond J. Foley
Division of Pulmonary/Critical Care, UConn Health, 263 Farmington Avenue, Farmington, CT 06030-1321, USA

Chun-Mao Juan, Shang-Yun Ho and Yuan-Chun Huang
Department of Medical Imaging, Changhua Christian Hospital, No. 135 Nanxiao St., Changhua 500, Taiwan

Mei-Ling Chen
Department of Pathology, Changhua Christian Hospital, No. 135 Nanxiao St., Changhua 500, Taiwan

Himaja Koneru, Monirul Islam and Debabrata Bandyopadhyay
Department of Thoracic Medicine, Geisinger Medical Center, Danville, PA, USA

Hesham Abdelrazek, Nikhil Madan, Sreeja Biswas Roy and Tanmay S. Panchabhai
Norton Thoracic Institute, St. Joseph's Hospital and Medical Center, Phoenix, AZ, USA

Pradnya D. Patil
Taussig Cancer Institute, Department of Hematology and Oncology, Cleveland Clinic, Cleveland, OH, USA

Samid M. Farooqui
Department of Internal Medicine, University of Oklahoma Health Sciences Center, Oklahoma City, OK, USA

Muhammad S. Khan and Viral Doshi
Department of Internal Medicine, University of Oklahoma Health Sciences Center, Oklahoma City, OK, USA
Section of Pulmonary, Critical Care and Sleep Medicine, University of Oklahoma Health Sciences Center, Oklahoma City, OK, USA

Laura Adhikari
Department of Pathology, University of Oklahoma Health Sciences Center, Oklahoma City, OK, USA

Tyler Pickell
Marian University College of Osteopathic Medicine, Indianapolis, IN, USA

Jamie Donnelly
Ameripath, Indianapolis, IN, USA

Francois Abi Fadel
Marian University College of Osteopathic Medicine, Indianapolis, IN, USA
Respiratory Institute, Cleveland Clinic, Cleveland, OH, USA

Mohamad Rachid, Khansa Ahmad, Meghan Saunders-Kurban, Aelia Fatima, Aditya Shah and Anas Nahhas
Internal Medicine, Advocate Christ Medical Center, Oak Lawn, IL, USA

Ali Zakaria, Bayan Al-Share and Khaled Al Asad
Istishari Hospital, Department of Internal Medicine, Division of Pulmonology, Amman 11183, Jordan

Sheila A. Habib
Department of Medicine, Division of Pulmonary Diseases and Critical Care Medicine, University of Texas Health at San Antonio (UTH-SA), San Antonio, TX 78229, USA
Medical Service, Division of Pulmonary Diseases and Critical Care Medicine, South Texas Veterans Health Care System (STVHCS), San Antonio, TX 78229, USA

Robert C. Vasko
Department of Pediatrics, Children's Hospital Los Angeles, Los Angeles, CA 90027, USA

Jack Badawy
Department of Medicine, Division of General and Hospital Medicine, UTH-SA, San Antonio, TX 78229, USA

Gregory M. Anstead
Department of Medicine, Division of Infectious Diseases, UTH-SA, San Antonio, TX 78229, USA
Medical Service, Division of Infectious Diseases, STVHCS, San Antonio, TX 78229, USA

Hussain Ibrahim, Adnan Khan, Shawn P. Nishi, Ken Fujise and Syed Gilani
University of Texas Medical Branch, 301 University Boulevard, 5.106 John Sealy Annex, Galveston, TX 77555-0553, USA

Serdar Şen, Nilgün Kanlıoğlu Kuman and Ekrem Şentürk
Thoracic Surgery Department, Faculty of Medicine, Adnan Menderes University, Aydın 09000, Turkey

Engin Pabuşcu
Thoracic Surgery Department, Osmaniye State Hospital, Toprakkale, Turkey

Ertan Yaman
Thoracic Surgery Department, C, orum State Hospital Corum, Turkey

Abhinav Agrawal, Braghadheeswar Thyagarajan, Sidney Ceniza and Syed Hasan Yusuf
Department of Internal Medicine, Monmouth Medical Center, Long Branch, NJ 07740, USA

M. C. Mirant-Borde M. M. Johnson
Division of Pulmonary Medicine, Mayo Clinic Florida, 4500 San Pablo Road, Jacksonville, FL 32224, USA

S. Alvarez
Division of Pulmonary Medicine and Infectious Disease, Mayo Clinic Florida, USA

Ching Hsueh, Shang-Yun Ho and Chiung-Ying Liao
Department of Medical Imaging, Changhua Christian Hospital, No. 135 Nanxiao Street, Changhua 500, Taiwan

Yuan-Chun Huang
Department of Medical Imaging, Changhua Christian Hospital, No. 135 Nanxiao Street, Changhua 500, Taiwan
Department of Radiology, Changhua Christian Hospital, Erlin Branch, No. 558, Section 1, Dacheng Road, Erlin Township, Changhua 526, Taiwan

Index